PROGRESS IN BRAIN RESEARCH

VOLUME 76

VESTIBULOSPINAL CONTROL OF POSTURE AND LOCOMOTION

Recent volumes in PROGRESS IN BRAIN RESEARCH

PROGRESS IN BRAIN RESEARCH

VOLUME 76

VESTIBULOSPINAL CONTROL OF POSTURE AND LOCOMOTION

EDITED BY

O. POMPEIANO

Dipartimento di Fisiologia e Biochimica, Università di Pisa, Pisa, Italy

and

J.H.J. ALLUM

Division of Experimental Audiology, Department of Otorhinolaryngology, University Hospital, Basel, Switzerland

ELSEVIER
AMSTERDAM – NEW YORK – OXFORD
1988

LC

© 1988, Elsevier Science Publishers B.V. (Biomedical Division)

ISBN 0-444-80976-7 (volume)
ISBN 0-444-80104-9 (series)

Published by:
Elsevier Science Pubishers B.V. (Biomedical Division)
P.O. Box 211
1000 AE Amsterdam
The Netherlands

Sole distributors for the U.S.A. and Canada:
Elsevier Science Publishing Company, Inc.
52 Vanderbilt Avenue
New York, NY 10017
U.S.A.

Library of Congress Cataloging-in-Publication Data

Vestibulospinal control of posture and locomotion.

  (Progress in brain research ; v. 76)
  Bibliography: p.
  Includes index.
  1. Posture.   2. Human locomotion.   3. Vestibular apparatus.   4. Afferent pathways.   I. Pompeiano, O.
II. Allum, J. H. J.   III. Series.
QP376.P7   vol.76   612'.82 s   [612'.76]   88-7119
[QP301]
ISBN 0-444-80976-7

Printed in the Netherlands

4-6-89

List of Contributors

V.C. Abrahams, Department of Physiology, Botterell Hall, Queen's University, Kingston, Ontario, K7L 3N6 Canada

J.H.J. Allum, Division of Experimental Audiology and Neurootology, Department of Otorhinolaryngology, University Hospital, CH-4031 Basel, Switzerland

B. Amblard, Laboratoire de Neurosciences Fonctionnelles, Unité de Neurosciences du Comportement, CNRS, 31 Chemin J. Aiguier, F-13402 Marseille CEDEX 9, France

J.F. Baker, Department of Physiology, Northwestern University Medical School, 303 East Chicago Avenue, Chicago, Illinois 60611, U.S.A.

J. Banovetz, Department of Physiology, Northwestern University Medical School, 303 East Chicago Avenue, Chicago, Illinois 60611, U.S.A.

G.R. Barnes, Vestibular Physiology Section, R.A.F. Institute of Aviation Medicine, Farnborough, Hantshire GU14 6SZ, U.K.

J. Berthélémy, Laboratoire de Psychophysiologie, Université de Provence, Centre de Saint-Jérome, Rue H. Poincaré, F-13397 Marseille CEDEX 13, France

A. Berthoz, Laboratoire de Physiologie Neurosensorielle, CNRS, 15 Rue de l'École de Médecine, F-75270 Paris CEDEX 06, France

F.O. Black, Department of Neurootology, Good Samaritan Hospital and Medical Center, 1015 N.W. 22nd Avenue, Portland, Oregon 97210, U.S.A.

L. Borel, Laboratoire de Psychophysiologie, Université de Provence, Centre de Saint-Jérôme, Rue H. Poincaré, F-13397 Marseille CEDEX 13, France

M.B. Carpenter, Department of Anatomy, F. Edward Hébert School of Medicine, Uniformed Services University of the Health Sciences, 4301 Jones Bridge Road, Bethesda, Maryland 20814-4799, U.S.A.

Y.S. Chan, Department of Physiology, Faculty of Medicine, University of Hong Kong, Li Shu Fan Building, 5 Sassoon Road, Hong Kong

Y.M. Cheung, Department of Physiology, Faculty of Medicine, University of Hong Kong, Li Shu Fan Building, 5 Sassoon Road, Hong Kong

J. Cremieux, Laboratoire de Neurosciences Fontionnelles, Unité de Neurosciences du Comportement, CNRS, 31 Chemin J. Aiguier, F-13402 Marseille CEDEX 9, France

I.S. Curtoys, Vestibular Research Laboratory, Department of Psychology, University of Sidney, Sidney 2006, New South Wales, Australia

C.L. Darlington, Vestibular Research Laboratory, Department of Psychology, University of Sidney, Sidney 2006, New South Wales, Australia

P. D'Ascanio, Dipartimento di Fisiologia e Biochimica, Università di Pisa, Via S. Zeno 31, I-56100 Pisa, Italy

D. Dememes, Laboratoire de Neurophysiologie Sensorielle, INSERM, U-254, Place E. Bataillon, F-34060 Montpellier CEDEX, France

J. Dichgans, Neurologische Klinik, Eberhard-Karls Universität Tübingen, Liebermeisterstrasse 18-20, D-7400 Tübingen, F.R.G.

H.-C. Diener, Neurologische Klinik, Eberhard-Karls Universität Tübingen, Liebermeisterstrasse 18-20, D-7400 Tübingen, F.R.G.

N. Dieringer, Physiologisches Institut, Universität München, Pettenkoferstrasse 12, D-8000 München 2, F.R.G.

M.B. Dutia, Department of Physiology, University Medical School, Teviot Place, Edinburgh EH8 9AG, U.K.

V.V. Fanardjian, Orbeli Institute of Physiology, Academy of Sciences of Armenian SSR, 22 Orbeli Brothers Street, 375028 Yerevan, U.S.S.R.

G.R. Fernie, Centre for Studies in Aging, Sunnybrook Medical Centre, Department of Surgery, University of Toronto, 2075 Bayview Avenue, Toronto, Ontario, M4N 3M5 Canada

H. Flohr, Abteilung für Neurobiologie, Universität Bremen, NW2, D-2800 Bremen 33, F.R.G.

H. Forssberg, Department of Physiology III, Karolinska Institute, Lidingövägen 1, S-114 33 Stockholm, Sweden

T. Futami, Department of Physiology, School of Medicine, Tokyo Medical and Dental University, 1-5-45 Yushima, Bunkyo-ku, Tokyo 113, Japan

Y. Gahéry, Laboratoire de Neurosciences Fonctionnelles, Unité de Neurosciences Intégratives, CNRS, 31 Chemin J. Aiguier, F-13402 Marseille CEDEX 9, France

J. Goldberg, Department of Physiology, Northwestern University Medical School, 303 East Chicago Avenue, Chicago, Illinois 60611, U.S.A.

V.S. Gurfinkel, Institute for Problems of Information Transmission, Academy of Sciences of the U.S.S.R., Ermolova Street 19, SU-101447 Moscow E24, U.S.S.R.

H. Hirschfeld, Department of Pediatrics, Karolinska Hospital/St. Görans Hospital, Lidingövägen 1, S-114 33 Stockholm, Sweden

F. Honegger, Division of Experimental Audiology and Neurootology, Department of Otorhinolaryngology, University Hospital, CH-4031 Basel, Switzerland

T. Hongo, Department of Neurophysiology, Institute of Brain Research, School of Medicine, University of Tokyo, 7-3-1 Hongo, Bunkyo-ku, Tokyo 113, Japan

F.B. Horak, Department of Neurootology and Neurological Sciences Institute, Good Samaritan Hospital and Medical Center, 1015 N.W. 22th Avenue, Portland, Oregon 97209, U.S.A.

J.C. Hwang, Department of Physiology, Faculty of Medicine, University of Hong Kong, Li Shu Fan Building, 5 Sassoon Road, Hong Kong

M. Igarashi, Department of Otorhinolaryngology and Communicative Sciences, Baylor College of Medicine, 1200 Moursund Avenue, Houston, Texas 77030-3498, U.S.A.

M. Ishii, Department of Otorhinolaryngology and Communicative Sciences, Baylor College of Medicine, 1200 Moursund Avenue, Houston, Texas 77030-3498, U.S.A.

K. Ishikawa, Department of Otorhinolaryngology and Communicative Sciences, Baylor College of Medicine, 1200 Moursund Avenue, Houston, Texas 77030-3498, U.S.A.

Y. Ito, Department of Otorhinolaryngology, Gifu University School of Medicine, 40 Tsukasamachi, Gifu 500, Japan

Y. Iwamoto, Department of Neurophysiology, Institute of Brain Research, School of Medicine, University of Tokyo, 7-3-1 Hongo, Bunkyo-ku, Tokyo 113, Japan

T. Kanaya, Department of Otolaryngology, Asahikawa Medical College, 4-5 Nishikagura, Asahikawa 078-11, Japan

E.A. Keshner, Department of Physiology, Northwestern University Medical School, 303 East Chicago Avenue, Chicago, Illinois 60611, U.S.A.

T. Kitama, Department of Physiology, Institute of Basic Medical Sciences, University of Tsukuba, Niihari-Gun, Ibaraki-Ken 305, Japan

M. Koizumi, Department of Otorhinolaryngology, Gifu University School of Medicine, 40 Tsukasamachi, Gifu 500, Japan

M. Lacour, Laboratoire de Psychophysiologie, Université de Provence, Centre de Saint-Jérôme, Rue H. Poincaré, F-13397 Marseille CEDEX 13, France

F. G. Lestienne, Laboratoire de Physiologie Neurosensorielle, CNRS, 15 Rue de l'École de Médecine, F-75270 Paris CEDEX 06, France

U. Lüneburg, Abteilung für Neurobiologie, Universität Bremen, NW2, D-2800 Bremen 33, F.R.G.

M. Maeda, Department of Neurosurgery and Casualty Center, School of Medicine, Juntendo University, 2-1-1 Hongo, Bunkyo-ku, Tokyo 113, Japan

B.E. Maki, Centre for Studies in Aging, Sunnybrook Medical Centre, Department of Surgery, University of Toronto, 2075 Bayview Avenue, Toronto, Ontario, M4N 3M5 Canada

D. Manzoni, Dipartimento di Fisiologia e Biochimica, Università di Pisa, Via S. Zeno 31, I-56100 Pisa, Italy

A. Marchand, Laboratoire de Neurosciences Fonctionelles, Unité de Neurosciences du Comportement, CNRS, 31 Chemin J. Aiguier, F-13402 Marseille CEDEX 9, France

K. Matsuyama, Department of Physiology, Asahikawa Medical College, 4-5 Nishikagura, Asahikawa 078-11, Japan

T. Mergner, Neurologische Universitätsklinik, Hansastrasse 9, D-7800 Freiburg i. Br., F.R.G.

H. Miyata, Department of Otorhinolaryngology, Gifu University School of Medicine, 40 Tsukasamachi, Gifu 500, Japan

S. Mori, Department of Physiology, Asahikawa Medical College, 4-5 Nishikagura, Asahikawa 078-11, Japan

L.M. Nashner, Neurological Sciences Institute, Good Samaritan Hospital and Medical Center, 1120 N.W. 20th Avenue, Portland, Oregon 97209, U.S.A.

A. Nieoullon, Laboratoire de Neurosciences Fonctionelles, Unité de Neurochimie, CNRS-BP 71, 31 Chemin J. Aiguier, F-13402 Marseille CEDEX 9, France

T. Ohgaki, Department of Otolaryngology, School of Medicine, Tokyo Medical and Dental University, 1-5-45, Yushima, Bunkyo-ku, Tokyo 113, Japan

A. Pellionisz, Department of Physiology and Biophysics, New York Universtity Medical Center, 550 First Avenue, New York, New York 10016, U.S.A.

B.W. Peterson, Department of Physiology, Northwestern University Medical School, 303 East Chicago Avenue, Chicago, Illinois 60611, U.S.A.

C.R. Pfaltz, Division of Experimental Audiology and Neurootology, Department of Otorhinolaryngology, University Hospital, Ch-4031, Basel, Switzerland.

O. Pompeiano, Dipartimento di Fisiologia e Biochimica, Università di Pisa, Via S. Zeno 31, I-56100 Pisa, Italy

J. Raymond, Laboratoire de Neurophysiologie Sensorielle, INSERM, U-254, Place E. Bataillon, F-34060 Montpellier CEDEX, France

F.J.R. Richmond, Department of Physiology, Botterell Hall, Queen's University, Kingston, Ontario, K7L 3N6 Canada

V.A. Sarkisian, Orbeli Institute of Physiology, Academy of Sciences of Armenian SSR, 22 Orbeli Brothers Street, 375028 Yerevan, U.S.S.R.

S. Sasaki, Department of Neurophysiology, Institute of Brain Research, School of Medicine, University of Tokyo, 7-3-1 Hongo, Bunkyo-ku, Tokyo 113, Japan

R.H. Schor, Departments of Otolaryngology and Physiology, University of Pittsburgh School of Medicine, Pittsburgh, Pennsylvania 15261, U.S.A.

Y. Shinoda, Department of Physiology, School of Medicine, Tokyo Medical and Dental University, 1-5-45, Yushima, Bunkyo-ku, Tokyo 113, Japan

C.L. Shupert, Department of Neurootology and Neurological Sciences Institute, Good Samaritan Hospital and Medical Center, 1015 N.W. 22th Avenue, Portland, Oregon 97209, U.S.A.

P.F. Smith, Vestibular Research Laboratory, Department of Psychology, University of Sydney, Sydney 2006, New South Wales, Australia

G. Stampacchia, Dipartimento di Fisiologia e Biochimica, Università di Pisa, Via S. Zeno 31, I-56100 Pisa, Italy

Y. Sugiuchi, Department of Otolaryngology, School of Medicine, Tokyo Medical and Dental University,. 1-5-45, Yushima, Bunkyo-ku, Tokyo 113, Japan

I. Suzuki, Department of Neurophysiology, Institute of Brain Research, School of Medicine, University of Tokyo, 7-3-1 Hongo, Bunkyo-ku, Tokyo 113, Japan

K. Takakusaki, Department of Physiology, Asahikawa Medical College, 4-5 Nishikagura, Asahikawa 078-11 Japan

U. Thoden, Neurologische Universitätsklinik, Hansastrasse 9, D-7800 Freiburg i. Br., F.R.G.

T. Tokita, Department of Otorhinolaryngology, Gifu University School of Medicine, 40 Tsukasamachi, Gifu 500, Japan

V.J. Wilson, Rockefeller University, 1230 York Ave., New York, New York 10021-6399, U.S.A.

C. Xerri, Laboratoire de Psychophysiologie, Université de Provence, Centre de Saint-Jérôme, Rue H. Poincaré, F-13397 Marseille CEDEX 13, France

H. Yamane, Department of Otorhinolaryngology and Communicative Sciences, Baylor College of Medicine, 1200 Moursund Avenue, Houston, Texas 77030-3498, U.S.A.

K. Yoshida, Department of Physiology, Institute of Basic Medical Sciences, University of Tsukuba, Niihari-Gun, Ibaraki-Ken 305, Japan

Preface

The attraction of the vestibular system to several generations of scientists has been its apparent neuronal simplicity, despite the fact that a quite complicated set of postural and motor deficits are observed when a peripheral lesion to this system occurs. For decades the function of the three neuronal vestibulo-ocular reflex arc has been investigated in detail as a prelude to understanding the mechanisms underlying the postural and motor abnormalities which occur when the receptors of, or nerve to, the peripheral vestibular system no longer function normally. The major challenge to the experimental skills of scientists, however, has been to understand the spinal motor regulation provided by vestibulospinal pathways, since these pathways are, to some extent, far more complex than those of the vestibulo-ocular reflex. This challenge acts as an intellectual stimulus for scientists working on different aspects of sensory neurophysiology, because at the level of spinal motoneurons labyrinthine, visual and muscle proprioceptive inputs interact. Thus it appears necessary to examine not just how labyrinthine signals enter the motor system and act at segmental and suprasegmental levels to ensure appropriate adjustments of the motoneuronal output. Rather, proprioceptive inputs from the limb and neck musculature and visual inputs must be taken into account as well.

The last ten years have seen a great development in this interdisciplinary field. In particular, detailed experiments from different groups of researchers have investigated the mechanisms by which labyrinthine signals intervene in the static and dynamic control of spinal motor activities. The spinal networks and supraspinal structures involved in the vestibular control of posture and movement have also been investigated, including the neurophysiological and neurochemical mechanisms involved in the gain regulation of vestibulospinal reflexes. Finally, the role that neck and visual inputs exert in the regulation of vestibulospinal reflexes has been studied in detail.

Work on vestibulospinal reflexes has also been extended to man's equilibrating reactions. The most significant aspect of this development is understanding how segmental and supraspinal mechanisms are used in the vestibular control of human posture and movement and how they are reflexly regulated. Interpretation of data from human experiments requires a detailed knowledge of animal studies and also suggests specific control experiments in animals. An in-depth treatment of the mechanisms underlying vestibulospinal reflexes in animals and humans is an important prerequisite to understanding the phenomena of vestibular deficits and adaptation required under abnormal (microgravity) or pathological conditions.

In 1985 a group of experts in the field discussed these scientific developments and decided to review in a comprehensive way with invited speakers the new information available. This review was organized as a satellite meeting to the Bárány Society meeting in Bologna during June 1987. The meeting was held in the Congress Hall of the Royal Carlton Hotel where the main Bárány Society meeting was also held. We are most grateful to the President of the Bárány Society Prof. J. Stahle, and the current vice-President

Prof. E. Pirodda, for having accepted our plans and putting at our disposal most of the facilities prepared for the main Bárány Society meeting.

The subject matter in this book, which contains the review articles provided by each selected lecturer, has been divided into 7 main sections. The first three sections present basic neuroanatomical neurophysiological aspects of vestibulospinal reflexes and document the neck afferent and visual influences on these reflexes. Following sections deal with the control of locomotion, posture (predominantly human posture), and eye-head-trunk coordination by vestibulospinal signals. The final section provides current knowledge on the processes underlying compensation of vestibulospinal deficits. For those wishing an overview of the matter an overall review preceding each main section has been added, so that the reader is informed as to which questions are still controversial and require further investigation for an ultimate answer. We hope in this way to provide a basis for those wishing a connected account of the field of vestibulospinal reflexes.

O. Pompeiano, Pisa
J.H.J. Allum, Basel

October 1987

Acknowledgements

The financial support of two companies – Tönnies Medical Electronics GmbH, Freiburg, Germany and Janssen Pharmaceutica AG, Baar, Switzerland – is gratefully acknowledged. Invaluable secretarial and organisational assistance was provided in three cities by Ms Wanda Brunetti (Basel), Ms Renata Petrucci (Bologna) and Ms Cristina Pucci (Pisa).

Contents

Section III — Neck Afferent and Visual Influences on Vestibulospinal Reflexes

SECTION I

Vestibular Nuclei: Projection Pathways, Neurotransmitters and Synaptology

O. Pompeiano and J.H.J. Allum (Eds.)
Progress in Brain Research, Vol. 76
© 1988 Elsevier Science Publishers B.V. (Biomedical Division)

Overview

V.J. Wilson

Rockefeller University, 1230 York Avenue, New York, NY 10021-6399, U.S.A.

This introductory section deals with connections of vestibular neurons: the inputs they receive from periphery and brainstem, the efferent projections they give rise to, the transmitters involved, and the related synaptic mechanisms. The experiments reviewed by Carpenter (Chapter 1) show how techniques such as transport of tritiated amino acids or horseradish peroxidase (HRP) have added to the earlier information on projections obtained with retrograde chromatolysis or degeneration studies. Knowledge of inputs to and outputs from the vestibular nuclei is now very comprehensive, but many specific questions remain unanswered even by the newer methods. For example, do commissural fibres interconnecting the bilateral vestibular nuclei issue from a specific population of neurons, or, more likely, are they collaterals of axons that project to other levels of the central nervous system? Questions such as these can be studied with the electrophysiological methods used by Dr. Fanardjian (Chapter 4) to map interconnections between the vestibular nuclei and other brainstem structures. They can also be answered by intra-axonal injection of HRP, the technique used by Dr. Shinoda (Chapter 2) to study the branching of vestibulospinal fibres. This work has confirmed that many of these fibres branch to different cord levels, and has revealed the apparent existence of synapses between lateral vestibulospinal fibres and forelimb motoneurons. As brought out in the discussion, however, there are neurons responding to natural stimulation in more dorsal spinal laminae, where vestibulospinal fibres do not seem to terminate. Is this because these neurons have dendrites that extend to regions where there are terminals, or because they are influenced by other descending systems? Finally, Dr. Raymond (Chapter 3) presents evidence that glutamate or aspartate is the transmitter liberated by vestibular afferent fibres. Important questions remain about the glutamate receptor types involved in various pathways, ipsilateral and commissural, impinging on vestibular neurons, and about denervation supersensitivity which may be used to identify receptor types: is it due to an increase in the number of receptors, or to an increase in binding characteristics?

O. Pompeiano and J.H.J. Allum (Eds.)
Progress in Brain Research, Vol. 76
© 1988 Elsevier Science Publishers B.V. (Biomedical Division)

CHAPTER 1

Vestibular nuclei: afferent and efferent projections

M.B. Carpenter

Department of Anatomy, F. Edward Hebért School of Medicine, Uniformed Services University of the Health Sciences, 4301 Jones Bridge Road, Bethesda, MD 20814-4799, U.S.A.

Vestibular ganglion cells innervating the utricle project upon neurons in the ventral LVN; cells innervating the saccule project upon ventral LVN, group y and lateral IVN, while ganglion cells innervating the cristae ampullaris of the SD project mainly upon MVN and SVN. Cerebellar afferents to the VN arise ipsilaterally from the anterior lobe vermis (LVN), the flocculus (SVN, MVN and y), the nodulus and uvula (MVN, IVN) and bilaterally from the fastigial nucleus (LVN, IVN). Commissural systems interconnect the MVN and peripheral SVN. The MVN, IVN and LVN receive modest projections from the dorsal regions of medullary and pontine RF. The SVN projects crossed and uncrossed fibres to TN and the OMC. The VST arises from the LVN and parts of other VN, provides collaterals to the LRN and projects preferentially upon cervical and lower lumbar segments by an elaborate collateral system. The MVN supplies the nuclei of the EOM and collaterals to cervical spinal segments. The IVN has diverse projections to the TN and the OMC, parts of the inferior olive, specific reticular nuclei, the cerebellum and the cervical spinal cord.

Introduction

Primary vestibular afferents constitute the major, but not the sole, input to the vestibular nuclei which in turn give rise to secondary vestibular fibres. Secondary vestibular projections play an important role in the maintenance of equilibrium, orientation in three-dimensional space and modification of muscle tone. This review concerns afferent projections to the vestibular nuclei and their projections within the neuraxis, except those to the thalamus.

Afferents to the vestibular nuclei

Inputs to the VN are derived from the VG, specific parts of the cerebellar cortex, the fastigial nuclei, a small number of brainstem nuclei and the spinal cord. Commissural connections interrelate the VN of the two sides and intrinsic connections exist among the VN of each side.

Primary vestibular fibres

Central projections of the VG terminate massively in the VN, in localized regions of the cerebellar cortex and in a few brainstem relay nuclei. Primary vestibular projections are ipsilateral and have aspartate/glutamate as their excitatory neurotrans-

---

Abbreviations: ACN, accessory cuneate nucleus; ACN, anterior canal nerve; AIN, abducens internuclear neuron; AN, abducens nucleus; EOM, extra-ocular muscle; FN, fastigial nucleus; GABA, γ-aminobutyric acid; GAD, glutamic acid decarboxylase; HRP, horseradish peroxidase; INC, interstitial nucleus of Cajal; INVN, interstitial nucleus of the vestibular nerve; IOS, inferior oblique subdivision; (Ri)MLF, (rostral interstitial nucleus of the) medial longitudinal fasciculus; ND, nucleus of Darkschewitsch; NIC, nucleus intercalatus; NPP, nucleus prepositus hypoglossi; NR, nucleus of Roller; NRgc, nucleus reticular gigantocellularis; OMC, oculomotor nuclear complex; PC, Purkinje cell; PPRF, pontine paramedian recticular formation; RF, reticular formation; (I/S/M)RS, (inferior/superior/medial) rectus subdivision; SCP, superior cerebellar peduncle; SD, semicircular duct; TN, trochlear nucleus; VG, vestibular ganglion; (L/I/M/S) VN, (lateral/inferior/medial/superior) vestibular nucleus; VOC, vestibulo-ocular cervical; (L/M)VST, (lateral/medial) vestibulospinal tract.

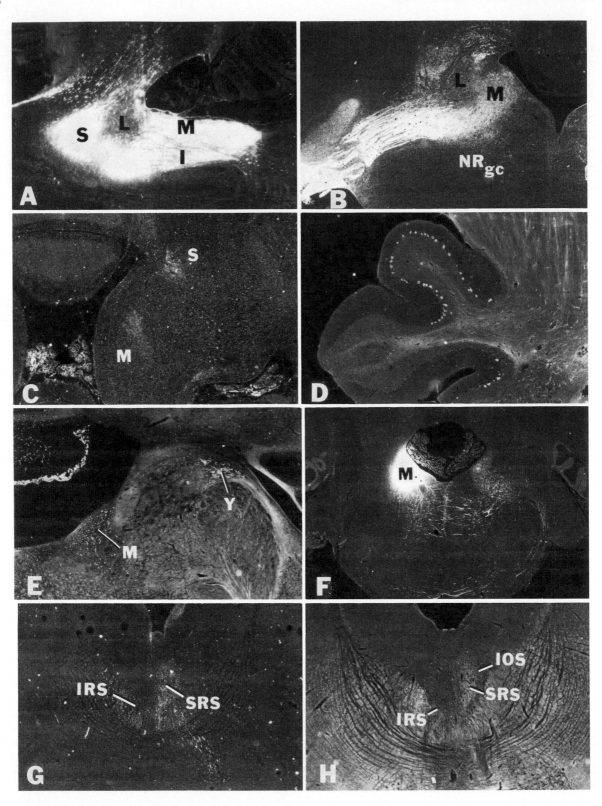

mitter [18]. Silver degeneration studies suggested a differential distribution of vestibular afferents within parts of each VN [47]. Portions of the VN not considered to receive primary afferents included: (1) the dorsal half of the LVN, (2) peripheral parts of the SVN, (3) caudal and medial parts of the MVN and (4) cell groups *f*, *x* and *z* in or near the IVN.

The central distribution of primary vestibular afferents was studied autoradiographically in monkeys in which gelfoam pledgets saturated with [³H]-amino acids (proline and/or leucine) were implanted in individual SDs [11]. The intention was to determine the central projections of VG cells innervating separate SDs, but in most instances uptake and transport occurred from VG cells innervating multiple receptors.

Labelling of all parts of the VG was associated with massive transport in all parts of the vestibular root (Fig. 1B). Ascending fibres projected dorsomedially and rostrally through portions of LVN to terminations in SVN and the cerebellum; descending branches provided terminals in the ventral LVN, and fibres which traversed the IVN. Terminal label in the VN was dense and widespread (Fig. 1A). In SVN, terminal label was distributed to all parts of the nucleus with the greatest density in the central large-celled region. In LVN, terminals were dense in ventral and rostral parts of the nucleus, while no terminals were present in dorsal and caudal regions (Fig. 1A,B). Terminal labelling in IVN formed two distinct pools of dense silver grains – one rostrally surrounding proximal root fibres and another in the caudal third of the nucleus – cells of group *f* were free of silver grains. MVN contained terminals

distributed homogeneously within its cytoarchitectonic borders. Projections to the so-called accessory vestibular nuclei were confined to the INVN and cell group *y* [8]. Larger cells located dorsal to *y*, designated as the infracerebellar nucleus by Gacek [22], contained no silver grains. Primary vestibular fibres projecting beyond the boundaries of the VN included punctate islands of terminals in rostral parts of the ACN and among cells in the subtrigeminal lateral reticular nucleus. Small numbers of fibres extended into the RF ventral to the VN, but terminals were not identified The most impressive reticular projections were distributed in dorsal portions of the nucleus NRgc caudally (Fig. 1B).

Isotope uptake in one animal, confined to cells of the inferior VG innervating the posterior duct, projected to terminals in medial parts of the SVN, the rostrolateral third of MVN and the oral pole of the IVN (Fig. 1C).

Transganglionic transport of HRP has been demonstrated from cut branches of the vestibular nerve innervating the ampulla of the lateral SD and the utricle in the cat [45]. VG neurons innervating the ampulla of the lateral SD provided collaterals to the superior part of the INVN and projected to terminations in all parts of the SVN, MVN and IVN. None of these fibres terminated in the LVN. Labelling of the utricular nerve distal to the VG produced central transport in small fibres terminating in ventral parts of the LVN and restricted adjacent regions of the MVN and IVN. HRP labelling of the macula of the saccule in the gerbil produced labelled terminals in the INVN, LVN, group *y*, lateral parts of IVN and the rostral ACN [29]. Termi-

Fig. 1. Monkeys H-1443 (A), U-55 (B) and U-91 (C). Cats U-254 (D,H), U-145 (E), U-138 (F) and U-196 (G). All dark-field photomicrographs. (A) Distribution of primary vestibular fibres in the VN as seen in a sagittal autoradiograph; S, L, M, and I indicate superior, lateral, medial and inferior vestibular nuclei. (B) Distribution of primary vestibular fibres in a transverse autoradiograph through the vestibular root; labelled fibres are seen extending into the NRgc. (C) Autoradiography of a horizontal section in a monkey with selective uptake of isotope in ganglion cells innervating the ampulla of the posterior semicircular duct; terminals are present in the rostral MVN and medial SVN. (D) Retrograde transport of HRP from the SVN to PCs in the rostromedial folia of the ipsilateral flocculus. (E) Retrograde labelling in MVN and group *y* (Y) cells from an HRP injection in the contralateral MVN. (F) Autoradiograph of commissural projections from an isotope injection in MVN to the opposite MVN. (G,H) Projections from the SVN to the OMC in an autoradiograph (G) and in an HRP-reacted section (H); fibres terminating in the SRS and IOS cross in the ventral tegmentum. Fibres terminating in the IRS ascend in the ipsilateral MLF. A–C, F and G, cresyl violet; D, E and H, neutral red. A–E and G–H, ×5; F, ×2.5.

nals were seen also in the uvula and in dorsal regions of the NRgc. VG cells innervating the crista of the posterior SD projected to medial parts of the MVN and SVN and to the uvula [29].

Cerebellar afferents

Afferents to the VN arise from the 'vestibulocerebellum' [6], the cerebellar vermis [49] and the fastigial nuclei [12].

Data concerning cerebellar projections to the VN were based upon HRP injections into individual VN in the cat and monkey [10,14,17]. Injections of HRP in the LVN produced retrograde transport in all folia of the ipsilateral anterior lobe vermis, labelling a narrow band of contiguous PCs; only scattered PCs were labelled in the posterior vermis and no cells were labelled in the ipsilateral flocculus. Cells in rostral and ventral regions of the ipsilateral FN were concomitantly labelled. Immunocytochemical data have shown GAD-reactive terminals in LVN, more intense dorsally than ventrally, and in group y [26]. Anterior lobe ablations reduced GAD-positive terminals in the LVN, but small GAD-positive cells and terminals persisted, suggesting intrinsic GABAergic neurons. Stimulation of the anterior lobe vermis produced inhibition in all regions of LVN, while fastigial neurons had excitatory influences upon neurons in the ventral LVN [4].

Injection of the IVN, including cell groups f and x, retrogradely labelled PC in the ipsilateral nodulus and uvula and cells in the middle third of the FN bilaterally with contralateral dominance. A meticulous retrograde study indicated that most projections to the IVN originated from PCs in the ipsilateral uvula, while the MVN received a projection mainly from the nodulus [31].

Cerebellar afferents to the MVN were derived mainly from a central band of PCs extending through all folia of the ipsilateral flocculus, although some PCs were labelled in the nodulus and uvula. Most of the floccular projection was to the rostral MVN. Observations were consistent with previous descriptions [42,55].

HRP injections confined to central and ventral peripheral regions of the SVN retrogradely labelled PCs only in the medial and rostral third of the ipsilateral flocculus (Fig. 1D). HRP injections in ventral peripheral parts of the SVN failed to label PCs in any part of the cerebellar cortex. These findings suggested that only cells in the central SVN receive cerebellar inputs derived from the rostromedial zone of the flocculus [43]. The SVN does not appear to receive afferents from the FN [12]. Cell group y, which receives afferents from the VG neurons innervating the saccule [20], received afferents from the most caudal zone of the flocculus [14,43].

Commissural connections

Clinical and experimental evidence indicate that the VN on the two sides function in an integrated manner, even though all primary vestibular and cerebellar cortical afferents are ipsilateral [23]. The anatomical substrate for this integrative function is a massive commissural system interconnecting portions of the VN (see [38]). Commissural fibres are of two types: (1) those that interconnect corresponding regions of the same nuclei, and (2) those that interconnect parts of different VN. The most massive commissural system interconnected virtually all parts of MVN (Fig. 1E,F). In addition, the MVN received contralateral projections from the peripheral SVN, group y and medial parts of IVN (Fig. 1E). The IVN received commissural fibres from the peripheral SVN, rostral MVN and y. The SVN received contralateral projections from the peripheral SVN, oral MVN, caudal MVN and IVN near their mutual border and group y. No cells of the LVN or groups f, x or y projected to their corresponding nucleus. Nearly all cells of group y are said to contribute to the vestibular commissural system [22]. Cells of the SVN and MVN on each side received large commissural projections interrelating corresponding regions of the nuclei. Commissural vestibular neurons receiving inputs from the ampullae have been considered to exert inhibitory effects contralaterally, while neurons with inputs from the otoliths were thought to mediate contralateral excitation [50]. The latter effect is probably mediated through the medullary RF (see [38]).

Intrinsic vestibular connections

Interconnections within the ipsilateral VN indicate interactions among component nuclei with distinctive projections. In the rat, reciprocal connections exist between the SVN and both the IVN and MVN, and less extensive connections interrelate the MVN and LVN [41]. HRP injections into the VN in the cat and monkey confirmed reciprocal projections between the MVN and IVN and the ipsilateral SVN, and demonstrated inputs to the LVN from the MVN.

Projections from brainstem nuclei

The only established descending projection to the VN arises from the INC, and provides collaterals to the ipsilateral MVN [15,37]. HRP injections into the MVN and SVN retrogradely labelled neurons in the ipsilateral INC, with the SVN receiving a smaller projection.

The perihypoglossal nuclei (i.e. the NPP, NIC and NR) project bilaterally to both the MVN and IVN [38]. The largest number of afferents, derived from the caudal NPP, were crossed (Fig. 2D).

Reticular projections

Attempts to assess reticular projections to the VN in degeneration studies have been unreliable. Localized HRP injections into individual VN in our studies indicated that reticular afferents were meagre. Modest numbers of reticular neurons were labelled bilaterally with contralateral dominance largely in dorsal regions of the pontine and medullary RF after HRP injections into the MVN, IVN and LVN. HRP injections into the SVN failed to label reticular neurons. No cells in the PPRF were labelled by any HRP injections of the VN in our studies. The only spinal afferents in our study originated from the central cervical nucleus and projected to contralateral MVN and IVN (Fig. 2F).

Projections of the vestibular nuclei

Secondary vestibular projections are more widely distributed in the neuraxis than similar secondary projections associated with other special sensory systems. This disposition reflects the multiplicity of vestibular functions related to maintenance of equilibrium, orientation in three-dimensional space and modifications of muscle tone. Observations reported here concerning efferent vestibular projections in the monkey and cat were based upon anterograde transport of [³H]amino acids and HRP injected into individual VN.

Superior vestibular nucleus

Efferent projections of the SVN were studied only in the cat. Tracer injections centred in the SVN produced ascending transport in the ipsilateral MLF and in a bundle ventral to the SCP which crossed at isthmus levels. Fibres entered the ipsilateral MLF rostral to the AN, and ascended to terminations in the TN and the IRS of the OMC (Fig. 2G,H). Smaller numbers of fibres projected beyond the OMC to terminations in the INC, the ND and the RiMLF [9]. Fibres identified near the ventral border of the SCP projected ventromedially and crossed the midline by arching over the interpeduncular nucleus. Almost all fibres crossed caudal and ventral to the decussation of the SCP, abruptly turned dorsally and projected through fibres of the SCP and MLF into the OMC (Fig. 2G,H). Fibres of this bundle terminated profusely in the SRS of the OMC; smaller numbers of fibres ended in the IOS of the OMC, the INC and ND. Isotope injections involving only dorsal, peripheral parts of the SVN produced mainly transport via the ventral tegmental bundle which was followed into the contralateral SRS and IOS of the OMC.

Crossed projections of the SVN originally were attributed to concomitant involvement of the SCP [21,32] the dentate nucleus or cell group y [46]. By combining lesions in the MLF or SCP with transport techniques, it was shown that HRP injections in the OMC selectively labelled either cells in the

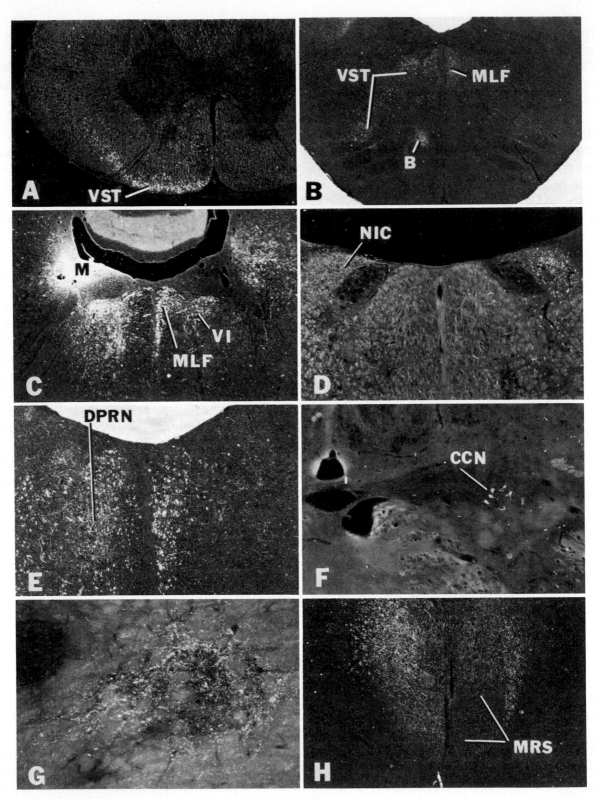

dorsal peripheral SVN (MLF lesions), or in the central SVN (SCP lesions) [56]. Cells in the peripheral SVN projected bilaterally to rostromedial folia of the flocculus with ipsilateral dominance. No fibres from the SVN descended in the VST or the MLF.

Lateral vestibular nucleus

Several fairly discrete HRP and isotope injections into the LVN were made in the cat and monkey. The principal anterograde transport was seen in the ipsilateral VST. Relatively coarse axons formed a loosely organized, oblique band in the brainstem, part of which could be followed into the ventral funiculus of the spinal cord (Fig. 2B). Collaterals of VST fibres arborized about neurons in the lateral reticular nucleus of the medulla. Anterograde transport of HRP from LVN injections could be followed in the VST only into upper cervical segments; with isotope injections, transport in the VST was evident throughout the cervical enlargement (Fig. 2A). Isotope injections into the LVN and IVN produced more extensive labelling of fibres in the VST and bilateral asymmetric transport in the descending MLF (Fig. 2B). Only large [³H]amino acid injections, involving multiple VN, produced transport in the VST which could be identified in lumbar spinal segments. Terminals of VST fibres were found mainly in medial parts of the anterior horn, i.e. in laminae VIII and VII [34].

The VST has been considered to arise exclusively from cells of the LVN, to be somatotopically organized, to extend ipsilaterally for the length of the spinal cord and to terminate on the somata and dendrites of cells in laminae VIII and VII [34,36]. Some evidence suggests that the VST may not arise exclusively from neurons in the LVN as indicated in our study; cells in the rostral IVN may contribute descending fibres [3, 35]. The somatotopic origin of the VST (cells in dorsocaudal regions projecting to lumbosacral segments and cells in the rostroventral region projecting to cervical segments) may be less precisely organized than originally considered, because some cells in the ventral LVN have been demonstrated to project to lumbar levels [3,35,52]. The somatotopic origin of the VST from the LVN is further blurred by evidence that fibres of the VST innervate more than one spinal segment [1,44] and the vestibulospinal system (LVST and MVST) has a 3–4-fold stronger influence upon cervical and lower lumbar regions than upon other spinal regions [3]. Intra-axonal HRP staining of VST axons in lower cervical segments revealed 1–7 collaterals emerging at right angles from stem axons with a restricted rostrocaudal, and extensive dorsoventral and mediolateral, terminal arborizations [44]. MVST collaterals projected into laminae VII and VIII and LVST collaterals projected to lamina IX. Cervical LVST collaterals made apparent synaptic contacts with proximal dendrites and/or somata of motoneurons and small numbers of collaterals crossed the midline and terminated in laminae VII and VIII. It seems probable that collaterals given off by the LVST in lumbar segments may have a similar disposition. In lumbosacral spinal segments the LVST has monosynaptic excitatory effects

Fig. 2. Monkeys U-177 (A), U-116 (B) and U-176 (H). Cats U-138 (C), U-122 (D), U-161 (E) and U-127 (F,G). All dark-field photomicrographs. (A) Autoradiograph of isotope transport via the VST at C₄. Following large injections of [³H]amino acids into the VN, transport could be traced in the VST to lumbar levels. (B) Autoradiograph of isotope transported via the VST and MLF in the medulla from an isotope injection in the LVN (L) and IVN (I); terminals from the IVN can be seen in nucleus β (B) of the ipsilateral inferior olive. (C) Autoradiograph of an isotope injection in the rostral MVN (M) with transport to the AN (VI) bilaterally, the opposite MLF and parts of the MVN and SVN contralaterally. (D) Anterograde and retrograde transport of HRP from the left MVN and IVN bilaterally to the NIC. (E) Autoradiograph of isotope transport via the descending MLF (bilateral) with terminals in the left dorsal paramedian reticular nucleus (DPRN). Isotope injection involved the LVN and IVN on the left. (F) Retrograde transport of HRP from the IVN to the contralateral CCN. (G) Anterograde transport of HRP from the IVN to profuse terminals in nucleus β. (H) Autoradiograph of isotope transported to the OMC from a large isotope injection involving all vestibular nuclei on the left; note the virtually clear area on the right which represents the MRS. A, B, C, E and H, cresyl violet; D, F and G, neutral red. A, E and F, ×15; B, ×5; C, D and H, ×9; G, ×63.

mainly upon extensor motoneurons that effect the ankle and knee [25,30].

Transport studies in the cat, but not in the monkey, revealed ascending ipsilateral projections via the ascending tract of Deiters' to the MRS of the OMC. Our studies provide no evidence that the LVN projects fibres to any part of the cerebellar cortex.

Inferior vestibular nucleus

Axoplasmic transport from injections into the IVN in the cat and monkey labelled terminals bilaterally in the dorsal paramedial reticular nuclei with ipsilateral dominance and terminals in the ipsilateral nucleus β of the inferior olive (Fig. 2B,E,G). Labelled axons descended bilaterally in the MLF to upper cervical spinal segments with the largest number of fibres ipsilateral; fibres could be traced into laminae VII and VIII. Ascending projections from the IVN entered the contralateral MLF and terminated in the TN and the IRS of the OMC. Cerebellar projections from the IVN were localized to the cortex of the ipsilateral nodulus and uvula.

Although degeneration studies indicated that descending spinal fibres in the MLF (MVST) originated only from MVN [33], physiological evidence suggested origins from the MVN, the IVN and a few cells in the LVN [39,53]. Stimulation of the VN has revealed that fibres in the MVST making monosynaptic connections with cervical α-motoneurons have both inhibitory and excitatory actions [5,51]. These effects, which could be evoked by stimulation of the labyrinth, acted upon cervical and thoracic motoneurons, but not on limb motoneurons. Inhibitory influences were mediated by subpopulations of neurons in the MVN, IVN and LVN [39]. A long vestibulospinal tract originating from the caudal MVN, IVN and group f could not be distinguished in our studies [35].

Medial vestibular nucleus

Projections from the MVN in the cat and monkey were similar in HRP and autoradiographic studies.

Terminals were present bilaterally in the NPP and the NIC with ipsilateral dominance (Fig. 2D). Bilateral descending fibres in the MLF were asymmetrically disposed; ipsilateral fibres were located dorsolaterally while contralateral fibres were ventromedial. Most of the crossed descending fibres in the MLF disappeared at lower medullary levels. Terminal arborizations were present around cells in the ipsilateral supraspinal nucleus and surrounding cells of the contralateral CCN. Fibres in the ipsilateral MLF were followed only into upper cervical segments. In the cat, ascending fibres emerged from the rostral MVN to enter the AN and the dorsomedial part of the opposite MLF. Terminals were profuse in all parts of the ipsilateral AN, but contralaterally were present only in dorsomedial regions of the AN (Fig. 2C). Fibres ascending in the opposite MLF terminated profusely in the TN and less numerously in the IRS of the OMC [2]. Fibres bypassing the OMC projected to the contralateral INC and modestly to the ND. A smaller number of fibres ascending in the ipsilateral MLF bypassed the TN and terminated in the MRS and IRS of the OMC.

Observations concerning ascending projections from the MVN in the monkey were flawed by isotope spread into the AN. Reliable observations could be made concerning ascending projections in the ipsilateral MLF, which were followed to terminations in the IRS, MRS and the IOS of the OMC. Fibres in the contralateral MLF, unquestionably arising from the MVN, terminated profusely in the TN and about cells of the INC. An autoradiographic comparison of ascending projections from the VN and AIN to the OMC in the monkey revealed virtually no projection to the contralateral MRS from the VN (Fig. 2H), but profuse endings around MRS neurons originated from the AIN [13]. Cerebellar projections from the MVN terminated mainly in a central band of the ipsilateral flocculus in the granular layer.

A physiological study indicated that projection neurons were most concentrated in the rostral MVN, and only about 17% of the MVN neurons had long descending axons [54]. Spinal projections of the MVN contained in the MLF had properties like other MVST fibres, although a larger number may have inhibitor actions upon motoneurons [40]. Since large numbers of neurons in the MVN project ascending and descending fibres in the MLF, it might be expected that collaterals of some cells would project in both directions. Injections of HRP in single axons of identified MVN neurons revealed bilateral terminals in the AN, bifurcating ascending and descending branches in the contralateral MLF and collaterals extending into the NPP and RF [27]. Dichotomizing axons of ventrolateral MVN neurons projected to the opposite AN and to motoneuronal pools at the C1–C2 spinal level [28]. About 60% of vestibulo-ocular neurons related to the ACN with projections to subdivisions of the OMC have been reported to send collaterals to contralateral extensor motoneurons in upper spinal segments [48]. These VOC neurons were located in the IVN, MVN and ventral LVN.

Cell groups x, y *and* z

Attempts to trace efferents from cell group *y* using HRP or isotope revealed only modest transport to parts of the ipsilateral MVN and IVN. These findings conflicted with our own retrograde studies indicating that cells of group *y* projected commissural fibres to parts of the MVN, IVN and SVN. Re-interpretation of our data leads to the conclusion that most of the cells of group *y* probably give rise to commissural fibres. Cells of the infracerebellar nucleus which do not respond to vestibular nerve stimulation project to the contralateral INC [19].

There has been some question as to whether groups *x* and *z*, which receive spinal afferents, should be considered vestibular nuclei. Cell group *z* projects to the contralateral thalamus and group *x* projects to the cerebellum [7,24]. In the monkey virtually all neurons in groups *x* and *z* are immunoreactive to choline acetyltransferase, while in the VN only modest numbers of cells in the caudal MVN and IVN are immunoreactive [16].

Acknowledgements

This work was supported by research grant C07005 from the Department of Defense, Uniformed Services University of the Health Sciences. The opinions and assertions contained herein are the private ones of the author and are not to be construed as official or reflecting the view of the Department of Defense or the Uniformed Services University of the Health Sciences. The experiments reported herein were conducted according to the principles set forth in the 'Guide for the Care and Use of Laboratory Animals', Institute of Laboratory Animal Resources, National Research Council NIH Pub. No. 80-23.

References

[1] Abzug, C., Maeda, M., Peterson, B.W. and Wilson, V.J. (1974) Cervical branching of lumbar vestibulospinal axons. *J. Physiol. London*, 243: 499–522.

[2] Akagi, Y. (1978) The localization of motor neurons innervating the extraocular muscles in the oculomotor nuclei of the cat and rabbit using horseradish peroxidase. *J. Comp. Neurol.*, 181: 745–762.

[3] Akaike, T. (1983) Neuronal organization of the vestibulospinal system in the cat. *Brain Res.*, 259: 217–227.

[4] Akaike, T. (1983) Electrophysiological analysis of cerebellar corticovestibular and fastigiovestibular projections to the lateral vestibular nucleus in the cat. *Brain Res.*, 272: 223–235.

[5] Akaike, T., Fanardjian, V.V., Ito, M. and Ohno, T. (1973) Electrophysiological analysis of the vestibulospinal reflex pathway of rabbit. II. Synaptic action upon spinal neurons. *Exp. Brain Res.*, 17: 497–515.

[6] Angaut, P. and Brodal, A. (1967) The projection of the 'vestibulocerebellum' onto the vestibular nuclei in the cat. *Arch. Ital. Biol.*, 105: 441–479.

[7] Brodal, A. (1974) Anatomy of the vestibular nuclei and their connections. In Kornhuber, H.H. (Ed.), *Handbook of Sensory Physiology, Vol. 6, Vestibular System*, Springer-Verlag, Berlin, pp. 239–352.

[8] Brodal, A. and Pompeiano, O. (1957) The vestibular nuclei in the cat. *J. Anat. London*, 91: 438–454.

[9] Büttner-Ennever, J.A. and Büttner, U. (1978) A cell group associated with vertical eye monuments in the rostral mesencephalic reticular formation of the monkey. *Brain Res.*, 151: 29–51.

[10] Carleton, S.C. and Carpenter, M.B. (1983) Afferent and efferent connections of the medial, inferior and lateral vestibular nuclei in the cat and monkey. *Brain Res.*, 278: 29–51.

[11] Carleton, S.C. and Carpenter, M.B. (1984) Distribution of primary vestibular fibres in the brainstem and cerebellum of the monkey. *Brain Res.*, 294: 281–298.

[12] Carpenter, M.B. and Batton, R.R. III (1982) Connections

14

of the fastigial nuclei in the cat and monkey. *Exp. Brain Res. Suppl.*, 6: 250–295.

[13] Carpenter, M.B. and Carleton, S.C. (1983) Comparison of vestibular and abducens internuclear projections to the medial rectus subdivision of the oculomotor nucleus in the monkey. *Brain Res.*, 274: 144–149.

[14] Carpenter, M.B. and Cowie, R.J. (1985) Connections and oculomotor projections of the superior vestibular nucleus and cell group 'y'. *Brain Res.*, 336: 265–287.

[15] Carpenter, M.B., Harbison, J.W. and Peter, P. (1970) Accessory oculomotor nuclei in the monkey: projections and effects of discrete lesions *J. Comp. Neurol.*, 140: 131–154.

[16] Carpenter, M.B., Chang, L., Pereira, A.B. and Hersh, L.B. (1987) Comparisons of the immunocytochemical localization of choline acetyltransferase in the vestibular nuclei of the monkey and rat. *Brain Res.*, 418: 403–408.

[17] Corvaja, N. and Pompeiano, O. (1979) Identification of cerebellar corticovestibular neurons retrogradely labelled with horseradish peroxidase. *Neuroscience*, 4: 507–515.

[18] Demêmes, D., Raymond, J. and Sans, A. (1984) Selective retrograde labelling of neurons of the cat vestibular ganglion with [^{3}H]D-aspartate. *Brain Res.*, 304: 188–191.

[19] Fukushima, K., Terashima, T., Kudo, J., Inoue, Y. and Kato, M. (1986) Projections of group y of the vestibular nuclei and the dentate and fastigial nuclei of the cerebellum to the interstitial nucleus of Cajal. *Neurosci Res.*, 3: 285–299.

[20] Gacek, R.R (1969) The course and central distribution of first order neurons supplying vestibular endorgans in the cat. *Acta Otolaryngol. Stockholm Suppl.*, 154: 1–66.

[21] Gacek, R.R. (1971) Anatomical demonstration of the vestibulo-ocular projections in the cat. *Acta Otolaryngol. Stockholm Suppl.*, 293: 1–63.

[22] Gacek, R.R. (1978) Location of commissural neurons in the vestibular nuclei of the cat. *Exp. Neurol.*, 59: 479–491.

[23] Galiana, H.L., Flohr, H. and Melvill Jones, G. (1984) A reevaluation of intervestibular nuclear coupling: its role in vestibular compensation. *J. Neurophysiol.*, 51 (1984): 242–259.

[24] Grant, G., Boivie, J. and Silfvenius, H. (1973) Course and termination of fibres from the nucleus z of the medulla oblongata. An experimental light microscopical study in the cat. *Brain Res.*, 55: 55–70.

[25] Grillner, S., Hongo, T. and Lund, S. (1970) The vestibulospinal tract. Effects on alpha-motoneurons in the lumbosacral spinal cord in the cat. *Exp. Brain Res.*, 10: 94–120.

[26] Houser, C.R., Barber, R.P. and Vaughn, J.E. (1984) Immunocytochemical localization of glutamic acid decarboxylase in the dorsal lateral vestibular nucleus: evidence for an intrinsic and extrinsic GABAergic innervation. *Neurosci. Lett.*, 47: 213–220.

[27] Ishizuka, N., Mannen, H., Sasaki, S.-I. and Shimazu, H. (1980) Axonal branches and terminations in the cat abducens nucleus of secondary vestibular neurons in the horizontal canal system. *Neurosci. Lett.*, 16: 143–148.

[28] Isu, N. and Yokata, J (1983) Morphophysiological study in the divergent projection of axon collaterals of medial vestibular nucleus neurons in the cat. *Exp. Brain Res.*, 53: 151–162.

[29] Kevetter, G.A. and Perachio, A.A. (1986) Distribution of vestibular afferents that innervate the sacculus and posterior canal in the gerbil. *J. Comp. Neurol.*, 254: 410–424.

[30] Lund, S. and Pompeiano, O. (1968) Monosynaptic excitation of alpha motoneurons from supraspinal structures in the cats. *Acta Physiol. Scand.*, 73: 1–21.

[31] Matsushita, M. and Wang, C.L. (1986) Cerebellar corticovestibular projections from lobule IX to the descending vestibular nucleus in the cat. A retrograde wheat germ agglutinin – horseradish peroxidase study. *Neurosci. Lett.*, 66: 293–298.

[32] McMasters, R.E., Weiss, A.H. and Carpenter, M.B. (1966) Vestibular projections to the nuclei of the extraocular muscles. Degeneration resulting from discrete partial lesions of the vestibular nuclei in the monkey. *Am. J. Anat.*, 118: 163–194.

[33] Nyberg-Hansen, R. (1964) Origin and termination of fibers from the vestibular nuclei descending in the medial longitudinal fasciculus. An experiment study with silver impregnation methods in the cat. *J. Comp. Neurol.*, 122: 355–367.

[34] Nyberg-Hansen, R. and Mascitti, T.A. (1964) Sites and mode of termination of fibers of the vestibulospinal tract in the cat. An experimental study with silver impregnation methods. *J. Comp. Neurol.*, 122: 369–388.

[35] Peterson, B.W. and Coulter, J.D. (1977) A new long spinal projection from the vestibular nuclei in the cat. *Brain Res.*, 122: 351–356.

[36] Pompeiano, O. and Brodal, A. (1957) The origin of vestibulospinal fibres in the cat. *Arch. Ital. Biol.*, 95: 166–195.

[37] Pompeiano, O. and Walberg, F. (1957) Descending connections to the vestibular nuclei: An experimental study in the cat. *J. Comp. Neurol.*, 108: 465–504.

[38] Pompeiano, O., Mergner, T. and Corvaja, N. (1978) Commissural, perihypoglossal and reticular afferent projections to the vestibular nuclei in the cat. *Arch. Ital. Biol.*, 116: 130–172.

[39] Rapaport, S., Susswein, A., Uchino, Y. and Wilson, V.J. (1977) Properties of vestibular neurons projections to neck segments of the cats spinal cord. *J. Physiol. London*, 268: 493–510.

[40] Rapoport, S., Susswein, A., Uchino, Y. and Wilson, V.J. (1977) Synaptic actions of individual vestibular neurons on cat neck motoneurons. *J. Physiol. London*, 272: 367–382.

[41] Rubertone, D.A., Mehler, W.R. and Cox, G.E. (1983) The intrinsic organization of the vestibular complex: evidence for internuclear connectivity. *Brain Res.*, 263: 137–141.

[42] Sato, Y., Kawasaki, T. and Ikarashi, K. (1982) Zonal organization of the floccular Purkinje cells projecting to the ves-

tibular nucleus in cats. *Brain Res.*, 232: 1–15.

[43] Sato, Y., Kawasaki. T. and Ikarashi, K. (1982) Zonal organization of the floccular Purkinje cells projecting to the group y of the vestibular nuclear complex and the lateral cerebellar nucleus in cats. *Brain Res*, 234: 430–434.

[44] Shinoda, Y., Ohgaki, T. and Futami, T. (1986) The morphology of single lateral vestibulospinal tract axons in the lower cervical spinal cord of the cat. *J. Comp. Neurol.*, 249: 226–241.

[45] Siegborn, J. and Grant, G. (1983) Brainstem projections of different branches of the vestibular nerve. An experimental study by transganglionic transport of horseradish peroxidase in the cat. I. The horizontal ampullar and utricular nerves. *Arch., Ital Biol.* 121: 237–248.

[46] Stanton, G.B. (1980) Afferents to oculomotor nuclei from area 'Y' in *Macaca mulatta*: an anterograde degeneration study. *J. Comp. Neurol.*, 192: 377–385.

[47] Stein, B.M. and Carpenter, M.B. (1967) Central projections of portions of the vestibular ganglia innervating specific parts of the labyrinth in the rhesus monkey. *Am. J. Anat.*, 120: 281–318.

[48] Uchino, Y. and Hirai, N. (1984) Axon collaterals of anterior semicircular canal-activated vestibular neurons and their coactivation of extraocular and neck motoneurons in the cat. *Neurosci. Res.*, 1: 309–325.

[49] Walberg, F. and Jansen, J. (1961) Cerebellar corticovestibular fibers in the cat. *Exp. Neurol.*, 3: 32–52.

[50] Wilson, V.J. and Melvill Jones, G. (1979) *Mammalian Vestibular Physiology*, Plenum Press, New York, 365 pp.

[51] Wilson, V.J. and Yoshida, M. (1969) Monosynaptic inhibition of neck motoneurons by the medial vestibular nucleus. *Exp. Brain Res.*, 9: 365–380.

[52] Wilson, V.J., Kato, M., Peterson, B.W. and Wylie, R.M. (1967) A single unit analysis of the organization of Deiters' nucleus. *J. Neurophysiol.*, 30: 603–619.

[53] Wilson, V.J., Wylie, R.M. and Marco, L.A. (1967) Projection to spinal cord from the medial and descending vestibular nuclei. *Nature*, 215: 429–430.

[54] Wilson, V.J., Wylie, R.M. and Marco, L.A. (1968) Organization of the medial vestibular nucleus. *J. Neurophysiol.*, 31: 166–175.

[55] Yamamoto, M. and Shimoyama, I. (1977) Differential localization of rabbit's flocculus Purkinje cells to the medial and superior vestibular nuclei, investigated by means of horseradish peroxidase retrograde axonal transport. *Neurosci. Lett.*, 5: 279–283.

[56] Yamamoto, M., Shimoyama, I. and Highstein, S.M. (1978) Vestibular nucleus neurons relaying excitation from the anterior canal to the oculomotor nucleus. *Brain Res.*, 148: 31–42.

O. Pompeiano and J.H.J. Allum (Eds.)
Progress in Brain Research, Vol. 76
© 1988 Elsevier Science Publishers B.V. (Biomedical Division)

CHAPTER 2

Vestibular projections to the spinal cord: the morphology of single vestibulospinal axons

Y. Shinoda[1], T. Ohgaki[2], T. Futami[1] and Y. Sugiuchi[2]

[1]*Department of Physiology and* [2]*Department of Otolaryngology, School of Medicine, Tokyo Medical and Dental University, 1-5-45, Yushima, Bunkyo-ku, Tokyo, 113, Japan*

The three-dimensional distribution of LVST and MVST axons was examined in the cat cervical spinal cord using an intra-axonal staining method. LVST and MVST axons were electrophysiologically identified by their responses to stimulation of the vestibular nucleus, bilateral vestibular primary afferents, the LVST and the MVST were stained with injection of HRP. The axonal trajectory was reconstructed from serial histological sections. LVST axons were found to have multiple axon collaterals in the cervical cord. The maximum number of the identified collaterals for one neuron was 7. These collaterals were observed in either LVST axons terminating at the cervical cord or those projecting below Th2. The rostrocaudal extension of terminals for each collateral was very restricted (mean = 760 μm) and much narrower than intercollateral intervals (mean = 1470 μm). In the gray matter, collaterals ramified successively, pursued a delta-like path, and terminated mainly in lamina VIII and in the medial part of lamina VII and many boutons made apparent contact with the cell bodies and the proximal dendrites of motoneurons in the ventromedial nucleus. Some terminals were also distributed to the ventrolateral part of lamina VII adjacent to lamina IX. One group of LVST axons projected to lamina IX in the lateral ventral horn and terminated on large neurons there, probably motoneurons of forelimb muscles. MVST axons had one to seven axon collaterals at C1–C3 within the range of the stained axon. Stem axons ran in the ventromedial funiculus and primary collaterals arose from them at right angles. Each collateral had a very narrow rostrocaudal spread as in LVST axons. Terminals were distributed in laminae VIII and IX, including the ventromedial nucleus, the spinal accessory nucleus, and the commissural nucleus. Many terminals seemed to make contact with retrogradely labelled motoneurons of neck muscles. Both crossed and uncrossed MVST axons had these characteristics.

Introduction

Vestibular influences on the spinal cord are mainly conveyed through two vestibulospinal tracts, the LVST and MVST. The LVST originates predominantly from Deiters' nucleus and descends to the sacral cord in the ventral funiculus [21,23], although a small number of the rostral descending nucleus neurons contribute to LVST cells [3,25]. The MVST mainly originates in the medial vestbular nucleus [19] and a minor contribution of neurons in the descending and lateral nuclei to this tract was recently found [3,14,25]. Some of the VS fibres in the LVST have monosynaptic connections with motoneurons for certain knee and ankle extensors, but they mainly exert di- and polysynaptic excitatory effects on extensor motoneurons and inhibitory effects on flexor motoneurons of the hindlimb [7,15,16]. Deiters' nucleus neurons have

---

Abbreviations: HRP, horseradish peroxidase; RS, reticulospinal; VS, vestibulospinal; (L/M)VST, (lateral/medial) vestibulospinal tract.

no monosynaptic connection with elbow, wrist and digit motoneurons, but they make polysynaptic excitatory connections with extensor forelimb motoneurons [41]. In contrast to these connections with forelimb motoneurons, LVST and MVST fibres make monosynaptic excitatory connections with neck [41] and trunk [42] motoneurons. Convergence of inputs from different semicircular canals and otolith organs [17,38,43] and interaction between vestibular inputs and peripheral somatic inputs [4,5,7] have been extensively analysed at different spinal neurons. But there is little information on its converse, divergent properties of single VS axons in the spinal cord. The descriptions of single vestibular nucleus neuron morphologies are based on studies using the Golgi impregnation method. These studies established the morphology of cell bodies and dendrites of vestibular nucleus neurons [9,18]. In Golgi-stained vestibular neurons, however, their axons could not be traced to the spinal cord.

This brief review will describe the intraspinal morphology of single LVST and MVST axons in the cervical spinal cord of the cat. VST axons were electrophysiologically identified and intra-axonally stained with HRP. HRP-stained axons were reconstructed three-dimensionally from serial sections [34].

Electrophysiological identification of VST axons

LVST axons were penetrated in the ventral funiculus between C1 and C8 at a depth of 4.0–6.6 mm (mainly 5.0–6.3 mm) from the dorsal cord surface and MVST axons in the ventromedial funiculus between C1 and C3 at a depth of 3.5–5.0 mm. Intra-axonal spikes were evoked from the ipsilateral vestibular nerve at a latency of 1.1 to 3.6 ms. When intra-axonal spikes were evoked by stimulation of the vestibular nerve, the axons were further examined by evaluating their direct responses to stimulation of the vestibular nucleus and the LVST and MVST at the medullary level. Since neurons activated with short latencies from the vestibular nerve can be either VS neurons or RS neurons [40], it was necessary to exclude RS axons from our sample. Latencies consistent with monosynaptic activation of second-order vestibular neurons range from 0.8 to 1.5 ms [39] or are shorter than 1.4 ms [24]. Therefore, the difference between the latencies of the vestibular-nerve-induced spikes and of the nucleus-induced spikes or the tract-induced spikes was calculated for each axon. When this difference was shorter than 1.3 ms (the longest value for monosynaptic activation (1.4 ms) minus a latent period for spike generation after stimulus onset (0.1 ms)), the axons were considered to be activated monosynaptically from the vestibular nerve. After electrophysiological identification of VS axons, HRP was injected iontophoretically through a recording electrode. Details of the injection and staining methods were described elsewhere [32,34].

Morphology of LVST axons in the lower cervical cord

Stem axons and primary collaterals

Stem axons of LVST neurons ran ventral to the ventral horn. The stem axons were stained over distances from 3.4 to 16.3 mm (mean ± S.D. 8.5 ± 3.7 mm) at a level between C4 and Th1. Over their course, multiple axon collaterals arose from single stem axons and all but one of the 19 axons examined had at least one axon collateral (Fig. 1). The maximum number of collaterals for a single LVST axon was 7 (mean ± S.D. 3.2 ± 2.0, n = 19). Intercollateral distances ranged from 400 to 4300 μm (mean ± S.D. 1490 ± 860 μm, n = 42) (Fig. 4). The collaterals were given off more or less at right angles from stem axons and entered the ventral horn at the ventral border of lamina VIII or lamina VII of Rexed [26, 27] and in some, at the lateral or ventrolateral border of lamina IX (Fig. 1). The diameter of stem axons ranged from 2.2 to 6.1 μm (mean ± S.D. 4.5 ± 1.1 μm, n = 20). In contrast, the diameter of the primary axon collaterals was very small, ranging from 1.0 to 2.1 μm (mean ± S.D. 1.6 ± 0.4 μm, n = 20).

Morphology of collaterals and their arborizations

Collaterals of LVST axons have a distinctive morphology and their branching patterns are very different from the patterns of other long descending tract axons [6,33]. LVST axons could be divided into two groups in terms of their collateral distribution in the gray matter; LVST axons of the medial type which had a main projection to laminae VII and VIII, and LVST axons of the lateral type which had a main projection to lamina IX. The more common of the two was the axon of the medial type. Although there were two main types, intermediate forms also existed.

LVST axons of the medial type

The stem axons of this type tended to descend in a more medial position in the ventral funiculus (Fig. 1), so that the primary collaterals ran almost vertically in a dorsal direction and entered the gray matter at the ventral border of lamina VIII or of lamina VII adjacent to lamina VIII. After entrance into the gray matter, the collaterals of the medial type continued to run in the dorsal direction and ramified successively 3 to 6 times through Rexed's laminae VII–VIII. Their main terminal arborizations were distributed to lamina VIII and the medioventral portion of lamina VII. On the way through la-

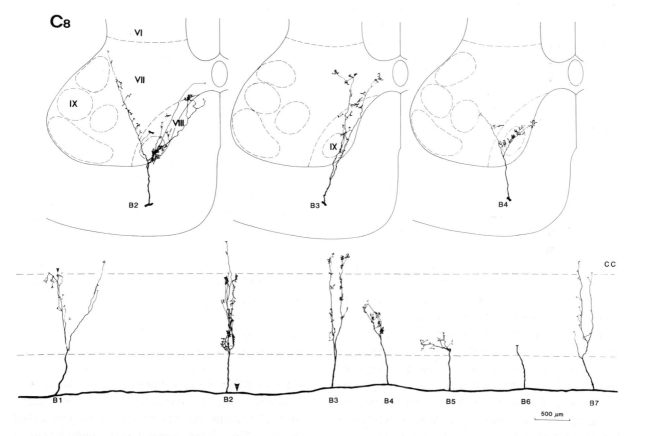

Fig. 1. Reconstructions of axon collaterals from a single LVST axon of the medial type at C8. Upper drawings are reconstructions in the transverse plane of B2–B4 axon collaterals shown in the sagittal plane in the lower drawing. The lower border of the central canal (CC) and the lower border of the ventral horn are indicated by the dashed lines. The arrow head indicates the injection site. The stem axon could be traced further rostrally (5.9 mm from B1) and caudally (2.7 mm from B7).

mina VIII, thin side branches were given off and terminal arborizations were distributed within the group of large cells (the nucleus ventromedialis) (Fig. 1, upper drawings). The collaterals then pursued a more-or-less straight course through lamina VIII or lamina VII close to the dorsal border of lamina VIII, occasionally subdividing as they ran in a dorsal direction. The collaterals then formed extensive terminal arborizations in the dorsal portion of lamina VIII or in the medial portion of lamina VII slightly ventral to the level of the central canal (Fig. 1, upper middle). In addition, some collaterals were also found to terminate in both these areas. These findings are in good agreement with the results of previous degeneration studies [20,21].

In contrast to the extensive dorsoventral and mediolateral extent of terminal arborizations, the rostrocaudal terminal field was very restricted. When viewed in the sagittal plane, collaterals formed a Y-shaped or delta-like path (Fig. 1). Usually, the terminal arborizations had the maximum rostrocaudal spread at the most dorsal portion which almost corresponded to a level of the central canal. The terminal arborizations of single collaterals extended rostrocaudally between 230 and 1560 μm (mean $\pm$ S.D. 760 $\pm$ 220 μm) for 16 collaterals that were particularly well stained and could, therefore, be traced to their terminals. Consecutive collaterals from a single axon were almost in line with one another in the sagittal plane, as is seen in Fig. 1. There were gaps between adjacent terminal arborizations from the same stem axon in a majority of LVST axons, since the intercollateral distances (1470 $\pm$ 880 μm, $n = 32$) were wider than the rostrocaudal lengths of individual collaterals (mean 760 μm). In rare cases, however, the terminal arborizations of adjacent collaterals overlapped each other. The branching patterns and collateral morphologies of adjacent collaterals from a single stem axon were essentially the same. This general feature of adjacent collaterals from single LVST axons is summarized in Fig. 4.

LVST axons terminate in the more dorsal portion of lamina VIII, where there are commissural cells sending their axons across the midline in the anterior commissure [37]. Some of these commissural interneurons terminate on contralateral motoneurons [8,29]. The contralateral effects following unilateral vestibular nucleus stimulation [10] might be exerted by way of these commissural cells. This was assumed to be the only pathway to convey contralateral effects, since a previous anatomical study reported that the VST was entirely uncrossed [21]. In the medial type of axons, however, there was a subgroup which had a contralateral as well as ipsilateral projection. This contralateral projection was not as extensive as the ipsilateral one and the main contralateral projection areas occupied lamina VIII and the ventromedial lamina VII at approximately the same rostrocaudal level as the ipsilateral projection area. Accordingly, some of the contralateral effects may be exerted by way of these axon collaterals of LVST axons.

LVST axons of the lateral type

About one-quarter of the examined axons which terminated at the brachial segments had a main projection to the lateral part of the ventral horn and terminated in lamina IX, so that they were grouped as the lateral type. A typical example of collaterals of the lateral type is shown in Fig. 3. The stem axons of the lateral type were usually located in the lateral portion of the ventral funiculus. Primary collaterals were given off approximately at right angles from the stem axons and ran vertically or slightly dorsolaterally to enter the gray matter at the ventral border of lamina IX or lamina VII adjacent to lamina IX.

Cervical collaterals of the LVST axons projecting to the thoracic or lumbar cord

Some LVST axons (4/11) projecting to the thoracic or lumbar cord had axon collaterals in the cervical cord. The maximum number of collaterals observed was two. This was in contrast to the finding that 22 out of 23 axons terminating above Th2 had 1 to 7 collaterals. The branching patterns of the axons in this group were essentially similar to those of the

21

axons of the medial type mentioned previously. Axon collaterals mainly projected to lamina VII and VIII (Fig. 4).

Morphology and distribution of synaptic boutons

Synaptic boutons of LVST axons are shown in the camera lucida drawings of Figs. 2 and 3. The total number of boutons per collateral varied from 38 to 262 (mean ± S.D. 161 ± 76, $n = 5$) for the medial type axons and from 98 to 271 (182 ± 69, $n = 5$) for the lateral type axons. In the transverse plane of the spinal cord, the synaptic boutons of LVST axons of the medial type were found mainly in laminae VII and VIII and very few were found in lami-

na IX in the lateral ventral horn (Fig. 2); those of the lateral type were mainly in lamina IX in the lateral ventral horn and lamina VII (Fig. 3). Abundant boutons were observed in the medial portion of lamina VII adjacent to the central canal (Fig. 2) and dorsal to lamina VIII in LVST axons of the medial type, but no substantial number of boutons was found in this region in LVST axons of the lateral type. Many synaptic boutons were also found in the ventrolateral or lateral portions of lamina VII adjacent to lamina IX. LVST axons of both the medial and the lateral type had a projection to this area. Boutons of LVST axons of the medial type were distributed over all of lamina VIII including the ventromedial nucleus (lamina IX within lamina

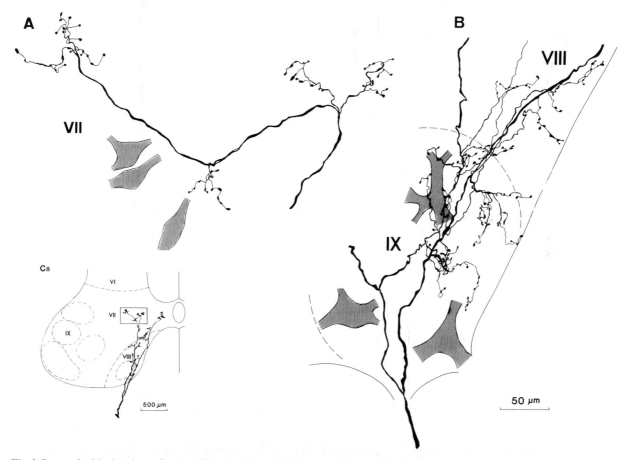

Fig. 2 Camera lucida drawings of synaptic boutons from LVST axons of the medial type, from transverse sections at C8. (A) Terminal axons in lamina VII of the axon collateral shown in the inset on the lower left. (B) Terminal axons in lamina VIII and lamina IX (the ventromedial nucleus) within lamina VIII. The calibration on the bottom right applies to A and B.

22

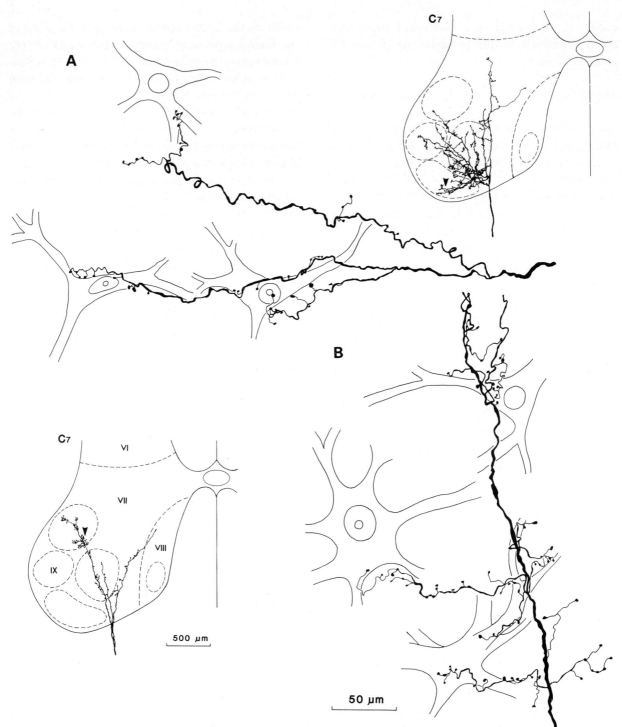

Fig. 3. Camera lucida drawings of synaptic boutons from two LVST axons of the lateral type, from transverse sections at C7. (A) Terminal axons in lamina IX of the axon collateral (indicated by an arrow head) shown in the inset on the right. (B) Terminal axons in lamina IX of the axon collateral (indicated by an arrow head) shown in the inset on the left. Note that boutons appear to make contact with motoneurons in lamina IX.

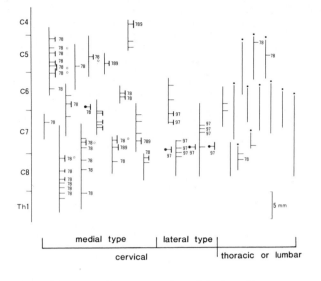

C4
C5
C6
C7
C8
Th1

medial type | lateral type
cervical | thoracic or lumbar

5 mm

Fig. 4. Diagrammatic representation of the branching patterns of LVST axons in the spinal cord. The total length of each stem axon stained is shown, together with the position of primary axon collaterals from the stem axon. The first 15 axons from the left were identified as belonging to the medial type. The next 6 axons belonged to the lateral type, and the next two axons were not identified. The numbers beside each collateral indicate the laminae where the collaterals terminate. The numbers from left to right indicate the prominence of termination. The stars (11 axons from the right) indicate the LVST axons projecting below Th2. Open circles indicate collaterals involving a contralateral projection. Closed circles indicate the axons in which collaterals were penetrated instead of stem axons.

VIII) (Fig. 2B). The terminal arborizations of LVST axons had boutons en passage and boutons terminals. Most synaptic boutons did not make contact with dendrites or cell bodies of the counter-stained cells but some boutons appeared to make contact with the proximal dendrites of neurons in laminae VII and VIII. This finding suggests that LVST axons mainly terminate on the more distal dendrites of cells in laminae VII and VIII. Apparent axosomatic and axodendritic contacts were also observed on some large (30–40 μm) and medium-sized (20–30 μm) neurons in the ventromedial nucleus within lamina VIII. A previous degeneration study reported that terminations of LVST axons were not found on motoneurons in the ventromedial

nucleus in the spinal enlargements, although a few terminations could be observed on this group of motoneurons of the thoracic cord [21]. The present study demonstrates the presence of synaptic contacts of LVST axons on the proximal dendrites and cell bodies of large cells in the ventromedial nucleus within lamina VIII, which are presumably motoneurons to axial muscles. In lamina IX, axon terminals were found in different motor nuclei of the lateral group and boutons appeared to make contact with cell bodies or the proximal dendrites of large neurons (30–50 μm) and sometimes small neurons. Synaptic boutons of LVST axons made apparent contact with proximal dendrites or somata of large neurons in lamina IX, presumably motoneurons to distal forelimb muscles. In previous degeneration studies no degeneration was seen in the lateral motor columns of the spinal enlargements following a lesion in the vestibular nuclei [20,21]. Grillner et al. [7], however, demonstrated monosynaptic excitation of quadriceps and gastrocnemius motoneurons by stimulation of Deiters' nucleus. Monosynaptic connections to forelimb motoneurons in the cat were absent [41], although LVST axons exerted monosynaptic effects on neck muscle motoneurons and thoracic back muscle motoneurons [41,42]. The present result gives morphological support to Grillner et al.'s physiological evidence, but does not fit with the data of Wilson's group.

Axon terminals were found in lamina VII adjacent to lamina IX in LVST axons of both medial and lateral type (Fig. 1 (upper left) and Fig. 2). LVST projection to this area has not yet been reported. This projection is important with regard to inhibitory postsynaptic potentials evoked disynaptically from Deiters' nucleus in hindlimb motoneurons [7]. By examining spatial summation between segmental and descending inputs, it has been shown that the LVST inhibits some hindlimb flexor motoneurons via the Ia inhibitory interneurons on the segmental reciprocal inhibitory pathway [11,12]. These Ia inhibitory interneurons are found to be located in lamina VII adjacent to lamina IX [13]. The present finding that LVST axons project to this same area at lower cervical levels may provide ana-

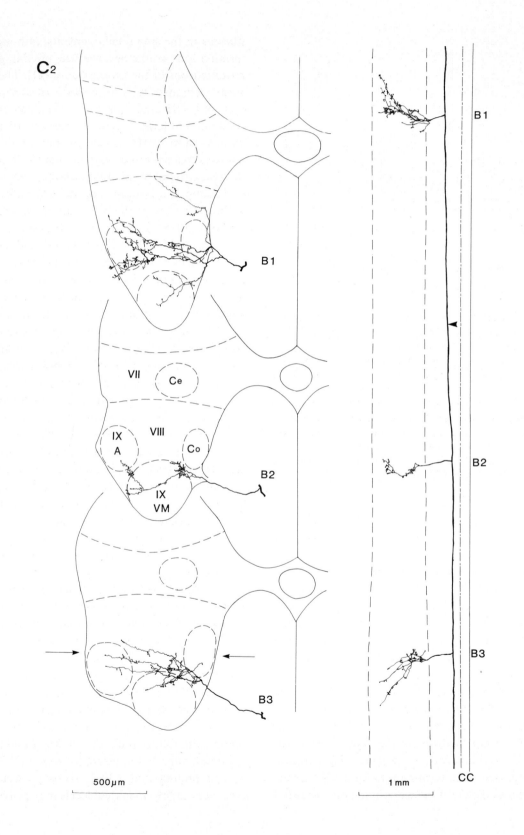

C₂

VII

Ce

IX
A

VIII

Co

IX
VM

B1

B2

B3

500μm

B1

B2

B3

CC

1 mm

tomical evidence for convergent inputs from Ia fibres and LVST axons onto Ia inhibitory interneurons.

Morphology of single MVST axons in the upper cervical cord

To compare the intraspinal branching patterns of MVST axons, a typical example of a MVST axon is shown in Fig. 5. The stem axon ran in the ventromedial funiculus and three axon collaterals arose from the stem axon at right angles. Collaterals entered into the grey matter at the medial border of the ventral horn and spread laterally in the lamina VIII in a delta-like fashion. Terminal boutons were most extensively distributed in the ventromedial and ventral parts of the ventral horn. This distribution pattern of terminal boutons confirms the degeneration study [19]. They were found in the ventromedial nucleus, the commissural nucleus and, in some MVST axons, in the spinal accessory nucleus. In these nuclei, many terminals made apparent contact with cell bodies and proximal dendrites. In the ventromedial nucleus of the upper cervical cord, motoneurons innervating M. splenius, M. biventer cervicis and M. complex are involved [28]. When these motoneurons were retrogradely labelled by injecting HRP into nerves of these muscles, terminal boutons of MVST axons were observed on the cell bodies and proximal dendrites of these labelled motoneurons. These findings give morphological support to the electrophysiological data [38,41]. As was the case in LVST axons, the rostrocaudal extension of individual axon collaterals was very narrow, ranging from 0.2 to 1.5 mm, and was much narrower than intercollateral intervals. One to 7 axon collaterals were identified in each axon. Both crossed and uncrossed MVST axons had common characteristics of branching patterns and terminal distribution described above.

Discussion

In previous studies of descending pathways, it has been tacitly assumed that long descending motor tract axons exert their effects only at one segmental level. Abzug et al. [1], however, first demonstrated that many axons of the LVST give off collaterals very rostral to their termination. RS axons also give off collaterals before terminating more caudally [22]. Further studies on corticospinal and rubrospinal axons have shown that single axons send multiple collaterals to widely separated segments in the cord [30,31,34]. Our morphological results have confirmed the physiological findings of Abzug et al. [2] and provide further evidence of the existence of multiple collaterals from single LVST axons.

Our present method allows us to stain axons for lengths of up to 25 mm [33]. Therefore, only a portion of the total trajectory of an axon in the spinal cord could be visualized. The question as to whether those LVST axons having axon collaterals to the lower cervical cord have also collaterals to the upper cervical cord remains open. However, we found that those LVST axons terminating in the brachial segments have axon collaterals in the higher cervical cord (C1–C4) (unpublished observations). These results suggest that a substantial proportion of LVST neurons have multiple axon collaterals and project to widely separated segments in the cervical cord. Since LVST axons of the medial type make synaptic contacts with motoneurons in the ventromedial nucleus within lamina VIII, this finding suggests that these neurons control excitability of various axial muscles, particularly Mm. dorsi proprii, concurrently at multisegmental levels. As was previously shown by Abzug et al. [2], another group of VS axons give off branches to both the cervical and the lumbar enlargements and influence both forelimb and hindlimb motoneurons. MVST axons also have multiple axon collat-

Fig. 5. Reconstruction of an uncrossed MVST axon in the upper cervical cord (C2). Dorsal view of the axon is shown on the right (dotted lines indicate the border of the grey matter at a level shown by two arrows). An arrow head shows an injection site. CC, central canal; VM, nucleus ventromedialis; A, nucleus accessorius; Co, nucleus commissuralis; Ce, nucleus cervicalis centralis. (Y. Shinoda, T. Ohgaki and Y. Sugiuchi, unpublished observations.)

erals and project to motoneurons of different neck muscles. These results indicate that single LVST axons have different combinations of target sites in the cord. Since some reflexes mediated by the VS system involve combined activation of the muscles of the neck, trunk and limbs, multiple branching of a single neuron might function to coordinate this type of widespread motor activity.

Acknowledgements

This research was supported by a grant from the Japanese Ministry of Education, Science and Culture for Scientific Research (59570052).

References

[1] Abzug, C., Maeda, M., Peterson, B.W. and Wilson, V.J. (1973) Branching of individual lateral vestibulospinal axons at different spinal cord levels. *Brain Res.*, 56: 327–330.

[2] Abzug, C., Maeda, M., Peterson, B.W. and Wilson, V.J. (1974) Cervical branching of lumbar vestibulospinal axons. *J. Physiol. London*, 243: 499–522.

[3] Akaike, T. (1983) Neuronal organization of the vestibulospinal system in the cat. *Brain Res.*, 259: 217–227.

[4] Aoyama, M., Hongo, T., Kudo, N. and Tanaka, R. (1971) Convergent effects from the bilateral vestibulospinal tracts on spinal interneurons. *Brain Res.*, 35: 250–253.

[5] Ten Bruggencate, G., Burke, R., Lundberg, A. and Udo, M. (1969) Interaction between the vestibulospinal tract, contralateral flexor reflex afferents and Ia afferents. *Brain Res.*, 14: 529–532.

[6] Futami, T., Shinoda, Y. and Yokota, J. (1979) Spinal axon collaterals of corticospinal neurons identified by intracellular injection of horseradish peroxidase. *Brain Res.*, 164: 279–284.

[7] Grillner, S., Hongo, T. and Lund, S. (1970) The vestibulospinal tract. Effects on alpha-motoneurones in the lumbosacral spinal cord in the cat. *Exp. Brain Res.*, 10: 94–120.

[8] Harrison, P.J., Jankowska, E. and Zytnick, D. (1986) Lamina VIII interneurones interposed in crossed reflex pathways in the cat. *J. Physiol. London*, 371: 147–166.

[9] Hauglie-Hanssen, E. (1968) Intrinsic neuronal organization of the vestibular nuclear complex in the cat. A Golgi study. *Ergeb. Anat. Entw. Gesch.*, 40: 1–105.

[10] Hongo, T., Kudo, N. and Tanaka, R. (1975) The vestibulospinal tract: crossed and uncrossed effects in hindlimb motoneurones in the cat. *Exp. Brain Res.*, 24: 37–55.

[11] Hultborn, H. and Udo, M. (1972) Convergence in the reciprocal Ia inhibitory pathway of excitation from descending pathways and inhibition from motor axon collaterals. *Acta Physiol. Scand.*, 84: 95–108.

[12] Hultborn, H., Illert, M. and Santini, M. (1976). Convergence on interneurones mediating the reciprocal Ia inhibition of motoneurones. III. Effects from supraspinal pathways. *Acta Physiol. Scand.*, 96: 368–391.

[13] Jankowska, E. and Lindström, S. (1972) Morphology of interneurones mediating Ia reciprocal inhibition of motoneurones in the spinal cord of the cat. *J. Physiol. London*, 266: 805–823.

[14] Kawai, N., Ito, M. and Nozue, M. (1969) Postsynaptic influences on the vestibular non-Deiters' nuclei from primary vestibular nerve. *Exp. Brain Res.*, 8: 190–200.

[15] Lund, S. and Pompeiano, O. (1965) Descending pathways with monosynaptic action on motoneurones. *Experientia*, 21: 602–603.

[16] Lund, S. and Pompeiano, O. (1968) Monosynaptic excitation of alpha motoneurones from supraspinal structures in the cat. *Acta Physiol. Scand.*, 73: 1–21.

[17] Maeda, M., Maunz, R.A. and Wilson, V.J. (1975) Labyrinthine influence on cat forelimb motoneurons. *Exp. Brain Res.*, 22: 69–86.

[18] Mannen. H. (1965) Arborisations dendritiques étude topographique et quantitative dans le noyau vestibulaire du chat. *Arch. Ital. Biol.*, 103: 197–219.

[19] Nyberg-Hansen, R. (1964) Origin and termination of fibers from the vestibular nuclei descending in the medial longitudinal fasciculus. An experimental study with silver impregnation methods in the cat. *J. Neurol.*, 122: 355–367.

[20] Nyberg-Hansen, R. (1969) Do cat spinal motoneurones receive direct supraspinal fiber connection? A supplementary silver study. *Arch. Ital. Biol.*, 107– 67–78.

[21] Nyberg-Hansen, R. and Mascitti, T.A. (1964) Sites and mode of termination of fibers of the vestibulospinal tract in the cat. An experimental study with silver impregnation methods. *J. Comp. Neurol.*, 122: 369–388.

[22] Peterson, B.W., Maunz, R.A., Pitts, N.G. and Mackel, R. (1975) Patterns of projection and branching of reticulospinal neurons. *Exp. Brain Res.*, 23: 333–351.

[23] Pompeiano, O. and Brodal, A. (1957) The origin of vestibulospinal fibres in the cat. An experimental–anatomical study with comments on the descending medial longitudinal fasciculus. *Arch. Ital. Biol.*, 95: 166–195.

[24] Precht, W. and Shimazu, H. (1965) Functional connections of tonic and kinetic vestibular neurons with primary vestibular afferents. *J. Neurophysiol.*, 28: 1014–1028.

[25] Rapoport, S., Susswein, A., Uchino, Y. and Wilson, V.J. (1977) Properties of vestibular neurons projecting to neck segments of the cat spinal cord. *J. Physiol. London*, 268: 493–510.

[26] Rexed, B. (1952) The cytoarchitectonic organization of the spinal cord in the cat. *J. Comp. Neurol.*, 96: 415–495.

[27] Rexed, B. (1954) A cytoarchitectonic atlas of the spinal

cord in the cat. *J. Comp. Neurol.*, 100: 297–379.

[28] Richmond, F.J.R., Scott, D.A. and Abrahams, V.C. (1978) Distribution of motoneurones to the neck muscles, biventer cervicis, splenius and complexus in the cat. *J. Comp Neurol.*, 181: 451–464.

[29] Scheibel, M.E. and Scheibel, A.B. (1969) A structural analysis of spinal interneurons and Renshow cells. In Brazier, M.A.B. (Ed.), *The Interneuron*, University of California Press, Berkeley/Los Angeles, pp. 159–208.

[30] Shinoda, Y., Arnold, A.P. and Asanuma, H. (1976) Spinal branching of corticospinal axons in the cat. *Exp. Brain Res.*, 26: 215–234.

[31] Shinoda, Y., Getz, C. and Arnold, A. (1977) Spinal branching of rubrospinal axons in the cat. *Exp. Brain Res.*, 30: 203–218.

[32] Shinoda, Y., Yokota, J. and Futami, T. (1981) Divergent projection of individual corticospinal axons to motoneurons of multiple muscles in the monkey. *Neurosci. Lett.*, 23: 7–12.

[33] Shinoda, Y., Yokota, J. and Futami, T. (1982) Morphology of physiologically identified rubrospinal axons in the spinal cord of the cat *Brain Res.*, 242: 321–325.

[34] Shinoda, Y., Ohgaki, T. and Futami, T. (1986) The morphology of single lateral vestibulospinal tract axons in the lower cervical cord of the cat. *J. Comp. Neurol.*, 249: 226–241.

[35] Shinoda, Y., Yamaguchi, T. and Futami, T. (1986) Multi-

ple axon collaterals of single corticospinal axons in the cat spinal cord. *J. Neurophysiol.*, 55: 425–448.

[36] Sprague, J.M. (1951) Motor and propriospinal cells in the thoracic and lumbar ventral horn of the rhesus monkey. *J. Comp. Neurol.*, 95: 103–123.

[37] Szenthágothai, J. (1951) Short propriospinal neurons and intrinsic connections of the spinal grey matter. *Acta Morph. Acad. Sci. Hung.*, 1: 81–94.

[38] Wilson, V.J. and Maeda, M. (1974) Connection between semicircular canals and neck motoneurons in the cat. *J. Neurophysiol.*, 37: 346–357.

[39] Wilson, V.J. and Melvill Jones, G. (1979) *Mammalian Vestibular Physiology*, Plenum Press, New York, 365 pp.

[40] Wilson, V.J. and Peterson, B.W. (1978) Peripheral and central substrates of vestibulospinal reflexes. *Physiol. Rev.*, 58: 80–105.

[41] Wilson, V.J. and Yoshida, M. (1969) Comparison of effects of stimulation of Deiters' nucleus and medial longitudinal fasciculus on neck, forelimb, and hindlimb motoneurons. *J. Neurophysiol.*, 32: 743–758.

[42] Wilson, V.J., Yoshida, M. and Schor, R.H. (1970) Supraspinal monosynaptic excitation and inhibition of thoracic back motoneurons. *Exp. Brain Res.*, 11: 282–295.

[43] Wilson, V.J., Gacek, P.R., Maeda, M. and Uchino, Y. (1977) Saccular and Utricular input to cat neck motoneurons. *J. Neurophysiol.*, 40: 63–73.

O. Pompeiano and J.H.J. Allum (Eds.)
Progress in Brain Research, Vol. 76
© 1988 Elsevier Science Publishers B.V. (Biomedical Division)

CHAPTER 3

Neurotransmitters in vestibular pathways

J. Raymond[1], D. Dememes[1] and A. Nieoullon[2]

[1]*Laboratoire de Neurophysiologie Sensorielle, INSERM U-254, Place E. Bataillon, F-34060 Montpellier CÉDEX, France and*
[2]*Laboratoire de Neurosciences Fonctionnelles, Unité de Neurochimie, CNRS–BP 71, 31 Chemin J. Aiguier, F-13402 Marseille CÉDEX 9, France*

Labyrinthic neurotransmitters. Afferent synapses: A Glu-like component may act as the endogenous transmitter of the vestibular hair-cell–afferent-fibre synapse. The proof of the synaptic origin of this component requires the identification of the adequate Glu synaptic receptors using more specific agonists or antagonists effects. A GABA-like component may also act as a modulator of the excitability of the postsynaptic neurons. Efferent synapses: ACh is the major efferent transmitter but the possibility remains that other additional transmitters or possibly cotransmitters are involved in the vestibular efferent pathways.

Central vestibular neurotransmission. Neurotransmitters of the vestibular nerve: Evidence from a variety of approaches supports the possibility that Glu or Asp are involved in the vestibular nerve transmission. These experiments include: (1) the localization of AAT, an enzyme interconverting Glu and Asp, in the vestibular ganglion neurons, (2) the selective retrograde labelling of vestibular ganglion neurons after high affinity uptake of D-[³H]Asp by the vestibular nerve terminals, (3) the selective labelling of vestibular nerve terminals following high-affinity uptake of [³H]Glu, and (4) biochemicals measurements of the high-affinity glutamate uptake in normal and deafferented vestibular nuclei. Nonlabyrinthic pathways neurotransmitters: Only a part of the neurotransmitters involved in the complex intrication of synapses devoted to each specific vestibular connection has been identified. For the commissural connections which are mainly inhibitory, GABA and Gly have been proposed from different data. In the frog, the excitatory commissural action involves an excitatory amino acid as transmitter. GABA and Glu have been proposed repectively as inhibitory and excitatory transmitters in vestibulo-ocular pathways. In the cerebello–vestibular interactions, one of the well-documented actions is the inhibitory GABAergic effect of the Purkinje cell terminals on the large Deiters' neurons. In the vestibulospinal pathways, it has been demonstrated that some direct vestibulospinal projections are cholinergic. Nevertheless, further studies are necessary to reveal the specific role of neuroactive substances which have been recently identified both in the vestibular nuclei and in other structures involved in the pathways.

Introduction

The vestibular labyrinth and its central pathways are of primary importance in the sensory control of behaviour. The various vestibular nuclei and their synaptic organization play a key role in the analysis of vestibular information and these nuclei can be subdivided not only according to their anatomical configurations but more particularly according to their specific connections with other brainstem regions involved in the control of posture and locomotion. The other main connections of the vestibular nuclei, such as those involved in vestibulospinal and vestibulo-ocular reflexes, have been extensively

Abbreviations: AAT, aspartate aminotransferase; ACh, acetyl choline; Asp, aspartate; ChAT, choline acetyltransferase; CNS, central nervous system; GABA, γ-aminobutyric acid; GAD, glutamic acid decarboxylase; Glu, glutamate; Gly, glycine; HAGU, high affinity glutamate uptake; NMDA, *N*-methyl-D-aspartate; VN, vestibular nucleus.

studied in both anatomical and physiological investigations (for review see [38]). However, data concerning the identity and function of neurotransmitters involved in the vestibular pathways were, until recently, quite sparse.

Study of transmitter identification and function in the CNS is becoming increasingly complex, since recent findings have shown that more than a single neuroactive substance can coexist in the same nerve terminal, that neurotransmitters may act at different postsynaptic receptors, and that, from the functional point of view, many of the neuroactive substances may act as neuromodulators rather than neurotransmitters. Definitive identification of a substance as a specific neurotransmitter of a particular synapse therefore involves obtaining multiple information on its synthesis, release, and interactions with specific receptors.

This review is related to some investigations concerning the possible identification of the primary afferent and efferent neurotransmitters effective in the vestibular sensory organs as well as to an attempt to identify the putative neurotransmitters acting in the vestibular nerve terminals. The involvement of putative neurotransmitters in nonlabyrinthic pathways in the central vestibular nuclei is also briefly considered.

Labyrinthic neurotransmitters

Neurotransmission of the afferent synapses between hair cells and vestibular fibres

Both morphological and physiological evidence were obtained that synaptic transmission from the vestibular hair cells to the afferent fibres is chemically mediated. Ultrastructural observations have revealed features such as presynaptic vesicles conforming to the structure of a chemical synapse [105]. Stimulation of the vestibular hair cells led to an excitation of the afferent terminals related to the release of excitatory neurotransmitter(s). Indeed, physiological investigations have demonstrated excitatory postsynaptic potentials in primary afferent fibres and synaptic delays related to chemical trans-

mission [41,78]. However, the nature of the primary afferent neurotransmitter remains unknown and is currently a matter of controversy. Until recently, very few studies have investigated synaptic pharmacology in the vestibular labyrinth. Some of the more recent studies support the hypothesis that the neurotransmitter in hair-cell–afferent-fibres synapses is the excitatory amino acid glutamate whereas other data suggest that GABA plays a physiological role in labyrinthic synaptic function.

Glutamate as a hair-cell neurotransmitter

The use of in-vitro preparations has made it possible to perform precise pharmacological studies on the effects of different substances on the activity of vestibular afferent fibres, thereby revealing a synaptic action of the putative neurotransmitter Glu and of its agonists and antagonists. Using the *Xenopus* lateral line as a model for understanding senso-

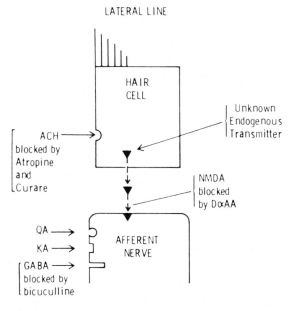

Fig. 1. Proposed sites of drug action at the hair-cell–nerve-fibre terminals in the lateral line of *Xenopus laevis*. NMDA was shown acting at the afferent transmitter site on the afferent nerve, and its effect appears to be blocked by D-α-aminoadipate (D-α-AA). Acetylcholine, a proposed efferent transmitter, was shown acting only at a hair-cell site; GABA, quisqualate (QA) and kainate (KA) were shown as acting at nerve-fibre sites. (From [10].)

ry transduction in the hair-cell system, various data [8,10] were consistent with the hypothesis that Glu is the endogenous neurotransmitter of the hair-cell–afferent-fibre synapse (Fig. 1). Glu also produced an increase in intra-axonal afferent fibre activities in the isolated membranous labyrinth of the frog blocked by selective Glu receptor antagonists [3,98]. Thus, although hair-cell–afferent-fibre synapses may be 'glutamatergic', it is not clear which sub-stance(s) represents the endogenous neurotransmit-ter, since the antagonists used or the postsynaptic receptors themselves are not selective enough to discriminate adequately between the agonists.

In-vivo investigations concerning Glu action in the cat labyrinth [19] concluded that L-Glu mimics the excitatory transmitter substance at the synaptic junction between hair cells and afferent terminals (Fig. 2). Glu is also a potent depolarizing agent [88]; hence it is difficult to definitively conclude on the specificity of its action on primary afferents and, since Glu can directly activate the sensory cells or induce secondary effects such as the release of other substances. Nevertheless, the application of very small concentrations of Glu (1 mM) in the endo-lymphatic space produced depolarization but no desensitization of primary afferents whose respon-siveness to a physiological stimulation of vestibular

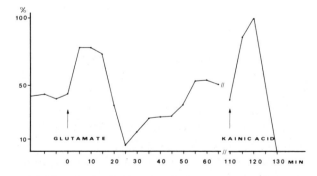

Fig. 2. Changes in firing rate of a superior vestibular nucleus unit after administration of glutamate (10^{-3} M) in the posterior semicircular canal. The activity increased for 10 min, and then decreased below the original spontaneous rate for the next 5 to 10 min, returning to the control level in 25 to 30 min. Kainic acid (10^{-4} M) transiently increased the spontaneous discharge, which was then abolished. (From [19]).

receptor was increased, and the return to the initial spontaneous firing rate took place rapidly without rinsing. So Glu action might have been ended by an endogenous renewal of endolymph or by specific physiological mechanisms that could implicate the existence of Glu receptors in the vestibular end-or-gans. The effect of kainate application supports this hypothesis.

This hypothesis was checked by in-vitro experi-ments testing for the presence of postsynaptic Glu receptors in the mouse vestibular epithelium. It has been proposed that excitatory amino acids, such as Glu and aspartate, can act on at least three types of pharmacologically distinguished receptors on the basis of their preferential activate by quisqualate, NMDA and kainate, respectively. These com-pounds are not present in nervous or sensory tissue but all are active in the lateral line [9], the identified receptor subclasses corresponding to NMDA and quisqualate being selectively associated with post-synaptic densities in the CNS [27]. The neurotoxic effects of these different excitatory amino acid agonists were studied using in-vitro preparations of embryonic and newborn mouse otic vesicles [74]. The onset and developmental pattern of their neu-rotoxic effects on the vestibular epithelium (Fig. 3) were related to the appearance of sites sensitive to excitatory amino acids on the corresponding vesti-bular afferent fibres which parallel the synaptogene-sis.

The apparent ubiquitous nature of the Glu recep-tor complicates efforts to identify the endogenous transmitter. The development of more specific exci-tatory amino acid agonists or antagonists might lead to a clearly selective action of the applied sub-stance on just the synaptic receptor.

GABA as a putative hair-cell neurotransmitter

Various data also suggested that GABA acts as an excitatory transmitter in vestibular hair cells. GABA synthesis from Glu was first reported in the fish vestibule [31] and more recently in chick vesti-bular cristae [54], implying the presence of the GABA-synthesizing enzyme, GAD. However the precise localization of the GABA synthesis in the

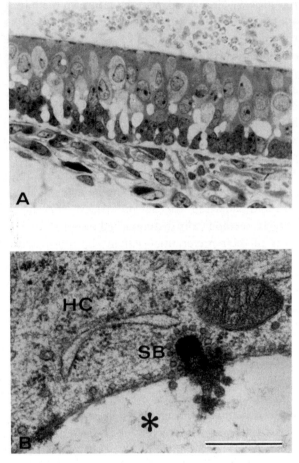

Fig. 3. (A) Light micrograph showing the reactions to kainate (20 μM) exposure (20 min, in-vitro incubation) of afferent fibres innervating the vestibular sensory cells of a newborn mouse utricular macula. Note the vacuolization of all afferent fibres and terminals and the contrasting good preservation of the sensory hair cells. × 800. (B) Electron micrograph of hair-cell–afferent synaptic junction. The presynaptic region of the hair cell (HC) is characterized by the presence of typical large synaptic bodies (SB) surrounded by synaptic vesicles. Hair cells are unaffected, but afferent nerve fibres(*) almost completely disappeared. Scale bar = 0.5 μm.

ous and GABA-induced irregular activity, does not apparently affect the discharge pattern of the regular activity. Similarly, GABA does not have an excitatory effect on evoked responses from the isolated crista ampullaris of the bullfrog [39] and neither GABA nor muscimol have any significant effect upon the resting membrane potential of the afferent in the frog labyrinth [3]. Finally, in the lateral line GABA was reported to have an inhibitory action [9].

Because of these often contradictory data, the role and origin of GABA in the vestibular epithelium require further investigation. GABA may have an excitatory effect by modulating the excitability of postsynaptic neurons in the vestibular ganglion, and rather than performing as the hair cells' transmitter, GABA may act as a facilitatory transmitter from one of the centrally arising efferents [3].

Neurotransmission in the vestibular efferent system

The origin and course of efferent vestibular pathways in mammals have been precisely described by the use of retrograde transport methods [20,36,37,101]. In the sensory epithelium, the vesiculated efferent endings contact either type II hair cells directly (axosomatic synapses) or the calices of type I hair cells and afferent fibres (axodendritic synapses). Regarding the functional role of the vestibular efferent system, initial studies indicated a predominant inhibitory efferent action [70,82]. However, in mammals, recent studies suggested that its peripheral action is more complex than hitherto suspected [18] and in the squirrel monkey, Goldberg and Fernandez [37] demonstrated an excitatory effect on vestibular afferents by stimulation of the efferent vestibular neurons.

Physiological and histochemical investigations involved ACh in vestibular efferent neurotransmission. However, histochemical evidence for acetylcholinesterase, the ACh-inactivating enzyme which is also known to be present in cells receiving a cholinergic input, is not a specific indication of cholinergic cells. Regarding the synthesis of ACh, ChAT was reported to be present in the isolated

vestibular tissue has so far not been determined. Further support for the GABA hypothesis has come from the work of Felix and Ehrenberger [28], reporting that microiontophoretic application of GABA increased the spontaneous activity of single units in the cat macula sacculi. However, bicuculline, a GABA-antagonist which blocks the spontane-

labyrinth [31,55]. Autoradiographic demonstration of retrograde transport of [³H]choline by efferent fibres in the cat labyrinth [22] further supports ACh participation in vestibular efferent transmission. Using [³H]choline, which is accepted to be selectively taken up through a high-affinity transport system in cholinergic nerve terminals, the authors found a selective retrograde labelling of vestibular efferent neurons in the brainstem following injections into the lateral semicircular canal of the cat labyrinth (Fig. 4). Because of such a transmitter-specific retrograde labelling was proposed for identifying different acidic amino acids, aminergic (for review see [16] and cholinergic [4,97,106] neuronal pathways, in the labyrinth the selectivity of the retrograde labelling of efferent neurons with [³H]choline may provide additional evidence that ACh is involved in the efferent vestibular control. However, since not all the efferent neurons were retrogradely labelled by [³H]choline, the possibility remains that other

additional neurotransmitters, or possibly cotransmitters, are involved. Biochemical and immunocytochemical data (Demêmes, E. Scarfone and A. Cupo, unpublished observations) have not revealed any enkephalins, indicating that these neuropeptides are probably not involved as transmitters in the vestibular efferent pathways. More recently, a ChAT immunofluorescence histochemistry study showed that, although ACh may act as a major efferent neurotransmitter, some efferent vestibular neurons may use other neuroactive substances as transmitters [85].

Central vestibular neurotransmission

Glutamate and aspartate as neurotransmitters of the vestibular nerve

Individual neurons within the VN are directly or indirectly innervated by vestibular ganglion neurons

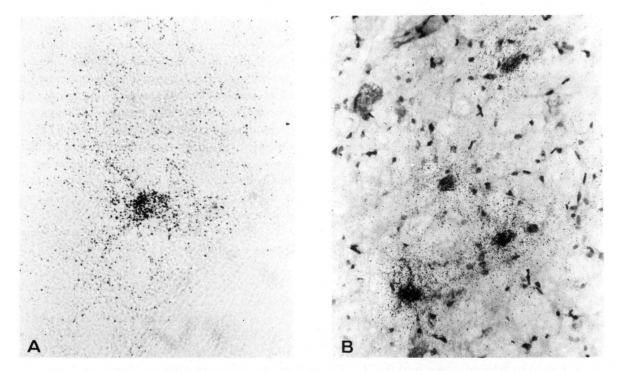

Fig. 4. Light microscopic autoradiographs on cryostat sections illustrating the selective labelling of cat efferent vestibular neurons after a [³H]choline injection into the ampulla of the lateral semicircular canal. (A) Focal accumulation of silver grains over the perikaryon and its processes. Unstained section. × 350. (B) A group of heavily labelled efferent neurons. Stained section. × 250.

associated with the sensory organs of the labyrinth. Afferents supplying the major vestibular receptors in mammals were located and exhaustively studied. The distribution of vestibular nerve endings was mapped in the cat and their synaptic actions were carefully examined [34,50,56,91,100]. Secondary vestibular neurons are subject to monosynaptic excitatory influence mediated by the vestibular nerve fibres constituting their main input [67,80,84,86].

In recent investigations, a variety of electrophysiological, histochemical and biochemical techniques were used to study putative excitatory neurotransmitter(s) in various brainstem areas [6]. Concerning the cochlear nerve terminals, the excitatory amino acids Asp and Glu were shown to be the most likely candidates [2,13,29,65,103]. Since the vestibular and cochlear nerves originate embryologically in the same stato-acoustic ganglion, we were led to hypothesize that the vestibular ganglion cells also use a Glu/Asp synaptic neurotransmitter.

Evidence from a variety of approaches supports the possibility that Glu or Asp are involved in the vestibular nerve transmission. These experiments include: (1) the localization of AAT, an enzyme interconverting Glu and Asp, in the vestibular ganglion neurons; (2) the selective retrograde labelling of vestibular ganglion neurons after high-affinity uptake of D-[^{3}H]Asp by the vestibular nerve terminals; (3) the selective labelling of vestibular nerve terminals following high-affinity uptake of [^{3}H]Glu, and (4) biochemicals measurements of the high-affinity Glu uptake in normal and deafferented vestibular nuclei.

Localization of AAT immunoreactivity in vestibular ganglion neurons

Glutaminase and/or AAT, two enzymes associated with the routine metabolism of Glu and Asp, may have an additional function in synthesis, regulating, and replenishing the neurotransmitter pools of these excitatory amino acids. In this case, these enzymes would be present in increased levels in glutamatergic or aspartatergic neurons and may be used as markers in immunocytochemical studies

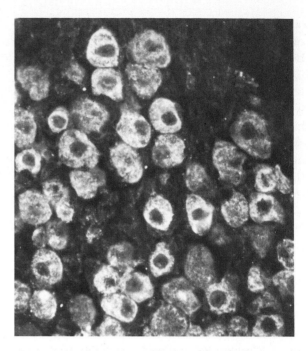

Fig. 5. Immunofluorescent localization of AAT immunoreactivity in the mouse vestibular ganglion neurons on a cryostat section. × 250.

[102]. Using antibodies against mitochondrial or cytosolic AAT [76] and immunocytochemical detection, we found heavy staining in vestibular ganglion neurons (Fig. 5). However, AAT is also involved in cellular energy metabolism and it was proposed that it complexes with malate dehydrogenase in a shuttle mechanism to transfer energy equivalents across the mitochondrial membrane [30]. Although these results show that Glu/Asp may be synthesized in vestibular neurons they do not provide definitive evidence that Glu/Asp act as neurotransmitters in the vestibular nerve.

Selective retrograde transport of D-[^{3}H]Asp in the vestibular nerve

Amino acid neurotransmitters are selectively taken up by high-affinity carriers in the presynaptic terminals of neurons from which they are released, and may be subsequently retrogradely transported in a specific manner from the terminal region to the somatodendritic part of the neurons [16]. Streit [94]

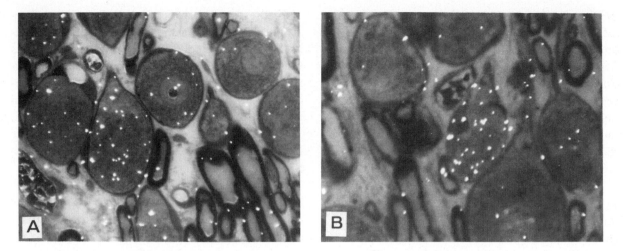

Fig. 6. Light microscopic autoradiographs of 1-µm semithin sections of vestibular ganglia 16 h after microinjections of D-[³H]Asp in the vestibular nuclei showing some heavily labelled perikarya. Transmitted bright-field (A) and reflected dark-field (B) illumination. × 600.

suggested that a selective transport of D-[³H]Asp could identify connections utilizing excitatory amino acids, i.e. L-Glu and/or L-Asp as neurotransmitters. In contrast with the L forms of Glu or Asp, D-Asp is a metabolically inert analogue of L-Glu and or L-Asp taken up through the same high- affinity transport system [5,17,52]. The possible retrograde transport to the vestibular ganglion neurons was therefore investigated following microinjections of D-[³H]Asp in the cat vestibular nuclei [23]. After uptake of D-[³H]Asp by vestibular nerve terminals, in-vivo autoradiographic labelling of ganglion cell bodies was observed and was more pronounced at 16 h survival time, than at 6 h (Fig. 6). This time-related progression of labelling was consistent with a retrograde axonal transport; some perikarya being heavily labelled and others only slightly. There is no evidence that this difference in labelling is related to the different morphological types of neurons described in the cat [90]. It could, in part, depend on the location of the axonal terminals of the ganglion neurons within the injected vestibular area and consequently on the uptake sites.

This retrograde labelling of vestibular ganglion neurons, a highly selective phenomenon for amino acid connections [106] therefore points to Glu or Asp as neurotransmitter(s) in afferent vestibular pathways. This data is in agreement with the role of these amino acids as vestibular excitatory neurotransmitters proposed on the basis of others investigations using electron microscope radioautography demonstrating in-vitro a selective uptake of [³H]Glu by the afferent nerve endings in the cat vestibular nuclei.

High-affinity Glu uptake in vestibular nerve terminals

Based on high-affinity Glu uptake, radioautographic and biochemical studies were devoted to the characterization of vestibular nerve terminals in the cat VN [74]. In the first part of the study, morphologically identified glutamatergic/aspartatergic terminals were characterized using [³H]Glu as a marker in electron microscopic autoradiography. However, since many other terminals innervate in the vestibular nuclei, a second biochemical approach was used to precisely determine the origin of putative glutamatergic nerve terminals. Sodium-dependent HAGU [57,59] was measured as an index of the presence and density of nerve terminals in normal and deafferented vestibular nuclei 8 to 11 days after unilateral lesion of the vestibular nerve, since the vestibular nerve is exclusively directed towards the ipsilateral vestibular nuclei.

Electron microscopic identification of nerve terminals labelled by [³H]Glu in cat vestibular nuclei. In addition to intrinsic cells and terminals originating from different pathways connecting the vestibular brainstem neurons, the main afferent projection of vestibular nuclei is provided by the ipsilateral vestibular nerve. We were able to label these axonal terminals by incubating sections of vestibular nuclei in the presence of 2 μM L-[³H]Glu, according with the method of Storm-Mathisen and Iversen [92].

The distribution of terminals labelled with [³H]Glu is consistent with the distribution of vestibular nerve endings in the vestibular nuclei. Electron microscopic examination of terminal patterns revealed that most of them exhibit synaptic contacts with unlabelled dendrites (Fig. 7). The density of labelled terminals was highest in the distal part of the dendritic trees. On the basis the ultrastructur-

al features, several types of labelled synapses correspond closely with the previously described vestibular nerve terminals [56,89]. Because of this similarity and the high density of the labelled terminals, the uptake of exogenous Glu appears to mainly occur in the vestibular nerve terminals although many other pathways contact the vestibular nuclei. These observations suggested that most putative Glu-containing nerve terminals originate in the vestibular nerve, but this has to be confirmed.

Biochemical measurements of HAGU in normal and deafferented vestibular nuclei. Glu uptake activity displayed by the vestibular nuclear complex is not very high. Compared to other cerebral structures dissected under similar experimental conditions, the mean vestibular HAGU was 4 to 8 times less than that of the striatal and thalamic areas exhibit-

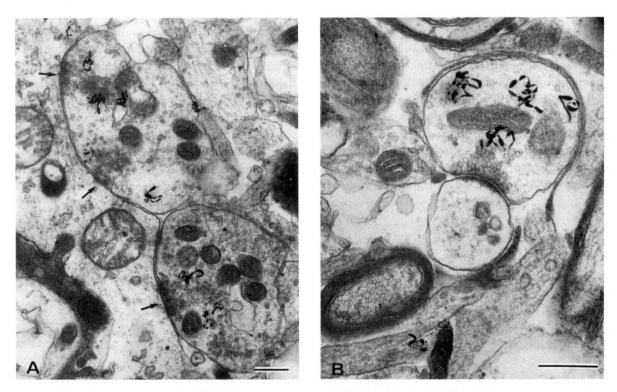

Fig. 7. Electron microscopic autographs of [³H]Glu-labelled nerve endings in the vestibular nuclei. (A) Two nerve endings with numerous mitochondria and synaptic vesicles which are crowded in front of one or two synaptic contacts, respectively (arrows). (B) Bouton-shaped nerve ending forming an asymmetric synaptic contact with a distal dendrite. Scale bar : 0.5 μm. (From [75].)

ing the highest CNS activities. However, HAGU level in the vestibular complex is similar to that of other brainstem nuclei such as the substantia nigra and at least 2 to 3 times that of the red nucleus, which has been reported to receive glutamatergic afferent pathways [49]. The HAGU level in the caudal part of the vestibular nuclei complex was about twice that measured in all of the remaining structure. Mean values were 4.06 ± 0.3 nmol/min/g prot. and 2.31 ± 0.1 nmol/min/g prot. In the central and rostral parts of the vestibular complex, no significant difference was detected between three arbitrarily separated areas, namely the dorsal, ventral, and lateral areas. The apparently uneven distribution of HAGU within the vestibular complex suggests an heterogeneous innervation of the various vestibular nuclei by glutamatergic or aspartergic nerve endings. Thus, the caudal part of the structure probably receives more amino acidic excitatory afferent fibres than its central and rostral parts.

Results of vestibular nerve deafferentation experiments have confirmed the heterogeneity of the glutamatergic or aspartatergic input to the VN (Fig. 8). In the caudal part of the structure, no significant change in HAGU was detected. In the remainder of the structure the mean decrease was 31% of that recorded on the side contralateral to the lesion. Mean HAGU in this area was 162 ± 0.1 nmol/min/g prot. Maximal decrease in HAGU following the lesion primarily occurred in the lateral and ventral parts of the two rostral thirds of the ipsilateral vestibular complex, suggesting that glutamatergic or aspartatergic fibres are contained in the vestibular nerve and contribute to the vestibular input. In the dorsal division of the rostral vestibular complex, HAGU only decreased by 12.5% and was not significantly different from control values. Individual cases confirmed these results. In the best case, HAGU decrease reached 58% in the lateral area of the central part; in the rostral part, the decrease was 46.3% ventrally and 19.7% dorsally.

Correlation of our biochemical results with the anatomical localization of the different vestibular nuclei shows that following vestibular nerve lesion the decrease in HAGU primarily occurred in the

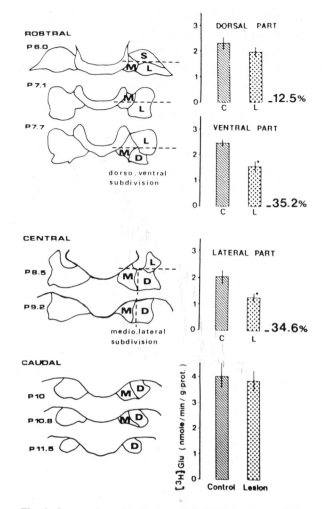

Fig. 8. Intranuclear distribution of HAGU in the vestibular complex of the cat. Effects of unilateral vestibular nerve lesion in 7 cats after a 8–11-day survival period. The standard diagrams on the left side illustrate the localization of each area examined from the caudal part of the structure (stereotaxic plane P.11.5, from [7]) the most rostral aspect (P.6). For each arbitrarily delimited area, from the caudal to rostral parts of the dissected structures, values of HAGU were measured in intact animals (control; C) and in animals subjected several days previously to a vestibular nerve lesion (lesion; L) are shown. Samples of the lateral part of the central portion of the vestibular nuclear complex comprise only the ventral subdivision. Data, expressed in nanomoles of L-[³H]Glu accumulated per minute and per gram protein, are the mean $\pm$ SD of a minimum of 8 samples assayed in the same brain area for each animal. Significance of differences from control: *$P < 0.05$ (Student's t-test). S, superior vestibular nucleus; M, medial vestibular nucleus; L, lateral vestibular nucleus; D, descending vestibular nucleus. (From [75].)

ventral lateral vestibular nucleus and in the rostral part of the descending vestibular nucleus. This projection pattern of putative glutamatergic or aspartatergic fibres of the vestibular nerve must be compared to the anatomical distribution of the primary vestibular afferent fibres into the vestibular complex [42,50,100]. Our quantitative findings are consistent with reports on the distribution and density of primary fibres and endings in the cat VN. HAGU decrease is highest in the subdivisions that receive the most primary innervation. The presence in the VN of nonvestibular endings that utilize Glu/Asp is, however, suggested by the fact that after destruction of the vestibular nerve, nonsignificant deficits in HAGU were reported in the caudal areas where the activity is highest. The caudal part of the descending nucleus receives multiple spinal excitatory inputs [70]. Because of the absence of a HAGU decrease in this area after vestibular nerve deafferentiation, one might suggest these spinovestibular fibres to be glutamatergic. Furthermore, in some other VN subdivisions, such as the dorsal part of the lateral VN, a moderate deficit ensued when the vestibular nerve was sectioned. These findings would be explicable if the total level of this amino acid contributed by the vestibular nerve is found to be small compared with levels contributed by other afferent systems also using Glu/Asp.

These data correlate electrophysiological findings on the characteristics of the vestibular unit firing patterns elicited by vestibular nerve stimulation [47,67,84]. The highest rate of monosynaptic excitatory inputs (50%) was found in the ventral, lateral, and rostral descending vestibular nuclei where, according to our biochemical results, putative glutamatergic vestibular nerve endings appear to be most dense. Electrophysiological studies have reported only 27% and 15% of such excitatory monosynaptic inputs in the superior and median vestibular nulei [80]. In these structures, neurons may receive only a few of their input from glutamatergic excitatory vestibular fibres and a relatively large input from interneurons or other brain structures known to project mostly to the various vestibular nuclei.

Nonlabyrinthic pathways neurotransmitters

Commissural connection putative neurotransmitters

An extensive system of commissural fibres interconnects the vestibular nuclei [35,51,71]. Its functional organization was defined by Shimazu and Precht [87] and was mainly characterized as a crossed inhibition. Concerning the nature of the neurotransmitter, some evidence has shown that one type of commissural unit may use GABA as a neurotransmitter whereas the other one may use Gly [24,72,73]. A contralateral excitatory commissural influence has been reported in the frog [25]. The increase in the commissural excitation and the alteration of cholinergic sensivity after hemilabyrinthectomy could mean that the commissural projection is cholinergic, but Cochran et al. [14] suggested that this excitatory action is mediated to a great extent through NMDA receptors involving an excitatory amino acid as neurotransmitter. Further studies will reveal the complex synaptic organization of these commissural connections.

Vestibulo-ocular pathway neurotransmitters

Electrophysiological studies have provided evidence for the existence of excitatory and inhibitory vestibulo-ocular pathways. Electrophysiological and neurochemical evidence supports the hypothesis that GABA is the inhibitory synaptic neurotransmitter in vestibular neurons projecting to ocular motoneurons [72,73]. The specific distribution of glutamatergic synapses on ocular motoneurons suggests that they probably have a vestibular origin and that Glu acts as a neurotransmitter in excitatory vestibulo-ocular pathways [21].

Cerebellovestibular pathways

Most physiological studies on neurotransmitters in the vestibular complex have focused on the lateral VN. One of the defined neurotransmitter actions concerns the inhibitory GABAergic effects on lateral VN neurons. The cerebellovestibular pathway originates in Purkinje cells of the anterior cerebellar vermis [15,99] and mediates monosynaptic inhibition on lateral VN neurons [44]. There is now good evidence that the neurotransmitter of this inhibition is GABA. GABA mimics the action of the inhibitory neurotransmitter released from Purkinje axon terminals and GABA levels in the dorsal lateral VN are greatly reduced after removal of the cerebellar vermis, whereas those of the ventral nucleus are unaffected [66]. GABA was also found in individual Purkinje cells of the cerebellar vermis as well as in their axon terminals in the lateral VN [32,63], and an immunocytochemical localization study of GAD [40], in conjunction with lesion of the Purkinje cell projection to the dorsal lateral VN, demonstrates the extent of GABAergic terminals on the somata and proximal dendrites of the large Deiters' neurons. Thus function of the dorsal lateral VN in the control of posture and movement could depend to a large extent upon the modulation of the cerebellum GABAergic inhibition. The persistence of GAD activity and GAD-positive terminals after isolation from Purkinje cells, however, suggests the existence of a second source which could be intrinsic to dorsal lateral VN neurons [32,40].

Vestibulospinal pathways

Vestibulospinal responses are in part mediated by disynaptic pathways including primary afferent synapses on vestibular neurons, which in turn project to spinal motoneurons. The lateral VN is known as the origin of the lateral vestibulospinal tract [12,43]. This pathway is considered to be related to a facilitatory action on extensor α motoneurons [53] and somatotopically organized [70]. Indeed, the medial and caudal vestibulospinal tracts originate in the medial, descending, ventrolateral VN [1,61,70] and in the descending VN, respectively [68,69]. Glycine was suggested to be associated with some vestibulospinal projections [104] but more recently an elegant study of the selective retrograde labelling of some vestibular neurons following injections of [^{3}H]choline into the rat spinal cord [46] suggested that some of the vestibulospinal neurons are cholinergic, although it remains to be established that these cells contain ChAT and therefore ACh.

The presence of some other neuroactive substances was revealed in the VN by immunocytochemistry, particularly for GAD and neuropeptides such as substance P, leuenkephalin, and calcitonin-gene-related peptide [11,48,60] but their actual presence and their effects have not yet been related to specific functional pathways. However, these substances may participate in vestibulospinal and/or vestibuloreticular interrelations.

Conclusions

This review summarizes our knowledge of substances which have been demonstrated to mediate synaptic transmission at specific sites along the vestibular pathways. It is obvious that this list is incomplete and that there are many gaps. With the advent of more sensitive analytical methods (immunocytochemistry, HPLC, pharmacology of postsynaptic receptors, in-situ hybridization), we are just beginning to be able to examine the neurochemical aspects of peripheral and central vestibular processing; further studies will quickly lead to a better characterization of the different roles of neurotransmitters and neuromodulators in generating the synaptic events involved in the coding of labyrinthic information and its integration in the various vestibular relays.

It is hoped that the understanding of this aspect of the vestibular function will contribute to specific pharmacological intervention in order to improve vestibular disorders in pathological or abnormal conditions of equilibration.

Acknowledgements

We are very grateful to several of our colleagues for substantial contributions to some of the studies presented in this chapter, especially Drs. Claude Dechesne, Gilles Desmadryl and Alain Sans. We also thank Dr. Max Recassens for kindly providing us with antisera against AAT, Jacqueline Boyer for her expert typing, and Joël Roudil for his competent photographic work.

References

[1] Akaike, T. (1983) Neuronal organization of the vestibulospinal system in the cat. *Brain Res.*, 259: 217–227.

[2] Altschuler, R.A., Neises, G.R., Harmisson, G.G., Wenthold, R.J. and Fex, J. (1981) Immunocytochemical localization of aspartate amino-transferase immunoreactivity in cochlear nucleus of guinea pig. *Proc. Natl. Acad. Sci. USA*, 78: 6553–6557.

[3] Annoni, JM., Cochran, S.L. and Precht, W. (1984) Pharmacology of the vestibular hair cell afferent fiber synapse in the frog. *J. Neurosci.*, 2106–2116.

[4] Bagnoli, P., Beaudet, A., Stella, M. and Cuénod, M. (1981) Selective retrograde labelling of cholinergic neurons with [³H]-choline. *J. Neurosci.*, 1: 691–695.

[5] Balcar, V.J. and Johnston, G.A.R. (1972) The structural specificity of the high affinity uptake of L-glutamate and L-aspartate by rat brain slices. *J. Neurochem.*, 19: 2657–2666.

[6] Beart, P.M. (1976) An evaluation of L-glutamate as the transmitter released from optic nerve terminals of the pigeon. *Brain Res.*, 110: 99–114.

[7] Berman, A.L. (1968) *The Brain Stem of the Cat. A Cytoarchitectonic Atlas with Stereotaxic Coordinates*, The University of Wisconsin Press, Milwaukee/London/Madison, 175 pp.

[8] Bledsoe, S., Bobbin, R.P., Thalmann, R. and Thalmann, I. (1980) Stimulus-induced release of endogenous amino acids from skins containing the lateral line organ in *Xenopus laevis. Exp. Brain Res.*, 40: 97–101.

[9] Bledsoe, S.C. Jr., Chibal, D.M., Bobbin, R.P. and Morgan, D.N. (1983) Comparative actions of glutamate and related substances on the lateral line of *Xenopus laevis. Comp. Biochem. Physiol.*, 75C: 119–206.

[10] Bobbin, R.P., Bledsoe, S.C., Winbery, S.L. and Jenison, G.L. (1985) Actions of putative neurotransmitters and other relevant compounds on *Xenopus laevis* lateral line. In D.G. Drescher (Ed.), *Auditory Biochemistry*, C.C. Thomas, Springfield, pp. 102–122.

[11] Bouras, C., Magistretti, P.J. and Morrison, J.H. (1986) An immunohistochemical study of six biologically active peptides in the human brain. *Human Neurobiol.*, 5: 213–226.

[12] Brodal, A., Pompeiano, O. and Walberg, F. (1962) *The Vestibular Nuclei and their Connexions. Anatomy and Functional Correlations*, Oliver and Boyd, Edinburgh, 198 pp.

[13] Canzek, V. and Reubi, J.C. (1980) The effect of cochlear nerve lesion on the release of glutamate, aspartate, and GABA from cat cochlear nucleus, in vitro. *Exp. Brain Res.*, 38: 437–441

[14] Cochran, S.L., Kasik, P. and Precht, W. (1987) Pharmacological aspects of excitatory synaptic transmission to second-order vestibular neurons in the frog. *Synapse*, 1: 102–123.

[15] Corvaja, N. and Pompeiano, O. (1979) Identification of cerebellar corticovestibular neurons retrogradely labeled with horseradish peroxidase. *Neuroscience*, 4: 507–515.

[16] Cuénod, M., Bagnoli, P., Beaudet, A., Rustioni, A., Wiklund, L. and Streit, I. (1982) Transmitter-specific retrograde labelling of neurons. In V. Chan-Palay and S.L. Palay (Eds.), *Cytochemical Methods in Neuroanatomy*, Alan R. Liss, New York, pp. 17-44.

[17] Davies, L.P. and Johnston, G.A.R. (1976) Uptake and release of D- and L-aspartate by rat brain slices. *J. Neurochem.*, 26: 1007–1014.

[18] Dechesne, C. and Sans, A. (1980) Control of the vestibular nerve activity by the efferent system in the cat. *Acta Otolaryngol. Stockholm, 90: 82–85.*

[19] Dechesne, C., Raymond, J. and Sans, A. (1984) The action of glutamate in the cat labyrinth. *Ann. Otol. Rhinol. Laryngol.*, 93: 163–165.

[20] Dechesne, C., Raymond, J. and Sans, A. (1984) The efferent vestibular system in the cat: a horseradish peroxidase and fluorescent retrograde tracer study. *Neuroscience*, 11: 893–901.

[21] Demêmes, D. and Raymond, J. (1982) Radioautographic identification of [³H]glutamic acid labeled nerve endings in the cat oculomotor nucleus. *Brain Res.*, 231: 433–437.

[22] Demêmes, D. Raymond, J. and Sans, A. (1983) Selective retrograde labelling of vestibular efferent neurons with [³H]-choline. *Neuroscience*, 8: 285–290.

[23] Demêmes, D., Raymond, J. and Sans, A. (1984) Selective retrograde labelling of neurons in the cat vestibular [³H] D-Aspartate. *Brain Res.*, 304: 188–191.

[24] Dieringer, N. and Precht, W., (1979) Mechanisms of compensation for vestibular deficits in the frog. I. Modification of the excitatory commissural system *Exp. Brain Res.*, 36: 311–328.

[25] Dieringer, N. and Precht, W. (1979) Mechanisms of compensation for vestibular deficits in the frog. II. Modification of inhibitory pathways. *Exp. Brain Res.*, 36: 329–341.

[26] Dohlman, G.F. (1965) Histochemical studies of vestibular mechanism. In G.L. Rasmussen and W.F. Windl (Eds.), *Neural Mechanisms of the Auditory and Vestibular Systems.* C.C. Thomas, Springfield, pp. 258–275.

[27] Fagg, G.E. and Matus, A. (1984) Selective association of N-methyl aspartate and quisqualate types of L-glutamate receptor with brain postsynaptic densities. *Proc. Natl. Acad. Sci. USA*, 81: 6876–6880.

[28] Felix, D. and Ehrenberger, K. (1982) The action of putative neurotransmitter substances in the cat labyrinth. *Acta Otolaryngol. Stockholm*, 93: 101–105.

[29] Fex, J. and Wenthold, R.J. (1976) Choline acetyltransferase, glutamate decarboxylase and tyrosine hydroxylase in the cochlea and cochlear nucleus of the guinea pig. *Brain Res.*, 109: 575–585.

[30] Fitzpatrick, S.M., Cooper, A.J.L. and Duffy, T.E. (1983) Use of β-methylene-D,L-aspartate to assess the role of

aspartate aminotransferase in cerebral oxidative metabolism. *J. Neurochem.* 41: 1370–1383.

[31] Flock, A. and Lam, D.M.K. (1974) Neurotransmitters synthesis in inner ear and lateral line sense organs. *Nature*, 249: 142–144.

[32] Fonnum, F., Storm-Mathisen, J. and Walberg, F. (1970) Glutamate decarboxylase in inhibitory neurons. A study of the enzyme in Purkinje cell axons and boutons in the cat. *Brain Res.*, 20: 259–275.

[33] Fonnum, F., Storm-Mathisen, J. and Divac, I. (1981) Biochemical evidence for glutamate as neurotransmitter in corticostriatal and corticothalamic fibers in rat brain. *Neuroscience*, 6: 863–873.

[34] Gacek, R.R. (1969) The course and central termination of first order neurons supplying vestibular endorgans in the cat. *Acta Otolaryngol. Stockholm, Suppl.* 254: 1–66.

[35] Gacek, R.R. (1978) Location of commissural neurons in the vestibular nuclei of the cat. *Exp. Neurol.* 59: 479–491.

[36] Gacek, R.R. and Lyon, M. (1974) The localization of vestibular efferent neurons in the kitten with horseradish peroxidase. *Acta Otolaryngol. Stockholm*, 77: 92–101.

[37] Goldberg, J.M. and Fernandez, C. (1980) Efferent vestibular system in the squirrel monkey: anatomical location and influence on afferent activity. *J. Neurophysiol.*, 43: 986–1025.

[38] Goldberg, J.M. and Fernandez, C. (1982) The vestibular system. In Darian-Smith (Ed.), *Handbook of Physiology. The Nervous System*, Vol. 3, American Physiological Society, Bethesda, pp. 977–1022.

[39] Guth, S.L. and Norris, C.H. (1984) Pharmacology of the isolated semicircular canal: effect of GABA and picrotoxin. *Exp. Brain Res.*, 56: 72–78.

[40] Houser, C.R., Barber, R.P. and Vaughn, J.E. (1984) Immunocytochemical localization of glutamic acid decarboxylase in the dorsal lateral vestibular nucleus: evidence for an intrinsic and extrinsic GABAergic innervation. *Neurosci. Lett.*, 47: 213–220.

[41] Ishii, Y., Matsuura, S. and Furukawa, T. (1971) Quantal nature of transmission at the synapse between hair cells and the eighth nerve fibers. *Jpn. J. Physiol.*, 19: 79–89.

[42] Ishizuka, N., Sasaki, S.I. and Mannen, H. (1982) Central course and terminal arborizations of single primary vestibular afferent fibers from the horizontal canals in the cat. *Neurosci. Lett.*, 33: 135–139.

[43] Ito, M., Hongo, T., Yoshida, M., Okada, Y. and Obata, K. (1964) Antidromic and trans-synaptic activation of Deiters' neurones induces from the spinal cord. *Jpn. J. Physiol.*, 14: 638–658.

[44] Ito, M., Kawai, N. and Udo, M. (1968) The origin of cerebellar-induced inhibition of Deiters' neurones. III. Localization of the inhibitory zone. *Exp. Brain Res.*, 4: 310–320.

[45] Iurato, S., Luciano, L., Pannese, E. and Reale, E. (1971) Histochemical localization of acetylcholinesterase (AChE) activity in the inner ear. *Acta Otolaryngol. Stockholm*, Suppl. 279: 1–50.

[46] Jones, B.E., Paré, M. and Beaudet, A. (1986) Retrograde labeling of neurons in the brain stem following injections of [³H]choline into the rat spinal cord. *Neuroscience*, 18: 901–916.

[47] Kawai, N., Ito, M. and Nozue, M. (1969) Postsynaptic influences on the vestibular non-Deiters nuclei from primary vestibular nerve. *Exp. Brain Res.*, 8: 190–200.

[48] Kawai, Y., Takami, K., Shiosaka, S., Emson, P.C., Hillyard, C.J., Girgis, S., MacIntyre, I. and Tohyama, M. (1985) Topographic localization of calcitonin gene-related peptide in the rat brain: an immunohistochemistry analysis, *Neuroscience*, 15: 747–763.

[49] Kerkerian, L., Nieoullon, A., Dusticier, N. (1982) Brain glutamate uptake: regional distribution study from sensorimotor areas in the cat. *Neurochem. Int.*, 4: 275–281.

[50] Korte, G.E. (1979) The brainstem projection of the vestibular nerve in the cat. *J. Comp. Neurol.*, 184: 279–292.

[51] Ladpli, R. and Brodal, A. (1968) Experimental studies of commissural and reticular formation projections from the vestibular nuclei in the cat, *Brain Res.*, 8: 65–96.

[52] Logan, W.J. and Snyder, S.H. (1972) High affinity uptake systems for glycine, glutamic and aspartic acids in synaptosomes of rat central nervous tissues. *Brain Res.*, 42: 413–431.

[53] Lund, S. and Pompeiano, O. (1965) Descending pathways with monosynaptic action on motoneurons. *Experientia*, 21: 602–603.

[54] Meza, G., Hernandez, C. and Ruiz, M. (1982) GABA synthesis in isolated vestibulary tissue of chick inner ear. *Brain Res.*, 241: 157–161.

[55] Meza, G., Lopez, I. and Ruiz, M. (1984) Possible cholinergic neurotransmission in cristae ampullares of chick inner ear. *Neurosci. Lett.*, 49: 93–98.

[56] Mugnaini, E., Walberg, F. and Hauglie-Hannsen, E. (1967) Observations of the fine structure of the lateral vestibular nucleus in the cat. *Exp. Brain Res.*, 4: 146–186.

[57] Nieouillon, A. and Dusticier, N. (1981) Increased glutamate decarboxylase activity in the red nucleus of the adult cat after cerebellar lesions. *Brain Res.*, 224: 129–139.

[58] Nieoullon, A. and Dusticier, N. (1981) Decrease in choline acetyl-transferase activity in the red nucleus of the cat after cerebellar lesions *Neuroscience*, 6: 1633–1641.

[59] Nieoullon, A. and Dusticier, N. (1983) Glutamate uptake, glutamate decarboxylase and choline acetyltransferase in subcortial areas after sensorimotor cortical ablations in the cat. *Brain Res. Bull.*, 10: 287–293.

[60] Nomura, I., Senba, E., Kubo, T., Shiraishi, T., Matsunaga, T., Tohyama, M., Shiotani, Y. and Wu, D.E. (1984) Neuropeptides and γ-aminobutyric acid in the vestibular nuclei of the rat: an immuno-histochemical analysis. I. Distribution. *Brain Res.*, 311: 109–118.

[61] Nyberg-Hansen, R. (1964) Origin and termination of fibers from the vestibular nuclei descending in the medial longitudinal fasciculus. An experimental study with silver

impregnation methods in the cat. *J. Comp. Neurol.*, 122: 355–367.

[62] Obata, K. and Highstein, S.M. (1970) Blocking by picrotoxin of both vestibular inhibition and GABA action on rabbit oculomotor neurones. *Brain Res.*, 18: 538–541.

[63] Okada, Y. and Shimada, C. (1976) Gamma-aminobutyric acid (GABA) concentration in a single neuron-localization of GABA in Deiters' neuron. *Brain Res.*, 107: 658–662.

[64] Obata, K., Ito, M., Ochi, R. and Sato, N. (1967) Pharmacological properties of the postsynaptic inhibition by Purkinje cell axons and the action of γ-aminobutyric acid on Deiters' neurones. *Exp. Brain Res.*, 4: 43–57.

[65] Oliver, D.L., Potashner, S.J., Jones, D.R. and Morest, D.K. (1983) Selective labeling of spiral ganglion and granule cells with D-aspartate in the auditory system of cat and guinea pig. *J. Neurosci.*, 3: 455–472.

[66] Otsuka, M., Obata, K., Miyata, Y. and Tanaka, Y. (1971) Measurement of γ-aminobutyric acid in isolated nerve cells of cat central nervous system. *J. Neurochem.*, 18: 287–295.

[67] Peterson, B.W. (1970) Distribution of neural response to tilting within the vestibular nuclei of the cat. *J. Neurophysiol.*, 33: 750–767.

[68] Peterson, B.W. and Coulter, J.D. (1977) A new long spinal projection from the vestibular nuclei in the cat. *Brain Res.*, 122: 351–356.

[69] Peterson, B.W., Maunz, R.A. and Fukushima, K. (1978) Properties of a new vestibulospinal projection, the caudal vestibulospinal tract. Exp. *Brain Res.*, 32: 287–292.

[70] Pompeiano, O. and Brodal, A. (1957) The origin of vestibulospinal fibers in the cat. An experimental–anatomical study, with comments on the descending medial longitudinal fasciculus. *Arch. Ital Biol.*, 95: 166–195.

[71] Pompeiano, O., Mergner, T. and Corvaja, N. (1978) Commissural, perihypoglossal and reticular afferent projections to the vestibular nuclei in the cat. An experimental anatomical study with the method of the retrograde transport of horseradish peroxidase. *Arch. Ital. Biol.*, 116: 130–172

[72] Precht, W., Baker, R. and Okada, Y. (1973) Evidence for GABA as the synaptic transmitter of the inhibitory vestibulo-ocular pathway. *Exp. Brain Res.*, 18: 415–428.

[73] Precht, W., Schwindt, P.C. and Baker, R. (1973) Removal of vestibular commissural inhibition by antagonists of GABA and glycine. *Brain Res.*, 62: 222–226.

[74] Raymond, J. and Desmadryl, G. (1985) In vitro effects of excitatory aminoacid analogues on embryonic and newborn mouse inner ear sensory structures. *Neurosci. Soc. Abstr.*, 11 (1): 448.

[75] Raymond, J., Nieoullon, A., Demêmes, D. and Sans, A. (1984) Evidence for glutamate as a neurotransmitter in the cat vestibular nerve. *Exp. Brain Res.*, 56: 523–531.

[76] Recasens, M. and Delaunoy, J.P. (1981) Immunological properties and immunohistochemical localization of cysteine sulfinate or aspartate aminotransferase isoenzymes in rat CNS. *Brain Res.*, 205: 351–361.

[77] Ross, C.D. and Godfrey, D.A. (1985) Distributions of aspartate aminotransferase and malate dehydrogenase activities in rat retinal layers. *J. Histochem. Cytochem.*, 33: 624–630.

[78] Rossi, M.L., Valli, P. and Casella, C. (1977) Post-synaptic potentials recorded from afferent nerve fibers of the posterior semicircular canal in the frog. *Brain Res.*, 135: 67–75.

[79] Rossi, M.L., Prigioni, I., Valli, P. and Casella, C. (1980) Activation of the afferent system in the isolated frog labyrinth, effects on the afferent EPSPs and spike discharge recorded from single fibers of the posterior nerve. *Brain Res.*, 185: 125–137.

[80] Rubin, A.M, Liedgren, S.R.C, Odkvist, L.M, Milne, A.C. and Fredriekson, J.M. (1977) Labyrinthine input to vestibular nuclei of the awake cat. *Acta Otolaryngol. Stockholm*, 84: 328–337.

[81] Russell, I.J. (1971) The pharmacology of efferent synapses in the lateral system of *Xenopus laevis*. *J. Exp. Biol.*, 54: 643–658.

[82] Russell, I.J. (1976) Amphibian lateral line receptors. In R. LLinas and W. Precht (Eds.), *Frog Neurobiology*. Springer-Verlag, New York, pp. 513–550.

[83] Sans, A. and Raymond, J. (1983) Fonction vestibulaire et équilibration. In Y. Guerrier and A. Uziel (Eds.), *Physiologie Neurosensorielle en O.R.L.*, Masson, Paris, pp. 130–165.

[84] Sans, A., Raymond, J. and Marty, R. (1972) Projections des crêtes ampullaires et de l'utricule dans les noyaux vestibulaires primaires. Etude microphysiologique et corrélations anatomo-fonctionelles. *Brain Res.*, 44: 337–355.

[85] Schwarz, D.W.F., Satoh, K, Schwarz, I.E., Hu, K. and Fibiger, H.C. (1986) Cholinergic innervation of the rat's labyrinth. *Exp. Brain Res.*, 64: 19–26.

[86] Shimazu, H. and Precht, W. (1965) Tonic and kinetic responses of cat's vestibular neurons to horizontal angular acceleration. *J. Neurophysiol.*, 28: 991–1013.

[87] Shimazu, H. and Precht, W. (1966) Inhibition of central vestibular neurons from the contralateral labyrinth and its mediating pathway. *J. Neurophysiol.*, 29: 467–492.

[88] Sonnhof, U. and Buhrle, C.P. (1980) On the postsynaptic action of glutamate in frog spinal motoneurons. *Pflügers Arch.*, 388: 101–109.

[89] Sotelo, C. and Palay, S.L. (1970) The fine structure of the lateral vestibular nucleus in the rat. II. Synaptic organization. *Brain Res.*, 18: 93–115.

[90] Spassova, I. (1982) Fine structure of the neurons and synapses of the vestibular ganglion of the cat. *J. Hirnforsch.*, 23: 657–669.

[91] Stein, B.M. and Carpenter, M.B. (1967) Central projections of portions of the vestibular ganglia innervating specific part of the labyrinth in the rhesus monkey. *Am. J. Anat.*, 120: 281–318.

[92] Storm-Mathisen, J. and Iversen, L.L. (1979) Uptake of ³H-glutamic acid in excitatory nerve endings: light and electron microscopic observations in the hippocampal formation of the rat. *Neuroscience*, 4: 1237–1253.

[93] Storm-Mathisen, J. and Wold, J.E. (1981) In vivo high affinity uptake and axonal transport of D-[2,3-³H]aspartate in excitatory neurons. *Brain Res.*, 230: 427–433.

[94] Streit, P. (1980) Selective retrograde labelling indicating the transmitter of neuronal pathways. *J. Comp. Neurol.*, 191: 429–463.

[95] Streit, P., Knecht, E. and Cuénod, M. (1979) Transmitter-specific retrograde labelling in the striato-nitral and raphe-nigral pathways. *Science*, 205: 306–308.

[97] Sugimoto, T. and Hattori, T. (1984) Organization and efferent projections of nucleus tegmenti pedunculopontinus pars compacta with special reference to its cholinergic aspects. *Neuroscience*, 11: 931–946.

[98] Valli, P., Zucca, G., Prigioni, I., Botta, L., Casella, C. and Guth, P. (1985) The effect of glutamate on the frog semicircular canal. *Brain Res.*, 330: 1–9.

[99] Walberg, F. and Jansen, J. (1961) Cerebellar corticovestibular fibers in the cat. *Exp. Neurol.*, 3: 32–52.

[100] Walberg, F., Bowsher, D. and Brodal, A. (1958) The termination of primary vestibular fibers in the vestibular nuclei in the cat. An experimental study with silver methods. *J. Comp. Neurol.*, 110: 391–419.

[101] Warr, W.B. (1979) Olivocochlear and vestibular efferent neurons of the feline brain stem: their location, morphology and number determined by retrograde axonal transport and acetylcholinesterase histochemistry. *J. Comp. Neurol.*, 161: 159-182.

[102] Wenthold, R.J. and Altschuler, R.A. (1982) Immunocytochemistry of aspartate aminotransferase and glutaminase. In L. Hertz, E. Kvamme, E.G. McGeer and A. Schouboe (Eds.), *Glutamine, Glutamate and GABA in the Central Nervous System*, Alan R. Liss, New York, pp 33–50.

[103] Wenthold, R.J. and Gulley, R.L. (1977) Aspartic acid and glutamic acid levels in the cochlear nucleus after auditory nerve lesion. *Brain Res.*, 138: 111–123.

[104] Werman, R., Davidoff, R.A. and Aprison, M.H. (1968) Inhibitory action of glycine on spinal neurons in the cat. *J. Neurophysiol.*, 31: 81–95.

[105] Wersall, J. (1956) Studies on the structure and innervation of the sensory epithelium of the cristae ampullares in the guinea pig. A light and electronmicroscopic investigation. *Acta Otolaryngol. Stockholm*, 126: 1–85.

[106] Wiklund, L.M. and Cuénod, M. (1984) Differential labeling of afferents to thalamic centromedian-parafascicular nuclei with [³H]choline and D-[³H]aspartate: further evidence for transmitter specific retrograde labelling. *Neurosci. Lett.*, 46: 275–281.

O. Pompeiano and J.H.J. Allum (Eds.)
Progress in Brain Research, Vol. 76
© 1988 Elsevier Science Publishers B.V. (Biomedical Division)

CHAPTER 4

Synaptic mechanisms of interaction of lateral vestibulospinal neurons with some brainstem structures

V.V. Fanardjian and V.A. Sarkisian

Orbeli Institute of Physiology, Academy of Sciences of the Armenian S.S.R., 22 Orbeli Brothers Street, 375028 Yerevan, U.S.S.R.

Effects of stimulation of some brainstem structures on Deiters' neurons were studied in cats using an intracellular recording technique. Stimulation of the rostral region of the inferior olive was shown to evoke mostly antidromic action potentials in Deiters' neurons, while stimulation of the caudal part of the same structure evoked predominantly synaptic responses. Messages from the rostral and particularly caudal regions of the inferior olive as well as from the nucleus reticularis tegmenti pontis evoked mono- and polysynaptic IPSPs in Deiters' neurons, while stimulation of the caudal part of the inferior olive evoked mono- and polysynaptic EPSPs. Axon collaterals of vestibular neurons projecting to the lateral, gigantocellular, parvicellular and paramedian reticular nuclei have been revealed. Stimulation of the lateral and particularly parvicellular reticular nuclei was found to evoke mono- and polysynaptic EPSPs and IPSPs in Deiters' nucleus. Stimulation of the gigantocellular and paramedian reticular nuclei evoked predominantly antidromic responses in these cells. Axon collaterals of the lateral vestibulospinal neurons to the caudal trigeminal, facial and hypoglossal nuclei have been revealed. Mono- and polysynaptic EPSPs were shown to arise in vestibular neurons following stimulation of the caudal trigeminal and facial nuclei, while IPSPs and disfacilitation could be elicited in the same cells by stimulation of the caudal trigeminal nucleus. In some vestibular neurons IPSPs were also observed following stimulation of the hypoglossal nucleus. Bilateral connections between Deiters' nucleus and the interstitial nucleus of Cajal and nucleus of Darkschewitsch have been detected. Stimulation of the latter two structures led to the rise of mono- and polysynaptic EPSPs and IPSPs in vestibular neurons. A topical correlation between Deiters' nucleus and the brainstem nuclei mentioned above was found. Convergence of influences from the stimulated structures on the vestibular neurons was revealed.

Introduction

It seems quite reasonable to divide all efferent vestibular nuclear neurons into six different functional groups: (1) vestibuloocular neurons, (2) vestibulospinal neurons, (3) vestibulocerebellar neurons, (4) vestibuloreticular neurons, (5) vestibular commissural neurons, (6) vestibulothalamic neurons [45]. One of the most powerful outputs is presented by the neurons of Deiters' nucleus, whose anatomical connections and functional relations with the vestibular apparatus [14, 46, 78, 86, 89, 92, 93], the cerebellum [2, 14, 25, 29, 47, 48, 88, 89, 91, 92] and the spinal cord [12, 14, 15, 69, 92] have been studied in detail; however, information about connections

---

Abbreviations: AP, action potential; CTN, caudal trigeminal nucleus; EPSP, excitatory postsynaptic potential; FN, facial nucleus; INC, interstitial nucleus of Cajal; IO(r/c), (rostral/caudal part of the) inferior olive; IPSP, inhibitory postsynaptic potential; LVN, lateral vestibular nucleus; ND, nucleus of Darkschewitsch; NRL, lateral reticular nucleus; NRG, nucleus reticularis gigantocellularis; NRParm, paramedian reticular nucleus; NRParv, nucleus reticularis parvicellularis; NRTP, nucleus reticularis tegmenti pontis; PH, nucleus hypoglossus; RF, reticular formation; VS, vestibulospinal.

of Deiters' nucleus with some brainstem structures is available from only a few morphological studies. Our investigation of synaptic processes of the lateral vestibulospinal neurons carried out on cats using the intracellular recording technique reveals some peculiarities of the interaction of Deiters' nucleus with a number of brainstem structures. Bilateral connections between those structures were found in many cases. Structures of the brainstem interacting with Deiters' nucleus could be divided into the following functional groups: (a) inferior olive and nucleus reticularis tegmenti pontis, (b) nuclei of the brainstem reticular formation, (c) cranial nerves nuclear complex, and (d) interstitial nucleus of Cajal and nucleus of Darkschewitsch.

Effects of stimulation of the inferior olive and nucleus reticularis tegmenti pontis

Morphological studies revealed olivocerebellar neurons with axon collaterals projecting into the Deiters' LVN [9, 19, 42, 43, 47]. Neurons of the NRTP were also found projecting to the medial vestibular nucleus [8]. Opposite connections from the vestibular nuclei to the IO [73] and from Deiters' nucleus to the NRTP [51] were also shown to exist.

From 169 cells sampled in Deiters' nucleus, 126 were activated by stimulation of the IO and NRTP.

Stimulation of the IOr evoked antidromic APs in 33 LVN neurons. Nine of them were VS cells (Fig. 1D). Antidromic APs were also recorded in LVN neurons following stimulation of the IOc (8 cells; Fig. 1A) and NRTP (4 cells, Fig. 1H).

The orthodromic APs were evoked in LVN neurons following single-shock stimulation of the IOr (10 cells, of which 5 were VS neurons), IOc (18 cells, 4 were VS neurons) and NRTP (8 cells, one was VS neuron) (Fig. 1I,J).

Latencies of antidromic and orthodromic APs, as well as EPSPs and IPSPs, following stimulation of the brainstem structures are presented in Table 1.

Orthodromic APs recorded from Deiters' neurons arose from EPSPs of a relatively simple form (Fig. 1E); EPSPs evoked by stimulation of the IOc

had amplitudes of 1.0–6.0 mV. In some EPSPs, a gradual increase in the intensity of IOr stimulation did not affect the latency and time-to-peak of depolarization, suggesting their mono- or oligosynaptic origin (Fig. 1B). EPSPs evoked by stimulation of the IOr were characterized by amplitudes of 1.0–4.0 mV. Excitatory postsynaptic potentials evoked by NRTP stimulation had the mean amplitude of 1.5 mV.

In some LVN neurons EPSPs were complicated by a late positive afterwave which probably occurred when an additional synaptic relay or fibres

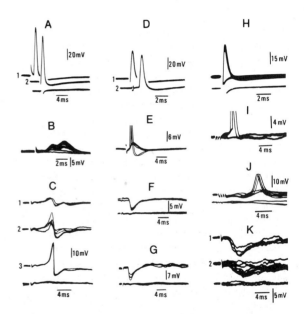

Fig. 1. Antidromic and synaptic activation of Deiters' neurons by stimulation of the IO and NRTP. (A,D,H) Antidromic APs of three Deiters' neurons evoked by stimulation of the caudal (A₁) and rostral (D₁) parts of the IO and NRTP (H). (A₂,D₂) Antidromic APs evoked by stimulation of lateral VS tract. (B,C,G) Mono- and polysynaptic EPSP (B), EPSP–IPSP sequence (C) and monosynaptic IPSP (G) of three Deiters' neurons evoked by stimulation of the caudal part of the IO with various intensities. (E,F) EPSP and IPSP of two Deiters neurons to stimulation of the rostral part of the IO. (I,J) Mono- (I) and (J) polysynaptic APs of two Deiters' neurons evoked by stimulation of the NRTP. (K) Monosynaptic IPSP of a Deiters neuron evoked by stimulation of the NRTP with various intensities. Here and in the following figures potentials are taken from 5 to 10 superimposed sweeps. Lower traces in A,C,F–H,K and in the following figures are extracellular controls.

TABLE 1.

Latencies of antidromic and orthodromic action potentials EPSPs and IPSPs of LVN neurons following stimulation of some brainstem structures

Structures stimulated	Antidromic AP			Orthodromic AP			EPSP			IPSP		
	n	Range	Mean ± S.D.	n	Range	Mean ± S.D.	n	Range	Mean ± S.D.	n	Range	Mean ± S.D.
IOr	33	0.2–0.7	0.4±0.14	10	1.5–5.0	2.0±1.61	3	2.8–3.6	mean 3.0	6	3.0–10.0	mean 6.5
IOc	8	0.2–0.5	mean 0.32	18	2.0–7.5	3.9±1.6	10	2.0–4.0	mean 3.2	9	2.8–9.2	mean 6.1
NRTP	4	0.25–0.4	mean 0.31	8	1.5–5.0	mean 2.5	4	1.0–5.2	mean 1.5	5	2.4–5.2	mean 3.1
NRL	212	0.15–1.0	0.33±0.16		—		5	0.5–2.5	mean 1.38	5	1.1–1.5	mean 1.3
NRParv	82	0.15–1.0	0.38±0.24	31	0.5–5.5	2.4±1.3	14	0.65–3.5	1.8±0.93	14	0.7–1.5	0.95±0.23
NRG	70	0.15–0.55	0.28±0.5		—			—			—	
NRParm	37	0.15–0.8	0.3±0.16	2	1.0–1.6	mean 1.3		—			—	
CTN	111	0.15–1.0	0.4±0.15	18	0.2–6.0	2.5±1.25	38	0.6–3.0	1.25±0.66	22	0.8–3.7	1.48±0.25
FN	107	0.15–0.8	0.3±0.15	8	1.0–3.7	mean 1.7	10	0.3–1.2	0.75±0.92		—	
PH	37	0.15–0.7	0.3±0.24		—			—		5	0.6–1.1	mean 0.94
INC	33	0.2–1.3	0.66±0.13	31	1.1–4.0	2.15±0.45	9	1.0–4.0	mean 1.35	6	1.0–3.0	mean 1.15
ND	20	0.2–1.5	0.85±0.3	25	1.1–3.5	2.0±0.4	4	1.2–2.2	mean 1.6	7	1.5–3.4	mean 1.9

of different calibre were involved (Fig. 1B). A succession of EPSP–IPSP was recorded in response to stimulation of the IOr (in 7 Deiters' neurons) and NRTP (in one Deiters' neuron) (Fig. 1C). Separate IPSPs were recorded in 20 Deiters' neurons following stimulation of the IO and NRTP. In a number of cases, gradual increase in the intensity of IOr, IOc and NRTP stimulation did not affect significantly the latency and time-to-peak of hyperpolarization of the short-latency IPSPs, suggesting their mono- or oligosynaptic origin (Fig. 1F,G,K).

Effect of stimulation of brainstem reticular formation nuclei

It has been shown that the sensory information from the labyrinth of one side can be transferred to the vestibular complex of the opposite side through the perihypoglossal nucleus [59] and the brainstem RF [51]. Such connections between vestibular structures of both sides and the RF are, apparently, necessary for coordinated movements of the eyes, neck muscles and extensors of the limbs during labyrin-

thine reflexes. Morphological features of RF projections to the vestibular nuclei have been studied in detail; less information, however, is available on the functional characteristics of the reticulo–vestibular relations.

Fibres projecting to the vestibular nuclei from the brainstem RF were revealed long ago by Cajal [22] and Lorente de Nó [53]. Collaterals of the VS tract projecting to the RF [22] as well as axon collaterals from the RF reaching Deiters' nucleus [75] were described. Experiments with lesioning of the descending and lateral vestibular nuclei predominantly revealed degenerating fibres in ipsilateral reticular pontine as well as medullary nuclei [24].

One of the main sources of efferent vestibular fibres to the NRParm is the LVN [33]. Morphological studies with anterograde degeneration technique [40, 44] and axon transport of horseradish peroxidase [70] revealed reticulovestibular fibres projecting to all main nuclei of the vestibular complex. Fibre collaterals of the VS tract to the NRL were found [23]. Antidromic activation of reticular neurons evoked by vestibular nuclear stimulation were also studied electrophysiologically (for references see [70]).

Intracellular potentials of 488 Deiters' neurons were recorded; 474 of these cells responded to stimulation of the NRL, NRParv, NRG and NRParm. Latencies of antidromic and orthodromic APs, as well as EPSPs and IPSPs following stimulation of these RF nuclei are shown in Table 1.

Stimulation of the NRL evoked antidromic APs in 212 Deiters' neurons. 108 of these cells were identified as VS neurons (Fig. 2A). Stimulation of the NRL evoked EPSPs in five Deiters' neurons. They had latencies of 0.5–2.5 ms (mean 1.38 ms); the values suggest the presence of both mono- and polysynaptic connections between the NRL and Deiters' neurons. Stimulation of NRL also gave rise to IPSPs in five LVN cells. Latencies of these IPSPs were 1.1–1.5 ms (mean 1.3 ms), evidently suggesting the presence of mono- and polysynaptic inhibitory influences from the NRL on Deiters' neurons. In some neurons IPSPs were followed by EPSPs which, at increasing intensities of NRL stimulation, were converted into grouped APs (Fig. 2B).

Single-shock stimulation of the NRParv evoked antidromic APs in 82 Deiters' neurons. 22 of these neurons were identified as VS units (Fig. 2C,D). Orthodromic APs were recorded in 31 Deiters' neurons in response to stimulation of the NRParv (Fig. 2F). The orthodromic APs appeared on the top of EPSPs with an amplitude of 2.0–11.0 mV (mean $\pm$ S.D. 4.75 ± 2.6 mV, $n = 14$) (Fig. 2E). Increasing intensities of NRParv stimulation did not change the latency of onset of some orthodromic APs, suggesting their monosynaptic origin. Gradual increase of NRParv stimulation intensity shortened the latencies of APs in some LVN neurons and, in 11 cells, led to a complete replacement of orthodromic APs with antidromic ones. These Deiters' neurons apparently have bilateral connections with NRParv cells. In 5 LVN neurons orthodromic potentials evoked by NRParv stimulation were based on a pronounced depolarization plateau, being represented by two and more spikes. These reactions of LVN neurons are similar to those appearing following stimulation of the caudal trigeminal nucleus. Stimulation of the NRParv evoked IPSPs in 14 LVN neurons.

In some LVN neurons, changing the NRParv stimulation intensity did not affect the latency or time-to-peak of de- and hyperpolarization indicating, apparently, their monosynaptic origin. Electrophoretic injection of chloride ions into the cell

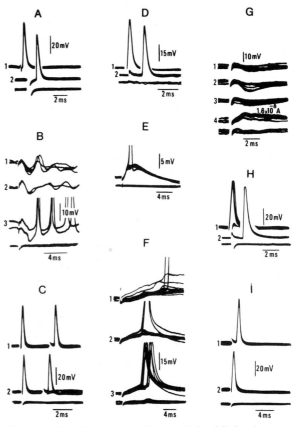

Fig. 2. Antidromic and synaptic potentials of Deiters' neurons evoked by stimulation of RF nuclei. (A,D,H,I) Antidromic APs of four Deiters' neurons evoked by stimulation of the NRL (A_1), NRParv (D_1), NRG (H_1) and NRParm (I_1). (A_2,D_2,H_2,I_2) Antidromic APs of the same cells evoked by stimulation of the lateral VS tract. ($C_{1,2}$) Collision of antidromic APs evoked by stimulation of the NRParv and lateral VS tract (spikes on the right). (B_{1-3}) IPSP with rebound facilitation of a neuron evoked by stimulation of the NRL with various intensities. (E,F) EPSPs and APs of two Deiters' neurons evoked in response of increasing intensity of NRParv stimulation. (G) IPSP of a Deiters' neuron to stimulation of the NRParv. Reversion of IPSP by hyperpolarizing current injection of 1.6×10^{-8}A.

changed the IPSP into a depolarizing potential, suggesting the inhibitory nature of these potentials (Fig. 2G).

Stimulation of the NRG led to antidromic excitation of 70 Deiters' neurons, 35 of them were identified as VS cells (Fig. 2H). Collision of antidromic APs evoked by stimulation of the lateral VS tract and NRG was observed. No excitatory or inhibitory potentials were observed in LVN neurons in response to NRG stimulation.

Antidromic APs were recorded in 37 LVN neurons following stimulation of the NRParm. 21 of them were VS units (Fig. 2I). In two cases stimulation of the NRParm evoked orthodromic responses appearing on the top of EPSPs. As in experiments with NRG stimulation, no inhibitory potentials were observed in LVN neurons in response to NRParm stimulation.

Analysis of the topographic distribution of LVN neurons responding to stimulation of RF nuclei showed that 86% of cells synaptically activated from NRL and NRParv were localized in the rostroventral half of the nucleus. The majority of LVN neurons antidromically activated from RF nuclei were distributed homogenously throughout the Deiters' nucleus.

Effects of stimulations of cranial nerve nuclei

Modification of the vestibular nystagmus by activation of the trigeminal nerve system was shown long ago by Lorente de Nó [54]. Changes in the spontaneous activity of vestibular neurons evoked by electric stimulation of the trigeminal nerve had been established [85]. Connections of the trigeminal nuclei with Deiters' nucleus were confirmed by morphological findings [17]. Trigeminal proprioceptive afferent fibres projecting to the vestibular nuclei and participating in the control of eye–head movements were also described [55]. Vestibular nuclei are shown to establish direct monosynaptic contacts with FN neurons [77]. It was also shown that vestibular neurons projecting to the oculomotor nucleus send axon collaterals to the FN [58]. Morphological studies revealed neurons in the ros-

tral part of the PH sending their axons to the LVN [47].

The intracellular activities of 419 LVN neurons responding to stimulation of the VIIIth nerve, CTN, FN and PH was recorded (see Table 1 for latency values).

Stimulation of the CTN evoked antidromic APs in 111 LVN cells, 33 of which were identified as VS neurons (Fig. 3A). In 18 LVN neurons, stimulation of the CTN also evoked orthodromic APs, which arose on the top of EPSPs. Four of these cells were identified as VS neurons. 38 Deiters' neurons responded with EPSPs to stimulation of the CTN (Fig. 3J, upper columns) with latencies ranging from 0.6 to 3.0 ms (mean $\pm$ S.D. 1.25 ± 0.66 ms, $n = 38$) and amplitudes ranging from 1.0 to 18 mV (mean $\pm$ S.D. 6.5 ± 5.46 mV, $n = 38$). In some EPSPs (Fig. 3B), gradual change of the stimulus intensity did not affect the latency and time-to-peak of the depolarization, suggesting their monosynaptic origin. In some LVN neurons, gradual intensification of CTN stimulation led to the increase of EPSP amplitude, shortening of its latency and onset of 3–5 APs on the top of a depolarizing wave (Fig. 3C,D). The origin of these grouped discharges in LVN neurons could be attributed, as for FN motoneurons [34], to gradual depolarization of the cell membrane due to summation of the high-frequency excitatory influences from the CTN on dendrites of the vestibular neurons.

Along with EPSPs, hyperpolarizing reactions to CTN stimulation were recorded in 51 LVN neurons. According to their characteristics they can be divided into two groups. Responses of the first group (22 cells) were IPSPs, the latencies of which ranged from 0.8 to 3.7 ms (mean $\pm$ S.D. 1.48 ± 0.25 ms, $n = 22$) (Fig. 3J, lower dark columns). Time-to-peak of hyperpolarization was 0.5–2.4 ms (mean $\pm$ S.D. 1.5 ± 0.39 ms, $n = 22$) and the total duration 2.0–12.0 ms (mean $\pm$ S.D. 5.75 ± 2.55 ms, $n = 22$). The amplitude of IPSPs was 1.5–14.0 mV (mean $\pm$ S.D. 6.32 ± 4.0 mV, $n = 22$). Electrophoretic injection of chloride ions into the cell reversed the IPSP into a depolarizing potential (Fig. 3F,G), revealing the inhibitory nature of the recorded po-

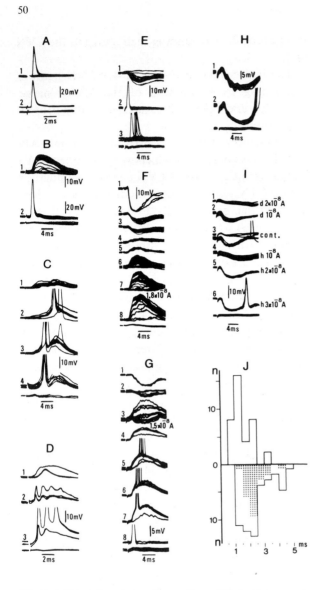

Fig. 3. Antidromic and synaptic reactions of Deiters' neurons to stimulation of the CTN and VIIIth nerve. (A) Antidromic APs of a Deiters' neuron evoked by stimulation of the CTN (A_1) and lateral VS tract (A_2). (B,C) EPSPs and APs of two Deiters' neurons evoked by CTN (B_1,C) and VIIIth nerve (B_2) stimulation. B_1 and C_{1-4} show gradual changes of stimulus intensity. (D) Bursting of a Deiters' neuron to CTN stimulation. (E–G) IPSPs, antidromic and orthodromic APs of three Deiters neurons evoked by stimulation of the CTN (E_1,F_1,G_1), lateral VS tract (E_2) and VIIIth nerve (E_3,G_8). (F_{1-8},G_{1-4}) Reversion of IPSPs by hyperpolarizing current injection of 1.8×10^{-8}A and 1.5×10^{-8} A. (G_{5-7}) Generation of APs on the top of the reversed IPSP by intensification of CTN stimulation. (H,I) Disfacilitatory hyperpolarization of two Deiters' neurons to CTN stimulation. (I_3) Control recording. Change of potentials by depolarizing (d) and

tentials. In some neurons change of the stimulus intensity did not alter the latency and time-to-peak of the hyperpolarization, suggesting their monosynaptic origin (Fig. $3E_1$).

Hyperpolarizing reactions of the second group of LVN neurons (29 cells) to CTN stimulation had latencies ranging from 1.2 to 4.5 ms (mean ± S.D. 2.5 ± 1.1 ms, $n = 29$) (Fig. 3H,J, lower white columns). The time-to-peak of hyperpolarization, total duration and amplitude of these potentials exceeded the equivalent parameters of IPSPs and were respectively 2.8–8.0 ms (mean ± S.D. 4.3 ± 1.4 ms, $n = 29$), 8.0–22.0 ms (mean ± S.D. 12.4 ± 4.64 ms, $n = 29$) and 3.0–20.0 mV (mean ± S.D. 10.7 ± 4.9 mV, $n = 29$). Intracellular injection of hyperpolarizing current and chloride ions did not lead to the distortion and reversal of the hyperpolarizing potential. Moreover, it became considerably larger following injection of hyperpolarizing currents and smaller during artificial depolarization of the membrane to the level of the equilibrium potential of EPSP (Fig. 3I). The described hyperpolarizing potentials were, in their characteristics, similar to the disfacilitatory hyperpolarization recorded first from the spinal extensor motoneurons under the inhibitory cerebellar influence [52, 83] and later in studies analyzing the cerebellar inhibitory influence on red nucleus neurons [84]. In this instance, the tonic excitatory influences on the red nucleus originated from neurons of the cerebellar interpositus nucleus, whose activity was inhibited by stimulation of Purkinje cells evoking disfacilitation of the rubral neurons. Disfacilitatory responses recorded from LVN neurons following CTN stimulation could be the result of removal of the tonic excitatory influences of the IO or FN on LVN neurons. Direct connections of the CTN with the IO [28,31], FN [26, 80] and vestibular nuclei [87] are well known. The possibility cannot be excluded that the

hyperpolarizing (h) current injections (values are given on the right of each record). (J) Latency distribution histograms of EPSPs (upper columns), IPSPs (lower dark columns) and disfacilitatory hyperpolarization (lower white columns) of Deiters' neurons evoked by CTN stimulation.

disfacilitatory potential that appears in LVN neurons is due to suppression of tonic excitatory influences from fastigial cells inhibited by activation of Purkinje cells through the trigeminal climbing fibre input [3].

Stimulation of the FN evoked antidromic APs in 107 neurons. 34 of them were VS neurons (Fig. 4B). Collison of antidromic APs evoked by FN and lateral VS tract stimulation was detected (Fig. 4B). In 8 LVN neurons orthodromic APs were recorded to FN stimulation. Four of them are found to be VS neurons; two neurons responded also to VIIIth nerve stimulation (Fig. 4A). In some cases, increase in the intensity of FN stimulation changed the orthodromic APs into antidromic ones (Fig. 4C,E), proving the existence of bilateral connections between LVN neurons and FN cells.

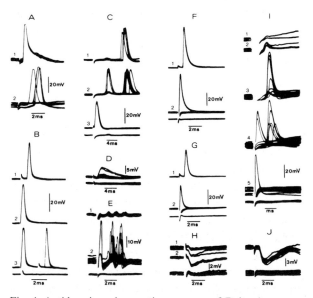

Fig. 4. Antidromic and synaptic responses of Deiters' neurons evoked by stimulation of the FN and PH. (A,C,E,I) Orthodromic APs of four Deiters' neurons evoked by stimulation of the VIIIth nerve (A_1), FN (A_2,C_2,E_2) and PH ($I_{3,4}$). In C and E_1 (from top to bottom) the stimulation intensity is gradually increased. (B,F,G) Antidromic APs of three Deiters' neurons evoked by over-threshold stimulation of the VS tract (B_1,F_1,G_1), FN (B_2), PH (F_2,G_2). (B_3) Collision of antidromic APs evoked by stimulation of the FN and VS tract. (D,H,J,) EPSP (D) and IPSPs (H,J) of three Deiters' neurons evoked by stimulation of the FN (D) and PH (H,J) with various intensities.

Stimulation of FN also evoked EPSPs in 10 Deiters' neurons with amplitudes of 1.5–6.0 mV (mean $\pm$ S.D. 3.6 ± 1.5 mV, $n = 10$). The stability of the latent period and time-to-peak of depolarization observed in some EPSPs to increasing intensities of FN stimulation indicates the presence of monosynaptic EPSPs (Fig. 4D). In none of the Deiters' neurons did stimulation of the FN evoke an inhibitory reaction.

Stimulation of the PH evoked antidromic APs in 37 LVN neurons. 13 of them were identified as VS (Fig. 4F,G) In one case stimulation of the PH evoked an EPSP with an orthodromic potential (Fig. 4I), which at a stronger intensity of stimulus was replaced by an antidromic potential. Stimulation of the PH evoked IPSPs in 5 LVN cells (Fig. 4H). They arose with latencies ranging from 0.6 to 1.1 ms (mean 0.94). Increase of stimulus intensity did not affect the latency and time-to-peak of hyperpolarization, thus suggesting their monosynaptic origin (Fig. 4H,J).

Analysis of the topographic distribution of LVN neurons responsive to stimulation of the CTN, FN and PH showed that the majority of cells (82%) affected by CTN stimulation were localized in the ventral half of Deiters' nucleus, whereas neurons responding to FN and PH stimulation were found predominantly in the dorsal half of the LVN.

Effects of stimulation of the interstitial nucleus of Cajal and nucleus of Darkschewitsch

Morphological data are available on the cerebellar projection to the vestibular nuclei through the INC and ND. These nuclei receive bilateral projections from the cerebellar nuclei (interpositus and dentatus) [27, 50] and in turn send efferent fibres to the vestibular nuclear complex [71]. In addition, there were vestibular neurons which could be antidromically activated by the INC [56, 57]. Recent electrophysiological studies have demonstrated the existence of interstitiospinal neurons sending collaterals to vestibular nuclei [36].

The intracellular activities of 168 LVN neurons were recorded; 133 cells responded to stimulation of the INC and ND (for latency values see Table 1).

In 33 Deiters' neurons, antidromic APs were evoked by stimulation of the INC (Fig. 5A,B). Five of these 33 neurons were identified as VS cells (Fig. 5C). Stimulation of the INC evoked orthodromic APs in 31 LVN neurons (Fig. 5J,K), 8 of which were VS cells. In 9 cells, stimulation of the INC evoked EPSPs with amplitudes varying from 0.5 to 5.0 mV. Latencies of EPSPs were 1.0–4.0 ms

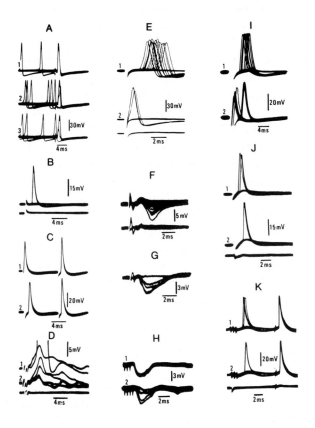

($n = 9$). This suggests the presence of mono- as well as polysynaptic excitatory connections between the INC and LVN neurons. In addition to isolated EPSPs, a succession of EPSP–IPSP was observed in three neurons, with IPSPs characterized by a greater amplitude (Fig. 5F). In 6 LVN neurons, stimulation of the INC evoked IPSPs with amplitudes of 1.0–6.0 mV. Some IPSPs had a complex configuration and consisted of two or more components. Change of INC stimulation intensity did not affect the latency or time-to-peak of the early component of hyperpolarization, indicating its monosynaptic origin (Fig. 5G). Monosynaptic IPSPs evoked by stimulation of the INC were revealed in motoneurons of the nucleus abducens [76].

Antidromic APs were observed in 20 LVN neurons on stimulation of the ND; 5 of these neurons were VS cells (Fig. 5C). In 25 LVN neurons, stimulation of the ND also evoked orthodromic APs on the top of EPSPs (Fig. 5D,J,K) with an amplitude of 1.0–3.0 mV. Stimulation of the ND evoked in 7 Deiters' neurons IPSPs with an amplitude of 1.0–6.0 mV. EPSPs and IPSPs in LVN neurons evoked in response to ND stimulation appeared separately and seldom. When compared to those evoked by INC stimulation they had a higher threshold. In a number of cases they consist of several components. Alteration of ND stimulation intensity had no effect on PSP latency or time-to-peak of the early component of depolarization (Fig. 5K) and hyperpolarization (Fig. 5H), suggesting the possibility of monosynaptic PSPs being evoked in LVN neurons in response to ND stimulation.

Among the neurons under study, 8 cells responded to INC and ND stimulation with anti- or orthodromic APs depending on the intensity of stimulation. Two of them are shown in Fig. 5 [E,I]; orthodromic responses were replaced by antidromic ones at increased stimulation intensities.

Convergence and divergence

In three Deiters' neurons convergence of influences from the rostral and caudal parts of the IO as well as from the NRTP was observed. One of them was

Fig. 5. Antidromic and synaptic potentials of Deiters' neurons evoked by stimulation of the INC and ND. (A,B,C) Intracellular antidromic APs of three Deiters' neurons evoked by stimulation of the INC (A,B,C₁) and ND (C₂). (A₁₋₃) Collision of antidromic AP with spontaneous activity. (B) Just-threshold stimulation. Potentials on the right of C and K are evoked to stimulation of the lateral VS tract. (D,J,K) Change of EPSPs into APs by stimulation of the INC (J₁, K₁) and ND (D₁,₂,J₂,K₂). (F–H) EPSP–IPSP sequence (F) and IPSPs (G,H) of three Deiters' neurons evoked by stimulation of the INC (F,G) and ND with various intensities. (E,I) Replacement of orthodromic APs by antidromic ones after intensification of INC (E) and ND (I) stimulation.

a VS neuron. Convergence of influences from the rostral and caudal parts of the IO was found in 5 LVN cells, 4 of which were VS neurons. Divergence of axons reaching the rostral and caudal parts of the IO was observed in 5 LVN neurons, 3 of them were VS neurons.

Among the LVN neurons under study there was a group of 136 VS cells which could, via their axon collaterals, also be antidromically driven from RF nuclei. Thus, in 12 (8.8%) LVN neurons antidromic APs were recorded following stimulation of all four reticular nuclei. 16 (11.7%) neurons of this group responded to stimulation of three reticular nuclei; 20 (14.7%) neurons to stimulation of two reticular nuclei, and 88 (64.7%) neurons to stimulation of one reticular nucleus. In some VS neurons of this group, stimulation of the reticular nuclei also evoked synaptic responses, suggesting convergent inputs from the reticular nuclei on neurons of Deiters' nucleus.

Convergence of infleunces from the CTN, FN and PH on LVN neurons was also observed. Stimulation of these nuclei led in some LVN neurons to antidromic activation, indicating the divergent effect of Deiters' neurons on those structures.

Convergence of influences from the INC and ND was observed in 26 of 133 LVN neurons (19.6%). 7 of these were VS cells. In 14 LVN neurons, stimulation of the INC and ND led to antidromic activation, suggesting the existence in these neurons of axon collaterals reaching both the INC and ND. Three cells of this group were identified as VS neurons. Two LVN neurons received convergent influences from the caudal and rostral parts of the IO, INC and ND.

Discussion

The experiments revealed some pecularities of neuronal interaction of Deiters' nucleus with brainstem structures, as mentioned above. General characteristics, as well as typical patterns of interaction of the lateral vestibulospinal neurons with various functional groups of brainstem nuclei, were described.

Inferior olive and nucleus reticularis tegmenti pontis

The following features of interaction of Deiters' nucleus with the IO and NRTP were observed:
(1) Stimulation of the rostral part of the IO evokes in Deiters' neurons mainly antidromic responses (antidromic 64%, synaptic 36%), whereas activation is mainly synaptic when the caudal part of the IO is stimulated (synaptic 85%, antidromic 15%).
(2) Stimulation of the NRTP produces synaptic responses in 82% of Deiters' neurons with only 18% of neurons responding antidromically.
(3) Stimulation of the rostral and particularly of the caudal parts of the IO and the NRTP evokes mono-, oligo- and polysynaptic IPSPs in Deiters' neurons; mono-, oligo- and polysynaptic EPSPs are evoked in some Deiters' neurons in response to stimulation of the caudal part of the IO.
(4) A EPSP–IPSP sequence was recorded from Deiters neurons to stimulation of the predominantly caudal part of the IO.

That antidromic APs were recorded from Deiters' neurons mainly in response to stimulation of the rostral part of the IO indicates that some LVN neurons send their axons mostly to this region of the IO. 21% of cells from this population of neurons occupied the dorsal part of Deiters' nucleus, 31% the middle part and 49% the ventral part of the nucleus. Moreover, 23% of Deiters' neurons could also be activated antidromically by stimulation of the lateral VS tract, which indicates the presence of VS neurons with axon collaterals projecting to the rostral part of the IO. Antidromic activation of Deiters' neurons was also observed with stimulation of the caudal part of the IO. Relevant in this connection is the study by Saint-Cyr and Courville [73], which suggests the possibility of retrograde transport of horseradish peroxidase from the IO to Deiters' neurons as well as to the other nuclei of the vestibular complex.

Unlike the rostral part of the IO, stimulation of the caudal region of this nucleus leads predominantly to the synaptic activation of Deiters' neurons. Neurons synaptically activated by stimulation of the caudal part of the IO were recorded mostly from the dorsal part of Deiters' nucleus (67%) as well as from its middle (22%) and ventral (11%) parts. Some recorded EPSPs were mono- or oligosynaptic origin. This agrees well with published data on the presence of a direct IO–LVN projection via the collaterals of olivocerebellar fibres [6, 41, 63, 65]. As to the polysynaptic EPSPs, they could possibly be caused by activation of the loop: climbing fibre collateral–nucleus fastigius–Deiters' nucleus (Fig. 6). The fact that antidromic and synaptic potentials could be recorded from Deiters' neurons in

response to NRTP stimulation is also in good accord with published data. Ladpli and Brodal [51] revealed a direct projection from Deiters' nucleus to the NRTP. Efferent fibres also extend from the NRTP to the medial vestibular nucleus [8]. Analysis of the distribution of the Deiters' neuron potentials recorded in our study following NRTP stimulation showed that antidromically activated neurons were localized in the ventral part of the nucleus, whereas neurons activated synaptically were found all over the Deiters' nucleus.

As mentioned above, mono- or oligosynaptic EPSPs and IPSPs were recorded from some Deiters' neurons. However, most of the inhibitory and excitatory postsynaptic influences from these structures on Deiters' nucleus utilized polysynaptic pathways.

The sequence of EPSP–IPSPs evoked by stimulation of the caudal part of the IO may possibly be explained by the involvement of climbing fibres projecting to the vermis of the cerebellar anterior lobe with collaterals reaching the LVN and the fastigial nucleus (Fig. 6). Neurons showing inhibitory responses to stimulation of the caudal part of the IO were localized in the dorsal part of Deiters' nucleus which is under a direct inhibitory influence of Purkinje cells from the parasagittal zone 'B' of the cerebellar anterior lobe [4, 5, 29, 35, 88].

Thus, inhibitory and excitatory influences of the IO and NRTP on Deiters' neurons should apparently be considered as a part of the mechanisms which participate in the coordination and integration of supraspinal information.

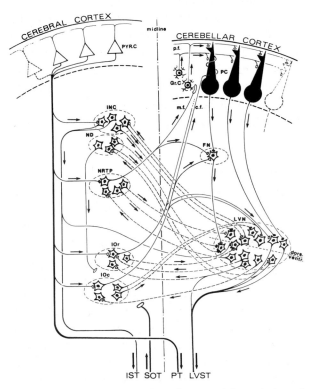

Fig. 6. Schematic representation of neuronal interrelation of Deiters' nucleus (LVN) with cerebellum, cerebral cortex, rostral and caudal parts of inferior olive (IOr and IOc), nucleus reticularis tegmenti pontis (NRTP), interstitial nucleus of Ramon y Cajal (INC) and nucleus of Darkschewitsch (ND). FN, fastigial nucleus; PYR.C, pyramidal cell; PC, Purkinje cell; Gr.C, granule cell; m.f., mossy fibre; c.f., climbing fibre; p.f., parallel fibre; IST, SOT, PT and LVST, interstitiospinal tract, spino-olivary tract, pyramidal tract and lateral vestibulospinal tract, respectively. Here and in the following diagrams arrows show direction of information flow. Inhibitory synapses are shown in black. Dotted lines represent pathways studied in the present work. (Modified from [1]; see also [74].)

Nuclei of the brainstem reticular formation

Stimulation of RF nuclei evoked in Deiters' neurons both antidromic and synaptic potentials. The results agree well with morphological [14, 33, 47, 51, 70] and physiological [66, 68, 79] findings published so far. It is known that a great number of different somatic and visceral signals converge on RF neurons before reaching the spinal motoneuronal pool [62, 72]; thus afferents are sent to the NRL not only from the LVN [51] but also from the spinal cord [13, 61], fastigial nucleus [90], red nucleus and cerebral cortex [16]. The NRL must be functionally considered as a relay station for command signals from the motor cortex (direct or mediated by the red nucleus) and ascending spinal impulses (through the bilateral ventral flexor reflex tract) [20, 21]. Information reaching the NRL is transferred further to the cerebellar cortex and from there to the intracerebellar and brainstem nuclei [16]. Being an important afferent input to the NRL, the bilateral ventral flexor reflex tract undergoes influences from the reticulocerebellar pathway (via the bulbospinal tract) and the VS tract [39, 64].

The NRParm receives some afferents from the

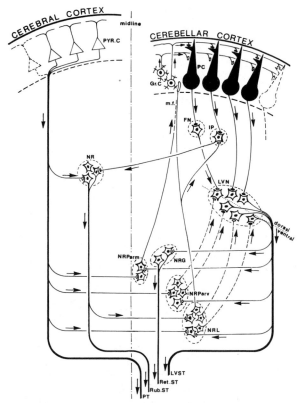

Fig. 7. Schematic representation of neuronal interrelation of Deiters' nucleus (LVN) with cerebellum, cerebral cortex and brainstem RF nuclei. NRL, lateral; NRParv, parvicellular; NRG, gigantocellular and NRParm, paramedian reticular nuclei; FN and IP, cerebellar fastigial and interposital nuclei; RN, red nucleus; PT, Rub.ST, Ret.ST and LVST, pyramidal, rubrospinal, reticulospinal and lateral vestibulospinal tracts, respectively.

sensorimotor cortex and spinal cord; almost all its projections are sent to the cerebellum [18]. The NRG, unlike the NRL and NRParv, is the main source of fibres of the reticulospinal tract and sends a very small number of projections to the cerebellum [7].

By modifying the activity of NRL and NRParm neurons, Deiters' nucleus provides a feed-back in the NRL – cerebellum – LVN – NRL and NRParm – cerebellum – LVN –NRParm loops, exerting an influence on the cerebellum and, via the NRL, also on the corticocerebellar functional loop (cerebral cortex – NRL – cerebellar cortex – fastigial, interpositus and red nuclei – NRL) [21] (Fig. 7). Analysis of the topographical distribution of Deiters' neurons responding to NRL and NRParv stimulation revealed their dominant localization in the rostroventral part of the nucleus. This agrees with morphological data [51, 70]. Inhibitory effects of rostroventral Deiters' neurons were evoked mainly by NRParv and NRL stimulation. Moreover, according to the somatotopical organization of the LVN, the rostroventral half of that nucleus is the representative zone of the neck, forelimb and afferents from the labyrinth and is under no direct inhibitory control of cerebellar anterior lobe Purkinje cells [35, 46, 49]. It is likely that the presence of inhibitory influences from the NRParv and NRL on rostroventral Deiters' neurons provides more delicately coordinated influences of these structures in the control of forelimb, neck and head movements.

Similar to Deiters' nucleus, the RF nuclei of the brainstem are considered to be an important relay station in the organization of motor control. Vestibulo- and reticulospinal systems may also provide presynaptic inhibition of afferents of Ia extensor motoneurons [10]. According to findings by Peterson and Felpel [67], RF nuclei are polysynaptically activated by the vestibular nerve. The results of our experiments revealed the presence of bilateral monosynaptic connection of the LVN with RF nuclei, apparently giving evidence of active participation and interaction of the reticulo- and vestibulospinal systems in the motor bulbo–spino–bulbar reflex.

Cranial nerve nuclei

Stimulation of the above-mentioned cranial nerve nuclei evoked in the majority of Deiters' neurons antidromic APs, suggesting the presence of vestibular neurons with axon collaterals projecting to these nuclei. It is known that the CTN, FN and PH participate in the realization of a large group of motor reactions including masticatory, mimic, blinking, swallowing and other reflexes. Axons of the secondary vestibular neurons carrying vestibular information to these structures are mainly involved in the regulation of movements of the head and eyes [58, 94]. It is assumed that the most probable role of interaction between these structures and the LVN is to coordinate the corresponding reflexes in integrated motor acts, thus providing specificity and functional pattern for each of the structures involved.

Stimulation of the CTN and FN evoked mono- and polysynaptic EPSPs in LVN neurons. EPSPs evoked by FN stimulation had a simple form and relatively small amplitude, whereas EPSPs evoked by CTN stimulation caused a depolarizing shift, often leading to generation of multiple discharges of LVN neurons. Modulation of activity of the vestibular neurons by the trigeminal complex was studied by Darian-Smith [32]. The results of this series of experiments showed that LVN neurons undergo an inhibitory influence from the CTN and FN. IPSPs evoked from these nuclei were both mono- and polysynaptic. Stimulation of the CTN also evoked a massive disfacilitatory hyperpolarization of LVN neurons. The average latency for such disfacilitation was 2.5 ms, which is sufficient for the involvement of the following structures and pathways in this process: (1) CTN – IO – LVN, (2) CTN – FN – LVN, (3) CTN – IO – climbing fibres – Purkinje cells – fastigial nucleus – LVN, and (4) CTN – trigeminal climbing fibres – Purkinje cells – fastigial nucleus – LVN (Fig. 8). It must be noted that the described disfacilitatory effects were mainly observed in the ventral half of the nucleus which, according to the somatotopic organization of the LVN, is the zone of representation of the neck, fore-limb and primary vestibular afferents and is out of the direct inhibitory control of the cerebellar anterior lobe Purkinje cells [35, 88]. The CTN is a sensory structure which has direct connections with the FN [26, 34, 80], and PH [60, 81] and, according to our experimental results, also with the LVN. Interaction of these nuclei must apparently be important for their coordinated functioning in the performance of complex motor reflex actions.

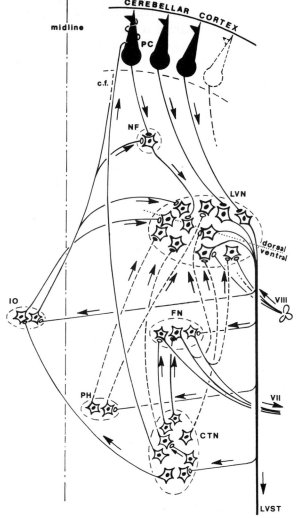

Fig. 8. Schematic representation of neuronal interrelation of Deiters' nucleus (LVN) with cerebellum and cranial nerves nuclei. CTN, caudal trigeminal nucleus; FN, facial nerve nucleus; PH, hypoglossal nerve nucleus; VII, facial nerve; VIII, vestibular nerve; LVST, lateral vestibulospinal tract; IO, inferior olive; NF, fastigial nucleus.

Interstitial nucleus of Cajal and nucleus of Darksche-witsch

Results of our experiments showed that LVN neurons establish bilateral connections with the INC and NP. Stimulation of these structures evoked both antidromic (52% to INC and 44% to ND stimulation) and orthodromic (48% to INC and 56% to ND stimulation) APs in LVN neurons. These results agree well with morphological data on INC and ND projections to vestibular nuclei, as well as direct ascending connections of the vestibular nuclei with the INC and ND [14, 71]. It is known from morphological observations that LVN neurons may have dichotomized axons, one branch of which extends rostrally to the brainstem structures and the other caudally to the spinal cord [14]. Such a type of neurons was also revealed in our experiments: about 1/5 of LVN cells antidromically activated by INC and ND stimulation were VS neurons.

Our findings on synaptic potentials recorded in LVN to INC stimulation agree with the results of electrophysiological studies in which interstitiospinal neurons were shown to send their axon collaterals to vestibular nuclei [36]. These neurons may actually establish monosynaptic contacts with neck motoneurons [38] and receive their main descending input from those regions of the frontal cortex [37] which are responsible for voluntary movements of the neck (Fig. 6). It is worth mentioning that most of the cells (86%) responding to INC and ND stimulation were localized in the ventral half of Deiters' nucleus, i.e. in the representation zone for the cervical section of the spinal cord.

One of the important results of these experiments is the recording of EPSPs and IPSPs from LVN neurons in response to INC and ND stimulation. Short latencies and other features observed in some of these PSPs suggest their monosynaptic origin. Similar effects of INC and ND stimulation were described by Schwindt et al. [76] for neurons of the trochlear nucleus. Monosynaptic EPSPs and IPSPs studied by them could be evoked by stimulation of any part of the INC and ND, so the latter were con-

sidered as homogeneous structures in which excitatory and inhibitory neurons are mixed. This conclusion may be also valid for the effects reported above.

Szentagothai and Schab [82] have shown that prolonged stimulation of the ND inhibits vestibularly evoked eye movements. Stimulation of the INC affects the activity of relay neurons of the horizontal and anterior canals [38]. It was found that vestibularly projecting interstitiospinal neurons control not only the vertical and circular neck movements, but also simultaneously send their motor impulses to the vestibular nuclei [36]. It was also demonstrated that some of the interstitiospinal neurons are influenced by the motor cortex representative zones of neck, back and shoulder [36, 37].

Thus, it seems possible that the INC and perhaps the ND (as a collector of input signals from the motor zones of the cerebral cortex, muscle afferents and labyrinth) exert a direct and mediated (via interneurons of the vestibular nuclei) modulatory influence on lateral VS neurons [56, 57]. Moreover, some of these VS neurons which are directly activated by stimulation of the INC and ND in return excite the neurons of these nuclei. This may be of special significance for correlation of the activity of both vestibulospinal and interstitiospinal systems during combined neck, head and limbs movements.

In conclusion, the results of the experiments revealed extensive connections of Deiters' nucleus with several brainstem structures. The most important function of these connections is to provide the LVN with various information determining and directing its integrative activity. They could also complement and complicate the comparatively simple functional organization of the lateral vestibulospinal neurons. This concerns most of all effects of cerebellar control. These vestibular nuclear neurons, receiving direct Purkinje cell projections, are considered equivalent to the cerebellar nuclear neurons. However, the neuronal connections around them are simpler than those around cerebellar nuclear neurons. Thus, vestibular nuclear neurons appear to constitute a simple or 'primitive' form of the corticonuclear complex [45]. Our experimental results revealed exceptionally large efferent projections of the LVN, particularly the axon collaterals of vestibulospinal neurons to different nuclear structures of the brainstem. The latter should provide systemic character of lateral vestibulospinal influences involving many brainstem structures in the organization of the specialized motor act.

References

[1] Allen, J.I. and Tsukahara, N. (1974) Cerebrocerebellar communication system. *Physiol. Rev.*, 54: 957–1006.

[2] Akaike, T., Fanardjian, V.V., Ito, M. and Nakamura, H. (1973) Cerebellar control of vestibulospinal tract cells in rabbit. *Exp. Brain Res.*, 18: 446–463.

[3] Andersson, G. and Eriksson, L. (1981) Spinal, trigeminal and cortical climbing fiber paths to the lateral vermis of the cerebellar anterior lobe in the cat. *Exp. Brain Res.*, 44: 71–78.

[4] Andersson, G. and Oscarsson, O. (1978) Projections to lateral vestibular nucleus from cerebellar climbing fiber zones. *Exp. Brain Res.*, 32: 549–564.

[5] Andersson, G. and Oscarsson, O. (1978) Climbing fiber microzones in cerebellar vermis and their projection to different groups of cells in the lateral vestibular nucleus. *Exp. Brain Res.*, 32: 565–579.

[6] Armstrong, D.M., Harvey, R.J. and Schilld, R.F. (1974) Topographical localization in the olivo-cerebellar projection: an electrophysiological study in the cat. *J. Comp. Neurol.*, 154: 287–302.

[7] Avanzino, G.L., Hösli, L. and Wolstencroft, J.H. (1966) Identification of cerebellar projecting neurons in nucleus reticularis gigantocellularis. *Brain Res.*, 3: 201–203.

[8] Balaban, C.D. (1983) A projection from NTRP of Bechterev to the medial vestibular nucleus in rabbits. *Exp. Brain Res.*, 51: 304–309.

[9] Balaban, C.D., Kawaguchi, Y. and Watanabe, E. (1981) Evidence of a collateralized climbing fiber projection from the inferior olive to the flocculus and vestibular nuclei in rabbits. *Neurosci. Lett.*, 22: 23–29.

[10] Barnes, C.D. and Pompeiano, O. (1971) Effects of muscle afferents on brain stem reticular and vestibular units. *Brain Res.*, 25: 179–183.

[11] Boyle, R. and Pompeiano, O. (1980) Responses of vestibulospinal neurons to sinusoidal rotation of neck. *J. Neurophysiol.*, 44: 633–649.

[12] Boyle, R. and Pompeiano, O. (1981) Convergence and interaction of neck and macular vestibular inputs on vestibulospinal neurons. *J. Neurophysiol.*, 45: 852–868.

[13] Brodal, A. (1949) Spinal afferents to the lateral reticular nucleus of the medulla oblongata in the cat. An experimental study. *J. Comp. Neurol.*, 91: 259–295.

[14] Brodal, A. (1974) Anatomy of the vestibular nuclei and their connections. In H.H. Kornhaber (Ed.), *Handbook of Sensory Physiology*, Vol. VIII, Springer, Berlin, pp 296–351.

[15] Brodal, A. and Angaut, P. (1967) The termination of spinovestibular fibers in the cat. *Brain Res.*, 5: 494–500.

[16] Brodal, P., Maršala, J. and Brodal, A. (1967) The cerebral cortical projection to the lateral reticular nucleus in the cat, with special reference to the sensorimotor cortical areas. *Brain Res.*, 6: 252–274.

[17] Brodal, A. and Saugstad, L. (1965) Retrograde cellular changes in the mesencephalic trigeminal nucleus in the cat following cerebellar lesions. *Acta Morph. Neerl. Scand.*, 6: 147–159.

[18] Brodal, A. and Torvik, A. (1957) Über den ursprung der sekundaren vestibulo-cerebellaren fasern bei der katze. Eine experimentell–anatomische studie. *Arch. Psychiat. Nervenkr.*, 195: 550–567.

[19] Brodal, A. and Walberg, F. (1977) The olivocerebellar projection in the cat studied with the method of retrograde axonal transport of horseradish peroxidase. IV. The projection to the anterior lobe. *J. Comp. Neurol.*, 172: 85–108.

[20] Brukmosser, P., Hepp, M.-R. and Wiesendanger, M. (1970) Cortical influence on single neurons of the lateral reticular nucleus of the cat. *Exp. Neurol.*, 26: 239–252.

[21] Brukmosser, P., Hepp, M.-R. and Wiesendanger, M. (1970) Effects of peripheral, ribral and fastigial stimulation on neurons of the lateral reticular nucleus of the cat. *Exp. Neurol.*, 27: 388–398.

[22] Cajal, S.R. (1909) *Histologie du Systéme Nerveux de l'Homme et des Vertébrés*, Vol I, Maloine, Paris.

[23] Carleton, S.C. and Carpenter, M.B. (1983) Afferent and efferent connections of the medial, inferior and lateral vestibular nuclei in the cat and monkey. *Brain Res.*, 278: 29–51.

[24] Carpenter, M.B. (1960) Fiber projections from the descending and lateral vestibular nuclei in the cat. *Am. J. Anat.*, 107: 1–22.

[25] Carpenter, M.B., Bard, D.S. and Alling, F.A. (1959) Anatomical connections between the fastigial nuclei, the labyrinth and the vestibular nuclei in the cat. *J. Comp. Neurol.*, 111: 1–25.

[26] Carpenter, M.B. and Hanna, G.R. (1961) Fiber projections from the spinal trigeminal nucleus in the cat. *J. Comp. Neurol.*, 117: 117–131.

[27] Chan-Palay, V. (1977) *Cerebellar Dentate Nucleus. Organization, Cytology and Transmitters*, Springer, Heidelberg, 548 pp.

[28] Cook, J.R. and Wiesendanger, M. (1976) Input from trigeminal cutaneous afferents of the inferior olive in cats. *Exp. Brain Res.*, 26: 193–202.

[29] Corvaja, N. and Pompeiano, O. (1979) Identification of cerebellar corticovestibular neurons retrogradely labelled with horseradish peroxidase. *Neuroscience*, 4: 507–515.

[30] Courville, J. (1966) Rubrobulbar fibers to the facial nucleus and the lateral reticular nucleus (nucleus of the lateral funiculus). An experimental study in the cat with silver impregnation methods. *Brain Res.*, 1: 317–337.

[31] Courville, J., Faraco-Contin, F. and Marcon, L. (1983)

Projections from the reticular formation of medulla, the spinal trigeminal and lateral reticular nuclei to the inferior olive. *Neuroscience*, 9: 129–139.

[32] Darian-Smith, I. (1973) The trigeminal system. In A.B. Iggo (Ed.), *Handbook of Sensory Physiology*, Vol. 11, Springer, Berlin, pp. 271–314.

[33] Elisevich, K.V., Hrysyshyn, A.W. and Flumerfelt, B.A. (1985) Cerebellar, medullary and spinal afferent connections of the paramedian reticular nucleus in the cat. *Brain Res.*, 332: 267–282.

[34] Fanardjian, V.V., Kasabyan, S.A. and Manvelian, L.R. (1983) Mechanisms regulating the activity of facial nucleus motoneurons. 2. Synaptic activation from the caudal trigeminal nucleus. *Neuroscience*, 9: 823–835.

[35] Fanardjian, V.V. and Sarkisian, V.A. (1980) Spatial organization of the cerebellar corticovestibular projection in the cat. *Neuroscience*, 5: 551–558.

[36] Fukushima, K, Murakami, S., Matsushima, J. and Kato, M. (1980) Vestibular responses and branching of interstitiospinal neurons. *Exp. Brain Res.*, 40: 131–145.

[37] Fukushima, K., Ohno, M., Murakami, S. and Kato, M. (1981) Effects of stimulation of frontal cortex, superior colliculus and neck muscle afferents on interstitiospinal neurons in the cat. *Exp. Brain Res.*, 44: 143–154.

[38] Fukushima, K., Pitts, N.G. and Peterson, B.W. (1978) Direct excitation of neck motoneurons by interstitiospinal fibers. *Exp. Brain Res.*, 33: 565–581.

[39] Gernandt, B.E., Igarashi, M. and Ades, H.W. (1966) Effects of prolonged caloric stimulation upon oculomotor, vestibulo-spinal and segmental spinal activity. *Exp. Neurol.*, 14: 249–263.

[40] Graybiel, A.M. (1977) Direct and indirect preoculomotor pathways of the brainstem: an autoradiographic study of the pontine reticular formation in the cat. *J. Comp. Neurol.*, 175: 37–38.

[41] Groenewegen, H.J. and Voogd, J. (1975) Afferent connections and efferent climbing fiber projections of the dorsal accessory olive in the cat, an Autoradiographic and degeneration study. *Exp. Brain Res.*, Suppl. 23: 80.

[42] Groenewegen, H.J. and Voogd, J. (1976) The longitudinal zonal arrangement of the olivocerebellar, climbing fiber projection in the cat. An autoradiographic and degeneration study. In O. Crentzfeldt (Ed.), *Afferent and Intrinsic Organization of Laminated Structures in the Brain*, *Exp. Brain Res.*, Suppl. 1: 65–71.

[43] Groenewegen, H.J. and Voogd, J. (1977) The parasagittal zonation within the olivocerebellar projection. I. Climbing fiber distribution in the vermis of cat cerebellum. *J. Comp. Neurol.*, 174: 417–488.

[44] Hoddevik, H.G., Brodal, A. and Walberg, F. (1975) The reticulovestibular projection in the cat. An experimental study with silver impregnation methods. *Brain Res.*, 94: 383–399.

[45] Ito, M. (1984) *The Cerebellum and Neural Control*, Raven Press, New York, pp. 149–163.

[46] Ito, M., Hongo, T. and Okada, Y. (1969) Vestibular evoked postsynaptic potentials in Deiters' neurons. *Exp. Brain Res.*, 7: 214–230.

[47] Ito, J., Sasa, M., Matsuoka, I. and Takaori, S. (1982) Afferent projection from reticular nuclei, inferior olive and cerebellum to lateral vestibular nucleus of the cat as demonstrated by horseradish peroxidase. *Brain Res.*, 231: 427–432.

[48] Ito, M., Udo, M, Mano, N. and Kawai, N. (1970) Synaptic action of the fastigiobulbar impulses upon neurons in the medullary reticular formation and vestibular nuclei. *Exp. Brain Res.*, 11: 29–47.

[49] Ito, M. and Yoshida, M. (1966) The origin of cerebellar-induced inhibition of Deiters neurons. I. Monosynaptic initation of the inhibitory postsynaptic potentials. *Exp. Brain Res.*, 2: 330–349.

[50] Kalil, K. (1981) Projection of the cerebellar and dorsal column nuclei upon the thalamus of the rhesus monkey. *J. Comp. Neurol.*, 195: 25–50.

[51] Ladpli, R. and Brodal, A. (1968) Experimental studies of commissural and reticular formation projection from the vestibular nuclei in the cat. *Brain Res.*, 8: 65–96.

[52] Llinas, R. (1964) Mechanisms of supraspinal actions upon spinal cord activities. Differences between reticular and cerebellar inhibitory actions upon alpha extensor motoneurons. *J. Neurophysiol.*, 27: 1117–1126.

[53] Lorente de Nó, R. (1933) Vestibulo-ocular reflex arc. *Arch. Neurol. Psychiat. Chicago*, 30: 245–291.

[54] Lorente de Nó, R. (1933) The interaction of the corneal reflex and vestibular nystagmus. *Am. J. Physiol.*, 103: 704–711.

[55] Manni, E. and Bortolomi, R. (1981) Peripheral and central organization of the extraocular proprioception in the Ungulata. In R. Granit and O. Pompeiano (Eds.), *Reflex Control of Posture and Movement, Progress in Brain Research*, Vol. 50, Elsevier, Amsterdam, pp. 291–299.

[56] Markham, C.H. (1968) Midbrain and contralateral labyrinth influences on brainstem vestibular neurons in the cat. *Brain Res.*, 9: 312–333.

[57] Markham, C.H., Precht, W. and Shimazu, H. (1966) Effect of stimulation of interstitial nucleus of Ramon y Cajal on vestibular unit activity in the cat. *J. Neurophysiol.*, 29: 493–507.

[58] McCrea, R.A., Yoshida, K., Evinger, C. and Berthoz, A. (1981) The location, axonal arborization and terminal sites of eye-movement-related secondary vestibular neurons demonstrated by intra-axonal HRP injection in the alert cat. In A. Fuchs and W. Becker (Eds.), *Progress in Oculomotor Research*, Elsevier, Amsterdam, pp. 378–386.

[59] Mergner, T., Pompeiano, O. and Corvaja, N. (1977) Vestibular projections to the nucleus interpositus of Staderini mapped by retrograde transport of horseradish peroxidase. *Neurosci. Lett.*, 5: 307–313.

[60] Mizuno, N. and Sauerland, E.B. (1970) Trigeminal proprioceptive projections to the hypoglossal nucleus and the cervical ventral gray column. *J. Comp. Neurol.*, 139: 215–226.

[61] Morin, F., Kennedy, D.T. and Gardner, E. (1966) Spinal

afferents to the lateral reticular nucleus. I. A histological study. *J. Comp. Neurol.*, 126: 511–522.

[62] Moruzzi, G. (1954) The physiological properties of the brain stem reticular system. In J.F. Delafresnaye (Ed.), *Brain Mechanisms and Consiousness*, Blackwell, Oxford, pp. 21–48.

[63] Oscarsson, O. (1973) Functional organization of spinocerebellar paths. In A. Iggo (Ed.) *Handbook of Sensory Physiology, Somatosensory System*, Vol. 2, Springer-Verlag, Berlin/Heidelberg/New York, pp. 339–380.

[64] Oscarsson, O. and Rosén, I. (1966) Response characteristics of reticocerebellar neurons activated from spinal afferents. *Exp. Brain Res.*, 1: 320–328.

[65] Oscarsson, O. and Sjülund, B. (1977) The ventral spinoolivocerebellar system in the cat. I. Identification of five paths and their termination on the cerebellar anterior lobe. *Exp. Brain Res.*, 28: 505–520.

[66] Peterson, B.W. and Abzug, C. (1975) Properties of projections from vestibular nuclei to medial reticular formation in the cat. *J. Neurophysiol.*, 38: 1421–1435.

[67] Peterson, B.W. and Felpel, L.P. (1971) Excitation and inhibition of reticulospinal neurons by vestibular, cortical and cutaneous stimulation. *Brain Res.*, 27: 373–376.

[68] Peterson, B.W., Fillion, M., Felpel, L.P. and Abzug, C. (1975) Responses of medial reticular neurons to stimulation of the vestibular nerve. *Exp. Brain Res*, 22: 335–350.

[69] Pompeiano, O. and Brodal, A. (1957) Spino-vestibular fibers in the cat. An experimental study. *J. Comp. Neurol.*, 108: 353–382.

[70] Pompeiano, O., Mergner, T. and Corvaja, N. (1978) Commissural perihypoglossal and reticular afferent projections to the vestibular nuclei in the cat. *Arch. Ital. Biol.*, 116: 130–172.

[71] Pompeiano, O. and Walberg, F. (1957) Descending connections to the vestibular nuclei. An experimental study in the cat. *J. Comp. Neurol.*, 108: 465–503.

[72] Rossi, J.F. and Zanchetti, A. (1957) The brainstem reticular formation. Anatomy and physiology. *Arch. Ital. Biol.*, 93: 199–438.

[73] Saint-Cyr, J.H and Courville, J. (1979) Projection from the vestibular nuclei to the inferior olive in the cat: an autoradiographic and horseradish peroxidase study. *Brain Res.*, 165: 189–200.

[74] Sarkisian, V.A. and Fanardjian, V.V. (1985) Neuronal mechanisms of the interaction of Deiters' nucleus with some brainstem structures. *Neuroscience*, 16: 957–968.

[75] Scheibel, M.E. and Scheibel, A.B. (1958) Structural substrates for integrative patterns in the brain reticular core. In H.H. Jasper and all (Eds.), *Reticular Formation of the Brain*, Little Brown and Co., Boston/Toronto, pp. 31–55.

[76] Schwindt, P.C., Precht, W. and Richter, A. (1974) Monosynaptic excitatory and inhibitory pathway from medial midbrain nuclei to the trochlear motoneurons. *Exp. Brain Res.*, 20: 223–238.

[77] Shaw, M.D. and Baker, R. (1983) Direct projections from vestibular nuclei to facial nucleus in cats. *J. Neurophysiol.*, 50: 1265–1280.

[78] Shimazu, H. and Precht, W. (1965) Tonic and kinetic responses of cat's vestibular neurons to horizontal angular acceleration. *J. Neurophysiol.*, 28: 991–1031.

[79] Spyer, K.M., Ghelarducci, B. and Pompeiano, O. (1974) Gravity responses of neurons in the main reticular formation. *J. Neurophysiol.*, 37: 705–721.

[80] Stewart, W.A. and King, R.B. (1963) Fiber projections from the nucleus caudalis of the spinal trigeminal nucleus. *J. Comp. Neurol.*, 121: 271–286.

[81] Sumino, R. and Nakamura, Y. (1974) Synaptic potentials of hypoglossal motoneurons and a common inhibitory interneuron in the trigemino–hypoglossal reflex. *Brain Res.*, 73: 439–454.

[82] Szentágothai, J. and Schab, R. (1956) A midbrain inhibitory mechanism of the oculomotor activity. *Acta. Physiol. Hung.*, 9: 89–98.

[83] Terzuolo, C.A. (1959) Cerebellar inhibitory and excitatory actions upon spinal extensor motoneurons. *Arch. Ital Biol.*, 97: 316–339.

[84] Toyama, K., Tsukahara, N. and Udo, M. (1968) Nature of the cerebellar influence upon the red nucleus neurons. *Exp. Brain Res.*, 4: 292–309.

[85] Troiani, D. and Petrosini, L. (1981) Neuronal activity in the vestibular nuclei after trigeminal stimulation. *Exp. Neurol.*, 72: 12–24.

[86] Walberg, F., Bowsher, O. and Brodal, A. (1958) The termination of primary vestibular fibers in the vestibular nuclei in the cat. An experimental study with silver methods. *J. Comp. Neurol.*, 110: 391–419.

[87] Walberg, F., Dietrichs, E. and Nordby, T. (1985) On the projections from the vestibular and perihypoglossal nuclei to the spinal trigeminal and lateral reticular nuclei in the cat. *Brain Res.*, 333: 123–130.

[88] Walberg, F. and Jansen, J. (1961) Cerebellar corticovestibular fibers in the cat. *Exp. Neurol.*, 3: 93–129.

[89] Walberg, F. and Mugnaini, E. (1969) Distinction of degenerating fibers in the cat. *Exp. Neurol.*, 3: 32–52.

[90] Walberg, F. and Pompeiano, O. (1960) Fastigiofugal fibers to the lateral reticular nucleus: an experimental study in the cat. *Exp. Neurol.*, 2: 40–53.

[91] Walberg, F., Pompeiano, O., Brodal, A. and Jansen, J. (1962) The fastigiovestibular projection in the cat. An experimental study with silver impregnation methods. *J. Comp. Neurol.*, 118: 49–76.

[92] Wilson, V.J. and Jones, G.M. (1979) *Mammalian Vestibular Physiology*, Plenum, New York, 356 pp.

[93] Wilson, V.J., Kato, M. Peterson, B.W. and Wylie, R.M. (1967) A single-unit analysis of the organization of Deiters' nucleus. *J. Neurophysiol.*, 30: 603–619.

[94] Yoshida, K., Berthoz, A., Vidal, P.P. and McCrea, R. (1981) Eye-movement-related activity of identified second order vestibular neurons in the cat. In A. Fuchs and W. Becker (Eds.), *Progress in Oculomotor Research*, Elsevier, Amsterdam, pp. 371–378.

SECTION II

Neurophysiology of
Vestibulospinal Reflexes

O. Pompeiano and J.H.J. Allum (Eds.)
Progress in Brain Research, Vol. 76
© 1988 Elsevier Science Publishers B.V. (Biomedical Division)

Overview

M.B. Dutia

Department of Physiology, University Medical School, Teviot Place, Edinburgh EH8 9AG, U.K.

The ongoing activity of vestibular afferent axons provides the central nervous system with continuous signals of head postion and the instantaneous direction and velocity of head displacement. This information is the foundation upon which the normal animal secures its postural stability, and builds its strategies for movement. Voluntary movements are always carried out in the context of the animal's attitude relative to the external forces acting upon it, usually of course the force of gravity. While the fundamental information of head orientation is provided by the vestibular system, extensive convergence occurs between this and the simultaneous visual, muscle proprioceptive and tactile afferent inputs from the neck and limbs. This gives the animal a complex multisensory framework in which to achieve postural stability and prepare for movement. There has been considerable progress over recent years in our understanding of the function and the neural substrate of this elaborate sensory-motor system. The five contributors to this session on the neurophysiology of vestibulospinal reflexes addressed several interesting aspects of the underlying neurophysiological mechanisms.

The first two chapters in this section, by Drs. Chan and Schor (Chapters 5 and 6), are concerned with the role of otolith afferents in vestibular reflexes. The central actions of these afferents have so far been studied in somewhat less detail than those of semicircular canal afferents, no doubt because of the practical difficulties of selective natural stimulation of the otoliths without canal stimulation. In the experiments of Dr. Chan and his colleagues this was achieved using slow OVAR of the animal at a constant velocity. Under these conditions the semicircular canal afferent discharge adapts to the constant rotational velocity, while the otolith afferents continue to be sinusoidally modulated as the orientation of the head changes with respect to gravity [5, 6]. In static-tilt-sensitive vestibular and fastigial neurons tested with OVAR, each neuron was maximally excited at a particular head position. The spatial location of this discharge maximum was independent of the amplitude of head tilt, but varied with clockwise or counter-clockwise rotation of the head. This is similar to the response of 'irregular' otolith afferents during OVAR [14]. An apparent difference between the response properties described by Dr. Chan and those reported by Schor et al. [16] was that the response vectors of the vestibular neurons were uniformly distributed in the roll and pitch planes, rather than predominantly aligned close to the roll plane. Chan et al.'s sample included units in the lateral, superior and rostral inferior vestibular nuclei, while Schor et al. concentrated specifically on the lateral nucleus. Thus the predominantly roll-oriented responses of lateral vestibular nucleus neurons correspond well with the responses to roll tilt of the forelimb extensors, while many of the neurons described by Chan et al. with response vectors away from the roll plane, may contribute to vestibulocollic or vestibuloocular reflexes.

In the experiments described by Dr. Schor

Abbreviations: Nrg, nucleus reticularis gigantocellularis; Nrpc, nucleus reticularis pontis caudalis; OVAR, off-vertical axis rotation.

(Chapter 6), selective otolith stimulation was achieved by inactivating all the semicircular canals by drilling through them ('canal-plugging' [15]). In canal-plugged decerebrate cats, roll tilting evokes reflex contractions in the forelimb extensors that are in phase with head position at low frequencies but develop a marked phase lag and increase in gain at higher frequencies around 1 Hz. Lateral vestibular nucleus neurons excited by side-up tilt (beta-type [7]) have similar frequency response dynamics, while those excited by side-down tilt (alpha-type) do not. Dr. Schor presented a model which described the transformation of the incoming otolith (head-position) signal into the beta-type muscle-like response. This involved the divergence of the afferent input into two paths, one carrying the head-position signal directly through to higher-order vestibular neurons while the other acted as an inhibitory, high-pass loop with high gain that also converged onto the higher-order neurons. The neural pathway mediating this feed-forward inhibition is likely to be through the cerebellum, and Dr. Schor reported that in cerebellectomized cats only a few beta-type responses remained. This suggests that the role of the cerebellum is to match the dynamics of the otolith system with those of the vertical semicircular canals which would also be stimulated by roll tilt, introducing a progressive phase lag in the otolith system response at higher frequencies where the head-velocity, phase-leading canal signals become available. By matching these two inputs, the cerebellum presumably ensures a stable gain and phase of the forelimb vestibulospinal reflexes over the middle frequency range (around 1 Hz), below which the reflex is driven predominantly by the otolith input and above which mainly by the canal inputs. Such integration of the afferent activity from different receptors extends the operating range of the vestibulospinal reflexes over a wide range of stimulus frequencies (cf. [8]).

In the third presentation in this section (Chapter 7), Professor Pompeiano described a series of experiments that demonstrated the relevance of the spinal Renshaw cells in regulating the vestibulospinal reflex response of fore- and hindlimb extensors to slow roll tilts. In addition to the lateral vestibulospinal tract which projects to the Renshaw cells indirectly, i.e. by utilizing the α extensor motoneurons and the corresponding recurrent collaterals, their excitability is regulated more directly by two other descending pathways during vestibulospinal reflexes [12, 13]. A reticulospinal pathway, originating from the medullary inhibitory reticular area of Magoun and Rhines (nucleus reticularis magnocellularis) excites Renshaw cells and thereby inhibits motor activity. Stimulation of the locus coeruleus has the opposite effect, suppressing Renshaw cell activity, presumably through a coerulospinal projection [9]. However, while these two pathways have opposite effects on the Renshaw cells, they are both activated by side-up tilting of the decerebrate animal. The possibility therefore exists that one of these pathways can be used simultaneously with the lateral vestibulospinal tract during vestibulospinal reflexes under different conditions. If the coerulospinal projection operates in conjunction with the vestibulospinal system, then its inhibitory influence on the Renshaw cells will decrease during side-down tilt, thus enhancing the recurrent inhibition of the motoneuron pools driven by the vestibulospinal volleys for that direction of animal orientation. In this instance, the gain of vestibular reflex will be reduced.

In contrast, if the reticulospinal system operates with the vestibulospinal system, then its excitatory influence on the Renshaw cells will decrease during side-down tilt. The resulting disfacilitation of Renshaw cells will enhance the motoneuronal responses to the excitatory vestibulospinal volleys driven by the same direction of animal orientation; in this instance the gain of the vestibular reflex will be enhanced. Indeed, by changing the balance of activity in the coerulear and reticular systems by means of systemically applied anticholinesterase, Professor Pompeiano showed that the gain of the vestibular reflex can be dramatically altered. The role of the Renshaw cell therefore appears to be rather more substantial than the traditional rate-limiting follower function generally assigned to it. It should be borne in mind that changes in excitability of the

Renshaw cells would affect the motoneurons' sensitivity not just to the vestibulospinal system specifically, but also to all other inputs converging upon them. Notwithstanding the complexity of these experiments, it would be very interesting to discover if other interneurons in the segmental spinal network are also subject to a similar supraspinal control, to allow a less global but equally subtle control of vestibulospinal reflex gain.

The next contribution, by Dr. Sasaki described an elegant series of experiments designed to locate and characterize the neural elements involved in the cortical and tectal control of the muscles of the neck (Chapter 8). Using electrophysiological and anatomical techniques, Dr. Sasaki and his colleagues have shown that the pyramidal (corticospinal) and tectospinal pathways to neck motoneurons share a common interposed neuron which is located in the brainstem reticular formation [1–3]. Cervical reticulospinal neurons activated monosynaptically by pyramidal and tectal stimuli are found in the Nrpc and the Nrg, and project monosynaptically to neck motoneurons. The former receive a large tectal and smaller pyramidal input and are presumably involved in reflex movements of the head, while the latter receive a large pyramidal input and smaller tectal input and presumably mediate voluntary cortical head movements. These neurons project to the spinal cord in a highly specific manner, as shown by spike-triggered averaging of their influence on splenius and biventer motoneurons. Nrpc neurons project specifically to splenius and also to abducens motoneurons, while Nrg neurones project specifically either to splenius or biventer motoneurons but never to both. The descending branches of these neurons terminate in laminae VI, VII and VIII in the lower cervical cord, and presumably mediate the integration of head-movement signals with the control of forelimb and shoulder muscles. These experiments reveal some of the mechanisms underlying the supraspinal control of the neck musculature at the cellular level, and further emphasize the high degree of organization within the brainstem projection to the cervical spinal cord [4, 11].

In the final presentation of the section (Chapter 9), Dr. Thoden discusses the differential effects of somatosensory afferent activity on the human vestibulo-ocular and vestibulospinal reflexes. The effects of somatosensory signals on the vestibulo-ocular reflex were examined by comparing the pattern of eye movements during sinusoidal rotation of a blindfolded subject who held on to a bar which either rotated with him or was fixed so that the arms rotated at the shoulders [10]. This stimulation of arm and shoulder proprioceptors had very little effect on the amplitude or velocity of the slow phase of nystagmus induced by rotation, but induced larger and more frequent saccades in the direction of body motion. In contrast, stimulation of neck proprioceptors by turning of the head caused a marked increase in body sway during galvanic labyrinthine stimulation. These results demonstrate the relatively greater importance of proprioceptive afferents in the vestibular control of the different body segments (head, neck, and trunk), each of which may move independently. In the vestibulo-ocular system, which is contained entirely within the head, the influence of somatosensory proprioceptive afferents in the intact awake subject appears to be much weaker.

References

[1] Alstermark, B., Pinter, M. and Sasaki, S. (1983) Brainstem relay of disynaptic pyramidal EPSPs to neck motoneurones in the cat. *Brain Res.*, 259: 147–150.

[2] Alstermark, B., Pinter, M. and Sasaki, S. (1983) Convergence on reticulospinal neurones mediating contralateral pyramidal disynaptic EPSPs to neck motoneurones. *Brain Res.*, 259: 151–154.

[3] Alstermark, B., Pinter, M. and Sasaki, S. (1985) Pyramidal effects on dorsal neck motoneurones in the cat. *J. Physiol. London*, 363: 287–302.

[4] Berthoz, A. and Grantyn, A. (1985) Burst activity of identified tecto-reticulo-spinal cells in the alert cat. *Exp. Brain Res.*, 57: 417–421.

[5] Chan, Y.S., Cheung, Y.M. and Hwang, J.C. (1985) Effect of tilt on the response of neuronal activity within the cat vestibular nuclei during slow and constant velocity rotation. *Brain Res.*, 345: 271–278.

[6] Chan, Y.S., Cheung, Y.M. and Hwang, J.C. (1987) Response characteristics of neurones in the cat vestibular nuclei during slow and constant velocity off-vertical axes rota-

66

tions in the clockwise and counterclockwise directions. *Brain Res.*, 406: 294–301.

[7] Duensing, F. and Schaeffer, K.-P. (1959) Uber die Konvergenz verschiedener labyrintharer Afferenzen auf einzelne Neurone des Vestibulariskerngebietes. *Arch. Psychiat. Nervenkr.*, 199: 345–371.

[8] Dutia, M.B. (1988) Interaction between vestibulocollic and cervicocollic reflexes: Automatic compensation of reflex gain by muscle afferents. In O. Pompeiano and J.H.J. Allum (Eds.), *Vestibulospinal Control of Posture and Locomotion, Progress in Brain Research, Vol. 76*, Elsevier, Amsterdam, pp. 172–180.

[9] Fung, S.J., Pompeiano, O. and Barnes, C.D. (1987) Suppression of the recurrent inhibitory pathway in lumbar cord segments during locus coerulus stimulation in cats. *Brain Res.*, 402: 351–354.

[10] Leopold, H.C., Mertinat, M. and Thoden, U. (1985) Modulation of vestibulo-ocular reflex by active stabilization of head to trunk. *Acta Ototalyngol. Stock.*, 99: 102–106.

[11] Peterson, B.W., Pitts, N.G., Fukushima, K. and Mackel, R. (1978) Reticulospinal excitation and inhibition of neck motoneurones. *Exp. Brain Res.*, 32: 471–489.

[12] Pompeiano, O., Wand, P. and Srivastava, U.C. (1985) Responses of Renshaw cells coupled with hindlimb extensor motoneurons to sinusoidal stimulation of labyrinth receptors in the decerebrate cat. *Pflügers Arch.*, 403: 245–257.

[13] Pompeiano, O., Wand, P. and Srivastava, U.C. (1985) Influence of Renshaw cells on the response gain of hindlimb extensor muscles to sinusoidal labyrinth stimulation. *Pflügers Arch.*, 404: 107–118.

[14] Raphan, T., Waespe, W. and Cohen, B. (1981) Vestibular nerve activity induced by off-vertical axis rotation. *Neurosci. Abstr.*, 7: 39.

[15] Schor, R.H. (1974) Responses of cat vestibular neurones to sinusoidal roll tilt. *Exp. Brain Res.*, 20: 347–362.

[16] Schor, R.H., Miller A.D. and Tomko, D.L. (1984) Responses to head tilt in cat vestibular neurones. I. Direction of maximum sensitivity. *J. Neurophysiol.*, 51: 136–146.

O. Pompeiano and J.H.J. Allum (Eds.)
Progress in Brain Research, Vol. 76
© 1988 Elsevier Science Publishers B.V. (Biomedical Division)

CHAPTER 5

Unit responses to bidirectional off-vertical axes rotations in central vestibular and cerebellar fastigial nuclei

Y.S. Chan, Y.M. Cheung and J.C. Hwang

Department of Physiology, Faculty of Medicine, University of Hong Kong, 5 Sassoon Road, Hong Kong

Extracellular recordings were made from tilt-sensitive units in the vestibular nuclei and the cerebellar fastigial nucleus of cats during slow constant-velocity rotations in the CW and CCW directions about different off-vertical axes (5–25°). Each unit showed modulation of discharge rate, with position-dependent discharge maximum and minimum during any 360° unidirectional rotation. The location of the CW discharge maximum differed from that obtained during CCW rotation while the response gain was not affected by the direction of rotation. Characterized directional axes of neurons could be found along the roll and pitch axes. Units were classified into either phase-lead or phase-lag groups based on the location of CW discharge maximum relative to the CCW counterpart along the rotatory locus. About two-third of the units showed phase-lead responses, while the remaining units showed phase-lag responses. In such off-vertical axis rotations, increase in the amplitude of head tilt resulted in an increase in the discharge modulation but did not result in significant fluctuation in the positions of the CW or CCW discharge maxima. It is suggested that these directional signals on head position in space would provide a framework for spatial coding in otolithic motor commands.

Introduction

The role of the otoliths in vestibular reflexes was extensively studied during roll and pitch tilt [1, 17, 30, 34], linear acceleration [2, 4, 28, 42] and rotations in sets of vertical or horizontal planes [5, 6, 15, 37]. The functional significance of the otoliths during continuous rotation of the head about an axis deviated from the earth's vertical (OVAR), though explored [12, 32], remains obscure. The problem was also addressed by Schor et al. [35, 36] using wobble rotations (at a constant tilt angle) which provides essentially the same positional stimulation to the vestibular apparatus as OVAR. With these head positional changes in space, the otolith organs would experience a sequential change in gravitational vector which could affect the vestibulo-ocular and/or vestibulospinal outputs. Continuous nystagmus during constant-velocity OVAR [14, 16, 46] and vestibulospinal reflexes acting on forelimb and shoulder muscles during wobble rotating stimulus [45] have been reported.

To understand how positional and directional information on the continuous excursion of the head during OVAR are processed in the vestibular system, it is important to know the contribution of the otolith inputs to neurons in the vestibular nuclei and fastigial nucleus, since some neurons in these regions are known to influence both the vestibulo-ocular [21, 23] and vestibulospinal pathways [43, 44]. Otolith afferents exhibited a directional difference in the head-position-dependent discharge rates for oppositely directed OVAR [32]. Similar positional and directional responses per 360° rotation cycle were observed in tilt-sensitive central vestibular neurons, receiving primarily if not exclusively otolith inputs during constant-velocity OVAR

Abbreviations: CW, clockwise: CCW, counter clockwise; OVAR, off-vertical axis rotation.

[12, 13]. In canal-plugged cats, central vestibular units have also been shown to demonstrate a phase difference in response peaks during bidirectional wobble rotating stimulus [35]. The response of neurons in the fastigial nucleus to OVAR, however, has never been studied, although cerebellar neurons have been shown to respond to static tilts [22] and sinusoidal roll tilts [8, 11, 38].

This report describes the directional responses of static-tilt-sensitive central vestibular and fastigial units to CW and CCW rotations about off-vertical axes of 5–25°.

Methods

Experiments were performed on adult cats precollicularly decerebrated under light ketamine anesthesia. Details of the methods for animal preparation, natural stimulation and data analysis have been described previously [10, 12, 23]. In brief, the head of the animal was mounted on a stereotaxic frame (Kopf) and maintained in the earth's horizontal plane (Fig. 1A). The cervical vertebral column was oriented perpendicular to gravity (the resting position of the cat as reported by Vidal et al. [40] with the C2 vertebra clamped to the stereotaxic frame, while the body and the extended limbs of the animal were secured rigidly to the tilt table. Relative movements of the head, neck and forelimbs was further miminized by means of a plaster cast.

Natural vestibular stimulations in the form of slow and constant-velocity rotations of the whole experimental set-up (1.75 or 4.7°/s) in both CW and CCW directions were applied about an axis (at 3 cm caudal to the midpoint of the interaural axis) tilted at variable angles (5–25°) from the earth's vertical axis. Table motion was monitored by the output of a potentiometer placed on the rotary axis of the table. Electrical stimulations applied through a microelectrode placed against the surface of the ipsilateral intact oval window were used to test for the latency of single units. Unitary activities from the vestibular nuclei and the fastigial nucleus on the left side were recorded extracellularly with tungsten microelectrodes inserted dorsoventrally

through the cerebellum. Only those units which were sensitive to ± 15° static tilts were analyzed during 2 or more successive complete 360° rotations in both the CW and CCW directions. The positions of the discharge maximum and the response gain (half peak-to-peak discharge modulation per degree of head tilt) were evaluated by spectral analysis performed off-line with a computer. Some units became silent during part of the 360° rotation cycle and their response gains were corrected [3]. Histological locations of all recorded units were reconstructed from serial sections.

Results

Neuronal responses of the vestibular nuclei

In this study, the spontaneous discharge of the population of tilt-sensitive units ($n = 77$) remained fairly stable when the head of the animal was held at a particular static head position. During any 360° unidirectional OVAR (at 1.75 °/s), each of these tilt-sensitive units exhibited a modulation of its discharge rate with maximal discharge at a specific position and minimal discharge at a position diametrically opposite to that of the maximum (Fig. 1B). There was only a very small difference among the response gains (mean ratio was 1.02) and the positions of discharge maxima (mean difference was 6°) in successive trials of unidirectional rotation. The response gain and the position of discharge maximum obtained during CW rotations were then compared with the corresponding patterns obtained from CCW rotations.

The spatial location of the discharge maxima for any one unit obtained during CW rotations differed from that obtained during CCW rotations. Such spatial difference in CW/CCW discharge maxima was arbitrarily defined in terms of phase difference ($\triangle \emptyset$). Neuronal response was thus classified into 2 groups based on the relative positions of the CW and CCW discharge maxima along the rotatory locus. The unitary response was arbitrarily described as $- \triangle \emptyset$ when the CW maxima as compared with the CCW maxima shifted in the CCW direction

(Fig. 1C$_1$); the response was defined as $+\triangle\varnothing$ when the CW maxima as compared with the CCW maxima shifted in the CW direction (Fig. 1C$_2$). (The $-$ and $+$ signs are not synonymous with phase lag and phase lead in the conventional sense). Fifty-one units showed a $-\triangle\varnothing$ response, while 26 units showed a $+\triangle\varnothing$ response (Fig. 1C$_3$). The gain values of the CW and CCW responses in the 2 groups of units were, however, similar (with a mean Grain$_{CCW}$/Grain$_{CW}$ ratio of 1.14 ± 0.06; mean $\pm$ SEM) (Fig. 1C$_3$, inset).

The gain and position of the discharge maxima for 10° OVAR in the CW direction was paired with that in the CCW direction in polar diagrams (Fig. 2B). For each responsive unit, the averaged position of the CW/CCW discharge maxima (in the small sector delimited by the responses) reflects the directional axis at which the plane of the functional polarization vector intersects at right angles to the rotatory locus employed in the present study. The spatial distribution of such directional axes revealed in the present population of central vestibu-

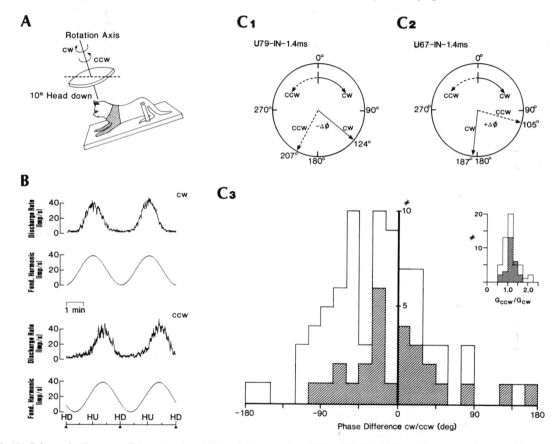

Fig. 1. (A) Schematic diagram of the animal at 10° head-down during CW and CCW OVAR. The plane of rotation is shown with respect to the earth's horizontal (dotted line). (B and C) Responses of central vestibular units to 10° OVAR. (B) Pattern of unitary response and its fundamental harmonic observed during 2 cycles of CW (upper set) or CCW (lower set) rotation. The distance between triangles along the abscissa signifies one complete 360° rotation. (C$_1$, C$_2$) Polar diagrams showing $\triangle\varnothing$ between CW and CCW responses for 2 monosynaptic inferior vestibular (IN) units: one shows $-\triangle\varnothing$ response pattern (C$_1$), while the other shows $+\triangle\varnothing$ response pattern (C$_2$). The solid line radiating from the centre represents the direction of CW discharge maximum, while the broken line represents the direction of CCW discharge maximum. The degree along the circumference indicate head positions: 0°, head-down; 90°, ipsilateral ear-down; 180°, head-up; 270°, ipsilateral ear-up. (C$_3$) Histogram showing distribution of the magnitude of $+$ and $-\triangle\varnothing$. Shading indicates the subpopulation of units receiving monosynaptic inputs. Inset: distribution of Grain$_{CCW}$/Grain$_{CW}$ ratio of the units showing $+\triangle\varnothing$ (shaded columns) and those showing $-\triangle\varnothing$ (white columns). C is modified from [13].

lar units (in the lateral, inferior and superior vestibular nuclei) is illustrated in Fig. 2A. For units with their characterized directional axes near roll (i.e. at 90° and 270° ± 45°), 22 were excited by ipsilateral ear-down (type α) and 13 by contralateral ear-down tilt (type β). Among those units with their characterized directional axes near pitch (i.e. at 0° and 180° ± 45°), 27 were excited by head-up tilt (type 1) and 15 by head-down tilt (type 2) [24, 31].

The relative behaviours of the CW and CCW responses to OVAR (1.75 °/s) at different head tilts (5–25°) was also studied in 29 central vestibular units. Units showed discharge modulations to bidirectional OVAR throughout this range of head dis-

placement. Though there was a slight fluctuation in the position of discharge maximum within the range of head displacements studied, 80% of the units had a persistent phase difference (either + or $- \triangle \varnothing$). For the remaining units, which demonstrated a reversal of phase difference with respect to head tilts, the $\triangle \varnothing$ for different head displacements was <30° (Fig. 3A). Within the given range of head tilts, the averaged positions of the CW/CCW discharge maxima (which represent the characterized directional axes) were not significantly modified by the amplitude of head displacements (Fig. 3B). As the amplitude of head displacement increased, the peak-to-peak modulation in response amplitude of

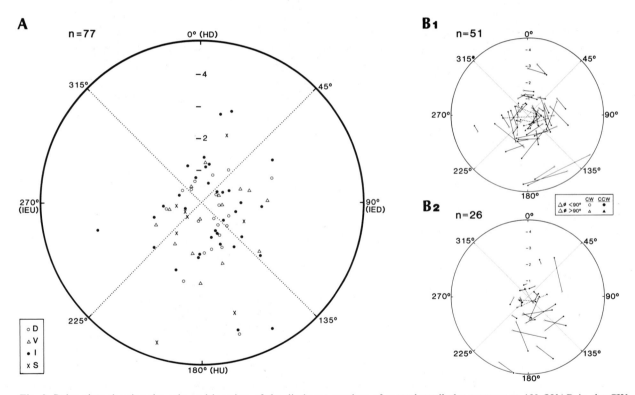

Fig. 2. Polar plots showing the gain and location of the discharge maxima of central vestibular neurons to 10° OVAR in the CW and CCW directions. The distance of each symbol from the centre of the diagram indicates either the mean gain value of the CW and CCW responses (A) or the response gain of each unit to individual input (B). Dotted lines arbitrarily divide the plane of rotation into 4 quadrants, that of head-down (HD), ipsilateral ear-down (IED), head-up (HU) and ipsilateral ear-up (IEU). A: Spatial distribution of the averaged positions of CW/CCW discharge maxima on the plane of rotation. D, dorsal part of lateral vestibular nucleus; V, ventral part of lateral vestibular nucleus; I, rostral part of inferior vestibular nucleus; S, superior vestibular nucleus. (B) Unitary responses for CW and CCW rotations plotted as a pair for units showing $- \triangle \varnothing$ (B₁) and $+ \triangle \varnothing$ (B₂) responses. Responses of the same unit to the CW and CCW rotations are connected by a straight line (solid lines for those showing $\triangle \varnothing$ <90°, broken lines for those showing $\triangle \varnothing$ >90°). B is from [13].

the units increased linearly. However, the gain values for each pair of CW/CCW responses at different head tilts exhibited no apparent difference.

Neuronal responses of the fastigial nucleus

Thirty-five units in the rostral fastigial nucleus responded to 10° OVAR (1.75 °/s) with modulation of discharge rate (a position-dependent maximum and minimum) during any 360° rotations in either the CW or CCW direction. Based on the classification of the unitary phase difference between CW and CCW discharge maxima as described in the preceding section for central vestibular units, 20 fastigial units exhibited $-\triangle\varnothing$, while 15 units showed $+\triangle\varnothing$. No apparent difference in response gain was observed between each pair of CW and CCW responses amongst the responsive units (mean Grain$_{CCW}$/Grain$_{CW}$ ratio was 1.05 ± 0.04;

mean ± SEM). However, the response gain of fastigial units to 10° OVAR was lower than that of central vestibular units. The spatial distribution of the directional axes indicating the plane of the functional polarization vector of the 35 fastigial units is illustrated in Fig. 4A; the characterized directional axes were found predominantly in the head-down and ipsilateral ear-down quadrants. The effect of head tilts (5–25°) on the responses of fastigial units to bidirectional OVAR was also examined ($n = 12$). Units were found to demonstrate persistent and/or reversal phase differences at different tilts (Fig. 4B). The characterized directional axis of each fastigial unit examined was not significantly modified with respect to changes in the amplitude of deviation from the earth's vertical.

Another group of fastigial units ($n = 9$) was sensitive to 10° OVAR (at 1.75 °/s) in only one direction (CW or CCW). However, on increasing

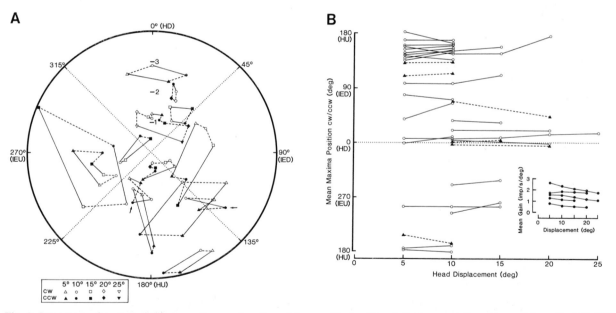

Fig. 3. Responses of central vestibular units as a function of the amplitude of head displacement from the earth's vertical (5–25°) during OVAR. (A) Polar diagram showing the gain and location of unitary discharge maxima to different head tilts. In this figure and in Fig. 4B, responses of the same unit within the excursion range of head tilts explored are joined by broken lines; those obtained at the two extreme positions of the head tilts are joined by solid lines. Units with reversal $\triangle\varnothing$ are marked with arrows. (B) Locations of the averaged positions of CW and CCW discharge maxima as a function of head tilts during OVAR. Responses of the same unit are joined: open symbols joined by solid lines indicate units with persistent $\triangle\varnothing$; filled symbols joined by broken lines indicate units with reversal of $\triangle\varnothing$. Inset: mean gain responses (for CW and CCW rotations) as a function of head displacement. Modified from [13].

either the amplitude of head displacement (to 15°) or the velocity of rotation (to 4.7 °/s), these units demonstrated comparable response gains in bidirectional rotations.

Discussion

Tilt-sensitive units in the vestibular nuclei and cerebellar fastigial nucleus of cats showed a difference in spatial location of the discharge maxima during slow OVAR in the CW and CCW directions. The modulation in neuronal discharge per 360° rotation reflects the sequential change in the gravitational vector acting on the otolith organs due to the instantaneous change of head position in space. Labyrinth inputs reach the vestibular nuclei and the fastigial nucleus via primary afferent fibres [7, 20], while the fastigial nucleus also receives indirect labyrinth inputs via the vestibular nucleus [27]. It is therefore not surprising that units in both the vestibular nuclei and the fastigial nucleus showed similar bidirectional OVAR response patterns although the response gain of the fastigial units was much lower than that of central vestibular units. However, unlike the central vestibular units which exhibited comparable gain to bidirectional OVAR of >5° head tilt, some fastigial units were sensitive to OVAR (<15° head tilt or <4.7 °/s) in only one direction, suggesting a differential threshold to bidirectional stimulation.

With the present mode of OVAR, the orientation of the functional polarization vector of each responsive neuron chould not be clearly defined because the rotary axis was limited to deviations of less than 25° from the vertical. Nevertheless, the general directional axis at which the plane of the functional polarization axis intersects at right angle to the rotatory locus could be deduced from the averaged position of the CW and CCW discharge maxima (within the small sector delimited by the CW and CCW discharge maxima). In otolith afferents, the functional polarization vectors were un-

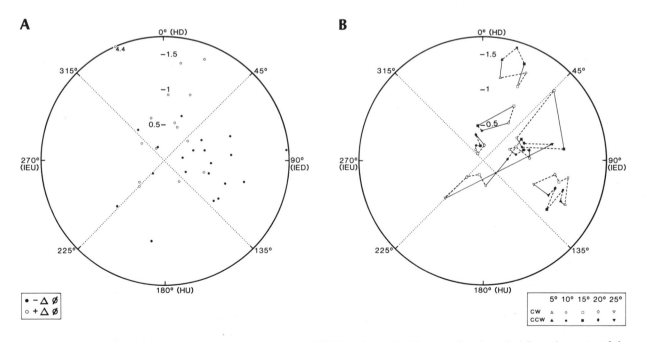

Fig. 4. Responses of fastigial units to OVAR in the CW and CCW directions. The distance of each symbol from the centre of the diagram indicates either the mean gain value of the CW and CCW responses (A) or the response gain of each unit to individual input (B). (A) Spatial distribution of the averaged positions of CW and CCW discharge maxima for units with − and + △∅ response patterns. (B) Unitary responses to different head tilts. Symbols and description as in Fig. 3A.

iformly distributed along the pitch and roll axes and angles in between [18, 39]. In this study, the spatial distribution of the characterized directional axis of units within the lateral, inferior and superior vestibular nuclei was in apparent agreement with the distribution of polarization vectors observed in otolith afferents (Fig. 2A). However, using bidirectional rotating wobble stimulus, Schor et al. [35] reported that in the population of lateral vestibular neurons studied there was a preponderance of response vectors near roll, with few vectors near pitch. The mounting of the animal is such that the orientation of the head and cervical column of the cat was different in the two laboratories: in our study, the head of the cat was horizontal and the cervical column was perpendicular to gravity (cf. Vidal et al. [40]) while Schor et al. [35] placed the head of the cat pitched down 25°, with the cervical column extended along the horizontal plane. The difference could also lie in the population of cells sampled as Schor et al. [35] used glass micropipettes (1–2 MΩ) whereas we used tungsten microelectrodes (9–12 MΩ) for recording. In this study, the fastigial neurons showed a predominance of the characterized directional axes in the head-down and the ipsilateral ear-down quadrants. Such a pattern within the rostral fastigial nucleus could conceivably be attributed to the relative lack of cerebellar Purkinje cell inhibition within the ipsilateral medial corticonuclear zone of the cerebellum during head-down and ipsilateral ear-down tilts [26, 38].

A directional difference in the location of the discharge maxima was observed in otolith afferents of monkeys in which 'regular' neurons demonstrated $\triangle\varnothing$ within 20° of each other, while 'irregular' neurons exhibited $\triangle\varnothing$ up to as much as 100° in response to bidirectional OVAR [32]. In the present study on cats, second- and higher-order neurons in the vestibular nuclei showed directional $\triangle\varnothing$ up to 160° and 172° respectively (Fig. 1B). The observation of a large directional $\triangle\varnothing$ in second-order neurons could imply further neural processing of inputs from otolith afferents, including recurrent collaterals of the second-order vestibular neurons. Based on the notion that the averaged position of

the CW and CCW discharge maxima of each responsive unit represents its characteristic directional axis, the response of $-\triangle\varnothing$ units (66% in the vestibular nuclei; 57% in the fastigial nucleus) would lead the stimulus, while the response of $+\triangle\varnothing$ units (34% in vestibular nuclei; 43% in fastigial nucleus) would lag behind the stimulus. A phase-lead response, though of a smaller value, was indeed observed in central vestibular neurons over a higher frequency range (0.01–0.02 Hz) than that used in this study [36].

Most responsive units showed a persistent phase difference (either $+$ or $-\triangle\varnothing$) with respect to oppositely directed OVAR at different head tilts with a small change in the locations of the unitary discharge maxima for either CW or CCW OVAR. The characterized directional axis of each neuron within the vestibular nuclei and fastigial nucleus remained relatively stable in space at different amplitudes of head displacement. The small changes in locations of discharge maxima may be due to converging inputs of otolith afferents or restricted branching patterns of the otolith afferents [29] which presumably innervate receptor hair cells with somewhat different but allied polarization vectors [19]. A change in head tilt may alter the relative contribution of shearing force acting on different hair cells and subsequently result in a shift in the spatial location of the unitary discharge maxima.

Though there is no apparent difference between the response gains for CW and CCW rotations, the discharge rate of each individual unit at a particular head position depends on the direction of rotation during OVAR. Based on the observation that the characterized directional axes of vestibular nuclear units were distributed over the entire plane of 360° rotation, each unit could respond to head movements in all directions, albeit at different discharge rates. The level of excitation among the whole population of neurons would vary at any one instant depending on the spatial head position during unidirectional OVAR. This spectrum of neuronal excitation would provide the necessary information for determining the spatial orientation and the direction of head movement. Some of these vestibular nuclear neurons are presumably involved in otolith-evoked modulation of oculomotor [9, 33, 46] and postural outputs [17, 45]. The fastigial nucleus would also constitute another processing station for motor adjustments via fastigiovestibular [25, 41] or fastigiospinal connections [44].

Acknowledgements

This work was supported in part by research grants from the Wing Lung Bank Medical Research Fund and the Research Grants Committee of the University of Hong Kong.

References

[1] Anderson, J.H. and Precht, W. (1979) Otolith responses of extraocular muscles during sinusoidal roll rotations. *Brain Res.*, 160: 150–154.

[2] Anderson, J.H., Soechting, J.F. and Terzuolo, C.A. (1977) Dynamic relations between natural vestibular inputs and activity of forelimb extensors in the decerebrate cat. I. Motor outputs during sinusoidal linear accelerations. *Brain Res.*, 120: 1–15.

[3] Anderson, J.H., Blanks, R.H.I. and Precht, W. (1978) Response characteristics of semicircular canal and otolith systems in cats. I. Dynamic responses of primary vestibular fibers. *Exp. Brain Res.*, 32: 491–507.

[4] Baarsma, E.A. and Collewijn, H. (1975) Eye movements due to linear accelerations in the rabbit. *J. Physiol. London*, 245: 227–247.

[5] Baker, J., Goldberg, J. and Peterson, B. (1985) Spatial and temporal response properties of the vestibulocollic reflex in decerebrate cats. *J. Neurophysiol.*, 54: 735–756.

[6] Baker, J., Harrison, R.E.W., Isu, N., Wickland, C. and Peterson, B. (1986) Dynamic of adaptive change in vestibulo-ocular reflex direction. II. Sagittal plane rotations. *Brain Res.*, 371: 166–170.

[7] Brodal, A. and Høivik, B. (1964) Site and mode of termination of primary vestibulocerebellar fibres in the cat. An experimental study with silver impregnation methods. *Arch. Ital. Biol.*, 102: 1–21.

[8] Boyle, R. and Pompeiano, O. (1980) Response characteristics of cerebellar interpositus and intermediate cortex neurons to sinusoidal stimulation of neck and labyrinth receptors. *Neuroscience*, 5: 357–372.

[9] Chan, Y.S., Hwang, J.C. and Cheung, Y.M. (1977) Crossed sacculo-ocular pathway via the Deiter's nucleus in cats. *Brain Res. Bull.*, 2: 1–6.

[10] Chan, Y.S., Hwang, J.C. and Cheung, Y.M. (1979) Vestibular function of saccule in cats as indicated by the response of Deiter's nucleus to static tilts. *Exp. Brain Res.*, 35: 591–594.

[11] Chan, Y.S., Manzoni, D. and Pompeiano, O. (1982) Response characteristics of cerebellar dentate and lateral cortex neurons to sinusoidal stimulation of neck and labyrinth receptors. *Neuroscience*, 7: 2993–3011.

[12] Chan, Y.S., Cheung, Y.M. and Hwang, J.C. (1985) Effect of tilt on the response of neuronal activity within the cat vestibular nuclei during slow and constant velocity rotation. *Brain Res.*, 345: 271–278.

[13] Chan, Y.S., Cheung, Y.M. and Hwang, J.C. (1987) Response characteristics of neurons in the cat vestibular nuclei during slow and constant velocity off-vertical axes rotations in the clockwise and counterclockwise rotations. *Brain Res.*, 406: 294–301.

[14] Cohen, B., Suzuki, J.-I. and Raphan, T. (1983) Role of the otolith organs in generation of horizontal nystagmus: effects of selective labyrinthine lesions. *Brains Res.*, 276: 159–164.

[15] Correia, M.J. and Money, K.E. (1970) The effect of blockage of all six simicircular canal ducts on nystagmus produced by dynamic linear acceleration in the cat. *Acta Otolaryngol. Stockholm*, 69: 7–16.

[16] Darlot, C., Cohen, B., Berthoz, A. and Denise, P. (1985) Off vertical axis rotation (OVAR): perception effects and eye movements induced by small angles of tilt. *Neurosci. Lett. Suppl.*, 22: S483.

[17] Dutia, M.B. and Hunter, M.J. (1985) The sagittal vestibulo-collic reflex and its interaction with neck proprioceptive afferents in the decerebrate cat. *J. Physiol. London*, 359: 17–29.

[18] Fernandez, C. and Goldberg, J.M. (1976) Physiology of peripheral neurons innervating otolith organs of the squirrel monkey. I. Response to static tilts and to long-duration centrifugal force. *J. Neurophysiol.*, 39: 970–984.

[19] Flock, Å. (1965) Electron microscopic and electrophysiological studies on the lateral line canal organ. *Acta Otolaryngol. Stockholm Suppl.*, 199: 1–90.

[20] Gacek, R.R. (1969) The course and central termination of first order neurons supplying vestibular endorgans in the cat. *Acta Otolaryngol. Stockholm*, 254: 1–66.

[21] Gardner, E.P. and Fuchs, A.F. (1975) Single-unit responses to natural vestibular stimuli and eye movements in deep cerebellar nuclei of the alert rhesus monkey. *J. Neurophysiol.*, 38: 627–649.

[22] Ghelarducci, B. (1973) Responses of the cerebellar fastigial neurons to tilt. *Pflügers Arch.*, 344: 195–206.

[23] Hwang, J.C. and Poon, W.F. (1975) An electrophysiology study of the sacculo-ocular pathways in cats. *Jpn. J. Physiol.*, 25: 241–251.

[24] Hwang, J.C., Or, T.H. and Cheung, Y.M. (1980) Response of central vestibular neurons to utricular stimulations in cats. *Exp. Brain Res.*, 40: 346–348.

[25] Ito, M., Udo, M., Mano, N. and Kawai, N. (1970) Synaptic action of the fastigiobular impulses upon neurones in the medullary reticular formation and vestibular nuclei. *Exp. Brain Res.*, 11: 29–47.

[26] Ito, M., Yoshida, M., Obata, K., Kawai, N. and Udo, M. (1970) Inhibitory control of intracerebellar nuclei by the Purkinje cell axons. *Exp. Brain Res.*, 10: 64–80.

[27] Kotchabhakdi, N. and Walberg, F. (1978) Cerebellar afferent projections from the vestibular nuclei in the cat: an experimental study with the method of retrograde axonal transport of horseradish peroxidase. *Exp. Brain Res.*, 31: 591–604.

[28] Lacour, M., Borel, L., Barthelemy, J., Harlay, F. and Xerri, C. (1987) Dynamic properties of the vertical otolith neck reflexes in the alert cat. *Exp. Brain Res.*, 65: 559–568.

[29] Lindeman, H.H. (1969) Studies on the morphology of the sensory regions of the vestibular apparatus. *Ergeb. Anat. Entw. Gesch.*, 42: 1–113.

[30] Lindsay, K.W., Roberts, T.D.M. and Rosenberg, J. (1976) Asymmetric tonic labyrinth reflexes and their interactions with neck reflexes in the decerebrate cat. *J. Physiol. London*, 261: 583–601.

[31] Peterson, B.W. (1970) Distribution of neural responses to tilting within vestibular nuclei of the cat. *J. Neurophysiol.*, 33: 750–767.

[32] Raphan, T., Waespe, W. and Cohen, B. (1981) Vestibular nerve activity induced by off vertical axis rotation. *Soc. Neurosci. Abstr.*, 7: 39.

[33] Reisine, H., Raphan, T. and Cohen, B. (1986) Activity in the vestibular nuclei during off-vertical axis rotation (OVAR). *Soc. Neurosci. Abstr.*, 12: 773.

[34] Schor, R.H. and Miller, A.D. (1981) Vestibular reflexes in neck and forelimb muscles evoked by roll tilt. *J. Neurophysiol.*, 46: 167–178.

[35] Schor, R.H., Miller, A.D. and Tomko, D.L. (1984) Responses to head tilt in cat central vestibular neurons. I. Direction of maximum sensitivity. *J. Neurophysiol.*, 51: 136–146.

[36] Schor, R.H., Miller, A.D., Timerick, S.J.B. and Tomko, D.L. (1985) Responses to head tilt in cat central vestibular neurons. II. Frequency dependence of neuronal response vectors. *J. Neurophysiol.*, 53: 1444–1452.

[37] Soechting, J.F., Anderson, J.H. and Berthoz, A. (1977) Dynamic relations between natural vestibular inputs and activity of forelimb extensors in the decerebrate cat. III. Motor output during rotations in the vertical plane. *Brain Res.*, 120: 35–47.

[38] Stanojevic, M., Erway, L., Ghelarducci, B., Pompeiano, O. and Willis, W.D. Jr. (1980) A comparison of the response characteristics of cerebellar fastigial and vermal cortex neurons to sinusoidal stimulation of macular vestibular receptors. *Pflügers Arch.*, 385: 95–104.

[39] Tomko, D.L., Peterka, R.J. and Schor, R.H. (1981) Responses to head tilt in cat eighth nerve afferents. *Exp. Brain Res.*, 41: 216–221.

[40] Vidal, P.P., Graf, W. and Berthoz, A. (1986) The orientation of the cervical vertebral column in unrestrained awake animals. I. Resting position. *Exp. Brain Res.*, 61: 549–559.

[41] Walberg, F. (1972) Cerebellovestibular relations: anatomy. In A. Brodal and O. Pompeiano (Eds.), *Basic Aspects of Central Vestibular Mechanisms, Progress in Brain Research, Vol. 37*, Elsevier, Amsterdam, pp. 361–376.

[42] Watt, D.G.D. (1976) Responses of cats to sudden falls: an otolith-originating reflex assisting landing. *J. Neurophysiol.*, 39: 257–265.

[43] Wilson, V.J. and Peterson, B.W. (1981) Vestibulospinal and reticulospinal systems. In V.B. Brooks (Ed.), *Handbook of Physiology, The Nervous System, Vol. 2, Motor Control*, American Physiological Society, Bethesda, pp. 667–702.

[44] Wilson, V.J., Uchino, Y., Maunz, R.A., Susswein, A. and Fukushima, K. (1978) Properties and connections of cat fastigiospinal neurons. *Exp. Brain Res.*, 32: 1–17.

[45] Wilson, V.J., Schor, R.H., Suzuki, I. and Park, B.R. (1986) Spatial organization of neck and vestibular reflexes acting on the forelimbs of the decerebrate cat. *J. Neurophysiol.*, 55: 514–526.

[46] Young, L.R. and Henn, V. (1975) Nystagmus induced by pitch and yaw rotation of monkeys. *Fortschr. Zool.*, 23: 235–246.

O. Pompeiano and J.H.J. Allum (Eds.)
Progress in Brain Research, Vol. 76
© 1988 Elsevier Science Publishers B.V. (Biomedical Division)

CHAPTER 6

Temporal transformation of signals from the otolith organs by the central nervous system of the cat

R.H. Schor*

Rockefeller University, 1230 York Avenue, New York, NY 10021-6399, U.S.A.

The otolith organs in the cat, which respond to linear accelerations of the head, can carry information about the position of the cat's head in space (with respect to gravity). During sinusoidal tilt, afferents continue to carry mainly head-position information, with gain flat or slowly increasing with frequency, and phase in the range 0°–30°. However, the dynamics of otolith reflexes in the forelimbs of decerebrate, canal-plugged cats show larger gain increases and phase lags of up to 180° at 1 Hz. Both afferent-like and reflex-like dynamic responses can be observed in second-order vestibular neurons. One mechanism to produce the response dynamics characteristic of the reflex in these neurons involves a parallel pathway from the eighth nerve to the vestibular nuclei; one branch would be a direct relay of afferent information, the other would amplify and filter the signal, and provide an inhibitory drive to the vestibular nuclei. Producing midline cerebellar lesions largely eliminates the observation of muscle-like responses in the vestibular nuclei, suggesting that the cerebellum may be involved in the inhibitory branch of this pathway.

Linear accelerations of the head result in the modulation of the activity in vestibular afferents innervating the otolith organs of the labyrinth. These signals convey information about the direction of head acceleration – if this acceleration is produced by tilting the head from the vertical, then the information corresponds to the orientation of the head with respect to gravity, or direction and size of head tilt.

We have been studying how the vestibular system of the decerebrate cat transforms the information about head orientation with respect to gravity, arriving from otolith afferents. The otolith system encodes two varieties of information – spatial information (in which direction the head is tilted) and temporal information (how head position is changing as a function of time). We have shown that, at the level of the vestibular nuclei, these two types of information from the otolith system are kept separate – neurons which respond best to a particular direction of tilt maintain their directional coding property over a broad range of stimulus frequencies [12]. We will therefore assume that temporal processing can be looked at in isolation, and will describe the type of temporal information available at various levels of the cat otolith–spinal reflex system.

To look at the function of the otolith organs, we have largely used the decerebrate cat preparation, with the semicircular canals inactivated by a plugging procedure, which renders the canals nonfunctional [6, 7]. Stimulation consisted of sinusoidal tilt in a vertical plane. In the early experiments, roll tilt (in the transverse plane) was employed [9, 10]; more recently, we first determined which direction of tilt best activates the neuron under study, then stimulate with a vertical plane aligned near such a best direction [11-13]. The stimulus frequency ranged from 0.01 to 2 Hz, with amplitudes typically of 10°

*Present address: Departments of Otolaryngology and Physiology, University of Pittsburgh School of Medicine, Pittsburgh, PA 15213, U.S.A.

(for frequencies below 0.2 Hz). This type of small-amplitude sinusoidal tilt induces a time-varying acceleration in the animal's frame of reference; the (animal) horizontal component varies sinusoidally, to a good approximation, while the vertical component consists of a constant plus a small second harmonic. Our analysis is based on the neural signals modulated at the frequency of sinusoidal tilt, which therefore arise due to the sinusoidal horizontal accelerations. Since the utricular macula tends to lie near the horizontal plane, these responses are more likely to be due to activation of the utricle, rather than the more vertical saccule.

The dynamic properties of the otolith system can be studied by observing how the response varies with the frequency of tilt. If response gain (measured with respect to the amplitude of tilt, or position of the animal) remains constant and phase (with respect to position) is near zero, the system is producing a pure 'position' response; if the gain grows linearly with frequency, and the phase leads by 90°, the response is a 'velocity' response (since the derivative of a sinusoid is proportional to its frequency, and peaks 90° earlier). Fernandez and Goldberg [5] demonstrated that while part of the afferent population in the squirrel monkey had 'position' response dynamics, another group of afferents had responses intermediate between 'position' and 'velocity' responses. Such response classes have also been observed in the cat ([1], R.H. Schor and B.R. Park, unpublished observations). Afferents appear to fall into two broad, overlapping groups – one has a fairly regular discharge, a somewhat low sensitivity to tilt, and in response to sinusoidal tilt, a constant gain and phase near zero. The other population has a more irregular discharge, is generally more sensitive to tilt, and exhibits a slight increase in gain and a small phase lead with respect to the stimulus [4, 5]. The difference in response dynamics is illustrated in Fig. 1 – from a population of 16 otolith afferents studied over a wide band of frequencies, eleven had flat gain and phase near zero (□) and five showed a gain increase and phase lead (△) (R.H. Schor and B.R. Park, unpublished observations). The response of these latter afferents

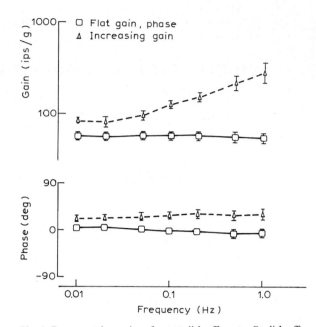

Fig. 1. Response dynamics of cat otolith afferents. Otolith afferents were divided into two groups, eleven afferents having similar gain at all tested frequencies and five having gain which increased at higher frequencies. Responses have been normalized by the response gain at 0.1 Hz, vectorially averaged, rescaled by the average gain, and plotted along with the standard error of gain and phase. Neurons with constant gain (□) show a constant phase near 0°, thus accurately signalling the position of the head with respect to the vertical, while neurons with increasing gain (△) show a constant phase lead, proportional to the slope of the gain increase.

can be modelled by a 'fractional differentiator' with exponent 1/3, a model which predicts a slope to the gain curve of 1/3 and a constant phase lead of 30°. Such a response lies between the 'position' (exponent 0) and 'velocity' (exponent 1) responses.

The signals arising from otolith afferents therefore largely encode the position of the animal, with perhaps some information as to velocity. However, if we look at one output of the otolith system, the response observed in forelimb extensor muscles, we see a different dynamic response pattern [9]. Fig. 2 shows (solid line) the average EMG response in the long head of triceps, recorded in decerebrate cats without functioning semicircular canals (the 'canal-plugged' preparation). For comparison, curves representing the two classes of afferent responses are

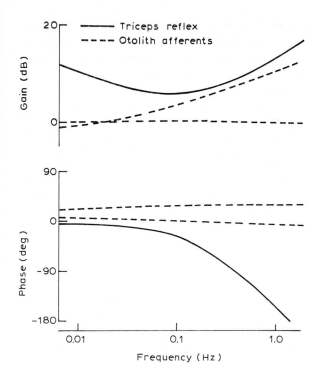

Fig. 2. Dynamic responses arising from otolith stimulation. The dashed lines represent the two classes of response dynamics seen in otolith afferents, as illustrated in Fig. 1. The solid line represents the averaged integrated EMG response from the triceps forelimb extensor muscle of decerebrate cats with nonfunctional canals (from [9]). It is characterized by a larger gain increase at high frequencies than that seen in the afferents, and a progressive phase lag which can reach 180° at 1 Hz.

illustrated as dashed lines. The reflex shows an increasing gain above 0.1 Hz which is somewhat steeper than that observed in the afferents. The phase response of the reflex departs radically from afferents, particularly at higher frequencies, where a significant phase lag, amounting to 180° at 1 Hz, can develop.

Where does the temporal transformation of the afferent signal take place? We first examined the response of neurons in the vestibular nuclei, with most of our recordings taken from the lateral and rostral inferior nuclei. We found two major classes of neural responses [10]. One group of neurons had response dynamics resembling those of otolith afferents (see Fig. 3), with flat or linearly-increasing

gain and phase near, or slightly leading, position. This type of response will be called an 'afferent-like' response. The other group of neurons had dynamics like the muscle, exhibiting both the large gain increase and progressive phase lag as frequency increased above 0.1 Hz; this can be called a 'muscle-like' response. We also noticed an interesting correlation between these temporal, dynamic, properties of the neurons and their spatial properties. Most neurons with afferent-like responses were excited by ear-down roll tilt and inhibited by ear-up roll, while neurons with muscle-like dynamics showed the opposite pattern, being excited by ear-up tilt. For convenience, we will call neurons excited by ear-down tilt α neurons and neurons excited by ear-up tilt β neurons, after Duensing and Schaefer [3]. Thus the two major classes of tilt-modulated neurons we

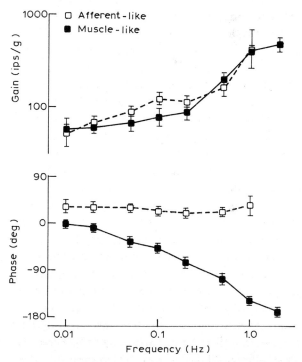

Fig. 3. Averaged responses of vestibular neurons. Responses from neurons best fit by a simple, afferent-like model (Model 3) or a more complex model which behaves more like the reflex muscle response (Model 2) were taken from the data of Schor et al. [12]. 26 afferent-like responses (□) and 24 muscle-like responses (■) were vectorially averaged.

found in the vestibular nuclei (of canal-plugged cats) were afferent-like α and muscle-like β neurons.

In an effort to understand the origin of these responses, we subsequently attempted to develop mathematical models which would provide good fits to the data we observed [8]. We found that the majority of our neurons could be fit by two models [12]. The afferent-like response, with its slow, almost-linear gain increase and phase near position, was fit by a model incorporating a fractional-differentiator ('fractional-s operator') and a low-pass filter. Note that such a fractional operator with a value of 1/3 represents the major feature of the afferent responses, illustrated in Fig. 1, exhibiting the increasing gain. The afferent-like response in Fig. 3 (□) represents the averaged response of 26 neurons best fit by this simple model.

The muscle-like response (Fig. 3, ■) required a more complex model, consisting of two parallel branches. One branch takes position information (present on otolith afferents) and simply relays the signal to second-order neurons. The other branch takes the same afferent signal, high-pass filters it to remove the low-frequency responses, and amplifies it by a factor of about ten. The branches converge onto second-order vestibular neurons, with the amplified, filtered input being inhibitory. At low frequencies, the high-pass filter effectively eliminates the inhibitory branch, and the system exhibits a position response, due to its direct afferent input. However, at high frequencies, the large inhibitory contribution dominates, producing a reflex with larger gain and reversed (180° lag) phase.

Most of the processing required to produce muscle-like responses therefore seems to take place at the level of neurons in the vestibular nuclei. We have also examined the response properties of cervical interneurons which may be relaying otolith information to forelimb motor pools [13]. These also show afferent-like or muscle-like responses – there is no evidence for significant further temporal processing of this signal within the spinal cord.

So how might the muscle-like response dynamics actually be produced? The parallel pathway model suggests looking for a structure which receives vestibular input and can inhibit second-order vestibular neurons: the cerebellum is an obvious candidate. We have recently begun experiments designed to investigate the possible role of the cerebellum in the production of these responses (R.H. Schor, A.D. Miller, and Y.S. Chan, preliminary findings). In a control sample of neurons taken in canal-plugged decerebrate cats, we found response dynamics consistent with our earlier studies [10, 12] – all eleven neurons with α responses (excited by ear-down tilt) had afferent-like responses, while five out of seven neurons with β responses had muscle-like responses. In contrast, after aspiration of the midline cerebellar vermis, only two neurons (one out of 23 neurons with an α response, one out of eight with β responses) exhibited a gain increase and phase lag at higher frequencies, and in both cases the phase lag only approached 90° at 1 Hz, instead of the more usual 180°. This finding is consistent with a cerebellar role in the production of the muscle-like vestibular responses; we are continuing these studies to obtain more direct evidence of cerebellar involvement.

The function of the increased gain and large phase lag at frequencies near 1 Hz observed in otolith-spinal reflexes is unclear, at present. In animals with intact labyrinths, the combined activation of the semicircular canals and otolith organs during sinusoidal roll tilt produces a response with phase lead at high frequencies, due to the velocity-proportional signal from the semicircular canals [2, 9]. Further experiments, perhaps utilizing horizontal translational movements, may provide more insight into the separate responsibility of the otolith organs in postural control.

Acknowledgements

This work has been supported in part by grants from NIH (NS02619, NS17808, NS24930 and BRSG S07 RR07065) and NASA (NSG2380).

References

[1] Anderson, J.H., Blanks, R.H.I. and Precht, W. (1978) Response characteristics of semicircular canal and otolith systems in cat. I. Dynamic responses of primary vestibular fibers. *Exp. Brain Res.*, 32: 491–507.

[2] Berthoz, A. and Anderson, J.H. (1971) Frequency analysis of vestibular influence on extensor motoneurons. I. Response to tilt in forelimb extensors. *Brain Res.*, 34: 370–375.

[3] Duensing, F. and Schaefer, K.P. (1959) Über die Konvergenz verschiedener labyrinthärer Afferenzen auf einzelne Neurone des Vestibulariskergebietes. *Arch. Psychiatr. Nervenkr.*, 199: 345–371.

[4] Fernandez, C. and Goldberg, J.M. (1976) Physiology of peripheral neurons innervating otolith organs of the squirrel monkey. I. Response to static tilts and to long-duration centrifugal force. *J. Neurophysiol.*, 39: 970–984.

[5] Fernandez, C. and Goldberg, J.M. (1976) Physiology of peripheral neurons innervating otolith organs of the squirrel monkey. III. Response dynamics. *J. Neurophysiol.*, 39: 996–1008.

[6] Money, K.E. and Scott J.W. (1962) Functions of separate sensory receptors of nonauditory labyrinth of the cat. *Am. J. Physiol.*, 202: 1211–1220.

[7] Schor, R.H. (1974) Responses of cat vestibular neurons to sinusoidal roll tilt. *Exp. Brain Res.*, 20: 347–362.

[8] Schor, R.H. (1985) Design and fitting of neural network transfer functions. *Biol. Cybern.*, 51: 357–362.

[9] Schor, R.H. and Miller, A.D. (1981) Vestibular reflexes in neck and forelimb muscles evoked by roll tilt. *J. Neurophysiol.*, 46: 167–178.

[10] Schor, R.H. and Miller, A.D. (1982) Relationship of cat vestibular neurons to otolith-spinal reflexes. *Exp. Brain Res.*, 47: 137–144.

[11] Schor, R.H., Miller, A.D. and Tomko, D.L. (1984) Responses to head tilt in cat central vestibular neurons. I. Direction of maximum sensitivity. *J. Neurophysiol.*, 51: 136–146.

[12] Schor, R.H., Miller, A.D., Timerick, S.J.B. and Tomko, D.L. (1985) Responses to head tilt in cat central vestibular neurons. II. Frequency dependence of neural response vectors. *J. Neurophysiol.*, 53: 1444–1452.

[13] Schor, R.H., Suzuki, I., Timerick, S.J.B. and Wilson, V.J. (1986) Responses of interneurons in the cat cervical cord to vestibular tilt stimulation. *J. Neurophysiol.*, 56: 1147–1156.

O. Pompeiano and J.H.J. Allum (Eds.)
Progress in Brain Research, Vol. 76
© 1988 Elsevier Science Publishers B.V. (Biomedical Division)

CHAPTER 7

The role of Renshaw cells in the dynamic control of posture during vestibulospinal reflexes

O. Pompeiano

Dipartimento di Fisiologia e Biochimica, Università di Pisa, Via S. Zeno 31, 56100 Pisa, Italy

Contraction of limb extensors during side-down tilt of the animal can be attributed to an increased discharge of lateral VS neurons which exert an excitatory influence on ipsilateral extensor motoneurons (α response). However, in addition to these neurons there are other neuronal systems, such as the CS and the medullary inhibitory RS neurons which also respond to animal tilt, but with a predominant response pattern characterized by a reduced discharge during side-down tilt (β response). This finding is surprising since the CS projection, which originates from the NE-containing LC neurons, is inhibitory on R cells linked with limb extensor (and flexor) motoneurons, while the medullary RS projection, which is driven presumably by cholinergic and cholinoceptive neurons located in the dorsal pRF, is excitatory on them. Experiments were performed in precollicular decerebrate cats to investigate the relative influence that the CS, as well as the RS, neurons exert on R cells coupled with limb extensor motoneurons in the following experimental conditions: (1) during the state of postural activity in which the LC neurons showed a steady discharge while the pRF neurons, as well as the related medullary inhibitory RS neurons, fired at a very low rate; in this instance the gain of the VS reflexes was quite low; and (2) during episodes of reduced postural activity following systemic administration of an anticholinesterase (0.05–0.10 mg/kg eserine sulphate), in which the discharge rate of LC neurons decreased, while that of the pRF neurons and the related medullary inhibitory RS neurons increased; in this instance the gain of the VS reflexes was greatly enhanced. In particular, the

activity of R cells monosynaptically linked with gastrocnemius–soleus motoneurons (GS R cells) was tested both in the animal at rest as well as during head rotation (at 0.026–0.15 Hz, $\pm 10°$) performed after bilateral neck deafferentation, thus leading to sinusoidal stimulation of labyrinth receptors. In control animals at rest the GS R cells were silent or fired at a low rate; moreover, the same units were either unresponsive or displayed only small-amplitude α responses to labyrinth stimulation. These responses were attributed to the fact that during side-down head rotation the increased discharge of VS neurons activated the GS motoneurons and, through their recurrent collaterals, the related R cells. However, the decrease in firing rate of the CS neurons for the same direction of head rotation would reduce the inhibitory influence that these noradrenergic neurons exert on the GS R cells, thus enhancing the functional coupling of these units with their own extensor motoneurons. This would explain why the response gain of hindlimb extensors to labyrinth stimulation was negligible or absent in these preparations. After systemic injection of the anticholinesterase, leading to an increased discharge of cholinoceptive pRF neurons and the related medullary RS neurons, the GS R cells increased their firing rate in the animal at rest; however, all the R cells which prior to the injection were either unresponsive or showed an α response to head rotation, now showed a β response for the same parameters of labyrinth stimulation. In particular, a reduced discharge of the GS R cells occurred during side-down head rotation, as shown for the majority of the RS neurons. It appears, therefore, that the

---

Abbreviations: AR, averaged response: CS, coeruleospinal; GS, gastrocnemius–soleus; LC, locus coeruleus; LVN, lateral vestibular nucleus; NE, norepinephrine; R cell, Renshaw cell; (m/p)RF, (medullary/pontine) reticular formation; RS, reticulospinal; VS, vestibulospinal.

same R cells which in the control situation responded to the excitatory VS volleys acting through the GS motoneurons were now decoupled from their input motoneurons and underwent the most efficient control of the RS pathway. The reduced discharge of the GS R cells during side-down head rotation would lead to disinhibition of limb extensor motoneurons, thus enhancing the response gain of the corresponding muscle to labyrinth stimulation. The R cells could then act as a variable gain-regulator at motoneuronal level during the VS reflexes.

Introduction

The VS reflexes elicited in decerebrate cats by sinusoidal stimulation of macular, utricular receptors are characterized by contraction of limb extensors during side-down tilt of the animal and relaxation during side-up tilt [10, 34, 60; cf. 28]. These postural changes were attributed to the activity of VS neurons originating from the LVN [3, 4, 61], which exert a monosynaptic and/or a polysynaptic excitatory influence on ipsilateral limb extensor motoneurons ([30]; for references see [43]). In fact, most of the lateral VS neurons projecting to the lumbosacral segments of the spinal cord respond to the positional signal during slow roll tilt of the animal (at 0.026 Hz, $\pm 10°$), the predominant response pattern being characterized by an increase in firing rate during side-down tilt and a decrease during side-up tilt (α response) [38, 63]. Surprisingly, in spite of the good decerebrate rigidity, the gain of the VS reflexes is very low in forelimb extensors and almost negligible or absent in hindlimb extensors.

It would be of interest to know whether in addition to the lateral VS tract, which activates directly the ipsilateral limb extensor motoneurons, there are other supraspinal descending pathways which may modify the response gain of these motoneurons to the excitatory VS volleys, by acting on R cells anatomically coupled with them. The hypothesis that R cells may serve as an adjustable gain-regulator acting at motoneuronal level during the VS reflexes is supported by the results of experiments showing that R cells interposed in the recurrent inhibitory circuit can be influenced not only by the cor-

responding motoneurons via the recurrent collaterals, but also by supraspinal sources acting directly upon them (for references see [46]). In these instances, excitation or inhibition of R cells might decrease or increase the amplitude of the motoneuronal responses to the excitatory volleys coursing along the lateral VS tract, as postulated also for other supraspinal descending systems [20].

The pathways which can be involved in the gain regulation of the VS reflexes are the CS tract, which originates from the NE-containing LC neurons and the RS tract, originating from the inhibitory area of the mRF. The following lines of evidence obtained in decerebrate cats support this hypothesis:

(1) Stimulation experiments have shown that the CS pathway exerts a facilitatory influence on ipsilateral limb extensor (and flexor) motoneurons [12, 13], an effect which can in part at least be attributed to suppression of the tonic discharge of inhibitory interneurons acting on spinal cord motoneurons [23]. Some of these interneurons could actually be R cells anatomically linked with extensor (and flexor) motoneurons. Indeed, there is evidence that stimulation of the LC antagonizes recurrent inhibition of monosynaptic reflexes by inhibiting the corresponding R cells, which would then be *decoupled* from the corresponding input motoneurons [14]. This is in accord with early findings that R cell activities were inhibited by iontophoretically applied NE [2, 9, 65], a putative transmitter of CS synapses. On the other hand, the medullary RS pathway, which exerts a postsynaptic inhibitory influence on limb extensor (and flexor) motoneurons ([21, 29, 42]; see [33]) may in part at least excite the corresponding R cells, which would then be *coupled* with the related input motoneurons ([15, 16, 25, 31]; see [46]).

(2) Experiments of unit recordings have shown that neurons located in the LC complex, i.e. the LC and the subcoeruleus area [1, 55] as well as in the inhibitory area of the mRF ([36, 52]; see [47]), some of which are antidromically activated by spinal cord stimulation at Th12–L1, respond to slow roll tilt of the animal (at 0.026–0.15 Hz, $\pm 10°$). In particular, the majority of these responses occurred

with an average phase lead with respect to the extreme animal position of $+26.4 \pm 25.6°$ (mean $\pm$ S.D.) for the LC complex neurons (i.e. 44 out of 49 units) and $+25.3 \pm 28.3°$ for the mRF neurons (i.e. 95 out of 113 units), thus being attributed to stimulation of macular receptors. Moreover, for both these populations of neurons, the predominant response pattern was characterized by a decrease in firing rate during side-down tilt and an increase during side-up tilt (β response), this pattern being just opposite to that found for the lateral VS neurons projecting to the same segments of the spinal cord. If the activity of the LC neurons predominated over that of the mRF neurons, then the limb extensor motoneurons would be excited by an increased discharge of VS neurons during side-down tilt, but this effect would be in part at least *attenuated* by the reduced discharge of CS neurons, leading to disinhibition of the related R cells. However, if the activity of the mRF neurons was more prominent than that of the LC neurons, then for the same direction of animal orientation the excitation of limb extensor motoneurons following the increased discharge of the VS neurons would be *enhanced* by a reduced discharge of the medullary RS neurons, leading to disfacilitation of the related R cells.

(3) Finally, lesion experiments have shown that electrolytic destruction of the LC, from which the CS pathway originates, increased the gain of the VS reflexes acting on ipsilateral limb extensors [6]. However, just the opposite result was obtained following lesion of the dorsal aspect of the pRF, whose neurons exert a direct excitatory influence on the inhibitory area of the mRF from which the RS pathway originates [7].

The experiments summarized in the present report were performed to find out whether reciprocal changes in posture as well as in gain of the VS reflexes occurred in the two opposite conditions in which either activity of LC neurons giving rise to the CS projection predominated over that of dorsal pRF neurons which drives the medullary RS system, or vice versa. Moreover, experiments were performed to study whether in these instances the R cells linked with limb extensor motoneurons behaved as if they were under the predominant control either of the CS or of the medullary RS neurons, thus intervening in the gain regulation of the VS reflexes.

Reciprocal discharge of locus coeruleus and pontine reticular neurons following activation of a cholinergic system

Experiments performed in precollicular decerebrate cats have shown that systemic injection of an anticholinesterase (0.10–0.15 mg/kg, i.v. of eserine sulphate) produced episodes of postural atonia which lasted on the average ten minutes ([32, 39-41]; for references see [24, 44, 45]). These episodes did not depend on a reduced discharge of LVN neurons leading to disfacilitation of spinal motoneurons, but rather on tonic activation of the medullary inhibitory RS system [44, 45]. Experiments of unit recordings have in fact demonstrated that selective changes in the discharge rate of brainstem neurons were involved in the appearance of these episodes [18, 48]. In particular, among 251 units recorded from different pontine regions before, during and after these episodes of postural atonia, 81 units (32.3%) were activated while 31 units (12.4%) were tonically inhibited throughout the cataplectic episodes. The first population of units, which fired at low rate in the control situation but selectively increased their discharge rate during these episodes, were found in the dorsal aspect of the pRF where presumably cholinergic and cholinoceptive neurons projecting to the inhibitory area of the mRF are located. On the other hand, the second population of units, which showed a steady discharge in the control situation but greatly decreased their firing rate during the induced episodes of postural atonia, were found particularly in the caudal part of the LC complex where noradrenergic neurons are located; some of these neurons could actually contribute to the CS pathway projecting to different segments of the spinal cord (for references see [11]).

The reciprocal rate profiles of the dorsal pRF neurons and the LC neurons during the state of postural activity and their reversal during the state of postural atonia suggest that a functional interaction occurs between the two cell groups [49]. In particular, it appears that the decerebrate rigidity was present as long as the LC neurons, in addition to their tonic facilitatory influence on limb extensor motoneurons via the CS pathway, exerted an inhibitory influence on the dorsal pRF neurons and the related medullary inhibitory RS system. As the LC activity began to wane, pRF neuronal discharge progressively increased, thus leading to tonic activation of the medullary inhibitory RS system as well as to suppression of the decerebrate rigidity. This hypothesis was supported by the fact that the discharge rate of RS neurons originating from the inhibitory area of the mRF tonically increased following injection of the anticholinesterase, thus leading to a decrease or suppression of postural activity [62]. The neurophysiological and the neurochemical mechanisms by which the LC neurons keep under their tonic inhibitory control the dorsal pRF neurons and thus the discharge of the related medullary RS neurons will be discussed in detail in another chapter [8].

It is of interest that the episodes of postural atonia induced by the anticholinesterase disappeared either spontaneously, or following somatosensory or acoustic stimulation. In these instances, the recovery of postural activity could be attributed to activation not only of the facilitatory structures of the brainstem, but also of LC neurons which would suppress the activity of the pRF, thus ending the discharge of the inhibitory RS system.

An interaction between LC neurons and pRF neurons might account for the suppression of postural activity which occurs not only in decerebrate cats following injection of an anticholinesterase, but also in intact animals during desynchronized sleep (for references see [17]).

Responses of limb extensor muscles to sinusoidal labyrinth stimulation following activation of a cholinergic system

In precollicular decerebrate cats, the multiunit EMG responses of limb extensors to roll tilt of the animal (at 0.026–0.15 Hz, $\pm 10°$) either displayed a very small gain, as demonstrated for the triceps brachii, or were almost absent, as shown for the triceps surae ([34, 37]; see also [5]). In the first instance the responses were characterized by an increased activity during side-down tilt of the animal and a decreased activity during side-up tilt (α responses).

Systemic injection of an anticholinesterase at a dose which in previous experiments abolished the decerebrate rigidity (0.10–0.15 mg/kg, i.v. of eserine sulphate), also suppressed the EMG responses of the limb extensors to animal tilt [35]. However, for a lower dose (0.05–0.10 mg/kg, i.v.) only a slight decrease in decerebrate rigidity as well as in the myotatic stretch reflexes occurred. In this instance, either a distinct modulation of the multiunit activity of extensor muscles occurred during animal tilt if the EMG response was absent prior to the injection, as for the triceps surae (Fig. 1, upper records) [37, 54], or else the gain of the EMG response to animal tilt greatly increased it the labyrinth input was only weakly effective, as for the triceps brachii (Fig. 1, middle and lower records) [51]. Moreover, no significant changes in pattern and phase angle of the responses were observed. These results did not depend on the decreased postural activity induced by the anticholinesterase, since they were still obtained when the reduced background discharge of the limb extensors following injection was compensated by an increased static stretch of the muscle. The increase in response gain induced by the anticholinesterase was observed 5–10 min after the injection, reached the highest value in about 1 hour and then slowly declined. Interestingly, somatosensory or acoustic stimulations produced a recovery of postural activity in the four limbs and a decrease or suppression of the EMG modulation of limb extensors during animal tilt [51, 54].

The effects described above did not depend on the peripheral but rather on the central action of the anticholinesterase, since no change in EMG modulation occurred following injection of neostigmine methylsulphate (0.05–0.30 mg/kg, i.v.) which does not cross the blood–brain barrier [51, 54]. Moreover, administration of the muscarinic blocker atropine sulphate (0.1–0.5 mg/kg, i.v.), which crosses the blood–brain barrier, but not of atropine methylnitrate (0.1–2.0 mg/kg, i.v.) suppressed the action of eserine [51, 54].

Electrolytic lesions limited to the dorsal aspect of the pRF, from which a tegmento-reticular tract ending on the medullary inhibitory area originates [22, 59], not only decreased the response gain of the tri-

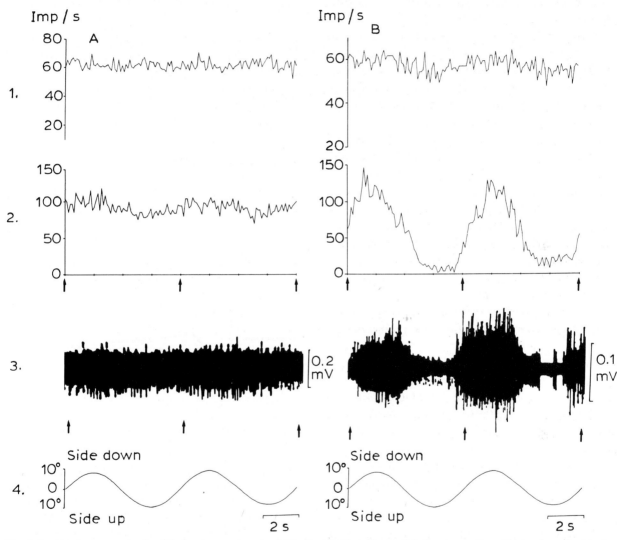

Fig. 1. Increase in response gain of limb extensors to animal tilt after injection of an anticholinesterase. Precollicular decerebrate cats. (1, 2) Sequential pulse density histograms (SPDHs) showing the averaged multiunit EMG responses of the left triceps surae (1) and the left triceps brachii (2) to roll tilt of the animal at 0.15 Hz, ± 10° (average of 7–12 sweeps, using 128 bins with 0.1 s bin width). The responses were recorded before (A) and after (B) individual or repetitive i.v. injection of 0.05–0.10 mg/kg of eserine sulphate. (3) Individual EMG traces of the triceps brachii contributing to the averaged responses illustrated in (2). (4) Animal displacement. Before injection of the anticholinesterase no modulation (A₁) or a slight modulation (A₂) of the EMG activity was observed. Injection of the anticholinesterase, which produced only a slight reduction of the spontaneous EMG activity of the limb extensors, brought to the light (B₁) or greatly increased (B₂) the amplitude of the EMG modulation to animal tilt. In particular, the mean gain of the first harmonic response of the triceps surae increased from 0 to 0.41 imp./s/deg, while that of the triceps brachii increased from 0.79 to 5.41 imp./s/deg. (From [51, 54]).

ceps brachii to labyrinth stimulation in normal decerebrate cats, but also prevented this gain from increasing after eserine injection [7]. This and other lines of evidence indicated that presumably cholinergic and cholinoceptive neurons activated by the anticholinesterase were located in the dorsal pRF [8].

If we combine these findings with those reported in the previous section, it appears that for the same labyrinth signal giving rise to excitatory VS volleys acting on extensor motoneurons, the amplitude of the EMG modulation of limb extensors depends on the relative resting discharge of both the LC neurons, from which the CS projection originates, and the dorsal pRF neurons, which drive the medullary inhibitory RS system. In particular, the higher the firing rate of the LC neurons in the animal at rest, the lower was the gain of the EMG responses of limb extensors to labyrinth stimulation. On the other hand, an increased discharge of the dorsal pRF neurons and the related medullary RS neurons led to an increased gain of the VS reflexes.

Responses of Renshaw cells to sinusoidal labyrinth stimulation following activation of a cholinergic system

Pompeiano et al. [53, 54] have recorded the response of R cells anatomically coupled with GS motoneurons during labyrinth stimulation in the two experimental conditions, i.e. before and after tonic activation of the cholinergic system. All the experiments were performed in precollicular decerebrate animals submitted to bilateral neck deafferentation, immobilized with pancuronium bromide (Pavulon, 0.6 mg/kg/h, i.v.; Organon, The Netherlands) and artificially ventilated. Moreover, both hindlimbs were denervated except for the nerves supplying the left GS muscle, which was de-efferented by section of the ventral roots L6-S2.

In the first group of experiments [53], the electrical activity of 47 R cells was recorded from L7 and upper S1 spinal-cord segments, both in the animal at rest as well as during bidirectional rotation of the head on the coronal plane (at 0.02–0.15 Hz, ± 10°)

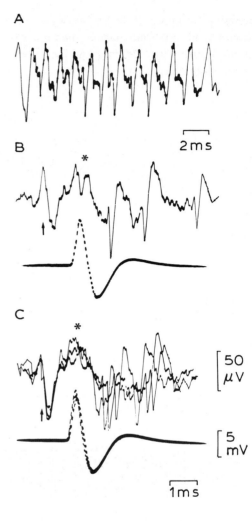

Fig. 2. Identification of a single Renshaw cell anatomically coupled with GS motoneurons (GS R cell). Precollicular decerebrate cat with bilateral neck deafferentation, paralyzed with pancuronium bromide. (A) Antidromic response of R cell following single-shock stimulation of the central end of L7 ventral root (0.2 ms pulse duration, 1.6 times the α threshold). (B, C) Single (B) and superimposed (C) orthodromic responses of the same R cell to stimulation of the ipsilateral GS nerve with 0.2 ms pulses, 2 times the threshold (T) for the group I afferents. The arrow indicates the field potential due to the orthodromic group I volley, and the asterisk indicates the field potential due to monosynaptic activation of the GS motoneurons, which coincides with the segmental monosynaptic reflex recorded from the ipsilateral ventral root L7 (lower record in B and C). The response of the R cell appears with a latency of 0.88 ms with respect to the peak of the segmental monosynaptic reflex, indicating that the reflex discharge of the GS motoneurons monosynaptically excited the R cell. (From [54].)

while the body remained fixed horizontally; due to neck deafferentation, this head displacement led to selective stimulation of labyrinth receptors. ARs of single units were recorded during successive cycles of head rotation. Among these R cells which responded monosynaptically to antidromic ventral root stimulation, 22 units were disynaptically excited by the orthodromic group I volleys induced by single-shock stimulation of the ipsilateral GS nerve, thus indicating that they were under the direct control of the recurrent collaterals of GS motoneurons monosynaptically driven by the orthodromic group Ia volleys (Fig. 2). It is of interest that these R cells increased their unit discharge in parallel with the amplitude of the GS monosynaptic reflex, the maximum activation being obtained at 1.6–2.0 T, i.e. when all the group Ia afferents contributing to the segmental monosynaptic reflex had been recruited by the stimulus (cf. [50, 58]). Moreover, the same units responded to static stretch of the corresponding muscle.

Among the 47 R cells tested, 9 units (2 of which coupled with GS motoneurons) were silent at rest and did not respond to head rotation, while the remaining 38 units (20 of which coupled with GS motoneurons), showed a spontaneous discharge at rest; moreover, among these spontaneously firing R cells, 31 units (16 of which coupled with GS motoneurons) responded to head rotation at either one or both the parameters indicated above. In resting animals with the ankle joint fixed at 90° dorsiflexion, all spontaneously active R cells fired at a low rate and their discharge rate closely corresponded to the mean firing rate (base frequency) evaluated during head rotation at 0.026 Hz, $\pm$ 10°. In particular, the base frequency evaluated for 24 spontaneously active units responsive to this stimulus (15 of which were coupled with GS motoneurons), corresponded to the average to 5.90 $\pm$ 5.35 imp./s (mean $\pm$ S.D.), while the gain and sensitivity of the first harmonic responses to head rotation at 0.026 Hz, $\pm$ 10° corresponded on the average to 0.075 $\pm$

0.059, imp./s/deg and 2.02 $\pm$ 2.08 %/deg (35 ARs). Moreover, the base frequency, as well as the gain and the sensitivity were on the average slightly higher for the 15 R cells coupled with the GS motoneurons (25 ARs) than for the 9 unidentified R cells (10 ARs).

As to the phase angle of the first harmonic responses of R cells to head rotation, most of the averaged responses (27 out of 35 ARs, i.e. 77.1%) recorded from 17 out of the 24 R cells were characterized by an increased discharge during side-down head rotation and a decreased discharge during side-up rotation and showed a phase angle which ranged from $\pm$ 90° to 0°, with a lead of + 3.1 $\pm$ 54.3° (mean $\pm$ S.D.) with respect to the extreme side-down head displacement (α responses). On the other hand, the responses recorded from the remaining 7 R cells (8 AR, i.e. 22.9%) showed a phase angle which varied from $\pm$ 90° to 180°, with a lag of $-$ 157.7 $\pm$ 69.6° (mean $\pm$ S.D.) (β responses). Similar results were also obtained from the averaged responses of R cells coupled with hindlimb extensor motoneurons, the majority of which (22 out of 25 AR, i.e. 88.0%) recorded from 13 out of 15 R cells showed α responses (Fig. 3A)*.

In addition to these findings, Pompeiano et al. [54] have recorded the activity of 9 R cells, 7 of which were anatomically coupled with the GS motoneurons, before and after systemic injection of an anticholinesterase. In the absence of drug injection, these R cells were either silent (1 unit) or fired at low rates at rest (8 units). The base frequency evaluated for the 9 R cells corresponded to 9.9 $\pm$ 9.6 imp./s (mean $\pm$ S.D.; 18 AR). Four out of 9 R cells (2 of which were coupled with the GS motoneurons) responded to head rotation at the parameters of 0.026–0.15 Hz, $\pm$ 10°; the remaining 5 R cells coupled with the GS motoneurons did not respond to the stimulus. The gain and the sensitivity of the first harmonic response of the R cells affected by head rotation corresponded to 0.074 $\pm$ 0.039 imp./s/deg and 1.62 $\pm$ 1.44 %/deg, respectively (mean $\pm$

---

*The results of these experiments can hardly be compared with those of more recent studies, in which responses of R cells elicited either by electrical stimulation of semicircular canal nerves [56] or during falling [57] were reported.

S.D.; 9 AR). Moreover, all these units displayed α responses with a phase lag of −10.4 ± 31.1° (mean ± S.D.) with respect to the extreme side-down head position as shown in the previous expe-

riments in which the activity of a larger population of R cells, particularly those coupled with GS motoneurons, was recorded [53].

After systemic injection of an anticholinesterase

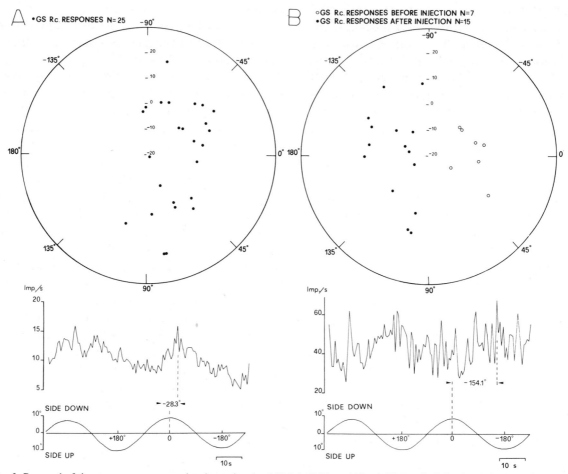

Fig. 3. Reversal of the response pattern to head rotation (at 0.026–0.15 Hz, ± 10°) of GS R cells following injection of an anticholinesterase under the same experimental conditions as in Fig. 2. (A, polar diagram) Dynamic characteristics of 25 ARs recorded from 15 GS R cells in normal decerebrate cats. (B, polar diagram) Characteristics of 7 ARs recorded from 2 GS R cells in the control situation (5 other GS R cells were unresponsive to head rotation), and 15 ARs recorded from 7 GS R cells after injection of an anticholinesterase (0.05–0.10 mg/kg, i.v. of eserine sulphate). The sensitivity of each response, defined as the percentage change of the mean firing rate per degree of displacement, is represented by the distance of the corresponding symbol from the centre of the diagram (see the scale along the vertical meridian in decibels). The relative position of the symbols with respect to the 0 meridian indicates in degrees the phase lead (positive values) or the phase lag (negative values) of responses with respect to the extreme side-down head displacement. Below each diagram, the upper record represents a SPDH (average of 8 sweeps, using 128 bins with 0.6 s bin width) showing the response of single GS R cells to head rotation at 0.026 Hz, ± 10°, while the lower trace indicates head position. In A the unit activity was recorded in a normal decerebrate cat and showed a base frequency of 11.0 imp./s; the response gain was 0.24 imp./s/deg, the sensitivity 2.15%/deg and the phase angle corresponded to a lag of −28.3° with respect to the extreme side-down head displacement. In B the unit activity was recorded 28 min after i.v. injection of 0.10 mg/kg eserine sulphate. In this instance the base frequency corresponded to 41.4 imp./s, the response gain was 0.39 imp./s/deg, the sensitivity 0.94%/deg, while the phase angle showed a lag of −154.1° with respect to the extreme side-down head displacement. (Modified from [53, 54].)

(0.05–0.10 mg/kg, i.v. of eserine sulphate), all the R cells which were silent or almost silent in normal decerebrate animals started to fire, whereas those which fired at a low rate prior to the injection increased their discharge rate later on. Therefore, the base frequency evaluated for the 9 R cells tested to head rotation (13.0 ± 12.7 imp./s (mean ± S.D.) for 20 AR) was higher than that obtained from the same units prior to the injection. All R cells tested, including those which did not respond to labyrinth stimulation, now showed a clearcut modulation of their firing rate to the parameters of head rotation reported above. In this instance, the gain and sensitivity of the first harmonic responses corresponded to 0.096 ± 0.087 imp./s/deg and 1.38 ± 1.19 %/deg, respectively (mean ± S.D.; 20 AR). The most striking finding, however, was that all units showed β responses, regardless of whether the R cells were either unresponsive or displayed an α response prior to the injection. There was a great scattering in the phase angle distribution, which ranged from ± 90° to 180°, the phase angle corresponding to a lag of − 179.0 ± 55.6° (mean ± S.D.) with respect to the extreme side-down head position. Similar results were also obtained if we considered only the AR recorded from R cells anatomically coupled with GS motoneurons (Fig. 3B).

The increase in mean firing rate as well as the reversal of the response pattern to head rotation in the spontaneously active units or the appearance of a β pattern of response in the silent units following injection of the anticholinesterase were on the average first detected 5 min after injection and persisted almost unmodified throughout the recording period (up to 35 min).

The effects elicited by injection of the anticholinesterase were state-dependent. In fact, a change in the 'waking' state of the animal following somatosensory or acoustic stimulation decreased the background discharge of the units and either suppressed the unit responses to head rotation or produced the reappearance of an α response. These findings can be related to the recovery of postural activity in the four limbs as well as to the reduced gain of the VS reflexes induced by the same stimuli in spite of injection of the anticholinesterase (see also [51]).

It is of interest that injection of the same doses of anticholinesterase performed after transection of the spinal cord at Th12 did not modify the activity of R cells anatomically linked with the GS motoneurons, which were silent or fired irregularly at a very low rate in the animal at rest; moreover, these units did not respond to head rotation at the parameters reported above [54].

Discussion

Experiments reported in the introduction have shown that the increased contraction of limb extensors which occurs during side-down animal tilt depends not only on the increased discharge of excitatory VS neurons (α responses [3, 4, 38, 61, 63]), but also on the reduced discharge of CS [1, 55] as well as of medullary RS neurons [36, 52] projecting to the corresponding segments of the spinal cord (β responses). This finding was apparently surprising, since both the CS and the medullary RS neurons exert an antagonistic influence on R cells linked with the limb motoneurons (see Introduction). The demonstration that in the decerebrate cat an increase or a decrease in postural activity depends on reciprocal changes in firing rate of LC neurons [48, 49] as well as of pRF neurons [18] and the related RS neurons originating from the inhibitory area of the mRF [62] led us to postulate that – in addition to changes in posture – changes in the VS reflexes may also occur, due to the predominant influence either of LC neurons and their direct projection to the spinal cord or of pRF neurons and the related medullary RS neurons. Experiments of unit recordings have in fact shown that during the state of postural rigidity occurring in precollicular decerebrate cats the LC neurons displayed a quite regular steady discharge [48, 49], while the pRF neurons [18] as well as the related medullary RS neurons [36, 52] fired at a very low rate; in this instance the gain of the VS reflexes, if present, was quite low [5, 34, 37, 54]. On the other hand the discharge rate of LC neurons decreased [48, 49] while that of pRF [18] and the related medullary RS neurons [62] increased during the episodes of postural hypotonia following i.v. administration of an anticholinesterase (0.05–0.10 mg/kg, i.v. of eserine sulphate); in this instance the gain of the VS reflexes greatly increased [37, 51]. These findings are of interest if we consider that the spontaneous discharge of LVN neurons did not change throughout these experiments [64]. It appears therefore that for the same labyrinth signal giving rise to excitatory VS volleys acting on ipsilateral limb extensor motoneurons, the gain of the corresponding VS reflexes depended on the predominant influence either of the CS or of the RS projection.

Let us examine first the results obtained in normal decerebrate cats, in which there is a prominent activity of LC neurons. In this instance the R cells anatomically linked with the GS motoneurons either fired at a low rate or were silent at rest [53]; this finding can be attributed to the tonic discharge of the CS neurons, leading to inhibition of R cell activity [14]. The same R cells either did not respond to standard parameters of head rotation or showed only a small-amplitude α response [53]. This response pattern can be attributed to the increased discharge of VS neurons during side-down rotation, which exerts an excitatory influence on GS motoneurons and, through their recurrent collaterals, on the related R cells. However, the simultaneous decrease in firing rate of the CS neurons for the same direction of head rotation [1, 55] would reduce the inhibitory influence that these neurons exert on R cells [14], thus enhancing the functional coupling of the R cells with their own extensor motoneurons. This finding explains why the response gain of limb extensors was negligible or absent in these preparations.

After systemic administration of the anticholinesterase, the resulting activation of pRF neurons and the related medullary RS neurons in the animal at rest increased the discharge rate of the R cells linked with the GS motoneurons [54]. The same R cells also responded to standard parameters of head rotation, but now all the tested units decreased their discharge during side-down head displacement (β responses), thus displaying a response pattern op-

posite to that obtained prior to the injection [54]. The increased discharge of the RS neurons and the related R cells following injection of the anticholinesterase would keep under the inhibitory control the limb extensor motoneurons in the animal at rest. However, the decrease in firing rate of the RS neurons during side-down head rotation would reduce the excitatory influence that these neurons exert on R cells ([15, 16, 25, 31]; for references see [46]). The increased disinhibition of limb extensor motoneurons which occurs for that direction of head displacement may thus increase the response gain of the corresponding extensor muscles to the same paremeters of rotation. We postulate, therefore that, following injection of the anticholinesterase, the R cells linked with the GS motoneurons escape the control of the VS pathway, thus being decoupled from their input motoneurons, and undergo the most efficient control of the RS pathway.

The great shift in the phase angle of R cells with respect to the extreme side-down (Fig. 3A) or side-up head displacement (Fig. 3B), as observed respectively in control experiments or after injection of the anticholinesterase, can still be attributed to stimulation of macular receptors if we assume that in both instances an interaction may occur at interneuronal level between the CS volleys exerting an inhibitory influence on R cells linked with GS motoneurons and the RS volleys exerting an excitatory influence on them. In fact, both these volleys acted in phase with respect to each other (β responses). However, while in the control experiments the CS influences would predominate over the RS influences, so that the reduced activity of CS neurons during side-down rotation would enhance the recruitment of R cells due to the motoneuronal discharge elicited by the VS volleys, after injection of the anticholinesterase the reduced activity of RS neurons for the same direction of head rotation would counteract the effects resulting from the increased discharge of GS motoneurons driven by the VS volleys, thus leading to derecruitment of the same R cells. It is likely that in this instance the small tonic motoneurons, which are more powerfully affected by recurrent inhibition [46], are more easily disinhibited during side-down tilt. Anatomical and physiological studies are required to find out whether the CS and the RS projections produce a higher number of synaptic contacts on the cell body and/or the proximal dendrites of R cells, than do the recurrent collaterals of the small-size tonic motoneurons ([26, 27]; for references see [46]).

A comparison between these findings and those obtained by recording the EMG responses of the triceps surae to animal tilt before and after injection of the anticholinesterase lead us to conclude that while in normal decerebrate cats the increased discharge of R cells during side-down head rotation would *limit the response gain* of the GS muscle to labyrinth stimulation, after injection of an anticholinesterase the reduced discharge of R cells for the same direction of head orientation would *enhance the response gain* of the GS muscle to the same labyrinth input.

The demonstration that, after injection of the anticholinesterase, the R cells coupled with GS motoneurons decreased their firing rate during side-down head rotation, while the EMG activity of the corresponding limb extensor muscle increased indicates that, under given conditions, the amount of motoneuronal activity and the related muscular force elicited during the VS reflexes may be determined by the activity of R cells.

There are a few other examples in the literature in which the activity of the two populations of α motoneurons and their target R cells may change reciprocally (cf. [46]). In our experiments it appears that the gain of the VS reflexes would decrease if the R cells are disinhibited by the CS mechanism, but would increase if the R cells are disfacilitated by the RS mechanism. The recurrent inhibition may thus act as a variable gain-regulator at the motoneuronal level (cf. [19]).

Acknowledgements

This study was supported by the NIH grant NS 07685-19 and a grant from the Ministero della Pubblica Istruzione, Roma, Italy.

References

[1] Barnes, C.D., D'Ascanio, P., Manzoni, D., Pompeiano, O. and Stampacchia, G. (1985) Responses of locus coeruleus neurons to sinusoidal stimulation of vestibular receptors. *Atti Soc. Ital. Biol., Soc. Ital. Fisiol., Soc. Ital. Nutr. um., Pisa*, Abstr. 164.

[2] Biscoe, T.J. and Curtis, D.R. (1966) Noradrenaline and inhibition of Renshaw cells. *Science*, 151: 1230–1231.

[3] Boyle, R. and Pompeiano, O. (1980) Reciprocal responses to sinusoidal tilt of neurons in Deiters' nucleus and their dynamic characteristics. *Arch. Ital. Biol.*, 118: 1–32.

[4] Boyle, R. and Pompeiano, O. (1981) Convergence and interaction of neck and macular vestibular inputs on vestibulospinal neurons. *J. Neurophysiol.*, 45: 852–868.

[5] Boyle, R. and Pompeiano, O. (1984) Discharge activity of spindle afferents from the gastrocnemius-soleus muscle during head rotation in the decerebrate cat. *Pflügers Arch.*, 400: 140–150.

[6] D'Ascanio, P., Bettini, E. and Pompeiano, O. (1985) Tonic inhibitory influences of locus coeruleus on the response gain of limb extensors to sinusoidal labyrinth and neck stimulations. *Arch. Ital. Biol.*, 123: 69–100.

[7] D'Ascanio, P., Bettini, E. and Pompeiano, O. (1985) Tonic facilitatory influences of dorsal pontine reticular structures on the response gain of limb extensors to sinusoidal labyrinth and neck stimulations. *Arch. Ital. Biol.*, 123: 101–132.

[8] D'Ascanio, P., Pompeiano, O. and Stampacchia, G. (1988) Noradrenergic and cholinergic mechanisms responsible for the gain regulation of vestibulospinal reflexes. In O. Pompeiano and J.H.J. Allum (Eds.) *Vestibulospinal Control of Posture and Locomotion, Progress in Brain Research, Vol. 76*, Elsevier, Amsterdam, pp. 361–374.

[9] Engberg, I. and Ryall, R.W. (1966) The inhibitory action of noradrenaline and other monoamines on spinal neurones. *J. Physiol. London*, 185: 298–322.

[10] Ezure, K. and Wilson, V.J. (1984) Interaction of tonic neck and vestibular reflexes in the forelimb of the decerebrate cat. *Exp. Brain Res.*, 54: 289–292.

[11] Foote, S.L., Bloom, F.E. and Aston-Jones, G. (1983) Nucleus locus coeruleus: new evidence of anatomical and physiological specificity. *Physiol. Rev.*, 63: 844–914.

[12] Fung, S.J. and Barnes, C.D. (1984) Locus coeruleus control of spinal cord activity. In C.D. Barnes (Ed.) *Brainstem Control of Spinal Cord Function, Research Topics in Physiology, Vol. 6*, Academic Press, Orlando, pp. 215–255.

[13] Fung, S.J. and Barnes, C.D. (1987) Membrane excitability changes in hindlimb motoneurons induced by stimulation of the locus coeruleus in cats. *Brain Res.*, 402: 230–242.

[14] Fung, S.J., Pompeiano, O. and Barnes, C.D. (1987) Suppression of the recurrent inhibitory pathway in lumbar cord segments during locus coeruleus stimulation in cats. *Brain Res.*, 402: 351–354.

94

[15] Haase, J. and Van der Meulen, J.D. (1961) Effects of supraspinal stimulation on Renshaw cells belonging to extensor motoneurones. *J. Neurophysiol.*, 24: 510–520.

[16] Haase, J. and Vogel, B. (1971) Direkte und indirekte Wirkungen supraspinaler Reizungen auf Renshaw-Zellen. *Pflügers Arch.*, 325: 334–346.

[17] Hobson, J.A. and Steriade, M. (1986) Neuronal basis of behavioral state control. In F.E. Bloom (Ed.) *Handbook of Physiology, Section 1, The Nervous System, Vol. IV, Intrinsic Regulatory Systems of the Brain*, American Physiological Society, Bethesda, pp. 701–823.

[18] Hoshino K, and Pompeiano, O. (1976) Selective discharge of pontine neurons during the postural atonia produced by an anticholinesterase in the decerebrate cat. *Arch. Ital. Biol.*, 114: 244–277.

[19] Hultborn, H., Lindström, S. and Wigström, H. (1979) On the function of recurrent inhibition in the spinal cord. *Exp. Brain Res.*, 37: 399–403.

[20] Hultborn, H. and Pierrot-Deseilligny, E. (1979) Input–output relations in the pathway of recurrent inhibition to motoneurones in the cat. *J. Physiol. London*, 297: 267–287.

[21] Jankowska, E., Lund, S., Lundberg, A. and Pompeiano, O. (1968) Inhibitory effects evoked through ventral reticulospinal pathways. *Arch. Ital. Biol.*, 106: 124–140.

[22] Jones, B.E. and Yang, T.-Z. (1985) The efferent projections from the reticular formation and the locus coeruleus studied by anterograde and retrograde axonal transport in the rat. *J. Comp. Neurol.*, 242: 56–92.

[23] Jordan, L.M., McCrea, D.A., Steeves, J.D. and Menzies, J.E. (1977) Noradrenergic synapses and effects of noradrenaline on interneurons in the ventral horn of the cat spinal cord. *Can. J. Physiol. Pharmacol.*, 55: 399–412.

[24] Jouvet, M. (1972) The role of monoamines and acetylcholine-containing neurons in the regulation of the sleep-waking cycle. *Ergebn. Physiol.*, 64: 166–307.

[25] Koizumi, K., Ushiyama, J. and Brooks, C. McC. (1959) A study of reticular formation action on spinal interneurones and motoneurones. *Jpn. J. Physiol.*, 9: 282–303.

[26] Lagerbäck, P.-A., Ronnevi, L.-O., Cullheim, S. and Kellerth, J.-O. (1978) Ultrastructural characteristics of a central cholinergic synapse in the cat. *Brain Res.*, 148: 197–201.

[27] Lagerbäck, P.-A., Ronnevi, L.-O., Cullheim, S. and Kellerth, J.-O. (1981) An ultrastructural study of the synaptic contacts of α_1-motoneuron axon collaterals. II. Contacts in lamina VII. *Brain Res.*, 222: 29–41.

[28] Lindsay, K.W., Roberts, T.D.M. and Rosenberg, J.R. (1976) Asymmetric tonic labyrinth reflexes and their interaction with neck reflexes in the decerebrate cat. *J. Physiol. London*, 261: 583–601.

[29] Llinás, R. and Terzuolo, C.A. (1964) Mechanisms of supraspinal actions upon spinal cord activities. Reticular inhibitory mechanisms on alpha extensor motoneurons. *J. Neurophysiol.*, 27: 579–591.

[30] Lund, S. and Pompeiano, O. (1968) Monosynaptic excitation of alpha-motoneurons from supraspinal structures in the cat. *Acta Physiol. Scand.*, 73: 1–21.

[31] MacLean, J.B. and Leffman, H. (1967) Supraspinal control of Renshaw cells. *Exp. Neurol.*, 18: 94–104.

[32] Magherini, P.C., Pompeiano, O. and Thoden, U. (1972) Cholinergic mechanisms related to REM sleep. I. Rhythmic activity of the vestibulo-oculomotor system induced by an anticholinesterase in the decerebrate cat. *Arch. Ital. Biol.*, 110: 234–259.

[33] Magoun, H.W. and Rhines, R. (1946) An inhibitory mechanism in the bulbar reticular formation. *J. Neurophysiol.*, 9: 165–171.

[34] Manzoni, D., Pompeiano, O., Srivastava, U.C. and Stampacchia, G. (1983) Responses of forelimb extensors to sinusoidal stimulation of macular labyrinth and neck receptors. *Arch. Ital. Biol.*, 121: 205–214.

[35] Manzoni, D., Pompeiano, O., Srivastava, U.C. and Stampacchia, G. (1983) Inhibition of vestibular and neck reflexes in forelimb extensor muscles during the episodes of postural atonia induced by an anticholinesterase in decerebrate cat. *Arch. Ital. Biol.*, 121: 267–283.

[36] Manzoni, D., Pompeiano, O., Stampacchia G. and Srivastava, U.C. (1983) Responses of medullary reticulospinal neurons to sinusoidal stimulation of labyrinth receptors in decerebrate cats. *J. Neurophysiol.*, 50: 1059–1079.

[37] Manzoni, D., Pompeiano, O., Srivastava, U.C. and Stampacchia, G. (1984) Gain regulation of vestibular reflexes in fore- and hindlimb muscles evoked by roll tilt. *Boll. Soc. Ital. Biol. Sper.*, 60, Suppl. 3: 9–10.

[38] Marchand, A., Manzoni, D., Pompeiano, O. and Stampacchia, G. (1987) Effects of stimulation of vestibular and neck receptors on Deiters neurons projecting to the lumbosacral cord. *Pflügers Arch.*, 409: 13–23.

[39] Matsuzaki, M. (1969) Differential effects of sodium butyrate and physostigmine upon the activities of para-sleep in acute brainstem preparations. *Brain Res.*, 13: 247–265.

[40] Matsuzaki, M., Okada, Y. and Shuto, S. (1968) Cholinergic agents related to para-sleep state in acute brain stem preparation. *Brain Res.*, 9: 253–267.

[41] Mergner, T., Magherini, P.C. and Pompeiano, O. (1976) Temporal distribution of rapid eye movements and related monophasic potentials in the brain stem following injections of an anticholinesterase. *Arch. Ital. Biol.*, 144: 75–99.

[42] Peterson, B.P., Pitts, N.G. and Fukushima, K. (1979) Reticulospinal connections with limb and axial motoneurons. *Exp. Brain Res.*, 36: 1–20.

[43] Pompeiano, O. (1975) Vestibulo-spinal relationships. In R.F. Naunton (Ed.), *The Vestibular System*, Academic Press, New York/San Francisco/London, pp. 147–180.

[44] Pompeiano, O. (1976) Mechanisms responsible for spinal inhibition during desynchronized sleep: experimental study. In C. Guilleminault, W.C. Dement and P. Passouant (Eds.), *Narcolepsy, Advances in Sleep Research, Vol. 3*, Spectrum, Flushing NY, pp. 411–449.

[45] Pompeiano, O. (1980) Cholinergic activation of reticular and vestibular mechanisms controlling posture and eye movements. In J. Hobson and M.A.B. Brazier (Eds.), *The Reticular Formation Revisited, IBRO Monograph Series, Vol. 6*, Raven Press, New York, pp. 473–512.

[46] Pompeiano, O. (1984) Recurrent inhibition. In R.A. Davidoff (Ed.), *Handbook of the Spinal Cord, Vol. 2-3*, Marcell Dekker, New York, pp. 461–557.

[47] Pompeiano, O. (1984) A comparison of the response characteristics of vestibulospinal and reticulospinal neurons to labyrinth and neck inputs. In C.D. Barnes (Ed.), *Research Topics in Physiology, Vol. 6. Brainstem Control of Spinal Cord Function*, Academic Press, New York, pp. 87–140.

[48] Pompeiano, O. and Hoshino, K. (1976) Tonic inhibition of dorsal pontine neurons during the postural atonia produced by an anticholinesterase in the decerebrate cat. *Arch. Ital. Biol.*, 114: 310–340.

[49] Pompeiano, O. and Hoshino, K. (1976) Central control of posture: reciprocal discharge by two pontine neuronal groups leading to suppression of decerebrate rigidity. *Brain Res.*, 116: 131–138.

[50] Pompeiano, O., Wand, P. and Sontag, K.-H. (1975) Response of Renshaw cells to sinusoidal stretch of hindlimb extensor muscles. *Arch. Ital. Biol.*, 113: 205–237.

[51] Pompeiano, O., Manzoni, D., Srivastava, U.C. and Stampacchia, G. (1983) Cholinergic mechanism controlling the response gain of forelimb extensor muscles to sinusoidal stimulation of macular labyrinth and neck receptors. *Arch. Ital. Biol.*, 121: 285–303.

[52] Pompeiano, O., Manzoni, D., Srivastava, U.C. and Stampacchia, G. (1984) Convergence and interaction of neck and macular vestibular inputs on reticulospinal neurons. *Neuroscience*, 12: 111–128.

[53] Pompeiano, O., Wand, P. and Srivastava, U.C. (1985) Responses of Renshaw cells coupled with hindlimb extensor motoneurons to sinusoidal stimulation of labyrinth receptors in the decerebrate cat. *Pflügers Arch.*, 403: 245–257.

[54] Pompeiano, O., Wand, P. and Srivastava, U.C. (1985) Influence of Renshaw cells on the gain of hindlimb extensor muscles to sinusoidal labyrinth stimulation. *Pflügers Arch.*, 404: 107–118.

[55] Pompeiano, O., Manzoni, D., Barnes, C.D., Stampacchia, G. and D'Ascanio, P. (1987) Labyrinthine influences on locus coeruleus neurons. *Acta Otolaryngol. Stock.*, 105: 576–581.

[56] Ross, H.-G. and Thewissen, M. (1987) Inhibitory connections of ipsilateral semicircular canal afferents to Renshaw cells in the lumbar spinal cord of the cat. *J. Physiol. London*, 388: 83–99.

[57] Ross, H.-G. and Wittrock, C. (1987) Renshaw cell activity in falling cats. *Pflügers Arch.*, 408 (Suppl. 1): R54.

[58] Ross, H.-G., Cleveland, S. and Haase, J. (1972) Quantitative relation of Renshaw cell discharges to monosynaptic reflex height. *Pflügers Arch.*, 332: 73–79.

[59] Sakai, K., Sastre, J.-P., Salvert, D., Touret, M., Tohyama, M. and Jouvet, M. (1979) Tegmentoreticular projections with special reference to the muscular atonia during paradoxical sleep in the cat: an HRP study. *Brain Res.*, 176: 233–254.

[60] Schor, R.H. and Miller, A.D. (1981) Vestibular reflexes in neck and forelimb muscles evoked by roll tilt. *J. Neurophysiol.*, 46: 167–178.

[61] Schor, R.H. and Miller, A.D. (1982) Relationship of cat vestibular neurons to otolith-spinal reflexes. *Exp. Brain Res.*, 47: 137–144.

[62] Srivastava, U.C., Manzoni, D., Pompeiano, O. and Stampacchia, G. (1982) State-dependent properties of medullary reticular neurons involved during the labyrinth and neck reflexes. *Neurosci. Lett. Suppl.* 10: S461.

[63] Stampacchia, G., Manzoni, D., Marchand, A.R. and Pompeiano, O. (1987) Convergence of neck and macular vestibular inputs on vestibulospinal neurons projecting to the lumbosacral segments of the spinal cord. *Arch. Ital. Biol.*, 125: 201–224.

[64] Thoden, U., Magherini, P.C. and Pompeiano, O. (1972) Cholinergic mechanisms related to REM sleep. II. Effects of an anticholinesterase on the discharge of central vestibular neurons in the decerebrate cat. *Arch. Ital. Biol.*, 110: 260–283.

[65] Weight, F.F. and Salmoiraghi, G.C. (1966) Adrenergic responses of Renshaw cells. *J. Pharmacol. Exp. Ther.*, 154: 391–397.

O. Pompeiano and J.H.J. Allum (Eds.)
Progress in Brain Research, Vol. 76
© 1988 Elsevier Science Publishers B.V. (Biomedical Division)

CHAPTER 8

Descending cortical and tectal control of dorsal neck motoneurons via reticulospinal neurons in the cat

Y. Iwamoto, S. Sasaki and I. Suzuki

*Department of Neurophysiology, Institute of Brain Research, School of Medicine, University of Tokyo, 7-3-1 Hongo, Bunkyo-ku,
Tokyo 113, Japan*

Dorsal neck motoneurons innervating SPL and BCC muscles received disynaptic exitatory effects after stimulation of the tectum and the pyramid in cats. These effects were mediated by RSNs in the NRPC and the NRG. While a majority of RSNs received monosynaptic excitatory inputs from the tectal and pyramidal volleys, RSNs in the NRPC and those in the NRG differed in the following points. The majority of RSNs in the NRPC received a larger input from the tectum than from the pyramid, and descended in the ipsilateral ventral funiculus in the C3 segment. RSNs in the NRG, in contrast, had a stronger input in general from the pyramid than from the tectum and descended in the ventrolateral or lateral funiculus of the ipsilateral side, or contralateral funiculi in the C3 segment. Studies of systematic threshold mapping for evoking antidromic spikes of RSNs in C2–C3 segments and intra-axonal staining of their descending axons in C1–C3 segments with horseradish peroxidase revealed the following. Among RSNs, those descending to brachial segments (C6–Th1) but not down to lumbar segments (C-RSNs) issued collaterals to the ventral horn of C1–C3 segments, while RSNs descending to the lumbar cord rarely gave off collaterals at C1–C3 segments. Direct monosynaptic excitatory connexions of C-RSNs in the NRPC and NRG with SPL and BCC motoneurons were demonstrated by the spike-triggered averaging method. Their connexions were muscle-specific. It was found that RSNs were last-order premotor relay neurons mediating descending commands from the cerebral cortex and the superior colliculus to neck motoneurons.

Introduction

Head movements play a key role in the orienting movements of directing and fixing the head and eyes toward a new target which has appeared in the periphery of the visual field [6]. This is especially important in the animals such as the cat in which the range of oculomotor movement is restricted to 15–20° [12].

Descending commands for the head movement have been considered to originate from the superior colliculus in visually triggered reflex movements and from the cerebral cortex (frontal eye field) in voluntary movements. With respect to neural pathways from these structures to neck motoneurons, stimulation of the superior colliculus and of the cerebral cortex has been shown to evoke disynaptic tectal and pyramidal EPSPs in the dorsal neck motoneurons, as shown in Fig. 1 [1, 2, 4]. Clear spatial facilitation of the EPSP from the tectal and pyramidal volleys (Fig. 1E) indicates that the two descending systems share common interneurons to evoke the EPSPs [1]. The tectal and pyramidal EPSPs and their spatial facilitation remain after interruption of the corticofugal fibres at the level of the obex, indicating that interneurons are located in the brainstem (Fig. 1). After interruption of corticofugal fibres at the level of mid-trapezoid body and the

---

Abbreviations: BCC, biventer cervicis and complexus; EPSP, excitatory postsynaptic potential; MLF, medial longitudinal fasciculus; NRG, nucleus reticularis gigantocellularis; NRPC, nucleus reticularis pontis caudalis; RSN, reticulospinal neuron; SPL, splenius.

obex, stimulation of corticofugal fibres between the two lesions still evoked the disynaptic EPSPs which were further facilitated by tectal stimulation. In contrast, stimulation of the cortifcofugal fibres at levels rostral to the mid-trapezoid body did not elicit any clear disynaptic EPSPs [1, 2]. This suggested that interneurons should be localized in the lower brainstem, i.e. in the pons and the medulla.

There have been abundant studies concerning the descending projections from the tectum and the cortex to the brainstem. Cortical efferent fibres terminate in the medial reticular formation and the trigeminal nucleus in the lower brainstem [5, 22, 23, 24, 26–29]. Tectal efferents from the deep layers terminate almost exclusively in the medial reticular formation in the pons and the medulla [3, 7, 8, 9, 15, 18, 20]. The above findings strongly suggested that medial RSNs are highly likely to be interneurons mediating the tectal and pyramidal disynaptic EPSPs of dorsal neck motoneurons. In fact, stimulation of the medial reticular formation of the pons and the medulla elicited monosynaptic EPSPs in the dorsal neck motoneurons [35]. However, the exact location of RSNs terminating on dorsal neck motoneurons, the course of their descending axons, and also the muscle specificity of their connexion with target motoneurons still remained to be studied. Thus, we attempted to identify the RSNs pro-

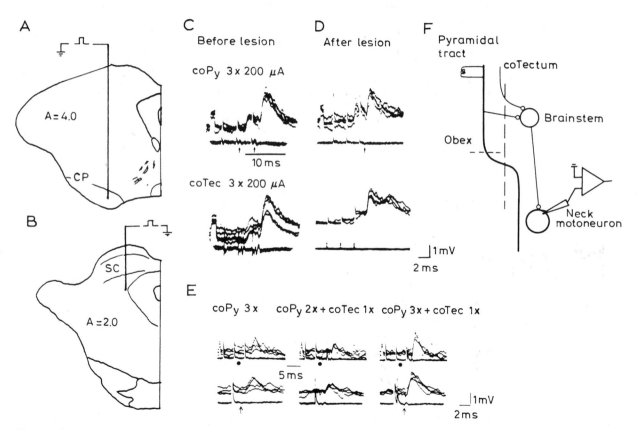

Fig. 1. Effects of lesions on pyramidal and tectal EPSPs of dorsal neck motoneurons. A and B indicate sites of stimulation in the cerebral peduncle (CP) and the tectum (SC), respectively. (C) Stimulation of the cerebral peduncle evoked disynaptic EPSPs before the pyramidal lesion (upper trace). The lower trace is a cord dorsum potential recorded near the glass micropipette. Arrows indicate the pyramidal direct volley. The lower trace is an example of tectal EPSP in the control cat. (D) Effects of a lesion of the pyramid at the level of the obex on the pyramidal (upper column) and tectal EPSPs (lower column). Note disappearance of the direct pyramidal volley (arrow). (E) Spatial facilitation of pyramidal EPSPs by the tectal volley. (F) A schematic diagram of pathways mediating the disynaptic pyramidal and tectal excitation.

jecting directly to neck motoneurons in cats using both anatomical and physiological methods.

Methods

Adult cats weighing 2.8–4.5 kg were anaesthetized with α-Chloralose (50 mg/kg) or Nembutal (40–50 mg/kg). Animals were immobilized by pancuronium bromide (Myoblock; Sankyo) and respired artificially.

Intracellular recordings were made with glass pipette microelectrodes filled with 2 M potassium citrate, having a resistance of 2–8 MΩ. Nerves supplying SPL and BCC muscles were dissected and stimulated bipolarly for identification of motoneurons. Various structures of the brain and spinal cord were stimulated monopolarly with tungsten needle electrodes insulated with lacquer except for at their tips. Efferent fibres from deep layers of the tectum were stimulated at the lateral border of the

central gray just before crossing to the contralateral side (A = 2.0, L = 2.5, H = −1.0, in Horsley-Clarke coordinates, Fig. 1B) to descend in the predorsal bundle. Corticofugal fibres were stimulated in the cerebral peduncle (A = 4.0, L = 4.0, H = −6.0, Fig. 1A).

Results

Descending pathways

Several lesion experiments were performed to define descending pathways to neck motoneurons. Fig. 2 shows the effects of a lesion of the MLF (A) through which most of the axons descending in the ventral funiculus pass down, and of a lesion of the lateral funiculus (B). Interruption of the MLF at 2–3 mm rostral to the obex reduced the tectal EPSPs by 70–90% in amplitude in all the 30 tested neck motoneurons supplying SPL and BCC muscles, while the pyramidal EPSPs decreased in amplitude

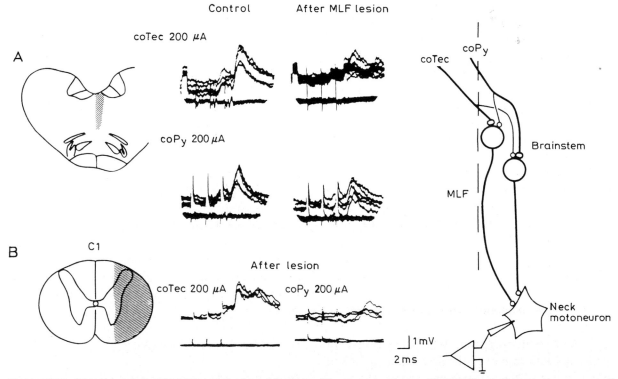

Fig. 2. Effects of lesions of the MLF (A) and the lateral funiculus (B) on tectal and pyramidal EPSPs. A diagram shows proposed neural circuits.

to only about a half of the control value (Fig. 2A). In contrast, tectal EPSPs were scarcely affected by a lesion of the lateral funiculus at C1, whereas pyramidal EPSPs were markedly reduced in amplitude down to 10–30% of those of intact cats in all the 30 motoneurons tested. Spatial facilitation between the two descending tracts in the lesioned cats was still observed as before the lesion. These results suggested that RSNs receiving large tectal and smaller pyramidal inputs descend in the ventral funiculus, while RSNs receiving a dominant input from the cerebral peduncle pass in the lateral funiculus (Fig. 2).

Descending volleys

To confirm the above interpretation, monosynaptic descending volleys elicited by stimulation of the tectum and the cerebral peduncle were explored systematically in the spinal funiculi in the C3 segment with a thick tungsten electrode (tip diameter, 100 μm). The volleys were recorded in a positive sign from the ends of axons which had been intentionally damaged by several up and down movements of the electrode. Stimulation of the superior colliculus evoked direct as well as monosynaptically evoked (P1 wave) volleys in the ventral funiculus. The amplitude of the P1 wave was largest in the ventromedial part of the ventral funiculus and became gradually smaller as the electrode was moved to more lateral or dorsal locations. In the ventromedial part of the ventral funiculus the monosynaptic volley evoked by stimulation of the cerebral peduncle was about one forth of the tectal monosynaptic volley at most. The pyramidal monosynaptic volley was, by contrast, recorded in wider areas extending from the ventral funiculus to the ventral half of the lateral funiculus.

Distribution of subgroups of reticulospinal neurons

The above results suggested that RSNs consist of subgroups with respect to the descending input and spinal course of their descending axons. The locations of individual RSNs in the pons and the medulla were systematically analysed in relation to their axonal course in the spinal funiculi and to inputs from the tectum and the cerebral peduncle.

While recording from single RSNs in the brainstem, the location of their descending axons in the C3 spinal cord was examined by finding low-threshold foci for their antidromic activation using an array of 5 tungsten electrodes inserted in the spinal funiculi as shown in Fig. 3A. Most of the RSNs were activated antidromically with the lowest threshold from one of the 5 electrodes as indicated in Fig. 3B, and thus the location of descending axons in the funiculi were unequivocally determined, except for in a few cases in which the thresholds were of similar value from two adjacent electrodes. They were classified into the following four groups: RSNs descending in the medial part of the ventral funiculus, those in the ventrolateral funiculus, those in the lateral funiculus and those in the contralateral funiculi, which are hereafter called RSNm, RSNml, RSNl and RSNc, respectively. Furthermore, RSNs projecting down to the C3 segment but not to C7 were defined as neck RSNs (N-RSNs), those descending up to C7 but not to the L1 were as cervical (C-RSNs) and those projecting down to L1 were as lumbar RSNs (L-RSNs). Fig. 3D shows the distribution of these subgroups of RSNs in the sagittal plane. RSNs in the NRPC almost invariably belonged to the RSNm, while those in the NRG belonged to the RSNml, RSNl or RSNc, which were intermingled in the NRG. There were no clear differences in the distribution between the N-, C- and L-RSNs, although the number of neurons sampled were numerous in the order of L-, C- and N-RSNs. In the frontal plane, their distribution was restricted within the medial two thirds of the reticular formation, extending from the midline to about 2 mm laterally, and dorsoventrally from 1 to 5.5 mm deep from the floor of the fourth ventricle.

Descending input to the RSNs

Stimulation of the contralateral tectum and of the cerebral peduncle evoked monosynaptic negative field potentials in the medial reticular formation in the pons and medulla. Rostrocaudally, the tectal field potential was large in the A2–P4 plane of Fig. 4A and progressively decreased in more caudal planes. Mediolaterally, it was almost restricted in the region extending from the midline to about 2 mm laterally. The pyramidal field potential was largest in the region extending from P4–P7 rostrocaudally and from the midline to 2 mm laterally in the mediolateral plane. However, it was about one third of the tectal field potential at most. In more rostral and caudal areas it was greatly reduced in amplitude.

Many of the RSNs in the above regions were excited by stimulation of the tectum and cerebral peduncle of the contralateral side with latencies of 1.0–2.8 ms, and 1.5–3.0 ms, respectively. Latencies less than 2.0 ms for tectal and 2.5 ms for pyramidal firing were taken as monosynaptic. More than 85% of RSNs in the NRPC which were located in the A2–P3 plane of Fig. 4A were activated monosynaptically from the tectum but only 20-30% were from the cerebral peduncle. In contrast, RSNs in the NRG (P4–P7) were activated more frequently from the cerebral peduncle (about 60% of RSNs) than from the tectum (about 30% of RSNs). This

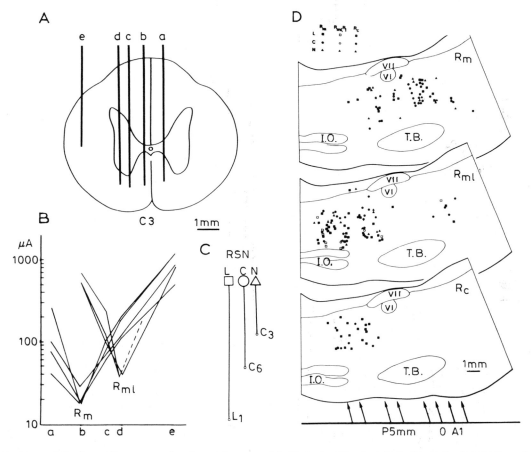

Fig. 3. Positions of the descending axons of various subgroups of RSNs in the C3 spinal funiculi and the distribution of subgroups of RSNs in the brainstem. (A) An array of 5 tungsten electrodes placed in C3 spinal funiculi. (B) Plots of the thresholds (ordinate) of antidromic spikes of each RSN against the 5 respective stimulating electrodes (a-e, abscissa). (C) A diagrammatic representation of N-, C- and L-RSNs. (D) Distributions of RSN subtypes in a parasagittal plane of the brainstem. Subtypes are indicated by different symbols. Rm, Rml and Rc refer to RSNs descended in the medial part of the ventral funiculus, in the ventrolateral funiculus and the contralateral funiculi, respectively.

is consistent with the idea that NRPC neurons receive input more from the tectum and less from the peduncle, while NRG neurons receive more pronounced input from the peduncle than from the tectum. This was further confirmed by recording intracellularly from many RSNs. As exemplified in Fig. 4B, larger EPSPs were evoked from the tectum than from the peduncle in RSNs in the NPRC, while the relation was reversed in NRG neurons (P5). A plot of the ratio of amplitudes of the tectal versus pyramidal EPSPs in many RSNs against their location revealed this relation clearly (Fig. 4C). These results were in good agreement with the findings described above.

Projection of C-RSNs to neck motoneurons

The latencies of the pyramidal and tectal EPSPs of neurons were compared with the sum of the latencies of the antidromic spikes from the C3 and that of orthodromic firing from the tectum and cerebral peduncle in each RSNs. The summed latencies were in the range of latencies of tectal (1.3–2.0 ms) EPSPs in C- and L-RSNs, but were longer than 2.0 ms in N-RSNs except for in two cells. This was also the case for pyramidal EPSPs. Thus only L- and C-RSN could contribute to the tectal and pyramidal EPSPs at the onset and the rising phase, while N-RSNs could contribute only to the very late part of the EPSPs.

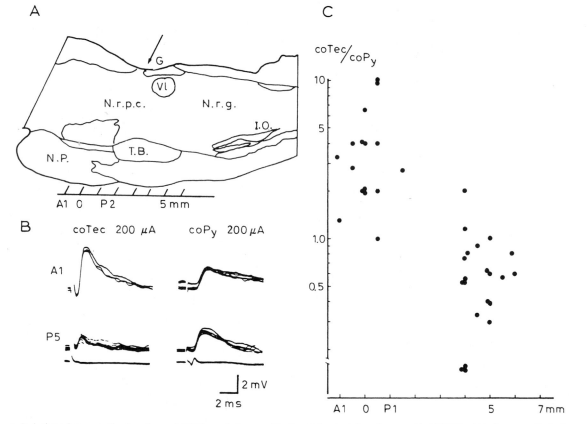

Fig. 4. Relations between the location of RSNs and the amplitude of the tectal and pyramidal EPSPs. (A) A presagittal plane of the brainstem 1 mm lateral from the midline. An arrow indicates a standard plane in the rostrocaudal coordinate. All electrodes were penetrated in parallel to the arrow. Each track was indicated by distances rostrally (A) or caudally (P) from the standard plane (AO/PO). (B) Examples of the tectal and pyramidal EPSPs of two RSNs located in A1 and P5 planes. (C) Plots of the ratio of the tectal versus pyramidal EPSP amplitude against the position of the recorded RSNs as a rostrocaudal coordinate. N.r.p.c, nucleus reticularis pontis caudalis; N.r.g., nucleus reticularis gigantocellularis; N.P., nucleus pontis; T.B, trapezoid body; I.O., inferior olive; G, genu facialis.

Stimulation of the C7 ventral funiculus evoked monosynaptic EPSPs of 2–5 mV in all the SPL and BCC motoneurons impaled, which were always larger than the disynaptic tectal and pyramidal EPSPs. The C7 evoked EPSPs cancelled out completely the tectal or pyramidal EPSPs in most of the cases when the two stimuli were given at proper intervals, indicating that most of the tectal and pyramidal EPSPs were mediated by RSNs projecting their descending axons down to the C7 segments. Stimulation of the ventral funiculus of L1 also induced monosynaptic EPSPs, but in only 35% of the motoneurons. The amplitude of L1 EPSPs were about 20–30% (range 5–55%) of the C7 evoked EPSPs. L1 evoked EPSPs also cancelled out tectal or pyramidal EPSPs. This shows that the contribu-

tion of L-RSNs, however, is likely to be small, since L1 evoked EPSPs were small both in the frequency of occurrence and in amplitude.

Branching of C-RSNs in the C2–C3 segments

To test whether C-RSNs in the NRPC and NRG project to the neck motor nucleus, systematic threshold mapping for evoking antidromic spikes was made in C2–C3 segments. In Fig. 5C, the size of circle indicates the threshold at each point and the numerals nearby indicate latencies of the antidromic spikes for a C-RSN in the NRPC (indicated by an asterisk in Fig. 5B). The stem axon is likely to descend in the ventral funiculus where the latencies were the shortest. Clear lengthening of latencies

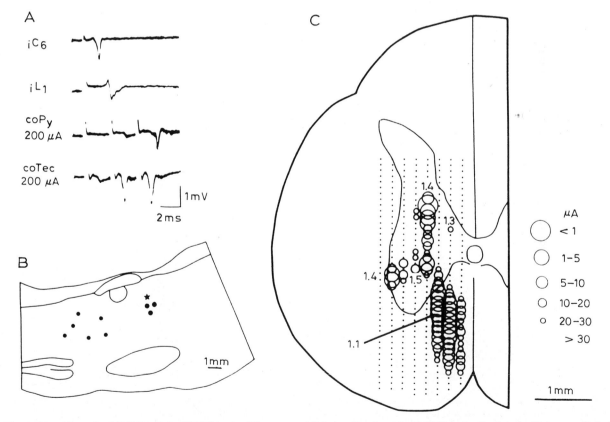

Fig. 5. Branching of a C-RSNm of the NRPC in the C3 segment. (A) Indentification of a C-RSN and orthodromic discharges elicited by the tectal volley. (B) Position of this RSN (asterisk) and other RSNs tested. (C) Threshold mapping for evoking antidromic spikes of the RSN shown in A. Thresholds are indicated by the sizes of the circles and numerals nearby are latencies of spikes elicited antidromically from the points.

in the gray matter and patch-like distribution of the low-threshold areas in the ventral horn strongly suggests that the axon projected there. Such branchings were obtained in all the ten C-RSNs in which more than 10 transverse planes were tested systematically. The analysed neurons distributed both in the NRPC and NRG, as shown in Fig. 5B.

Axonal trajectory of C-RSNs

To obtain a detailed picture of their axonal trajectory, intra-axonal staining of the C-RSNs was performed. C-RSNs were identified by the location of the descending axons, antidromic invasion from the C7 but not from the L1 segment and monosynaptic excitation from both the tectum and the cerebral peduncle of the contralateral side.

Fig. 6 shows the trajectories of two C-RSN axons. The axon in A passes in the medial part of the ventral funiculus, and therefore is likely to originate from the NRPC. Collaterals are given off from the stem axon toward the ventral horn, entering the gray matter from its medial border. Within the ventral horn many collaterals are given off, and terminals are distributed mainly in lamina IX, where neck motor nuclei are located [38]. Many terminals were observed to be closely apposed to the soma and proximal dendrites of large motoneuron-like neurons. Five other axons in the ventral funiculus were successfully stained. Their spinal trajectories were similar to that in Fig. 6A in principle. Fig. 6B exemplifies an axon which passes in the ventrolateral funiculus, and thus is most likely to originate from a C-RSN in the NRG. It gives off terminals

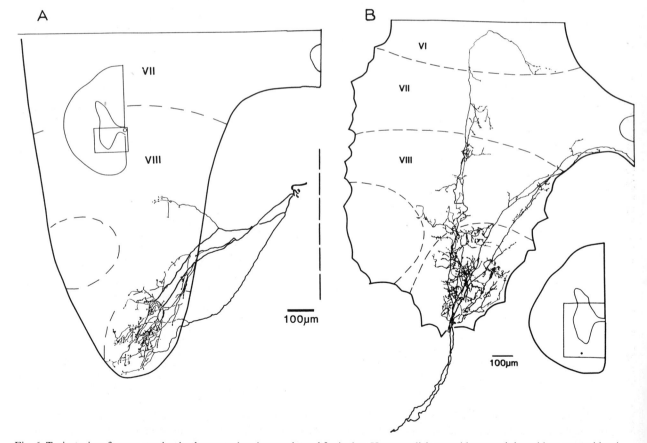

Fig. 6. Trajectories of axons passing in the ventral and ventrolateral funiculus. Horeseradish peroxidase was injected into axons identified physiologically. The drawings were reconstructed from the serial sections of 100 μm.

chiefly in lamina IX, where neck motor nuclei are situated, but scarcely in lamina IX of the spinal accessory nucleus. In two other C-RSNs whose stem axons were located similarly, terminals were distributed predominantly in the spinal accessory nucleus but rarely in lamina IX of neck motoneurons. These findings suggest a highly specific projection of single axons to different motor nuclei. Axons passing in the lateral funiculus terminated either in laminae VII and VIII, or predominantly in the spinal accessory nucleus. In each case, many boutons were observed to be closely apposed to the proximal dendrite or soma of neurons of various size.

Monosynaptic excitatory connexions of RSNs with dorsal neck motoneurons

Direct monosynaptic connexions of C-RSNs with dorsal neck motoneurons were verified by the spike-triggered averaging method. The experimental arrangement is shown in Fig. 7C. The cell shown in Fig. 7 was located in the NRG (asterisk in B), antidromically activated from C6 but not from L1 (A, hence C-RSN), and monosynaptically activated from the tectum (A, coTec) and the cerebral peduncle (not illustrated). The axon descended in the ventrolateral funiculus as revealed by low threshold

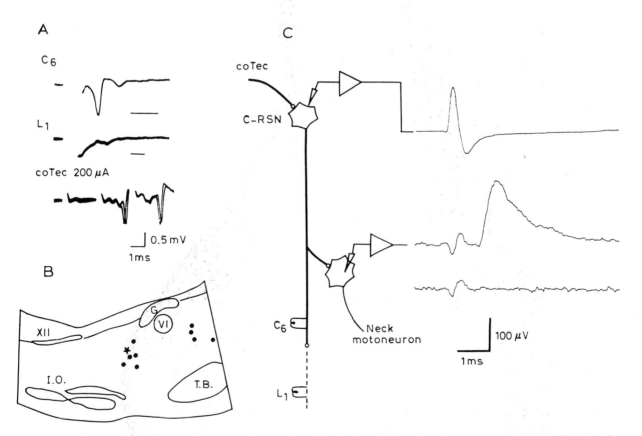

Fig. 7. A direct evidence of monosynaptic excitatory connexion of a C-RSN with dorsal neck motoneurons. (A) Identification of a C-RSN, and orthodromic firing from the tectal volley. (B) The position of this C-RSN (asterisk) and other C-RSNs which had monosynaptic connexions with neck motoneurons: T.B., trapezoid body; I.O., inferior olive; G, genu facialis. (C) Experimental arrangements of the spike-triggered averaging and a unitary EPSP. The lowest trace is the extracellular unitary field potential. The positive–negative waves in the middle and the lowest trace which appear in close relation with the triggered spike are cross-talk of the latter to the intracellular recording system.

(less than 5 μA) foci therein. Computer averaging of synaptic noise of a SPL motoneuron triggered by spontaneous spikes of the C-RSN showed that a unitary EPSP was evoked. The latency of the EPSP was 0.8 ms from the onset of the triggering spike, and hence was in the range of monosynaptic connexion. Such unitary EPSPs were obtained in 32 pairs of motoneurons (32 cells) and C-RSNs (10 cells). The amplitude of unitary EPSPs ranged between 10 and 200 μV. The latencies varied between 0.8 and 1.7 ms. The ten C-RSNs which made monosynaptic excitatory connexions with SPL and/or BCC motoneurons were located both in the NRPC and NRG, as shown in Fig. 7B.

Muscle specificity of the connexion

The spike-triggered averaging technique was applied to many motoneurons to answer the question of how single C-RSNs make specific connexion with motoneurons of functionally different dorsal neck muscles: SPL as the lateral head flexor and BCC as the head elevator. Most C-RSNs examined were found to make connexion preferentially with either SPL or BCC motoneurons. C-RSNs in the NRPC were connected predominantly with SPL motoneurons, while C-RSNs in the NRG made connexion with BCC motoneurons as frequently as SPL motoneurons, where the muscle specificity of connexion was kept in each cell.

Discussion

There have hitherto been many studies suggesting connexion of RSNs of the pontomedullary reticular formation with motoneurons supplying axial muscles including neck muscles. Studies using anterograde degeneration methods [32, 36] and anterograde transport of labelled amino acid [17] have revealed that RSNs in the pontomedually reticular formation densely project to motor nuclei supplying axial muscles including neck muscles as well as laminae VII and VIII of Rexed [37] in cats. It is also known that stimulation of various sites of pontomedullary reticular formation induces monosy-

naptic EPSPs in many species of motoneurons supplying neck, forelimb and hindlimb muscles [19, 34, 35].

The present study has provided evidence of the monosynaptic excitatory connexion of RSNs of the NRPC and NRG with dorsal neck motoneurons supplying SPL and BCC muscles. Noteworthy is the muscle specificity of the connexion of RSNs with dorsal neck motoneurons. The muscle specificity of RSN connexions would make it possible for higher centres to have access to individual muscles and to specify a proper group of muscles in particular movements. This is of great importance with respect to the function of RSNs, since SPL and BCC muscles differ in their actions. The SPL muscle is active when a cat turns the head ipsilaterally, while it is silent during elevation of the head. The BCC muscles are tonically active in the normal standing position and show burst activity during head elevation, and usually depression prior to lateral flexion of the head in the cat (T. Isa and S. Sasaki, unpublished observations).

With respect to the cortical origin of the input to RSNs, projection from the area 6aβ and the medial part of area 4γ [16] of the anterior sylvian gyrus have been shown by retrograde transport of horseradish peroxidase injected in the pontomedully reticular formation in the cat [19, 21]. These regions correspond to the frontal eye field [13, 14, 41, 42] and neck and trunk areas [31] in the cat. Stimulation of the respective areas is shown to elicit coordinated eye and head movements [13, 14] and movements of the head or the trunk in the cat [31]. Stimulation of the tectum has also been shown to produce organized eye and head movements in the cat [11, 40]. Since descending tracts from these centres is now shown to converge on neurons of the NRPC and the NRG (cf. also [33]), it is tempting to consider that the NRPC and NRG form the centre of eye–head coordination.

Movements are usually associated with a shift in the centre of gravity of the body, and therefore it seems absolutely necessary to adjust posture prior to and during movements. This was, in fact, clearly demonstrated during tactile limb placing reactions in the cat by Massion [30]. In this connexion descending collaterals of C-RSNs to the brachial segment and more lower segments is of great interest. These descending collaterals have been shown to terminate predominantly in laminae VIII and VII, less in lamina VI and very little in lamina IX of limb motor nuclei (S. Sasaki, unpublished observations). This would imply that when the head moves, the same descending commands are transmitted in parallel to these spinal neuronal circuitries. Since neurons in lamina VIII–VI receive inputs from vestibulospinal tracts and polysynaptic inputs from primary afferents, they could provide the spinal reflex centres with information about the head position in space and about peripheral conditions of the limb. Thus, spinal motor centres of laminae VIII–VI could integrate all the information required for postural adjustment during head movements. In this way descending collaterals of C-RSNs may be involved in the postural control of the body during head movements.

Acknowledgements

The authors wish to express their gratitude to Prof. H. Shimazu for continuous support during the course of this study. This study was supported by Grants from the Ministry of Education, Science and Culture of Japan (Project Nos. 58570051, 59570051, 60480104) and the grant provided by the Ichiro Kanehara Foundation.

References

[1] Alstermark, B., Pinter, M. and Sasaki, S. (1983) Convergence on reticulospinal neurons mediating contralateral pyramidal disynaptic EPSPs to neck motoneurons. *Brain Res.*, 259: 151–154.

[2] Alstermark, B., Pinter, M.J. and Sasaki, S. (1985) Pyramidal effects in dorsal neck motoneurones of the cat. *J. Physiol. London*, 363: 287–302.

[3] Altman, J. and Carpenter, M.B. (1961) Fiber projections of the superior colliculus in the cat. *J. Comp. Neurol.*, 116: 157–177.

[4] Anderson, M.E., Yoshida, M. and Wilson, V.J. (1971) Influence of superior colliculus on cat neck motoneurons. *J. Neurophysiol.*, 34: 898–907.

[5] Astruc, J. (1971) Corticofugal connections of area 8 (frontal eye field) in *Macaca mulatta. Brain Res.*, 33: 241–256.

[6] Bizzi, E., Kaili, R.E. and Tagliasco, V. (1971) Eye-head coordination in monkeys: evidence for centrally patterned organization. *Science*, 173: 452–454.

[7] Edwards, S.B. and Henkel, C.K. (1978) Superior colliculus connections with the extraocular motor nuclei in the cat. *J. Comp. Neurol.*, 179: 451–467.

[8] Graham, J. (1977) An autoradiographic study of the efferent connections of the superior colliculus in the cat. *J. Comp. Neurol.*, 173: 629–654.

[9] Grantyn, A. and Grantyn, R. (1982) Axonal patterns and sites of termination of cat superior colliculus neurons projecting in the tecto-bulbo-spinal tract. *Exp. Brain Res.*, 46: 243–256.

[10] Grillner, S. and Lund, S. (1968) The origin of a descending pathway with monosynaptic action on flexor motoneurones. *Acta Physiol. Scand.*, 74: 274–284.

[11] Guitton, D., Crommelinck, M. and Roucoux, A. (1980) Stimulation of the superior colliculus in the alert cat. I. Eye movement and neck EMG activity evoked when the head is restrained. *Exp. Brain Res.*, 39: 63–73.

[12] Guitton, D., Douglas, R.M. and Volle, M. (1984) Eye-head coordination in cats. *J. Neurophysiol.*, 52: 1030–1050.

[13] Guitton, D. and Mandl, G. (1978) Frontal 'oculomotor' area in alert cat. I. Eye movements and neck activity evoked by stimulation. *Brain Res.*, 149: 295–312.

[14] Guitton, D. and Mandl, G. (1978) Frontal 'oculomotor' area in alert cat. II. Unit discharges associated with eye movements and neck muscle activity. *Brain Res.*, 149: 313–327.

[15] Harting, J.K. (1977) Descending pathways from the superior colliculus: An autoradiographic analysis in the rhesus monkey (*Macaca mulatta*). *J. Comp. Neurol.*, 173: 583–612.

[16] Hassler, R. and Muhs-Clement, K. (1964) Architektonischer Aufbau des sensorimotorischen und parietalen Cortex der Katze. *J. Hirnforsch.*, 6: 377–420.

[17] Holstege, G. and Kuypers, H.G.J.M. (1982) The anatomy of brain stem pathways to the spinal cord in cat. A labeled amino acid tracing study. In H.G.J.M. Kuypers and G.F. Martin (Eds.), *Descending Pathways to the Spinal Cord, Progress in Brain Research, Vol. 57*, Elsevier, Amsterdam, pp. 145–175.

[18] Huerta, M.F. and Harting, J.K. (1982) Tectal control of spinal cord activity: Neuroanatomical demonstration of pathways connecting the superior colliculus with the cervical spinal cord grey. In H.G.J.M. Kuypers and G.F. Martin (Eds.), *Descending Pathways to the Spinal Cord, Progress in Brain Research, Vol. 57*, Elsevier, Amsterdam, pp. 293–328.

[19] Isa, T. and Sasaki, S. (1986) Input organization of reticulospinal neurons from the cerebral cortex and tectum in the cat. *J. Physiol. Soc. Jpn.*, 48: 297.

[20] Kawamura, K., Brodal, A. and Hoddevik, G. (1974) The projection of the superior colliculus onto the reticular formation of the brainstem. An experimental study in the cat. *Exp. Brain Res.*, 19: 1–19.

[21] Keizer, K. and Kuypers, H.G.J.M. (1984) Distribution of corticospinal neurons with collaterals to lower brainstem reticular formation in cat. *Exp. Brain Res.*, 54: 107–120.

[22] Künzle, H. and Akert, K. (1977) Efferent connections of cortical area 8 (frontal eye field) in *Macaca fascicularis*. A reinvestigation using the autoradiographic technique. *J. Comp. Neurol.*, 173: 147–164.

[23] Kuypers, H.G.J.M. (1958) An anatomical analysis of corti-co-bulbar connexions to the pons and lower brainstem in the cat. *J. Anat. London*, 92: 198–218.

[24] Leichnetz, G.R. (1980) An anterogradely-labeled prefrontal cortico-oculomotor pathway in the monkey demonstrated with HRP gel and TMB neurohistochemistry. *Brain Res.*, 198: 440–445.

[25] Leichnetz, G.R. (1982) Connections between the frontal eye field and pretectum in the monkey: an anterograde/retro-grade study using HRP gel and TMB neurohistochemistry. *J. Comp. Neurol.*, 207: 394–402.

[26] Leichnetz, G.R (1985) The frontal eye field projects to the nucleus prepositus hypoglossi in the monkey. *Neurosci. Lett.*, 54: 185–188.

[27] Leichnetz, G.R., Smith, D.J. and Spencer, R.F. (1984) Cortical projections to the paramedian tegmental and basilar pons in the monkey. *J. Comp. Neurol.*, 228: 388–408.

[28] Leichnetz, G.R., Spencer, R.F., Hardy, S.G.P. and Astruc, J. (1981) The prefrontal corticotectal projection in the monkey: an anterograde and retrograde horseradish peroxidase study. *Neuroscience*, 6: 1023–1041.

[29] Leichnetz, G.R., Spencer, R.F. and Smith, D.J. (1984) Cortical projections to nuclei adjacent to the oculomotor complex in the medial dien-mesencephalic tegmentum in the monkey. *J. Comp. Neurol.*, 228: 359–387.

[30] Massion, J. (1979) Role of motor cortex in postural adjustments associated with movement. In H. Asanuma and V.J. Wilson (Eds.), *Integration in the Nervous System*, Igakushoin, Tokyo, pp. 239–258.

[31] Nieoullon, A. and Rispal-Padel, L. (1976) Somatotopic localization in cat motor cortex. *Brain Res.*, 105: 405–422.

[32] Nyberg-Hansen, R. (1965) Sites and mode of termination of reticulo-spinal fibers in the cat. An experimental study with silver impregnation methods. *J. Comp. Neurol.*, 124: 71–100.

[33] Peterson, B.W., Anderson, M.E. and Filion, M. (1974) Responses of ponto-medullary reticular neurons to cortical, tectal and cutaneous stimuli. *Exp. Brain Res.*, 21: 19–44.

[34] Peterson, B.W., Pitts, N.G., Fukushima, K. and Mackel, R. (1978) Reticulospinal excitation and inhibition of neck motoneurons. *Exp. Brain Res.*, 32: 471–489.

[35] Peterson, B.W., Pitts, N.G. and Fukushima, K. (1979) Reticulospinal connections with limb and axial motoneurons. *Exp. Brain Res.*, 36: 1–20.

[36] Petras, J.M. (1967) Cortical, tectal and tegmental fiber connections in the spinal cord of the cat. *Brain Res.*, 6: 275–324.

[37] Rexed, B. (1954) A cytoarchitectonic atlas of the spinal cord in the cat. *J. Comp. Neurol.*, 100: 297–379.

[38] Richmond, F.J.R., Scott, D.A. and Abrahams, V.C. (1978) Distribution of motoneurones to the neck muscles, biventer cervicis, splenius and complexus in the cat. *J. Comp. Neurol.*, 181: 451–464.

[39] Rossi, G.F. and Brodal, A. (1956) Corticofugal fibres to the brainstem reticular formation. An experimental study in the cat. *J. Anat. London*, 90: 42–63.

[40] Roucoux, A., Guitton, D. and Crommelinck, M. (1980) Stimulation of superior colliculus in the alert cat. II. Eye and head movements evoked when the head unrestrained. *Exp. Brain Res.*, 39: 75–85.

[41] Schlag, J. and Schlag-Rey, M. (1970) Induction of oculomotor responses by electrical stimulation of the prefrontal cortex in the cat. *Brain Res.*, 22: 1–13.

[42] Tamai, Y., Fujii, T., Nakai, M., Komai, N. and Tsujimoto, T. (1983) Eye movements evoked by electrical stimulation of the frontal cortex in the coronary sulcus of the cat. *Jpn. J. Physiol.*, 33: 305–308.

[43] Valverde, F. (1962) Reticular formation of the albino rat's brainstem: cytoarchitecture and corticofugal connections. *J. Comp. Neurol.*, 119: 25–54.

[44] Walberg, F. (1957) Do the motor nuclei of the cranial nerves receive corticofugal fibers? An experimental study in the cat. *Brain*, 80: 597–605.

O. Pompeiano and J.H.J. Allum (Eds.)
Progress in Brain Research, Vol. 76
© 1988 Elsevier Science Publishers B.V. (Biomedical Division)

CHAPTER 9

Effects of proprioceptive inputs on vestibulo-ocular and vestibulospinal mechanisms

U. Thoden and T. Mergner

Neurologische Universitätsklinik, Hansastrasse 9, D-7800 Freiburg i. Br., F.R.G.

Effects of proprioceptive inputs on the oculomotor and the skeletomotor system in general, and on the vestibular reflexes of these systems in particular, are considered. As concluded from the literature and from our own experimental data, proprioceptive effects on gaze stabilization appear to be weak and equivocal in normal adults as concerns the slow components of the eye reflex. By contrast, given a certain behavioural set, proprioceptive effects on saccadic gaze shifts were found to be prominent and unequivocal. It is postulated that the proprioceptive input in normal adults is involved in mechanisms that select between two different behavioural states, one being related to the maintenance of spatial orientation of the self relative to the outer world, the other to a re-orientation. With respect to the vestibulospinal system, preliminary evidence for a gating of this system by proprioceptive inputs is presented.

Introduction

It is known that posture and gaze are rather effectively stabilized even in the absence of vision. An essential contribution to these mechanisms stems from the vestibular system that informs the brain about movements of the head in space. Other inputs are known to originate from proprioceptors. Proprioceptors in the neck, conceivably, provide information on the relative movement between head and trunk, and, at least theoretically, they could complete the vestibular information to also allow the control of trunk position in space. The message from proprioceptors in the limbs could be used to evaluate the relative movement between the trunk and its ground support and thus could deliver additional information on self-motion. However, little is known so far on how this sensory information is transformed into the appropriate outputs, despite the fact that a considerable amount of experimental data on these issues has been collected in the last decades. In the following we shall look at some of these data and emphasise particular findings that we think to be of relevance in the intact and mature individual.

Contributions of arthrokinetic information to eye movements

In humans, movements of the extremities relative to the trunk may induce self-motion sensation and nystagmus. In experiments of Brandt et al. [1], blindfolded subjects were sitting upright on a stationary turning chair that was surrounded by a drum rotating with constant velocity. When subjects firmly placed their hands on the inner wall of the drum, such that their arms were passively rotated in the shoulder joints for about ninety degrees, after a latency of one to several seconds a sensation of self-rotation counter to, and a nystagmus slow

---

Abbreviations: COR, cervico-ocular reflex; EMG, electromyograph; EOG, electro-oculogram; SA, saccadic amplitude; SF, saccadic frequency; SPV, slow-phase velocity; VOR, vestibulo-oculomotor reflex.

phase in the direction of, the arm rotation could a- rise. At the lowest stimulus velocity, 10 deg/s, the 'gain' reached about 0.5, but it rapidly saturated at higher velocities, not exceeding 10–15 deg. Eye po- sition in the orbit ('Schlagfeld') was shifted towards the perceived self-rotation, obviously due to large nystagmus quick phases. The effects showed a high intra- and interindividual variability and, if promi- nent, were followed by positive after-effects. They were said to occur neither with corresponding ac- tive arm movements nor with the tactile movement stimulus that arose when subjects let the drum slip over the palm of their hands if the latter were held stationary.

The authors interpreted their findings as being in line with a functionally significant somatosensory– vestibular convergence in the central vestibular sys- tem. Indeed, convergence of arthrokinetic and ves- tibular inputs have been observed in unidentified neurons of the vestibular nuclei of the cat [2] and in neurons that project into the medial longitudinal fasciculus [3]. The input mainly stems from proxi- mal joints, i.e. from the hip and shoulder as well as from the knee and elbow joints [4]. Such convergen- ces have also been observed in vestibular neurons of the thalamus [5] and the cortex of the monkey [6] as well as of the cortex of the cat [7–9]. Thus, the question arises whether we are dealing with some kind of somatosensory reflex on the eyes, which is comparable to and, under certain circum- stances, interacts with, the VOR.

However, nystagmus and/or the sensation of self- motion may also be observed in a variety of condi- tions which we hardly would consider as reflexes. Such conditions may consist of moving sound sour- ces that give the impression of relative motion be- tween the self and the 'acoustic surround' [10, 11], of the hypnotic suggestion [12] or the imagination [13] of seen motion, and of tactile motion cues ap- plied to the sole of the feet and the palms of the hands [14]. Furthermore, the effects may occur dur- ing 'apparent stepping around', i.e. if subjects are walking on a moving platform, thereby maintain- ing an almost constant position in space, as re- ported by Bles and coworkers [15, 16]. These au-

thors attribute the latter finding to the somatosensory input that arises during walking, while Lackner and DiZio [14], who compared passi- ve and active conditions, attribute them, at least in part, to efferent signals. The great variety of effec- tive 'inputs' for nystagmus and self-motion sensa- tion sheds some doubts on a theory according to which all the 'inputs' simply converge on the vesti- bulo-oculomotor system and the perceptual system for self-motion.

Under most 'normal' conditions one would ex- pect that the proprioceptive input is activated in combination with the vestibular input. One could therefore speculate that the role of the propriocepti- ve input is to compensate for the known deficiency of the VOR, which, with passive horizontal rota- tions in the dark, has a gain clearly below unity, and which deteriorates even more at stimulus fre- quencies below 0.1 Hz. However, a detailed and complete study on this question is missing so far. The effect of an arthrokinetic input to the VOR in subjects who actively stabilized their heads on their trunks, has recently be investigated by the group of one of the authors (Thoden; [17, 18]). Essential points of this study will be described in the follow- ing.

In particular, 15 subjects (male and female stu- dents) were seated blindfolded on a rotation chair. In order to have a constant baseline of vigilance a- cross the different experimental conditions, they performed controlled mental arithmetics through- out the tests. Eye movements were recorded by DC electro-oculography and analysed from a strip chart recorder. Whole body rotations were applied sinusoidally about the vertical axis with a constant amplitude of $\pm 20°$, the frequencies were 0.05, 0.1, 0.2 and 0.33 Hz. Subjects wore a light helmet, which was attached to a rotatable axis suspended from an earth-fixed frame. The axes of the helmet and the turning chair were co-linear. Helmet rota- tion in space was recorded with the help of a poten- tiometer and compared to the chair rotation in spa- ce in order to assure that subjects did not actively turn their head.

Nystagmus was compared across the following

three conditions:

A. *Passive VOR*. Subjects leaned their heads against a neck support fixed to the turning chair.

B. *Active VOR*. This condition differed from A by the following two modifications: (1) subjects' heads were without neck support. They were instructed to actively ensure that, with the imposed body rotation, the head was turned in space as to be constantly aligned to the trunk in the primary (straight ahead) position; the potentiometer readings showed that they performed only minor if any head (-to-trunk) movements. (2) They were holding bimanually a bar that was fixed to, and thus rotated with, the chair.

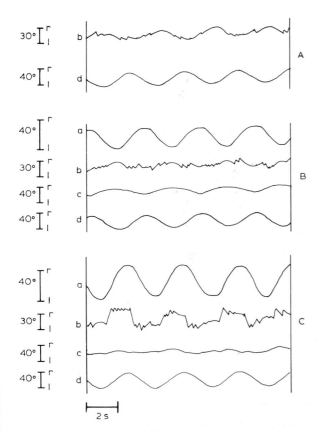

C. *Active VOR combined with synergistic arthrokinetic input*. This condition differed from B in one respect: the bar held by the subjects was kept space-stationary by fixing it to a ground-based support. As a result, their arms were passively rotated in the shoulder joints to and fro, counter to the body oscillations.

Representative examples of the nystagmus obtained in conditions A–C are given in Fig. 1. Note that the slow component of the nystagmus is somewhat enhanced in B as compared to A, and that there is only little if any further increment in C. Even more pronounced is the 'activation' of the saccades in conditions B and C. Moreover, there is a difference in the eye-movement patterns between B and C, mainly due to the saccades; particularly large saccades occur in C shortly after the reversal of the stimulus direction, which shift the eyes into the direction of the body rotation.

Fig. 2 gives average values of all subjects at 0.1 Hz stimulus frequency for the gain of peak *SPV*, *SF*, and the mean SA measured successively over time periods of 1 s. There is an increase of all three measures in B and C as compared to A (statistically significant). Thus, the active head stabilization in condition B as well as head stabilization plus the synergistic arthrokinetic input in condition C enhance both the VOR and the saccadic activity. Remarka-

Fig. 1. Representative examples of nystagmus obtained in the 'passive VOR' condition (A) and in the 'active VOR' conditions with the subjects bimanually holding a chair-fixed bar (B) and a space-fixed bar (synergistic arthrokinetic input; C). *a*, head position in space; *b*, horizontal eye movements; *c*, head re trunk position (*a* minus *d*); *d*, chair position in space.

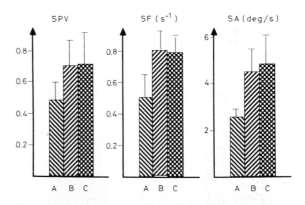

Fig. 2. Mean values of 15 subjects. Gain of peak slow-phase velocity (SPV), saccadic frequency (SF), and saccadic amplitudes measured successively over time periods of 1 s (SA) for the three conditions A, B, C in Fig. 1. Frequency: 0.1 Hz; $\pm 20°$. Vertical bars indicate S.D.

bly, the latter effect appears to be more prominent than the former; the increase of SF and SA is larger than that of SPV. These effects were also observed at the other frequencies tested. The effect on the SPV was more marked at the low than at the high frequencies. By contrast, the effects on SF and SA were larger at the high than at the low frequencies.

When comparing the conditions B and C, the differences of the three measures were, on the average, only minor (Fig. 2) and statistically not significant, despite the obvious difference of the overall nystagmus pattern in the examples of Fig. 1 (B and C). We therefore evaluated two further measures: the *amplitude* and the *instant* (relative to the cycle of chair position, 2π) of the *maximum shifts of eye position* in the orbit ('Schlagfeld'). The results are shown in Fig. 3. There is a difference between B and C as concerns the instant of peak eye shift (right panel); in B, it occurs *prior* to the reversal of rotation direction (1.5π; note that only nystagmus in one direction is considered), and *after* the reversal in C. By contrast, the amplitudes in B and C (left panel) are about the same. Note also that there is some eye shift in A (also in the direction of body rotation), the amplitude of which is small, however, as compared to that in B and C. The instant of this eye shift in A does not occur at the time of chair rever-

sal (peak of both angular position and acceleration) as in B and C, but at the time of peak angular velocity (1π).

In summary, when adding a synergistic arthrokinetic input to the VOR in subjects who actively stabilize their heads, there is no considerable change as concerns the slow component and the saccadic activity apart from some shift in the temporal occurrence of the saccades. Unfortunately, the arthrokinetic effects on the 'passive VOR' has not yet been tested. We find it remarkably, however, that the active stabilization of the head with respect to the trunk enhanced the VOR. Similarly, Barr et al. [19] observed an increase of the VOR gain when their subjects imagined a visual target stationary in space, and a decrease when they imagined it as moving with their heads. The authors postulated that there exists, in addition to and interacting with the VOR, a system that, even in the absence of vision, 'calculates' the head motion relative to the spatial reference, which is selected as a goal for gaze stabilization.

In the experiments of Barr et al. [19], however, the increase in VOR gain was associated with a decrease in number of saccades, and, vice versa, the decrease of the VOR gain with an increase in the number of saccades. In our experiments with the additional somatosensory input, there was an excessive 'activation' of the saccades along with the enhancement of the VOR. Conceivably, the latter effect is functionally different from the former. We assume that in our conditions a mechanism was acting on the saccadic system, which is not due to a change in vigilance that we tried to keep constant. Interestingly, a similar influence on saccades as observed with the arthrokinetic input has also been found with neck proprioceptive input (see below).

Influences of neck proprioceptive input on the VOR

Neck proprioceptive stimulation during rotation of the trunk relative to the stationary head in the rabbit has long been known to elicit eye movements [20, 21]. This 'cervico-ocular reflex' (COR) was found to be 'compensatory', i.e. its direction is such

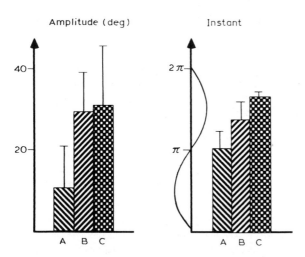

Fig. 3. Amplitude and instant of the maximum shifts of eye position in the orbit for the three conditions A, B and C in Fig. 1.

as to aid gaze stabilization in space when the head is rotated relative to the stationary trunk. Thus, this COR acts synergistically with the VOR. DeKleijn [21] found it to depend critically on the integrity of the cervical dorsal roots C1–C2. Furthermore, with isolated head rotations, he found it to sum linearly with the tonic eye reflex (presumably the tonic VOR) that arises with vestibular stimulation in the vertical planes, and to substitute, although insufficiently, the missing tonic vestibular eye reflex upon horizontal stimulation. Barmack et al. [22], who studied the dynamic aspects of these reflexes, observed comparable summation effects, the neck effect being most prominent with low-frequency stimulation in the horizontal plane, where the VOR is poor. Remarkably, the saccades arising with the neck stimulation had the same direction as the COR; thus they were counter to those arising with vestibular stimulation. With combined stimulation of the two inputs during isolated head rotation, the saccades were virtually absent. According to these findings, the cervical input may be considered to be almost ideal to aid the VOR in gaze stabilization during horizontal head rotation (in the following we shall restrict ourselves to this plane of rotation) with respect to both the COR and the neck-induced saccades.

These findings in the rabbit and corresponding, although less convincing findings in other experimental animals [23] are in line with a number of observations on the COR in man. It has been reported that the COR is also compensatory and most prominent at low frequencies [24]. Furthermore, in patients with labyrinthine lesions, a COR of considerable gain may be found, which aids gaze stabilization during head rotation [25]. This is in line with earlier reports on a prominent compensatory COR in such patients [26–29] and with findings in labyrinthine-lesioned monkeys [30].

Evidence for a cervical input to the oculomotor system and for a cervicovestibular convergence also comes from a number of electrophysiological studies. In the decerebrate cat, vestibular reponses of abducens motor neurons were modified by electrical stimulation of upper cervical dorsal roots, and, as judged from brainstem lesions, the effect appeared to be conveyed via the vestibular nuclei [31]. Also, two types of convergence of vestibular and neck inputs have been oberved in abducens neurons, one with the two inputs being approximately in phase with each other, the other almost representing a counter-phase combination [32]. In the vestibular nuclei of the cat, cervicovestibular convergence has been found in a few neurons with vestibulo-oculomotor projection and with presumed vestibulo-oculomotor function [33]. Summing up all of the above studies, there is no doubt about the existence of a neck input to the oculomotor system, and about its *potential* in aiding the VOR in the stabilization of gaze during head rotation.

Yet the matter appears to be more complex. Barany [34] produced COR-like eye movements in newborn and premature infants, but the effect was only prominent in the first days after birth. In normal adults the existence of a COR was doubted by Barany [35] and even denied by DeKleijn and Stenvers [36]. Thus, it is possible that in the normal adult this reflex has undergone an involution and/or is obscured by a superstructure of other mechanisms? In favour of this assumption is the observation that a prominent COR may be found in patients with labyrinthine deficits (see above) and with cerebral lesions [36].

Nevertheless, with the use of more elaborated stimulation and recording techniques, a weak COR can even be found in normal adults. Still controversial is, however, the direction of this COR. It has been described as compensatory by some authors [24, 37], and anticompensatory by others [38]. Also, there are observations of an anticompensatory COR in experimental animals [39, 40]. And, as pointed out by Fuller [40] and by Barlow and Freedman [38], a compensatory COR, that aids the VOR in the cervicovestibular combination of isolated head rotation, would counteract it in a combination with the two inputs having opposite signs (i.e. when there is a trunk excursion in the same direction as head excursion in space, but with larger amplitude). The latter combination, which certainly belongs to our behavioural repertoire, would in fact call for an anticompensatory COR in order to aid the VOR. Following this line of thought, it is still an open question whether the weak COR in normal adults is (a) functionally relevant only with one cervicovestibular combination, (b) is functionally irrelevant, or (c) is modified in its direction according to the combination and the required function.

A further possibility is that there is a functionally relevant neck effect on the oculomotor activity of normal adult which exists independently of the COR, but concerns the saccades. In normal adults, it has been shown that neck stimulation induces prominent saccades, which are oriented in an anticompensatory direction. And the saccades occurring with the cervicovestibular combination during head rotation are larger than those with whole body rotation, leading to a shift of gaze in the direction of rotation [28, 41, 41]. Functionally, as originally stressed by Frenzel [28], this neck effect would aid gaze re-orientation in the direction of head rotation rather than its stabilization.

In a recent study, Jürgens et al. [43] investigated the influence of two different mental sets on the eye-movement patterns evoked by neck, horizontal canal, and in phase as well as counter-phase canal-neck combinations in normal adults. The point of departure for this study was the observation that the same neck stimulus does not only elicit a sensation of head-to-trunk rotation, but also a sensation of trunk rotation in space (in the direction of the actual trunk excursion) and an illusion of head rotation of opposite direction in space (i.e. in the direction of the relative head-to-trunk displacement), depending on what the subjects focused their attention ([44, 45]; also [42, 46]). With various combinations of neck and canal stimulations at 0.2 Hz stimulus frequency, the trunk-turning sensations obtained could be described as the result of a linear subtraction of the two individual effects, and the head-turning sensation as the result of an addition. We wondered whether the discrepant results reported earlier on the COR may depend on the fact that the subjects may perceive different turning sensations, and also, how this might influence the sac-

cades. We therefore repeated part of this study, evaluating in addition to the subjects' turning sensations their eye movements. The most relevant results will be described in the following.

Blindfolded subjects were seated on a rotation chair that was equipped with a head-rotation device. The set up allowed independent rotations of body in space and head to trunk. By appropriate combinations of these rotations the following four stimuli were generated (cf. Fig. 4A): (a) Canal stimulation (C). (b) Neck stimulation (N). (c) Canal 'plus' neck stimulation (C, + N; 'in-phase combination'). (d) Canal 'minus' neck stimulation (C, − N; 'counter-phase combination'). Sinusoidal rotations of 10 deg/s with a frequency of 0.2 and 0.05 Hz were applied. In one set of trials, subjects estimated their trunk-turning sensation in space, and in another their head-turning sensation in space. They were further instructed not to actively participate in

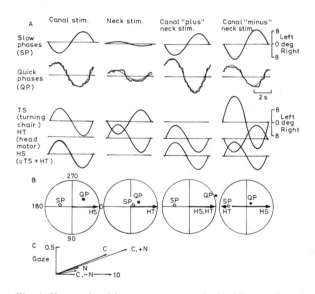

Fig. 4. Slow and quick eye movements obtained by canal, neck and combined canal-neck stimulations (stimulus frequency: 0.2 Hz; head-turning sensation). (A) Example taken from one subject. Upper panels: averaged cumulative eye positions, separated for slow and quick phases. Lower panels: position curves of trunk in space (TS), head-versus-trunk (HT), and head-in-space (HS). (B) Median values for slow and quick phases (SP and QP, respectively) taken from 20 subjects, in polar coordinates. (C) Median gaze shifts in the four stimulus conditions as a polar plot.

the imposed rotations, but to remain passive. Horizontal eye movements were recorded with conventional EOG and fed, together with the position reading of head and chair, into a laboratory computer. With the help of the computer, the cumulative eye position of slow eye movements (slow phases) were separated from that of saccades (quick phases) and averaged independently from each other ($n = 8$ with the 0.2 Hz and $n = 4$ with the 0.05 Hz stimulus). Phase and gain of the fundamental contained in the responses was extracted by Fourier analysis, added to the eye position curves and plotted in polar coordinates.

Fig. 4A shows, as an example, the averaged slow phases and quick phases recorded from one subject in the four stimulus conditions. Stimulus frequency was 0.2 Hz, the instruction was to estimate head rotation. Note that in this example the neck stimulus elicited a small COR response (slow phase) in the direction of the head-to-trunk excursion ('anticompensatory' direction), and a more prominent saccadic response (quick phase), roughly in the same direction. On the whole, however, there was a great variation in gain and phase of the averaged (and even more of the individual) COR and saccadic responses across the 20 subjects tested, at both stimulus frequencies. The median gain of the COR obtained at 0.2 Hz was 0.1, and the median phase showed a lag of 336° re head-to-trunk position (SP in the second polar plot of Fig. 4B). The corresponding values for the 0.05 Hz stimulus are 0.13 and 274°. Very similar data were obtained for the trunk-turning sensation, and, again, the gain of the COR at 0.05 Hz was slightly larger than that at 0.2 Hz. Thus, remarkably, the COR in our group of normal adults was, on the average, very weak. We consider it as too poor to attribute any functional meaning to it.

The median values for the *slow phases* obtained at 0.2 Hz (head-turning sensation) are given in Fig. 4B ($\diamond$ SP). With either of the two canal-neck combinations, they are somewhat larger as compared to canal stimulation alone. The same effect was also observed for the 0.05 Hz stimulations and for the experiments where subjects estimated the trunk-turning sensation. In a more detailed analysis we extracted, by vector summation, presumed neck effects on the VOR ($N' = C, + N - C; - N' = C, - N - C$) and compared them to the actual measured neck responses (N); the gains of the former were larger than those of the latter, and the phases clearly different. However, when doing the same accross the two combination responses ($2N' = C, + N - C, - N$), the resulting vectors were close to what could be expected from the corresponding N. This allowed us to describe the neck effect on the VOR by two distinct mechanisms, one being a linear summation of the two inputs, the other a nondirection-specific facilitation.

The neck effects on the *saccades* obtained with the canal-neck combinations were clearly more prominent. The median values for the saccades also are given in Fig. 4B ($\blacksquare$ QP; 0.2 Hz; head-turning sensation). It is immediately obvious that the summation of the median canal- and neck-induced saccades gives roughly the values as the median saccades obtained with the combinations. Due to the neck-induced saccades, there is a clear gaze shift in the direction of head rotation in space. The gaze was calculated by summing the vectors of slow phases, quick phases, and of the head in space rotation. The results are shown in Fig. 4C. The fact that the vector obtained with canal stimulation has a gain of about one indicates that the eyes keep, on the average, close to their primary position in the orbit and are taken along with the head rotation in space. With the in-phase combination (head rotation on stationary trunk), the gaze is shifted beyond the primary position in the direction of head rotation. Thus, in this condition, the neck effect would be apt to facilitate the acquisition of a new visual target in space. With the counter-phase combination (trunk rotation in the same direction as the head rotation but with twice the amplitude), the gaze is hardly shifted in space, due to the fact that the reset of the VOR in the orbit by saccades is suppressed. In this condition, gaze is stabilized in space fairly well, even in the absence of a visual target. At 0.05 Hz, canal- and neck-induced saccades had smaller gains, but otherwise the summation effects with the saccades and the gaze shifts were similar. Remarkably, such consistent patterns were *not* observed when subjects estimated trunk rotation either at 0.2 or at 0.05 Hz. This makes us believe that these neck effects are distinct from the COR, involving high-level mechanisms as it is the perception of how the head is moved in space.

It is possible, that not only the perception of passive head movements, but also an intentional or motor 'efference' of active head movements can induce such changes of the eye-movement patterns. One problem with the interpretation of the eye-movement pattern obtained with active head movements is to distinguish between the afferent and the efferent neck effects. A first step in this direction has been undertaken in experiments of Doerr and Thoden [47], which will be presented in the following.

Their subjects were sitting blindfolded on a turning chair and performed actively sinusoidal head movements in the horizontal plane of about $\pm 20°$ in space. They wore a light helmet, which was rotatably fixed to a chair-based support. Head (helmet) rotation re chair was recorded with the help of a potentiometer, head rotation in space was extracted from trunk (chair) rotation in space and head-to-trunk rotation. The frequency of the head movement, given by a metronome, was 0.1 or 0.2 Hz. Two sets of experiments were performed. In A the chair was stationary, so that the head-to-trunk and head-in-space excursions were identical. In B the trunk was passively rotated along with the active head movement in space, the head-to-trunk excursion thus being only a fraction of the head-in-space movement. This was done by feeding the helmet output in the appropriate way into the chair input and training the subjects to build up slowly the desired head movement. The chair followed the head with a phase lag of not more than a few degrees. The profile and amplitude of the head rotation in space closely resembled those obtained in A. Horizontal eye movements were recorded with conventional EOG and analysed from strip-chart recordings.

When comparing the eye-movement responses obtained in A (normal head movements) with those in B (head movement with 'minimized' head-to-trunk excursion), no statistically significant difference was found as concerns the gain of slow phase velocity, the mean saccadic amplitude, and the peak amplitude of eye shift in the orbit. The only difference we noticed concerned the temporal distribution of the saccades in the stimulus cycle. As a measure of the distribution, we evaluated the mean saccadic amplitude successively over time periods of 0.4 and 0.8 s. The results obtained from 5 subjects and 10 cycles of 0.1 Hz head movements per subject are shown in Fig. 5. Note that mean saccadic amplitude shows a direction reversal and abrupt peak roughly at the time of peak head displacement

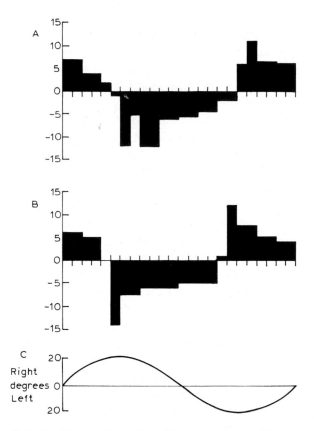

Fig. 5. Distribution of saccadic amplitudes over sinusoidal active head movements (0.1 Hz) with normal and 'minimized' head-to-trunk excursion (A and B, respectively). Means of 10 cycles in 5 subjects. (C) Head-in-space position.

(acceleration), and that the saccadic peak in B occurs slightly earlier than that in A. We tend to attribute this difference to the phase difference between head and chair (at the time when subjects reversed the head movement, the head motion in space imposed by the chair rotation was not yet reversed). Taken together, the findings indicate that the volition of a head movement, i.e. the efference signal alone, is enough to induce the observed change in saccadic activity and thus the gaze shift.

Coming back to the general topic, i.e. to the influence the neck input has on the oculomotor system, we would like to make two points. Firstly, what is considered to be a COR in normal adults appears to be weak and highly variable. We see no common denominator for a functional role of this COR in a collective of normal adults. This does not exclude the possibility that certain individuals, or patients with labyrinthine or cerebral lesions, make use of it in some way. If one considers not only head movements on a stationary trunk, but the whole repertoire of possible head and trunk movements in space and relative to each other, the information supplied by the neck input on head position in space is equivocal. Therefore, reflexive stabilization of gaze in physical space appears to us to be a matter mainly of the vestibular input (in visual space, accordingly, mainly of the visual input). The canal information is frequency deficient in the horizontal plane, but at least it is unequivocal. Secondly, there is a prominent neck effect on saccades and thus on gaze. This effect, given the appropriate mental set, is able to re-orient gaze with head movements on the one hand, and to suppress gaze shifts with counter-phase canal–neck combinations on the other. The influence of mental set and volition indicates that high-level cerebral functions are involved. We deem it unlikely that the effect simply resulted from the subjects' imagination of visual targets in space. Rather, we assume that we are dealing with a genuine effect that switches, without representing a reflex in the classical sense, between two internal modes of behaviour, one dealing with the stabilization of orientation, the other with the reorientation of oneself relative to the surround.

Proprioceptive effects on vestibulospinal mechanisms

According to the neuroanatomical and neurophysiological literature, signals from semicircular canals and otoliths are transmitted to the spinal cord via various distinct pathways and interfere with mechanisms of posture and locomotion. Vice versa somatosensory afferents from the neck, trunk and limbs are known to exert a strong influence onto the vestibular system [48]. These two sets of inputs appear to interact with each other not only at the level of the spinal cord [49] and in centres of the brainstem [2, 4, 33, 50–58] but also in higher cerebral structures [5–9]. The postural reflexes upon vestibular and proprioceptive stimulation that are prominent early in ontogenesis or after extensive cerebral lesions appear to be replaced in normal adults by 'postural reactions' that involve more global aspects like the consideration of all sensory information, the knowledge of the overall situation, and volition.

Already at basic levels, one may possibly distinguish between two different modes of vestibular-somatosensory interaction. First, there appears to be a complementory mode. As an example, tonic vestibular and neck inputs interact in such a way that the combined stimulation that would occur during head tilt on the stationary trunk leads to a cancellation of the individual vestibular and neck effects on extensor muscles in the forelimb of cat [59, 60]. The more general notion is that the brain, summing linearly the two inputs, is able to 'calculate' trunk excursion in space from the vestibular information on head-in-space and the neck information on head-versus-trunk. Second, there may be a kind of competitive mode, where the proprioceptive input gates the vestibular input. Evidence for such a mechanism has been obtained in a recent study by Kasper et al. [61], of which some details will be reported in the following.

A modulating influence of limb somatosensory input on single vestibular nuclear neurons was obtained in chronically prepared, awake cats. In particular, the responses of vestibular neurons to horizontal canal stimulation with whole-body rotation

118

(0.2 Hz, ± 17°) and with head tilt in roll (0.1 Hz, ± 7°) was compared across the following two conditions: (a) The animals' limb were without support from beneath. (b) A platform was propped against the limbs from below (addition of deep somatosensory input). The neurons to be reported responded neither to superficial somatosensory stimulation, nor to neck stimulation as tested by corresponding rotations of the trunk versus the stationary head. Eleven out of 29 vestibular cells that responded to horizontal rotation were clearly affected by the somatosensory input in that the mean discharge rate was decreased, and the gain of the canal response was diminished. Also, 19 out of 28 tilt-modulated cells showed pronounced effects with the additional somatosensory input; mean discharge rate was increased, however, and the gain decreased. Fig. 6 shows an example of such a tilt-sensitive neuron. Further experiments are necessary to show whether the observed effects are related to the vestibulospinal system, as in our assumption. Indeed, it was recently demonstrated that changes in gain of vestibulospinal reflexes acting on forelimb extensor muscles occurred in decerebrate cats following dorsiflexion or plantar flexion of the forepaw [62].

What could be the functional role of this hypothetical gating mechanism? It is conceivable that the vestibulospinal responses depend, to a certain extent, on the proprioceptive information about the status of the limb support on the ground. It could well be that postural stabilization is related to two different reference systems. One could be the immediate surround as experienced by the somatosensory inputs. The other could be the 'physical space' in which self-motion is registered by the vestibular input. As long as the surround is assumed to be stable in space, the somatosensory cues might suffice. However, as soon as the surround is not reliably perceived or even continuously moving in physical space, the vestibular information becomes indispensable. This idea could be related to the postural responses upon external pertubations in normal adults, where the vestibular contribution comes into play mainly with prolonged oscillations of the ground support ([63]; see also Chapter 22).

It is open to question whether this presumed mechanism uses the efferent vestibular system or convergences onto central vestibular neurons. However, it appears likely that higher levels are normally also involved, as was postulated above for the proprioceptive effects on the oculomotor system.

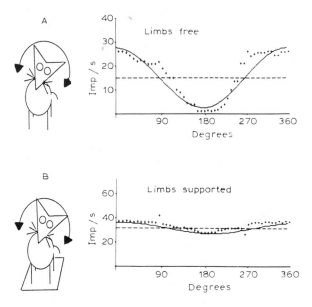

Fig. 6. The effect of limb support on the tilt response of a vestibular nuclear neuron. Averaged discharge rate ($n = 10$) as a function of sinusoidal head tilt in roll (0.1 Hz, 7°). Crosses give discharge rate, full lines the fundamental extracted by Fourier analysis. The neuron showed no neck input (trunk rotation versus the stationary head). (A) Without limb support. (B) Platform propped against the limbs.

References

[1] Brandt, T., Buchele, W. and Arnold, F. (1977) Arthrokinetic nystagmus and egomotion sensation. *Exp. Brain Res.*, 30: 331–338.

[2] Fredrickson, J.M., Schwarz, D. and Kornhuber, H.H. (1966) Convergence and interaction of vestibular and deep somatic afferents upon neurons in the vestibular nuclei of the cat. *Acta Otolaryngol. Stockholm*, 51: 168–188.

[3] Rubin, A.M., Liedgren, S.R.C., Odkvist, L.M., Milne, A.C. and Fredrickson, J.M. (1978) Labyrinthine and somatosensory convergence upon vestibuloocular units. *Acta Otolaryngol. Stockholm*, 85: 54–62.

[4] Mackert, A., Kasper, J. and Thoden, U. (1984) Responses to corneal stimulation in vestibulospinal units of nucleus Deiters. *Exp. Neurol.*, 83: 24–32.

[5] Deecke, L., Schwarz, D.W.F. and Fredrickson, J.M. (1977) Vestibular responses in the rhesus monkey ventroposterior thalamus. II. Vestibuloproprioceptive convergence at thalamic neurons. *Exp. Brain Res.*, 30: 219–232.

[6] Schwarz, D.W.F. and Fredrickson, J.M. (1971) Rhesus monkey vestibular cortex: a bimodal primary projection field. *Science*, 172: 289–291.

[7] Kornhuber, H.H. and Aschoff, J.C. (1964) Somatisch-vestibulare integration an Neuronen des motorischen Cortex. *Naturwissenschaften*, 51: 62–63.

[8] Odkvist, L.M., Liedgren, S.R.C., Larsby, B. and Jervall, L. (1975) Vestibular and somatosensory inflow to the vestibular projection area in the postcruciate dimple region of the cat cerebral cortex. *Exp. Brain Res.*, 22: 185–196.

[9] Deecke, L., Mergner, T. and Becker, W. (1979) Neuronal responses to natural vestibular stimuli in the cat's anterior suprasylvian gyrus. *Adv. Oto-Rhino-Laryngol.*, 25: 74–81.

[10] Von Stein, St. (1910) *Schwindel (Autokinesis externa et interna)*. Lessier, Leipzig.

[11] Doge, R. (1972) Threshold of rotation. *J. Exp. Psychol.*, 6: 107–137.

[12] Brady, J.P. and Levitt, E.E. (1964) Nystagmus as a criterion of hypnotically induced visual hallucinations. *Science*, 146: 85–86.

[13] Zikmund, V. (1966) Oculomotor activity during visual imagery of a moving stimulus pattern. *Stud. Psychol. Praha*, 8: 254–272.

[14] Lackner, J.R. and DiZio, P. (1984) Some efferent and somatosensory influences on body orientation and oculomotor control. In: L. Spillmann and B.R. Wooten (Eds.), *Sensory Experience, Adaptation and Perception*, Lawrence Erlbaum, London, pp. 281–301.

[15] Bles, W. (1981) Stepping around: circular vection and coriolis effects. In: J. Long and A. Baddeley (Eds.), *Attention and Performance, Vol. IX*, Lawrence Erlbaum, London, pp. 47–61.

[16] Bles, W., Klören, T., Büchele, W. and Brandt, T. (1983) Somatosensory nystagmus: physiological and clinical aspects. *Adv. Oto-Rhino-Laryngol.*, 3: 30–34.

[17] Leopold, H.C., Mertinat, M. and Thoden, U. (1984) Modulation of vestibuloocular reflex (VOR) by somatosensory input from the arm. In: A. Neetens (Eds.), *Proceedings Ophthalmology* pp. 95–98.

[18] Leopold, H.C., Mertinat, M. and Thoden, U. (1985) Modulation of vestibulo-ocular reflex (VOR) by active stabilization of head to trunk. *Acta Otolaryngol. Stockholm*, 99: 102–106.

[19] Barr, C.C., Schultheis, L.W. and Robinson, D.A. (1976) Voluntary, non visual control of the human vestibulo-ocular reflex. *Acta Otolaryngol. Stockholm*, 81: 365–375.

[20] Barany, R. (1906) Augenbewegungen, durch Thoraxbewegungen ausgelost. *Zbl. Physiol.*, 20: 298–302.

[21] DeKleijn, A. (1921) Tonische Labyrinth- und Halsreflexe auf die Augen. *Pflügers Arch.*, 186: 82–97.

[22] Barmack, N.H., Nastros, M.A. and Pettorossi, V.E. (1981) The horizontal and vertical cervico-ocular reflex of the rabbit. *Brain Res.*, 224: 261–278.

[23] Magnus, R. (1924) *Körperstellung*, J. Springer, Berlin, pp. 173–195.

[24] Meiry, J.L. (1971) Vestibular and proprioceptive stabilisation of eye movements. In P. Bach-y-Rita, C.C. Collins and J.E. Hyde (Eds.), *The Control of Eye Movements*, Academic Press, New York, pp. 483–493.

[25] Kasai, T. and Zee, S.D. (1978) Eye-head coordination in labyrinthe defective human beings. *Brain Res.*, 144: 123–141.

[26] Bikeles, G. and Ruttin, E. (1915) Über die reflektorischen kompensatorischen Augenbewegungen bei beiderseitiger Ausschaltung des N. Vestibularis. *Neurol. Zbl.*, 34: 807–810.

[27] Fischer, M.H. (1926) In Sachen des Drehnystagmus. *Acta Otolaryngol., Stock.*, 7: 495–504.

[28] Frenzel, H. (1928) Rucknystagmus als Halsreflex und Schlagfeldverlagerung des labyrintharen Drehnystagmus durch Halsreflexe. *Z. Hals-Nasen-Ohrenheilk.*, 21: 177–187.

[29] Frenzel, H. (1930) Halsreflektorisches Augenrucken von vestibularer Schlagform bei vollständig oder nahezu vollständig Labyrinthlosen (Drehunerregbaren). *Passow-Schafer Beitr. Hals-, Nasen-, Ohrenheilk.*, 28: 177–187.

[30] Dichgans, J., Bizzi, E., Morasso, P. and Tagliasco, V. (1973) Mechanisms underlying recovery of eye-head coordination following bilateral labyrinthectomy in monkeys. *Exp. Brain Res.*, 18: 548–562.

[31] Hikosaka, O. and Maeda, M. (1973) Cervical effects on abducens motoneurons and their interaction with vestibuloocular reflex. *Exp. Brain Res.*, 18: 512–530.

[32] Thoden, U. and Schmidt, P. (1979) Vestibular-neck interaction in abducens neurons. In R. Granit and O. Pompeiano (Eds.), *Reflex Control of Posture and Movement, Progress in Brain Research, Vol, 50*, Elsevier/North-Holland, Amsterdam, pp. 561–566.

[33] Anastasopoulos, D. and Mergner, T. (1982) Canal-neck interaction in vestibular nuclear neurons in the cat. *Exp. Brain Res.*, 46: 269–280.

[34] Barany, R. (1918/19) Uber einige Augen- und Halsmuskelreflexe bei Neugeborenen. *Acta Otolaryngol. Stockholm*, 1: 79–102.

[35] Barany, R. (1924) Gibt es Schwindel resp. Nystagmusanfälle als Halfsreflex? *Acta Otolaryngol. Stockholm*, 7: 1–2.

[36] DeKleijn, A. and Stenvers, H.W. (1941) Tonic neck reflexes on the eye muscles in man. *Proc. K. Ned. Akad. Wet.*, 44: 385–396.

[37] Barnes, G.R. and Forbat, L.N. (1979) Cervical and vestibular afferent control of the oculomotor response in man. *Acta Otolaryngol. Stockholm*, 88: 79–87.

[38] Barlow, D. and Freedmann, W. (1980) Cervico-ocular reflex in the normal adult. *Acta Otolaryngol. Stockholm*, 89: 487–496.

[39] Gresty, M.A. (1976) A reexamination of 'neck reflex' eye movements in the rabbit. *Acta Otolaryngol. Stockholm*, 81: 386–394.

[40] Fuller, J.H. (1980) The dynamic neck eye reflex in mammals. *Exp. Brain Res.*, 41: 29–35.

[41] Doerr, M., Leopold, H.C. and Thoden, U. (1981) Vestibulo-ocular reflex (VOR), cervico-ocular reflex (COR) and its interaction in active head movements. *Arch. Psychiatr. Nervenkr.*, 230: 117–127.

[42] Bles, W. and de Jong, J.M.B.V. (1982) Cervico-vestibular and visuo-vestibular interaction. *Acta Otolaryngol. Stockholm*, 94: 61–72.

[43] Jurgens, R., Mergner, T. and Schmid-Burgk, W. (1982) Modification of VOR slow and quick components by neck stimulation and turning sensation. In R. Roucoux and M. Crommelinck (Eds.), *Physiological and Pathological Aspects of Eye Movements*, Junk, The Hague/Boston/London, pp. 365–370.

[44] Mergner, T., Anatasopoulos, D., Becker, W. and Deecke, L. (1981) Discrimination between trunk and head rotation: A study comparing neuronal data from the cat with human psychophysics. *Acta Psychol.*, 48: 291–302.

[45] Mergner, T., Nardi, G.L., Becker, W. and Deecke, L. (1983) The role of canal-neck interaction for the perception of horizontal trunk and head rotation. *Exp. Brain Res.*, 49: 198–208.

[46] Thoden, U., Doerr, M. and Leopold, H.C. (1983) Motion perception of head or trunk modulates cervico-ocular reflex (COR). *Acta Otolaryngol. Stockholm*, 96: 9–14.

[47] Doerr, M. and Thoden, U. (1987) Eye movements during voluntary head motion with minimized cervical input. *Arch. Otorhinolarygol.* (in press).

[48] Wilson, V.J. and Peterson, B.W. (1978) Peripheral and central substrates of vestibulospinal reflexes. *Physiol. Rev.*, 58: 80–105.

[49] Lundberg, A. (1979) Multisensory control of spinal reflex pathways. In R. Granit and O. Pompeiano (Eds.), *Reflex Control of Posture and Movement, Progress in Brain Research, Vol. 50*, Elsevier/North-Holland, Amsterdam, pp. 11–28.

[50] Wilson, V.J., Kato, M., Thomas, R.C. and Peterson, B.W. (1966) Excitation of lateral vestibular neurons by peripheral afferent fibers. *J. Neurophysiol.*, 29: 508–529.

[51] Rubin, A.M., Liedgren, S.R.C., Ödkvist, L.M., Milne, A.C. and Fredrickson, J.M. (1978) Labyrinthine and somatosensory convergence upon vestibulospinal neurons. *Acta Otolaryngol. Stockholm*, 86: 251–259.

[52] Rubin, A.M., Liedgren, S.R.C., Ödkvist, L.M., Larsby, B. and Aschan, G. (1979) Limb input to the cat vestibular nuclei. *Acta Otolaryngol. Stockholm*, 87: 113–122.

[53] Boyle, R. and Pompeiano, O. (1980) Responses of vestibulospinal neurons to sinusoidal rotation of neck. *J. Neurophysiol.*, 44: 633–649.

[54] Boyle, B. and Pompeiano, O. (1981) Convergence and interaction of neck and macular vestibular inputs on vestibulospinal neurons. *J. Neurophysiol.*, 45: 852–868.

[55] Srivastava, U.C., Manzoni, D., Pompeiano, O. and Stampacchia, G. (1984) Responses of medullary reticulospinal neurons to sinusoidal rotation of neck in the decerebrate cat. *Neuroscience*, 11: 473–486.

[56] Pompeiano, O., Manzoni, D., Srivastava, U.C. and Stampacchia, G. (1984) Convergence and interaction of neck and macular vestibular inputs on reticulospinal neurons. *Neuroscience*, 12: 111–128.

[57] Marchand, A.R., Manzoni, D., Pompeiano, O. and Stampacchia, G. (1987) Effects of stimulation of vestibular and neck receptors on Deiters' neurons projecting to the lumbosacral cord. *Pflügers Arch.*, 409: 13–23.

[58] Stampacchia, G., Manzoni, D., Marchand, A.R. and Pompeiano, O. (1987) Convergence of neck and macular vestibular inputs on vestibulospinal neurons projecting to the lumbosacral segments of the spinal cord. *Arch. Ital. Biol.*, 125: 201–224.

[59] Lindsay, K.W., Roberts, T.D.M. and Rosenberg, J.R. (1976) Asymmetric tonic labyrinth reflexes and their interaction with neck reflexes in the decerebrate cat. *J. Physiol. London*, 261: 583–601.

[60] Manzoni, D., Pompeiano, O., Srivastava, U.C. and Stampacchia, G. (1983) Responses of forelimb extensors to sinusoidal stimulation of macular labyrinth and neck receptors. *Arch. Ital. Biol.*, 121: 205–214.

[61] Kasper, J., Pascal-Leone, A., Mackert, A. and Thoden, U. (1986) Influence of standing on vestibular neuronal activity in awake cats. *Exp. Neurol.*, 92: 37–47.

[62] D'Ascanio, P., Bettini, E., Pompeiano, O. and Stampacchia, G. (1985) Effects of passive flexion of the forepaw on the response gain of limb extensor to sinusoidal stimulation of labyrinth receptors. *Arch. Ital. Biol.*, 123: 195–221.

[63] Diener, H.C., Dichgans, J., Guschlbauer, B. and Bachner, M. (1986) Role of visual and static vestibular influences on dynamic posture control. *Human Neurobiol.*, 5: 105–113.

Neck Afferent and Visual Influences on Vestibulospinal Reflexes

O. Pompeiano and J.H.J. Allum (Eds.)
Progress in Brain Research, Vol. 76
© 1988 Elsevier Science Publishers B.V. (Biomedical Division)

Overview

R. H. Schor[*]

Rockefeller University, 1230 York Avenue, New York, NY 10021-6399, U.S.A.

The majority of the chapters in this section dealt with neck afferent information and its contribution to postural reflexes acting on the neck and limbs. Several issues were raised by the papers, and further elaborated in the discussion periods: What are the neck afferents providing input to the postural control systems? Through what pathways is this information transmitted? How is the spatial and temporal information from the various receptors organized by the central nervous system to produce meaningful reflex responses?

The first two contributions, by Drs. Abrahams and Richmond (Chapter 10) and by Dr. Wilson (Chapter 11), demonstrated that muscle spindles in the neck probably provide the major afferent input to the central nervous system: Dr. Abrahams demonstrated that the neck is richly endowed with spindles, arranged in complex patterns whose function is not yet completely understood, and Dr. Wilson showed that afferents with properties characteristic of spindles are activated by passive head movements, and appear to provide afferent input for the tonic neck reflex. The response of these afferents, in the decerebrate cat, can provide the head-position information necessary for the production of a meaningful postural reflex. The question arose whether spindles are the most appropriate sensor for head position, if they are providing a load-dependent signal to the central nervous system, and how can they also provide an accurate signal of head position? Probably under most conditions, the head provides a relatively constant, largely inertio-elastic, load to the neck, so that head-position change directly translates into a changing (elastic) load. When an external load is applied, for example when an animal carries prey in its mouth, the additional load is time-invariant; any changes in spindle output would therefore again correspond largely to head-position changes. Gamma efferent control of neck spindles may perhaps play a role in compensation for such load changes, but this awaits further study.

How does neck information reach and influence various postural reflex systems? Dr. Wilson demonstrated (Chapter 11) that the tonic neck reflex probably involves a direct relay through medial propriospinal neurons. Dr. Manzoni showed (Chapter 12) that neck influence on hindlimb postural reflexes may be relayed through vestibulospinal and reticulospinal neurons. Neck signals are also present in other brainstem structures, such as the lateral reticular nucleus. How does this proprioceptive information reach higher levels? Yoshida (Chapter 13) showed that one route may involve the central cervical nucleus, which receives neck afferent information as well as signals from the vertical semicircular canals, and provides a relay to the cerebellum. Another question is: Under what sort of descending control are these neck receptors?

Neck afferent information, taken as a whole, presents a fairly complex set of data: neck muscle spindles are arranged in various morphological ar-

---

[*]*Present address*: Departments of Otolaryngology and Physiology, School of Medicine, University of Pittsburgh, Pittsburgh, PA 152213, U.S.A.

rays which will probably show different responses to stretch, the muscles themselves span different joints, with their fibres arranged in a variety of spatial orientations, and finally the neck, as a mechanical structure, imposes constraints on the types of movements which can be produced, and sensed, by these muscles. How is this spatially diverse information organized, and combined with other sensory information in the production of coordinated reflex responses?

Dr. Peterson (Chapter 14) presented one possible scheme for explaining the responses observed in the cervicocollic and vestibulocollic reflexes of the cat. He and his colleagues approximated the pulling direction of fifteen pairs of neck muscles, assumed that the primary sensory signals were from muscle receptors activated by stretch in the same pulling direction, that muscles acted independently, and that the motor control strategy was to expend the least amount of (muscle) energy when compensating for a stretch or vestibular disturbance along any direction. Under these assumptions, they found that there is fairly good agreement between the direction of vestibular or cervical stimulation which produces the maximal electromyograph response in the muscle and the direction predicted by the model. However, such directions for optimal activation are often not at all aligned with the muscle's pulling direction, a natural consequence of combining muscle actions when the muscles are not pulling at right angles to each other. However, the organizational principle of 'least energy' does not seem to apply for voluntary movements. Dr. Richmond noted that, in fact, muscles do not seem to act independently: certain synergies seem to be brought into play, perhaps to stabilize parts of the vertebral column.

The functional role of neck input to the postural control system, especially to the hind limbs, is still unclear. While Dr. Manzoni showed that neck rotation modulates vestibulospinal and reticulospinal neurons projecting to the lumbosacral levels, at the level of the gastrocnemius muscle, little modulation is observed in the decerebrate cat, perhaps due to altered descending tonic drive in this preparation.

How do signals from various neck muscles interact with each other, and with signals from the vestibular organs? Dr. Manzoni demonstrated that both neck and vestibular signals are present, and sum linearly, in vestibulospinal and reticulospinal neurons. Furthermore, as shown by Drs. Dutia (Chapter 15), Wilson, and Peterson, the vestibulocollic and cervicocollic reflexes, when activated simultaneously (such as by moving the head on a stationary body), appear to combine linearly, since the gain, phase, and directional properties of the combined response can be predicted from the vectorial addition of the responses to cervical and vestibular inputs applied in isolation.

How might other postural control signals interact with the neck/vestibulospinal system? Dr. Gahéry (Chapter 16) examined postural adjustments accompanying limb movements induced by cortical stimulation. He demonstrated that the postural deficits following lesions of the lateral reticular nucleus was similar to those following neck deafferentation, and concluded that adjustments to cortically evoked movements probably share a common pathway with labyrinth- and neck-evoked postural responses. The final presentation in this section examined the interaction of visual and vestibular information during vertical movements. Dr. Lacour (Chapter 17) demonstrated that, within the vestibular nuclei, neurons tend to respond in an opposite fashion to vestibular and visual input, so that when moving vertically in a stationary visual world, the two inputs augment each other. Such visual/vestibular interaction provides an extended frequency range of vertical head movements capable of evoking postural reflexes, a direct analogy to the much-studied interaction of the horizontal vestibulo-ocular reflex and the optokinetic system.

O. Pompeiano and J.H.J. Allum (Eds.)
Progress in Brain Research, Vol. 76
© 1988 Elsevier Science Publishers B.V. (Biomedical Division)

CHAPTER 10

Specialization of sensorimotor organization in the neck muscle system

V.C. Abrahams and F.J.R. Richmond

Department of Physiology, Queen's University, Kingston, Ontario, Canada K7L 3N6

The receptors of neck muscles are present in large numbers, and form receptor complexes within the muscles. One of the simplest complexes is a dyad in which a muscle spindle and a Golgi tendon organ lie side-by-side. Muscle spindles that form a dyad are characteristically small and have only a single bag fibre. The bag fibre continues into a second spindle encapsulation which has a normal complement of 2 bag fibres. This complex of two muscle spindles and a tendon organ gives rise to 5 to 6 sensory axons and is one of the simplest receptor complexes. In the deep muscles of the neck, complexes may involve up to 12 spindles as well as other receptors. The large dorsal neck muscles are compartmentalized and are crossed by tendinous inscriptions. Receptor complexes are organized within compartments and inscriptions are the insertion point for many of the tendon spindle/Golgi tendon organ complexes. Receptor complexes in neck muscles mainly give rise to ascending connections. The segmental spinal reflexes initiated by such receptors are usually weak and are frequently inhibitory in nature.

Introduction

Neck muscles, like most skeletal muscles, play two roles in the control of movement. The muscles serve as effectors by developing the forces required to stabilize or move different parts of the skeleton. They also contain neural elements which provide information about body position and muscle perfor-

mance. The neck muscles have many features that are basic to all skeletal muscles, and some of these features have recently been reviewed elsewhere in some detail [1, 2]. This account will deal with certain specializations of sensorimotor organization that are characteristic of neck muscles. These specializations influence the way that neck muscles function in monitoring and executing head movements.

Specializations in the sensory apparatus

Muscle receptors occur in very high densities

It has been known for more than 50 years that neck muscles are particularly rich in muscle receptors. Voss [3–5] counted the number of muscle spindles present in a variety of neonatal human muscles. He found that neck muscles, and in particular deep neck muscles close to the vertebral column, contained a high density of muscle spindles. More recent quantitative studies of shoulder muscles, dorsal neck muscles and intervertebral muscles in the cat have shown that all neck muscles are relatively rich in receptors, but receptor densities were highest in muscles investing the vertebral column. For example, spindle densities in the clavotrapezius muscle were 30 to 35/g [6], those in biventer cervicis

---

Abbreviations: CCN, central cuneate nucleus; ECN, external cuneate nucleus; EMG, electromyograph; GTO, Golgi tendon organ; HRP, horseradish peroxidase.

75 to 100/g [7], and those in deep intervertebral muscles 150–500/g [8]. Comparable densities are only found elsewhere in the small muscles of the digits. However, digital muscles generally weigh less than 1 g so that their absolute content of spindles is relatively low [9]. More proximal muscles such as the large muscles of the cat hindlimb generally have spindle densities of 10–30/g and an overall content of 30–80 spindles [10].

In addition to their dense content of muscle spindles, neck muscles contain substantial numbers of other receptors, including Golgi tendon organs, paciniform corpuscles and undifferentiated free nerve endings [11]. Golgi tendon organs are richly distributed throughout intervertebral muscles and dorsal muscles [11]. For example, the dorsal neck muscle biventer cervicis contains more than 100 tendon organs distributed not only at the muscle insertion, but also along the faces of the many tendinous inscriptions that divide the muscle into a series of linked compartments (F.J.R. Richmond and S. Villeneuve, unpublished observations). Much less information is available concerning the numbers and distribution of the smaller receptors that are served by fine myelinated or unmyelinated axons. However, analyses of fibre spectra in neck muscle nerves have shown that the majority of axons have diameters of less than 6 μm [12]. Axons of this calibre are likely to supply paciniform corpuscles and a number of undifferentiated free endings. The endings supplied by Group III axons have the response properties of high-threshold mechanoreceptors [13]. Detailed studies of receptors served by unmyelinated (Group IV) fibres have not yet been conducted. However, Group IV axons are very common in neck muscle nerves and what little evidence exists suggests that they serve receptors with nociceptive properties.

Muscle receptors exist in a range of configurations not commonly found in most limb muscles

The numerous receptors in neck muscles assume a range of structures and interrelationships that are quite uncommon in most other skeletal muscles.

The muscle spindle is generally described as a single isolated receptor (e.g. [14, 15]). However, work by Cooper and Daniel [16, 17] on human neck muscles, described the presence of muscle spindles that were linked together. In the cat, anatomical studies have shown that only a minority of neck muscle spindles exist as single isolated receptors [7, 8]. Instead, they are grouped in arrays consisting of 2 to 5 spindles. The linked receptors lie in close contact with one another and in many instances they share capsular or intrafusal fibre elements. One interesting form of conjunction between spindle units that is commonly seen in the neck is the tandem spindle. In this compound receptor at least two spindle encapsulations are linked in series by a common intrafusal fibre. These linkages sometimes occur between two spindles with similar intrafusal fibre contents and similar patterns of innervation. More commonly, linked spindle units have different structural features. One spindle unit with a conventional intrafusal fibre content and nerve supply is joined by way of a shared intrafusal fibre to a second smaller encapsulation that contains a reduced number of intrafusal fibres and a much sparser nerve supply [18, 19] (Fig. 1). The specialized features of the smaller spindle suggest that its transductive mechanisms may differ from the larger spindle unit to which it is linked. Most notably, the smaller encapsulation lacks a nuclear bag$_1$ fibre. In typical spindles the bag$_1$ fibre is thought to play a major role in transducing the velocity-sensitive response of the primary ending [20]. In addition, the smaller unit (called a b$_2$c unit because it contains only a bag$_2$ fibre (b$_2$) and a grouping of chain fibres (c) has a greatly reduced fusimotor innervation (Fig. 1). This fusimotor innervation appears to come only from axons with anatomical features typical of static fusimotor axons [19]. No anatomical evidence could be found that the smaller b$_2$c units were innervated by any of the other fusimotor axons such as skeletofusimotor or dynamic fusimotor axons.

In physiological studies of spindles in neck muscles, Richmond and Abrahams [21] identified a substantial number of afferent endings from spindles which could not be classified as primary or secondary endings on the basis of their responses to muscle stretch. The so-called 'intermediate responses' demonstrated by these endings suggested that they originate from primary-like afferents with a reduced sensitivity to the velocity phase of a muscle stretch. Such characteristics are consistent with responses that might be expected from b_2c spindle units. All of this work suggests that muscle spindles from neck muscles supply the nervous system with

at least three different varieties of sensory signal rather than the customary two. However, the uses to which these signals are put remains to be explored.

Muscle spindles in the neck also occur in close physical connection with other receptors including GTOs and paciniform corpuscles. The relationship between a GTO and a muscle spindle is of particular interest. It has been suggested that such relation-

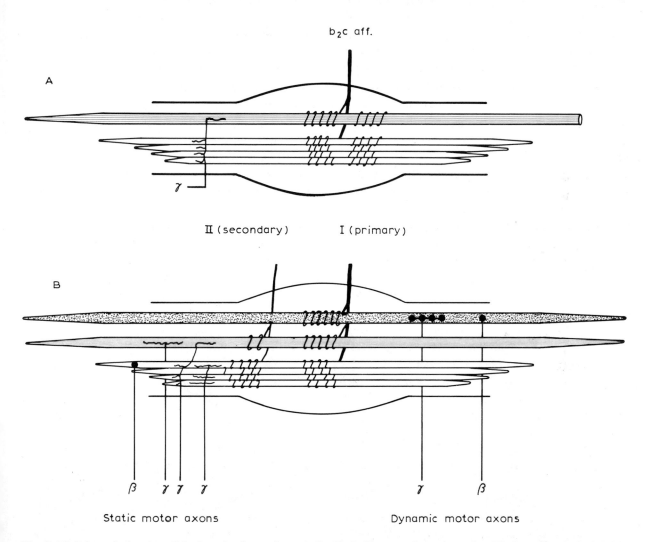

Fig. 1. (A) Schematic drawing of the bc unit of a tandem spindle. Chain fibres are shown in outline. The bag_2 fibre is shaded. The receptor is supplied by a single sensory axon (b_2c aff.) and by 1–3 motor axons with terminals typical of static fusimotor axons (γ). (B) Schematic drawing of a conventional spindle. The spindle contains a bag_1 fibre (stippled) as well as a bag_2 fibre (shaded) and chain fibres. These spindles have both primary and secondary sensory endings, and are supplied by at least four types of motor axons, including static and dynamic axons.

128

ships will occur occasionally on a random basis in muscles which contain high densities of receptors [14], but anatomical studies in hindlimb [22] and neck muscles (F.J.R. Richmond and S. Villeneuve, unpublished observations) have shown that as many as one-third of GTOs lie alongside a muscle spindle or a muscle spindle complex. The common occurrence of the dyad suggests that it may not be a chance arrangement. Together these two receptors are in a position to provide detailed information about length and force development in a small number of motor units immediately surrounding the dyad. Once again the morphological analyses have preceded physiological studies and it is not yet clear whether or how the signals from these simple receptor complexes are processed at higher levels of the nervous system. Interestingly, spindle units that are found close to musculotendinous insertions are most commonly the smaller b_2c units of tandem spindles [19], so that the tandem spindles are polarized with the smaller encapsulation located close to a muscle attachment.

The organization of receptor groupings has also been studied in neck muscles close to vertebrae [8]. In keeping with their much higher spindle densities, these muscles contain elaborate receptor complexes that have large numbers of individual elements.

Some aggregates of receptors may contain as many as ten or more muscle spindles and additionally include a small terminal element that has the morphological features of a small GTO. Such receptor complexes can supply sensory information from more than a dozen afferent fibres that originate from the many spindles.

Muscle receptors have non-uniform but predictable patterns of intramuscular distribution

When three-dimensional maps of muscle receptors are made, it is clear that receptors in individual muscle have a specific pattern of distribution. Because GTOs are only found at musculotendinous junctions, they are confined to the ends of those muscles which lack intramuscular tendons. However, large neck muscles such as the biventer cervicis and splenius are crossed by tendinous inscriptions. These muscles have tendon organs at many sites in the bellies of the muscles as well as the muscle origin and insertion. Since tandem spindles are polarized in their orientation the larger encapsulation of a tandem spindle in biventer cervicis or splenius generally sits within the mass of the muscle whereas the smaller b_2c encapsulation is attached to a tendon or tendinous inscription [18, 19]. Thus

Rostral   Caudal

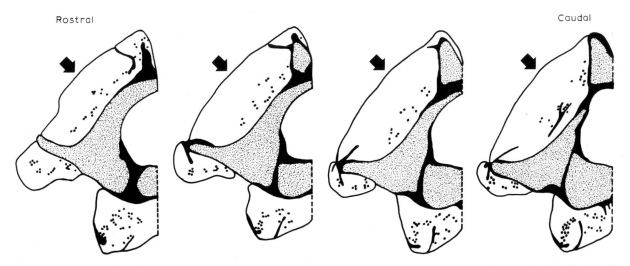

Fig. 2. Distribution of muscle spindles (dots) shown in a series of transverse sections cut at intervals through the decalcified C1–C2 joint of a cat. Bones are shown stippled. Spindles in intervertebral muscles are not distributed uniformly. In obliquus capitis caudalis (arrows) the receptors are typically located in muscle regions that contain the highest proportions of type SO fibres.

each receptor type appears to provide information about a specific part of the substance of the muscle, particularly those parts of the muscle where fibres insert into tendon.

There is a further aspect of the distribution of muscle receptors that is related to the distribution of different motor unit types. Both muscle spindles and GTOs are primarily restricted to those muscle regions that have the highest proportion of slow fibres. Thus, even in deep neck muscles which have exceptionally high overall contents of receptors, some regions of the muscle are receptor-free and receptors are concentrated into particular parts of the muscle. As Fig. 2 shows, the superficial regions of some intervertebral muscles seldom contain muscle receptors. The large aggregates of muscle spindles and their associated receptors that are present in these muscles are confined to a narrow subvolume deep in the muscle which contains the highest proportion of type SO fibres.

Neck muscle spindles have weak excitatory connections onto neck motoneurons

Despite the abundance of muscle spindles in the neck muscles, segmental monosynaptic excitatory connections to neck motoneurons are not strong. In the hindlimb it is possible to excite all motoneurons in a pool by stimulation of the appropriate dorsal roots [23]. This is not the case in the upper cervical cord [24]. Part of the explanation has been found in recent experiments in which 1A afferents of dorsal neck muscles were injected intra-axonally with HRP [25]. These studies showed that spindle afferents from neck muscles have infrequent collaterals and make contacts with only a small number of motoneurons located in a restricted rostrocaudal zone.

In recent experiments reflex effects in the neck were explored in alert cats chronically instrumented with electrodes for nerve stimulation and EMG recording (Fig. 3) (G.E. Loeb and F.J.R. Richmond, unpublished observations). C1 nerve bundles supplying rectus capitis posterior or C3 nerve bundles supplying splenius or biventer cervicis were stimulated electrically. In keeping with the earlier studies

Intact

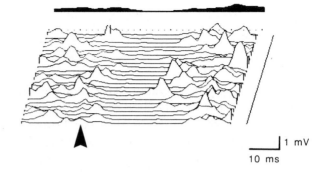

Deafferented

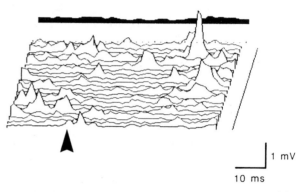

Fig. 3. Raster diagrams of EMG activity from biventer cervicis. R (top) and L (bottom) recorded while the cat lapped milk. At arrows a single stimulus at 4–10 T was delivered to the C1 rectus capitis posterior nerves. Top record: intact side, EMG activity is inhibited. Bottom record: C1 ganglion has been removed, no inhibition.

on decerebrate and anaesthetized intact cats, little evidence could be found that single stimuli produced excitatory reflexes even between synergistic muscles. In contrast, a modest inhibitory effect occurred within 5 ms of stimulating C1 nerves from rectus capitis posterior. This inhibition primarily affected motor-unit activity of those extensor muscles that are synergistic to rectus capitis major, particularly biventer cervicis (Fig. 3). That this effect originated from sensory receptors (rather than any kind of Renshaw inhibition) was confirmed by examining the reflexes in animals which had been unilaterally deafferented by removal of one C1 ganglion at the time of electrode implantation. Inhibitory effects were lost on the side of dorsal root extirpation.

Neck muscle receptors project extensively to precerebellar nuclei

From the earliest degeneration experiments, it has been obvious that afferent fibres entering the upper cervical dorsal roots project to the central cervical nucleus and the ECN, both identified as precerebellar nuclei [26–28]. This is not to say that the projections of afferents from cervical segments are exclusively precerebellar; afferent terminations were also reported in other regions, including the deep layers of the main cuneate nucleus and the intermediate nucleus of Cajal [29]. In more recent years projections of neck muscle nerves have been studied more specifically using the transganglionic transport of HRP. These experiments have emphasized that many of the precerebellar projections originate from neck muscle afferent fibres [30–32]. In the ECN the projection is 'musculotopic', i.e. individual muscles project to separate subvolumes of the nucleus [30–32]. The musculotopic nature of the projection has been established in electrophysiological experiments by Murakami and Kato [33] and more recently confirmed by Abrahams et al. [41]. The latter experiments have also shown that there are at least 3 classes of second-order cells in the ECN. About one-third of the neurons examined can only be activated from the nerves supplying one muscle compartment. About one-third of the neurons may be activated by stimulation of nerves supplying more than one compartment. The remaining class of neurons can only be activated by a nerve supplying one compartment, but their activation is facilitated by the stimulation of nerves from a number of other compartments.

The other precerebellar nucleus, the CCN has been thoroughly studied electrophysiologically by Hirai et al. [27]. The CCN also shows great specificity of input. Thirty of 69 neurons tested received input from only a single segment of a single muscle. The remaining neurons, particularly those in caudal segments, received excitatory effects from more than one segment. Although in the primate the ECN projects to both the cerebellum and the thalamus [26, 28], no evidence as yet exists that the ECN and the CCN in the cat have any targets other than cerebellar structures. The significance of this dual disynaptic pathway to the cerebellum remains to be explained.

Specializations in the effector apparatus

The neck contains many muscles that have complementary functions

The necks of quadrupeds and humans contain more than 20 pairs of muscles that can participate in the execution of head movements. Many muscles may potentially contribute to a single head movement in any given direction. For example, biventer cervicis, occipitoscapularis, rectus capitis major, complexus and spinalis dorsi all run in parallel to the vertebral column and thus are suited to roles in head extension. Recent EMG studies in alert, freely moving cats [34, 35] have demonstrated that all of these muscles show increased activity during behaviours that require lifting of the head (Fig. 4).

Nevertheless, there is some specialization within this synergistic muscle grouping as the activity of muscles with similar pulling directions is not identical during the execution of many movements. Each of the 20 pairs of muscle has its own unique attachments and its own biomechanical properties. In the head extensor grouping, biventer cervicis spans 8 cervical joints and runs from an origin on the thoracic vertebrae to an insertion on the lambdoidal crest of the skull. In contrast, rectus capitis posterior crosses only the suboccipital joints and spinalis dorsi crosses only the lower cervical joints between C3 and C7. The relative actions of each of these head extensors depends upon the initial posture of the animal and upon the joint(s) across which the movement must take place. For example, Fig. 4 shows the EMG patterns in several muscles when the head is lifted rapidly across the suboccipital joints as the cat licks its paw. In this movement,

EMG   Cross-correlograms

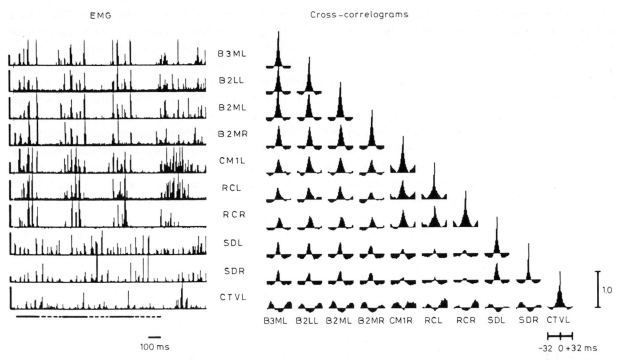

Fig. 4. EMG activity and associated cross-correlograms. The EMG records were made during grooming behaviour in which the cat licked its paws. The bars at the bottom of the left-hand record indicate head extension. These movements are associated with rhythmic EMG bursts. The matrix of cross-correlograms shown on the right give a measure of the synchronization of the activity in the muscle pairs indicated. Note that the plot at the right-hand end of each line is the autocorrelation function. Narrow, strongly positive peaks indicate strong synchronization. Negative correlation (below the base line) indicates alternation of EMG spike bursts.
Abbreviations: CTVL, left centrotransversarius; SDL, spinalis dorsi, left; SDR, spinalis dorsi, right; RCL, rectus capitis posterior major, left; RCR, rectus capitis posterior major, right; CMIL, complexus, compartment 1, left; B3ML, biventer cervicis, compartment 3 medial, left; B2LL, biventer cervicis, compartment 2 lateral, left; B2ML, biventer cervicis, compartment 2 medial, left; B2MR, biventer cervicis, compartment 2 medial, right.

EMG activity in rectus capitis major and biventer cervicis is strongly modulated and occurs only during the extension phase of the movement. However, spinalis dorsi shows a more consistent pattern of EMG activity with little modulation. Similarly, some large movements that appear to be made across lower cervical joints elicit strongly modulated EMG activity in spinalis dorsi, but little or no change in the activity of suboccipital muscles.

An understanding of the biomechanics and functions of a single neck muscle depends on good data concerning its anatomical relationships with skeletal structures, its fibre-type distribution, its motor unit organization and its physical dimensions. It also depends upon a knowledge of the sites at which joint movement is occurring because the forces produced by muscle action will depend on the joints at which the movement must be made. Understanding the actions of neck muscles is particularly complicated because many movements are made simultaneously across a number of cervical joints which can move in one direction or another. Further, the actions of single muscles may be part of a motor program involving the concurrent activation of many muscles. EMG studies have already shown that most head movements are produced by the composite action of many, but not all, of the muscles present in the neck. The synergistic relationships between muscles are further complicated by the temporal sequence with which muscles are recruited. Head movement, must thus involve a complex pattern of orchestration of motor unit activity by the nervous system.

The architecture and innervation of a single neck muscle can be surprisingly complex

Architectural specializations are present both in the muscle-fibre and tendon organization of neck muscles and in their patterns of innervation. The large dorsal neck muscles in the cat have been subjected to the most detailed studies [1, 7, 36]. Each of these muscles is supplied by a series of separate nerve bundles originating from different cervical segments. Each nerve bundle supplies motor units that are compartmentalized in a predictable manner within the muscle mass. In some muscles, such as biventer cervicis, the serially ordered compartments of motor units are defined and separated by the interposition of bands of tendinous material called tendinous inscriptions, through which no muscle fibres pass [37]. In other long muscles, such as splenius, some motor units can maintain an in-series organization without the presence of tendinous inscriptions [36]. The fibres of in-series motor units are arranged so that their constituent muscle fibres interdigitate extensively, as shown in Fig. 5. The series organization of motor units in the long neck muscles have significant implications for their functional properties. If tension is to be developed efficiently in these muscles, the motor units that lie in series with one another must be recruited concurrently. Contraction of a single compartment of motor units in isolation would simply stretch the neighbouring passive muscle subvolume and minimal tension will be developed between the two ends of the muscle. EMG experiments in alert, freely moving animals suggest that motor units in contiguous compartments are recruited in a highly synchronized manner [38] (Fig. 4). Functionally, this requires the simultaneous recruitment of motoneurons whose cell bodies lie at different segmental levels and are somewhat widespread in the spinal cord [39, 40].

In neck muscle, as in all other muscles, the basic functional unit is the single motor unit. These have been shown in some muscles to have an unusual columnar arrangement. Glycogen depletion experiments in biventer cervicis have shown, as expected, that individual motor units are confined to a single compartment. However, these motor units are further restricted to a small subvolume so that they form a narrow column within the compartment [37]. Motor units are thus arranged as a series of in-parallel strips. This elaborate in-series and in-parallel organization must be an important factor in determining the way in which the muscle can operate and motor commands must be exercised, but the significance of these arrangements is still not understood.

Motor units are commonly recruited in periodic bursts whose frequency and timing are synchronized from one muscle to another

Studies of cat limb muscles have given rise to the view that motor units in a muscle are recruited asynchronously in order to smooth out the force production of the individual motor units. However, EMG studies in alert cats show that the recruitment of motor units in neck muscles can be synchronized. Synchronization is particularly obvious in movements involving head extension, such as head elevation associated with orientation or grooming. EMG spike activity occurs in 30–40 Hz bursts, each burst separated from the next by a silent period. Similar bursts occurs simultaneously in most other active muscles in the dorsal neck. An inverse phasing of recruitment has been seen in a few ventral muscles. These are muscles that normally have antagonistic actions to the dorsal extensors, but are sometimes recruited with them during certain types or behaviour. For example, Fig. 4 shows a bursting pattern in the muscle centrotransversarius (which lies on the ventral surface of the venteral column and presumably acts as a vertebral flexor) that alternates with bursts in the vertebral extensors, spinalis dorsi, complexus and biventer cervicis. The inverse phasing can be most clearly seen in cross-correlograms of EMG activity. The central mecha-

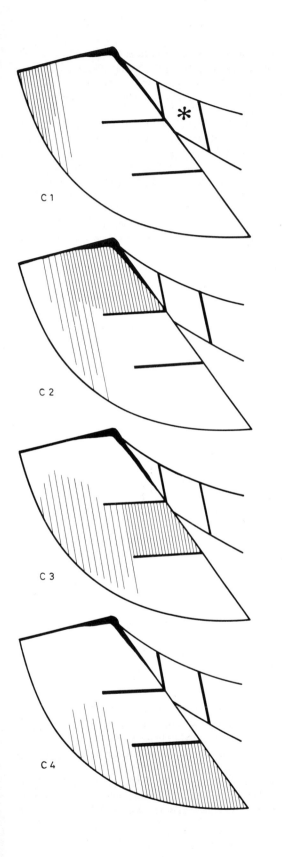

Fig. 5. Motor territories in splenius supplied by different segmental nerve bundles. Each territory (hatched area) was mapped using the method of glycogen depletion. In lateral parts of splenius (right), motor domains are separated by tendinous inscriptions. In medial parts (left) depleted and nondepleted motor units supplied by adjacent nerves maintained an in-series organization, but interdigitated extensively. The slip of muscle attaching to the lateral tendon of splenius (marked with an asterisk) is longissimus capitis. (From Richmond et al. [36].)

nisms responsible for these unusual patterns of motor unit synchrony and the functional significance of these activity patterns remain to be explained.

Loeb et al. [38] have suggested that propriospinal circuits may be involved in the synchronization of these patterns of motoneuron recruitment. Whatever the mechanisms involved, the synchronization of motor unit firing in cervical segments suggests that recruitment patterns may follow substantially different rules than those observed in other motor systems.

Acknowledgements

Supported by MRC of Canada and by the Laboratory of Neural Control N.I.N.C.D.S., N.I.H., Bethesda.

References

[1] Richmond, F.J.R. and Vidal, P.P. (1988) The motor system: joints and muscles of the neck. In B. Peterson and F.J.R. Richmond (Eds.), *Control of Head Movement*, Oxford University Press, New York, pp. 1–21.

[2] Richmond, F.J.R., Bakker, D.A. and Stacey, M.J. (1988) The sensorium: receptors of neck muscles and joints. In B. Peterson and F.J.R. Richmond (Eds.), *Control of Head Movement*, Oxford University Press, New York, pp. 49–62.

[3] Voss, H. (1937) Untersuchungen über Zahl, Anordnung und Lange der Muskelspindeln in den Lumbricalmuskeln des Menschen und einiger Tiere. *Z. Mikr. Anat. Forsch.*, 42: 509–524.

[4] Voss, H. (1956) Zahl und Anordnung der Muskelspindeln in den oberen Zungenbeinmuskeln, im M. trapezius und M. litissimus dorsi. *Anat. Anz.*, 103: 443–446.

[5] Voss, H. (1958) Zahl und Anordnung der Muskelspindeln in den unteren Zungenbeinmuskeln, dem M. sternocleidomastoideus und den bauchund tiefen Nackenmuskeln. *Anat. Anz.*, 105: 265–275.

[6] Keane, J.M. (1981) *Peripheral Organization of the Trapezius Muscle Complex in the Cat*, M.Sc. Thesis, Queen's University, Kingston, 178 pp.

[7] Richmond, F.J.R. and Abrahams, V.C. (1975) Morphology and distribution of muscle spindles in dorsal muscles of the cat neck. *J. Neurophysiol.*, 38: 1322–1339.

[8] Bakker, D.A. and Richmond, F.J.R. (1982) Muscle spindle complexes in muscles around upper cervical vertebrae in the cat. *J. Neurophysiol.*, 48: 62–74.

[9] Ip, M.C. (1961) *The Number and Variety of Proprioceptors in certain Muscles of the Cat*, M.Sc. Thesis, University of Hong Kong, Hong Kong.

[10] Chin, N.K., Cope, M. and Pang, M. (1962) Number and distribution of spindle capsules in seven hindlimb muscles of the cat. In D. Barker (Ed.), *Symposium on Muscle Receptors*, University Press, Hong Kong, pp. 241–248.

[11] Richmond, F.J.R. and Bakker, D.A. (1982) Anatomical organization and sensory receptor content of soft tissues surrounding upper cervical vertebrae in the cat. *J. Neurophysiol.*, 48: 49–61.

[12] Richmond, F.J.R., Anstee, G.C.B., Sherwin, E.A. and Abrahams, V.C. (1976) Motor and sensory fibres of neck muscle nerves in the cat. *Can. J. Physiol. Pharmacol.*, 54: 294–304.

[13] Abrahams, V.C., Lynn, B. and Richmond, F.J.R. (1984) Organization and sensory properties of small myelinated fibres in the dorsal cervical rami of the cat. *J. Physiol., Lond.*, 347: 177–187.

[14] Matthews, P.B.C. (1972) *Mammalian Muscle Receptors and their Central Actions*, Edward Arnold, London, 630 pp.

[15] Hulliger, M. (1984) The mammalian muscle spindle and its central control. *Ergebn. Physiol.*, 101: 1–110.

[16] Cooper, S. and Daniel, P.M. (1956) Human muscle spindles. *J. Physiol. London*, 133: 1–3P.

[17] Cooper, S. and Daniel, P.M. (1963) Muscle spindles in man; their morphology in the lubricals and the deep muscles of the neck. *Brain*, 86: 563–586.

[18] Bakker, G.J. and Richmond, F.J.R. (1981) Two types of muscle spindles in cat neck muscles: a histochemical study of intrafusal fiber composition. *J. Neurophysiol.*, 45: 973–986.

[19] Richmond, F.J.R., Bakker, G.J., Bakker, D.A. and Stacey, M.J. (1986) The innervation of tandem muscle spindles in the cat neck. *J. Comp. Neurol.*, 245: 483–497.

[20] Boyd, I.A. (1981) The action of the three types of intrafusal fibre in isolated cat muscle spindles on the dynamic and length sensitivities of primary and secondary sensory endings. In A. Taylor and A. Prochazka (Eds.), *Muscle Receptors and Movement*, MacMillan, London, pp. 17–32.

[21] Richmond, F.J.R. and Abrahams, V.C. (1979) Physiological properties of muscle spindles in dorsal neck muscles of the cat. *J. Neurophysiol.*, 42: 604–617.

[22] Marchand, R., Bridgman, C.F., Shumpert, E. and Eldred, E. (1971) Association of tendon organs with spindles in muscles of the cat's leg. *Anat. Rec.*, 169: 23–32.

[23] Clamann, H.P., Gillies, J.D., Skinner, R.D. and Henneman, E. (1974) Quantitative measurements of output of a motoneuron pool during monosynaptic reflexes. *J. Neurophysiol.*, 37: 1328–1337.

[24] Abrahams, V.C., Richmond, F.J.R. and Rose, P.K. (1975) Absence of monosynaptic reflex in dorsal neck muscles in the cat. *Brain Res.*, 92: 130–131.

[25] Keirstead, S.A. and Rose, P.K. (1983) Projections of muscle spindle afferents intra-axonally stained with horseradish peroxidase in the upper cervical spinal cord of the cat. *Can. J. Physiol. Pharmacol.*, 61: Axiii, p. XIII.

[26] Somana, R. and Walberg, F. (1980) A re-examination of the cerebellar projections from the gracile, main and external cuneate nuclei in the cat. *Brain Res.*, 186: 33–42.

[27] Hirai, N., Hongo, T., Sasaki, S., Yamashita, M. and Yoshida, K. (1984) Neck muscle afferent input to spinocerebellar tract cells of the central cervical nucleus in the cat. *Exp. Brain Res.*, 55: 286–300.

[28] Berkley, K.J., Budell, F.J., Blomqvist, A. and Bull, M. (1986) Output systems of the dorsal column nuclei in the cat. *Brain Res. Rev.*, 11: 199–225.

[29] Imai, Y. and Kusama, T. (1969) Distribution of the dorsal root fibres in the cat. An experimental study with the Nauta method. *Brain Res.*, 13: 338–359.

[30] Abrahams, V.C., Richmond, F.J.R. and Keane, J. (1984) Projections from C2 and C3 nerves supplying muscles and skin of the cat neck: a study using transganglionic transport of horseradish peroxidase. *J. Comp. Neurol.*, 230: 142–154.

[31] Bakker, D.A., Richmond, F.J.R. and Abrahams, V.C. (1984) Central projections from cat suboccipital muscles: a study using transganglionic transport of horseradish peroxidase. *J. Comp. Neurol.*, 228: 409–421.

[32] Bakker, D.A., Richmond, F.J.R., Abrahams, V.C. and Courville, J. (1985) Patterns of primary afferent termination in the external cuneate nucleus from cervical axial muscles in the cat. *J. Comp. Neurol.*, 241: 467–479.

[33] Murakami, S. and Kato, M. (1983) Central projection of nuchal group I muscle afferent fibres of the cat. *Exp. Neurol.*, 79: 472–487.

[34] Richmond, F.J.R., Loeb, G.E. and Reesor, D. (1985) Electromyographic activity in neck muscles during head movement in the alert, unrestrained cat. *Soc. Neurosci. Abstr.*, 11: 85.

[35] Roucoux, A. and Crommelinck, M. (1988) Control of head movement during visual orientation. In B. Peterson and F.J.R. Richmond (Eds.), *Control of Head Movement*, Oxford University Press, New York, pp. 208–223.

[36] Richmond, F.J.R., MacGillis, D.R.R. and Scott, D.A. (1985) Muscle-fiber compartmentalization in cat splenius muscles. *J. Neurophysiol.*, 53: 868–885.

[37] Armstrong, J.B., Richmond, F.J.R. and Rose, P.K. (1982) Compartmentalization of motor units in the muscle biventer cervicis. *Soc. Neurosci. Abstr.*, 8: 330.

[38] Loeb, G.E., Yee, W.J., Pratt, C.A., Chanaud, C.M. and Richmond, F.J.R. (1987) Cross-correlation of EMG reveals widespread synchronization of motor units during some slow movements in intact cats. *J. Neurosci. Methods*, 21: 239–249.

[39] Richmond, F.J.R., Scott, D. and Abrahams, V.C. (1978) Distribution of motoneurons to the neck muscles biventer cervicis, splenius and complexus in the cat. *J. Comp. Neurol.*, 181: 451–463.

[40] Abrahams, V.C. and Keane, J. (1984) Contralateral, midline and commissural motoneurons of neck muscles: a retrograde HRP study in the cat. *J. Comp. Neurol.*, 223: 448–456.

[41] Abrahams, V.C., Downey, E.D. and Hammond, C.G.M. (1988) Organisation of sequential input from neck muscles to the external cuneate nucleus of the cat. *Exp. Brain Res., in press.*

O. Pompeiano and J.H.J. Allum (Eds.)
Progress in Brain Research, Vol. 76
© 1988 Elsevier Science Publishers B.V. (Biomedical Division)

CHAPTER 11

Convergence of neck and vestibular signals on spinal interneurons

V.J. Wilson

The Rockefeller University, 1230 York Avenue, New York, N Y 10021-6399, U.S.A.

The activity of interneurons in the cat cervical spinal cord, some in the enlargement and others in the upper cervical segments, is modulated by both whole body and body-on-head rotation. The two inputs, vestibular and neck, invariably oppose each other. The neurons, which include propriospinal neurons, presumably play a role in vestibulospinal and tonic neck reflexes. The dynamics of responses to sinusoidal stimulation indicate that for individual interneurons vestibular activity may originate in semicircular canals, otolith organs, or both receptor types. One source of neck input is from muscle spindles whose axons enter the spinal cord in the upper cervical segments. Response dynamics of these spindle afferents are very similar to those of interneurons.

Introduction

Rotation of the head with respect to the body evokes vestibulospinal and tonic neck reflexes acting on the limbs; reflexes important in the control of posture [19, 26]. Sinusoidal analysis with roll tilt as the stimulus has shown that in the decerebrate cat the two reflexes have similar gain and phase up to frequencies of about 0.2 Hz [11, 28]. In addition, the reflexes oppose each other, whether the stimulus is only roll [12, 17, 20] or a combination of roll and pitch [38]. For example, when the head is rolled to one side the vestibulospinal reflex excites the extensors of the limbs on the ear-down side, whereas the tonic neck reflex inhibits these extensors and excites those in the contralateral limbs. The result of these spatial and dynamic properties is that, at least at low frequencies, the reflexes tend to cancel each other.

Convergence and cancellation of neck and vestibular inputs occurs at premotor levels and also may take place at motoneurons themselves. One locus of convergence is in the vestibular nuclei. The activity of neurons in Deiters' nucleus, including many identified as vestibulospinal neurons, is modulated by both whole body and trunk rotation, i.e. by stimuli that activate vestibular and neck receptors respectively (e.g. [5]). When low-frequency roll stimulation is used, responses to neck and vestibular stimuli are out of phase (i.e. oppose each other) in more than half of the neurons [5]. Responses typically oppose each other when the stimulus consists of combined roll and pitch [16]. These latter experiments also show that, whereas some Deiters' neurons responding to neck rotation respond to stimulation of both canals and otoliths, others have only canal or otolith input. That is, neck input converges on neurons whose vestibular responses range from very tonic to very phasic.

Neck–vestibular convergence also takes place at spinal interneurons, where, as is the case with the reflexes themselves, the two inputs invariably oppose each other. Neurons with such convergence have been studied in the cervical enlargement [35] and in

---

Abbreviations: EMG, electromyograph; EPSP, excitatory postsynaptic potential; HRP, horseradish peroxidase; (L/M)VST, (lateral/medial) vestibulospinal tract.

segments rostral to the cervical and lumbar enlargements known to contain propriospinal neurons [6, 7, 33, 35]. As illustrated for the cervical cord in Fig. 1, the neurons in question are usually located medially in the gray matter. The remainder of this review will deal with the properties of vestibular and neck inputs to medial cervical neurons, concentrating on those in the C3–C4 segments, and will briefly consider the role these neurons may play in vestibular and tonic neck reflexes acting on the forelimbs.

Response of cervical interneurons to vestibular stimulation

Wilson et al. [35] studied neurons in C4–C8 that responded to roll tilt of the body with respect to the head and found that many also responded to vestibular stimulation (Fig. 1). Some were classified as receiving otolith or canal input, others as receiving a combination of the two. These experiments have recently been extended by Schor et al. [31] who also studied neurons in both the enlargement and in C4. Stimuli consisted of combined roll and pitch ('wobble' [30]), making it possible to determine the preferred direction of tilt for each neuron, and to study

the neuron's dynamics with stimuli oriented as closely as possible to that direction. The types of dynamics observed are illustrated in Fig. 2. 'Velocity' responses, indicating the presence of canal input (sometimes alone, sometimes in combination with otolith input), are shown in Fig. 2A, which also shows typical dynamics of vestibular reflexes acting on forelimb extensor muscles in the decerebrate cat. Fig. 2B illustrates 'position' responses, which are probably due to otolith input only. Some neurons were studied in preparations in which the semicircular canals had been inactivated by plugging, preparations in which the usual reflex response is replaced by a 'complex' one which manifests increasing gain and phase lag at frequencies above 0.1 Hz [28]. As shown in Fig. 2C, neurons in such preparations had position responses, and reflex-like complex behaviour was rare. This is a surprising observation, because in canal-plugged cats many vestibulospinal neurons do have complex responses [29].

Neurons in C4 may receive vestibular input via the LVST and MVST, or reticulospinal fibres (see [37]). Most MVST fibres end in the upper cervical

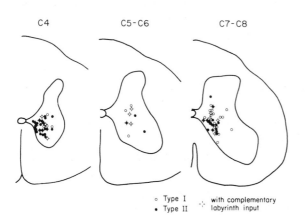

Fig. 1. Location of recording points determined either by dye marks or by reference to dye marks in the same track. Circular symbols represent neurons for which only neck information was available; symbols with crosses show neurons tested for and receiving vestibular input. Type I neurons are excited by roll jaw rotation to the ipsilateral side, type II neurons by contralateral jaw rotation. Complementary labyrinth input opposes (i.e. is out of phase with) neck input. (From [35]).

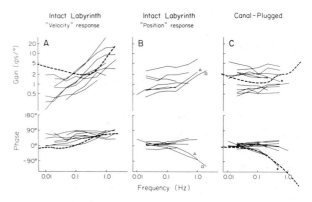

Fig. 2. Response dynamics of cervical interneurons to vestibular stimulation. Responses in animals with intact labyrinth have been grouped into 'velocity' (A) and 'position' (B) responses, with the former having larger phase leads and gain increases at high frequencies. The heavy dashed line in A illustrates the roll reflex response dynamics observed in the forelimb extensor muscle triceps brachii, the heavy line in C illustrated the forelimb reflex in the canal-plugged preparation (adapted from [28]). The gain and phase curves of three 'complex' responses are identified by symbols. (From [31]).

segments, and therefore only LVST or reticulospinal axons can act on neurons in the enlargement monosynaptically. The MVST, however, could influence these cells disynaptically via propriospinal neurons. For example, although few of the C4 neurons whose responses to vestibular stimulation were studied by Schor et al. [31] were tested for the presence of a caudally projecting axon, it is likely, because of their locations in the grey matter, that many were propriospinal neurons with axons terminating in the cervical enlargement where they may make synapses with segmental interneurons or with motoneurons. (Fig. 4B [7]). In any case, monosynaptic input from the vestibular nuclei does not seem to play a major role in determining interneuron response to natural stimulation. Erulkar et al. [10] first showed that some spinal interneurons responded at disynaptic latency to stimulation of the vestibular nerve. Many of our neurons were also excited disynaptically by such stimuli, but their responses to natural stimulation did not differ from those of neurons lacking such short-latency input [31].

Response of cervical interneurons to neck stimulation

When the body is rotated while the head is kept stationary the activity of many medially located cervical interneurons is strongly modulated. The dynamics of this modulation, i.e. gain slope and phase, resemble the dynamics of the response of forelimb extensor muscles, with the one difference that, on the average, the interneuron response has a phase advance of about 30–40° with respect to EMG modulation [35]. As already indicated, the interneurons are found in the enlargement and at upper cervical levels (Fig. 1) and many of those in the latter group are propriospinal neurons [7]. The question is: What receptors are activated by neck rotation, and how does this activity reach interneurons?

It has long been believed that the tonic neck reflex is due to excitation of neck-joint afferents [21]. A role for such receptors remains a possibility, but there is little anatomical evidence for the presence of slowly adapting receptors in the neck joints [25].

Even if such receptors were present it is by no means certain that their responses would code joint angle and be a suitable input for the tonic neck reflex [9]. Lately much attention has been devoted to the numerous muscle spindles in perivertebral neck muscles [4, 24, 25], which may provide some of the afferent input that evokes the tonic neck reflex. In recent experiments we have studied the behaviour of primary afferents whose activity is modulated by head rotation by taking advantage of the fact that the C2 dorsal root ganglion lies outside the spinal column and is easily accessible [8]. The C2 segment is known to provide afferent input which is important for the tonic neck reflex [19]. Floating electrodes were used to record from spontaneously firing afferents, most of which were identified as spindle afferents. Because input to the ganglion was restricted by nerve section, the spindles were probably located in lateral and ventral perivertebral muscles, as well as in sternocleidomastoid and, to a lesser extent, trapezius. The wobble stimulus was used to determine the best direction of head tilt (neck muscle stretch) for every afferent, and the dynamics were then studied with sinusoidal stimuli oriented close to this direction. In this way we identified two groups of spindle afferents with different properties. Type A afferents had a highly nonlinear response, great sensitivity to small sinusoidal stimuli and a strong dynamic response to trapezoidal stretch: these were probably mainly primary receptors. Type B afferents typically responded fairly linearly, had lower sensitivity and a less dynamic response than type A afferents. This group of receptors probably consisted in part of spindle secondaries, but could have included type A receptors relatively insensitive to roll and pitch and most sensitive to yaw rotation, which was not available for these experiments. More recently we were able to rotate the head in roll, pitch and yaw. Some type B receptors turned out to be most sensitive to yaw and, when stimulated in that direction, did respond more like type As, but the behaviour of the majority did not change qualitatively [36]. It therefore becomes more likely that the remaining type B receptors include many spindle secondaries.

Fig. 3 shows the similarity between the dynamics of the responses of neck spindle afferents and of C4 neurons to neck rotation. This similarity in behaviour, coupled with the great number of spindles in the neck musculature, supports the hypothesis that these receptors contribute to the responses of the interneurons discussed above, and to the tonic neck reflex.

Neck afferent input may get to the interneurons by two routes. Firstly, neck afferents can act on spinal neurons by a loop through the brainstem, of which vestibulospinal and reticulospinal neurons are the descending limb [5, 20]. Secondly, they may excite the neurons via intrinsic spinal pathways. The existence of such pathways is revealed by electric stimulation of the C2 ganglion, which excites some C4 neurons at latencies too short to allow a side path through the brainstem [34]. Furthermore, degeneration experiments have shown that afferents entering the spinal cord at the C2 level can be

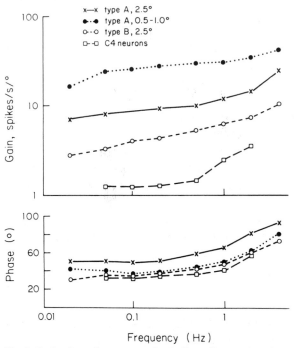

Fig. 3. Bode plots of responses of spindle endings and C4 interneurons to sinusoidal stimulation. The C4 neuron data ($n = 35$) is from the labyrinthectomized, decerebrate cats of Wilson et al. [35]. The n for type A spindle afferents was 15 at 2.5°, 5 at 1.0° and 0.5°, and 13 for type B afferents. (From [8]).

traced caudally as far as C6 [15, 18], and stimulation of the C2 dorsal root evokes monosynaptic EPSPs in some long propriospinal neurons in C3–C5 [3]. None of these experiments identified the afferents involved. We have recently determined the caudal extent of the descending collaterals of C2 spindle afferents by stimulating them antidromically with a moveable electrode on the surface of the dorsal columns while recording from the C2 ganglion [39]. Approximately a third of the spindle afferents have decending collaterals that extend as far as C4 or further, and the latency of their response to antidromic stimulation is appropriate to allow monosynaptic transmission to neurons at the C4 level. Evidence from HRP injection of primary spindle-like afferents shows that, at least in the segment in which they enter the spinal cord, these afferents terminate medially in the grey matter [14, 27], including the region where propriospinal neurons modulated by neck rotation and projecting to different levels of the spinal cord are found (Fig. 4). There is thus reasonable evidence for spindle activity reaching cervical propriospinal neurons in the same, or more caudal, segments.

Reflex role of propriospinal neurons

Until recently there has been no anatomical or physiological evidence for monosynaptic connections between neurons in the vestibular nuclei and forelimb motoneurons (see [37] for review), thus emphasizing the role of interneurons in vestibulospinal reflexes acting on the forelimbs. Connections between upper cervical afferents and forelimb motoneurons also are polysynaptic [22]. It seems very likely that some of the interneurons that we studied in the cervical enlargement project to motoneurons and play a role in neck and vestibular reflexes. It is tempting to suggest that the same is true for propriospinal neurons. Laterally located propriospinal neurons in C3–C4 provide one route for pyramidal impulses to forelimb motoneurons and are required for target reaching, as opposed to food taking, movements [2]. Medially located neurons in these, and perhaps more caudal, segments may be impor-

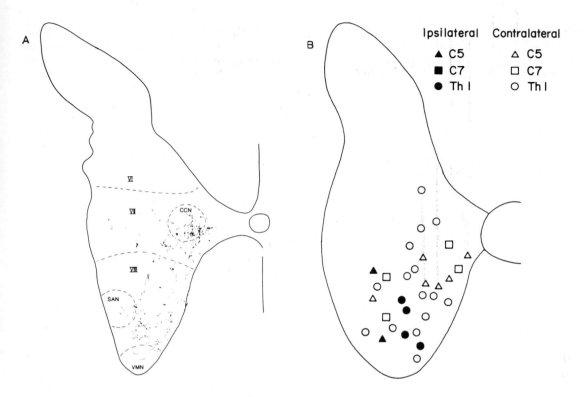

Fig. 4. (A) Distribution in C2, in the sagittal plane, of boutons from a primary spindle-like afferent injected intra-axonally with HRP. This afferent, innervating the biventer cervicis–complexus muscle, entered the spinal cord in C2. Each dot shows the position of a single bouton. SAN, spinal accessory nucleus; CCN, central cervical nucleus; VMN, ventral medial nucleus. (From [27]). (B) Location in C4 of propriospinal neurons whose activity was modulated by neck rotation. These neurons were activated antidromically by electrodes placed ipsi- or contralaterally in the ventral white matter at the segmental levels indicated. (Unpublished observations of E.E. Brink, I. Suzuki, S.J.B. Timerick and V.J. Wilson).

tant in neck and vestibular reflexes. This, however, remains a hypothesis. It must still be demonstrated that propriospinal neurons belonging to this population make synapses with forelimb motoneurons, although experiments using retrograde transneuronal transport of wheat germ agglutinin-HRP, such as those of Alstermark and Kummel [1], and corresponding ones in the lumbar cord by Harrison et al. [13], suggest that some of them do. Furthermore, in some situations there are differences between the behaviour of interneurons and muscle. In the case of neck reflexes, it is not known whether the phase difference between the responses of interneurons and muscle referred to above is due to the difference in preparations in which the two were studied (e.g. paralysed vs. nonparalysed) or indicates the

presence of additional elements in the pathway. In the case of vestibulospinal reflexes, the responses of interneurons and muscle to natural stimulation that activates the whole labyrinth are often similar (Fig. 2A). However, the complex response characteristic of pure otolith reflexes, found in vestibulospinal neurons, is elusive at the interneuronal level, suggesting that another route to motoneurons must exist. Recently Shinoda et al. [32] have produced evidence that some LVST axons terminate in lamina IX in the cervical enlargement and make synapses with limb motoneurons. Perhaps as far as some vestibulospinal reflexes acting on the limb are concerned, such connections between LVST axons and motoneurons are more important than previously believed.

142

Acknowledgement

Work in the author's laboratory supported by grants from NIH (NS02619) and NASA (NSG2380).

References

[1] Alstermark, B. and Kummel, H. (1986) Transneuronal labelling of neurones projecting to forelimb motoneurones in cats performing different movements. *Brain Res.*, 376: 387–391.

[2] Alstermark, B., Lundberg, A., Norsell, U. and Sybirska, E. (1981) Integration in descending motor pathways controlling the forelimb in the cat. 9. Differential behavioural defects after spinal cord lesions interrupting defined pathways from higher centres to motoneurones. *Exp. Brain Res.*, 42: 299–318.

[3] Alstermark, B., Lundberg, A., Pinter, M. and Sasaki, S. (1987) Long C3–C5 propriospinal neurones in the cat. *Brain Res.*, 404: 382–388.

[4] Bakker, D.A. and Richmond, F.J.R. (1982) Muscle spindle complexes in muscles around upper cervical vertebrae in the cat. *J. Neurophysiol.*, 48: 62–74.

[5] Boyle, R. and Pompeiano, O. (1981) Convergence and interaction of neck and macular vestibular inputs on vestibulospinal neurons. *J. Neurophysiol.*, 45: 852–868.

[6] Brink, E.E., Suzuki, I., Timerick, S.J.B. and Wilson, V.J. (1984) Directional sensitivity of neurons in the lumbar spinal cord to neck rotation. *Brain Res.*, 323: 172–175.

[7] Brink, E.E., Suzuki, I., Timerick, S.J.B. and Wilson, V.J. (1985) Tonic neck reflex of the decerebrate cat: a role for propriospinal neurons. *J. Neurophysiol.* 54: 978–987.

[8] Chan, Y.S., Kasper, J. and Wilson, V.J. (1987) Dynamics and directional sensitivity of neck muscle spindle responses to head rotation. *J. Neurophysiol.*, 57: 1716–1729.

[9] Darian-Smith, I. (1984) The sense of touch: performance and peripheral neural processes. In I. Darian-Smith (Ed.), *The Nervous System, Vol. 3, Sensory Processes*, Williams and Wilkins, Baltimore, pp. 739–788.

[10] Erulkar, S.D., Sprague, J.M., Whitesel, B.L., Dogan, S. and Jannetta, P.J. (1966) Organization of the vestibular projection to the spinal cord of the cat. *J. Neurophysiol.*, 29: 626–664.

[11] Ezure, K. and Wilson, V.J. (1983) Dynamics of neck-to-forelimb reflexes in the decerebrate cat. *J. Neurophysiol.*, 50: 688–695.

[12] Ezure, K. and Wilson, V.J. (1984) Interaction of tonic neck and vestibular reflexes in the forelimb of the decerebrate cat. *Exp. Brain Res.*, 54: 289–292.

[13] Harrison, P.J., Jankowska, E. and Zytnicki, D. (1986) Lamina VIII interneurones interposed in crossed reflex pathways in the cat. *J. Physiol. London*, 371: 147–166.

[14] Hirai, N., Hongo, T., Sasaki, S., Yamashita, M. and Yoshida, K. (1984) Neck muscle afferent input to spinocerebellar tract cells of the central cervical nucleus in the cat. *Exp. Brain Res.*, 55: 286–300.

[15] Imai, Y. and Kusama, T. (1969) Distribution of the dorsal root fibers in the cat. An experimental study with the Nauta method. *Brain Res.*, 13: 338–359.

[16] Kasper, J., Schor, R.H. and Wilson, V.J. (1987) Convergence of neck and vestibular influences on neurons in the vestibular nuclei of the decerebrate cat. *Soc. Neurosci. Abstr.*, 13: 1224.

[17] Lindsay, K.W., Roberts, T.D.M. and Rosenberg, J.R. (1976) Asymmetric tonic labyrinth reflexes and their interaction with neck reflexes in the decerebrate cat. *J. Physiol. London*, 261: 583–601.

[18] Liu, C.N. (1956) Afferent nerves to Clarke's and the lateral cuneate nuclei in the cat. *Arch. Neurol. Psychiat.*, 75: 67–77.

[19] Magnus, R. (1924) *Korperstellung*, Springer-Verlag, Berlin.

[20] Manzoni, D., Pompeiano, O., Srivastava, U.C. and Stampacchia, G. (1983) Responses of forelimb extensors to sinusoidal stimulation of macular, labyrinth and neck receptors. *Arch. Ital. Biol.*, 121: 205–214.

[21] McCouch, G.P., Deering, I.D. and Ling, T.H. (1951) Location of receptors for tonic neck reflexes. *J. Neurophysiol.*, 14: 191–195.

[22] Nakajima, K., Maeda, M., Ishii, S. and Miyazaki M. (1981) Neuronal organization of the tonic neck reflex. *Equilibrium Res.*, 40: 195–201.

[23] Pompeiano, O., Manzoni, D., Srivastava, U.C. and Stampacchia, G. (1984) Convergence and interaction of neck and macular vestibular inputs on reticulospinal neurons. *Neuroscience*, 12: 111–128.

[24] Richmond, F.J.R. and Abrahams, V.C. (1979) Physiological properties of muscle spindles in dorsal neck muscles of the cat. *J. Neurophysiol.*, 42: 604–617.

[25] Richmond, F.J.R. and Bakker, D.A. (1982) Anatomical organization and sensory receptor content of soft tissues surrounding upper cervical vertebrae in the cat. *J. Neurophysiol.*, 48: 49–61.

[26] Roberts, T.D.M. (1978) *Neurophysiology of Postural Mechanisms* (2nd edn.), Butterworths, London, 415 pp.

[27] Rose, P.K. and Keirstead, S.A. (1986) Segmental projections from muscle spindles: a perspective from the upper cervical spinal cord. *Can. J. Physiol. Pharmacol.*, 64: 505–508.

[28] Schor, R.H. and Miller, A.D. (1981) Vestibular reflexes in neck and forelimb muscles evoked by roll tilt. *J. Neurophysiol.*, 46: 167–178.

[29] Schor, R.H. and Miller, A.D. (1982) Relationship of cat vestibular neurons to otolith-spinal reflexes. *Exp. Brain Res.*, 47: 137–144.

[30] Schor, R.H., Miller, A.D. and Tomko, D.L. (1984) Responses to head tilt in cat central vestibular neurons. I. Direction of maximum sensitivity. *J. Neurophysiol.*, 51: 136–146.

[31] Schor, R.H., Suzuki, I., Timerick, S.J.B. and Wilson, V.J. (1986) Responses of interneurons in the cat cervical cord to vestibular tilt stimulation. *J. Neurophysiol.*, 56: 1147–1156.

[32] Shinoda, Y., Ohgaki, T. and Futami, T. (1986) The morphology of single lateral vestibulospinal tract axons in the lower cervical spinal cord of the cat. *J. Comp. Neurol.*, 249: 226–241.

[33] Suzuki, I., Timerick, S.J.B. and Wilson, V.J. (1985) Body position with respect to the head or body position in space is coded by lumbar interneurons. *J. Neurophysiol.*, 54: 123–133.

[34] Suzuki, I., Park, B.R. and Wilson, V.J. (1986) Directional sensitivity of, and neck afferent input to, cervical and lumbar interneurons modulated by neck rotation. *Brain Res.*, 367: 356–359.

[35] Wilson, V.J., Ezure, K. and Timerick, S.J.B. (1984) Tonic neck reflex of the decerebrate cat: response of spinal interneurons to natural stimulation of neck and vestibular receptors. *J. Neurophysiol.*, 51: 567–577.

[36] Wilson, V.J., Kasper, J., Yates, B.J. and Schor, R.H. (1987) Three-demensional directional sensitivity of neck muscle spindle responses to head rotation. *Soc. Neurosci. Abstr.*, 13: 1693.

[37] Wilson, V.J. and Melvill Jones, G. (1979) *Mammalian Vestibular Physiology*, Plenum, New York, 365 pp.

[38] Wilson, V.J., Schor, R.H., Suzuki, I. and Park, B.R. (1986) Spatial organization of neck and vestibular reflexes acting on the forelimbs of the decerebrate cat. *J. Neurophysiol.*, 55: 514–526.

[39] Yates, B.J., Kasper, J. and Wilson, V.J. (1987) Descending projections of neck muscle spindle afferents in the dorsal columns. *Soc. Neurosci. Abstr.*, 13: 1694.

O. Pompeiano and J.H.J. Allum (Eds.)
Progress in Brain Research, Vol. 76
© 1988 Elsevier Science Publishers B.V. (Biomedical Division)

CHAPTER 12

Convergence of macular vestibular and neck inputs on vestibulospinal and reticulospinal neurons projecting to the lumbosacral cord

D. Manzoni

Dipartimento di Fisiologia e Biochimica, Università di Pisa, Via S. Zeno 31, 56100 Pisa, Italy

The activity of excitatory LVN neurons as well as of reticular neurons located in the inhibitory area of the medullary RF, the majority of which were antidromically identified as projecting to the lumbosacral segments of the spinal cord, was recorded in decerebrate cats. These neurons were tested during sinusoidal stimulation of macular vestibular, neck or combined receptors by using sinusoidal rotations about the longitudinal axis at the standard parameters of 0.026 Hz, $\pm 10°$. A large proportion of LVN neurons as well as of medullary RF neurons responded with a periodic modulation of their firing rate to individual stimulation of vestibular and neck receptors. For both populations of convergent neurons the gain of the neck responses was higher on the average than that of the macular responses; moreover, the neck responses showed a larger phase lead with respect to position than the responses of the same neurons to the macular input at the standard parameters of stimulation. As to the response pattern, the majority of the convergent vestibular (53/58, i.e. 91.4%) and reticular neurons (58/71, i.e. 81.7%) showed reciprocal ('out of phase') responses to the two inputs. However, while the VS neurons were mainly excited during side-down animal tilt and side-up neck rotation, the RS neurons showed the opposite response patterns. The response characteristics of vestibular and medullary reticular neurons to the combined macular and neck inputs, elicited during head rotation, closely corresponded to those predicted by a vectorial summation of the individual macular and neck responses. The findings are discussed in relation to the possibility that both excitatory VS neurons as well as presumably inhibitory RS neurons contribute to the postural adjustments of the limb musculature during the vestibular and neck reflexes.

Introduction

Experiments performed in decerebrate cats have shown that displacement of the head after neck deafferentation [14] or slow sinusoidal tilt about the longitudinal axis of the whole animal on the one hand ([9, 20, 34]; for references see [3]), and displacement of the neck with a stationary head on the other [7, 8, 9, 14, 17, 18, 20, 23] produced opposite patterns of responses in limb extensors, due to stimulation of macular labyrinth and neck receptors. In particular, side-down rotation of the head or of the animal produced contraction, whereas side-up rotation resulted in relaxation of ipsilateral limb extensors; these reciprocal patterns of response, however, reversed for the same directions of neck rotation. These findings could explain why directional changes in head position in the intact preparation, i.e. when both tonic labyrinth and neck reflexes act in opposition, leave the position of the limbs unmodified [9, 20, 24, 32, 33, 40].

Abbreviations: LVN, lateral vestibular nucleus; RF, reticular formation; (l)RS, (lumbosacral) reticulospinal; (l)VS, (lumbosacral) vestibulospinal.

The responses of limb extensors to independent or combined labyrinthine and neck stimulations, as described above, can in part at least be attributed to an integration of opposite influences arising from macular and neck receptors, converging through independent or common channels on either spinal motoneurons and propriospinal neurons [41] or neurons of supraspinal pathways. This last hypothesis has been tested at the level of two main populations of neurons: the VS neurons originating from the LVN, which exert an excitatory influence on ipsilateral extensor motoneurons ([16]; for references see [26, 42]) and the RS neurons originating from the medial aspect of the medullary RF, which exert an inhibitory influence on the same motoneurons [10, 15, 19, 25].

Observations originally made by Boyle and Pompeiano [3–5] demonstrated that most of the LVN neurons received convergence from both types of receptors, as shown by the appearance of responses which were mainly in phase with animal position and neck displacement; however, not all these units were excited by side-down animal tilt (cf. also [35]) and side-up neck rotation. In these experiments, the majority of the recorded units were not antidromically identified as projecting to specific segments of the spinal cord; moreover, these units were found to be histologically distributed throughout the whole extent of the LVN, which controls not only the limb extensors but also the dorsal neck musculature. Therefore, the units which did not show the reciprocal pattern of responses to the two inputs described above could be involved in some synergistic influence that the same inputs exert on motoneurons controlling neck and/or axial muscles [28].

The hypothesis that changes in firing rate of LVN neurons contribute to the postural adjustments of limb extensors during natural stimulation of macular labyrinth and neck receptors is supported by the results of recent experiments showing that VS neurons originating from the LVN and antidromically activated as projecting to the lumbosacral segments of the spinal cord (lVS neurons) were mainly excited during side-down tilt of the whole animal and side-up neck rotation [22, 30, 39].

In addition to these findings, experiments were performed in which the response characteristics of presumably inhibitory RS neurons originating from the medial aspect of the medullary RF and projecting to the lumbosacral segments of the spinal cord (lRS neurons) were recorded during independent or combined stimulation of labyrinth and neck receptors. In particular, it was shown that most of these neurons increased their firing rate during side-up animal tilt and side-down neck rotation [21, 28, 29, 38]. These response patterns were just opposite to those displayed by the lVS neurons for the same directions of animal tilt and neck displacement, thus contributing to the postural responses of limb extensors during the vestibular and neck reflexes.

The experiments reviewed in this chapter were performed to study the degree of convergence of both macular and neck inputs on these two populations of neurons, as well as the characteristics of their response to individual or combined stimulations of labyrinth and neck receptors. The results were obtained by the author in collaboration with Drs. O. Pompeiano and G. Stampacchia (Pisa), A.R. Marchand (Marseille) and U.C. Srivastava (Allahabad).

Convergence of macular and neck inputs on lateral vestibulospinal neurons

Marchand et al. [22] and Pompeiano et al. [30] have recorded the activity of 119 histologically identified LVN neurons, 106 of which were activated antidromically by electrical stimulation of the spinal cord between Th12 and L1 (lVS neurons: conduction velocity of the corresponding axons, 90.5 $\pm$ 20.8 m/s, mean $\pm$ S.D). Of the 119 neurons, 77 (64.7%) responded to roll tilt of the whole animal at the standard parameters of 0.026 Hz, $\pm 10°$; moreover 65 out of these 77 units were antidromically activated by spinal cord stimulation. If we consider the same population of 119 neurons, 81 (68.1%) were modulated during neck rotation at the same parameters reported above; moreover, 74 out of these 81 units projected to the lumbosacral cord.

Among the 119 units tested during sinusoidal

stimulation of macular and neck receptors, 58 (48.7%) received convergent input from both types of receptors [39]. Histological controls indicated that these convergent units were mainly located within the dorsocaudal part of the LVN (43 out of 58 units), the remaining units being located within the rostroventral part of the LVN (15 out of 58 units). Moreover, most of the convergent units (52 out of 58 units) were lVS units.

The base frequency of all the lateral vestibular neurons receiving convergent input from both macular and neck receptors corresponded on the average to 17.9 ± 16.7 imp./s (mean $\pm$ S.D., $n = 58$), if evaluated during stimulation at standard parameters of labyrinth or neck receptors. The average gain of these units was higher for the neck responses (0.58 ± 0.45 imp./s/deg, mean $\pm$ S.D.) than for the macular responses (0.52 ± 0.49 imp./s/deg) (paired t-test, $p < 0.01$), as shown also in Fig. 1A, where for each convergent unit the gain of the neck response was related to that of the macular response. Moreover, the ratio between the response

gains to the neck input and the macular input (G_N/G_M) averaged 1.66 ± 1.55 (mean $\pm$ S.D.) for the 58 convergent units, corresponding to 1.52 ± 1.26 (mean $\pm$ S.D.) for the 52 lVS neurons. It is of interest that the gain values obtained for the convergent units were higher than those obtained for the units responding only to labyrinth ($n = 19$ units; 0.33 ± 0.35 imp./s/deg, mean $\pm$ S.D.) or neck stimulation ($n = 23$; 0.24 ± 0.12 imp./s/deg) (t-test between the means, $p > 0.05$ and $p < 0.001$ for gain differences of the units responding only to the macular input or to the neck input).

The distribution of the phase angle of the macular and the neck responses for the convergent vestibular nuclear neurons is shown in the upper histograms of Fig. 2A and B, respectively. Most units were grouped in two main populations, indicated by horizontal bars, which responded preferentially to the direction of stimulus orientation, and showed an average phase lead with respect to the extreme side-down ($0°$) or side-up ($180°$) displacement of $+21.9 \pm 25.9°$ (mean $\pm$ S.D.) for the macular re-

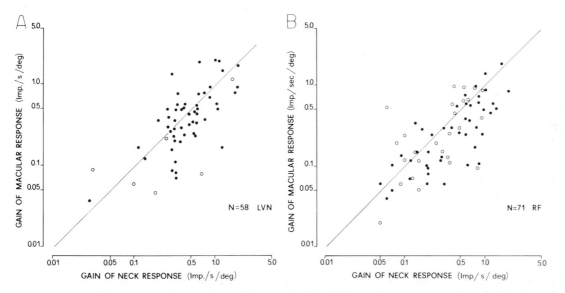

Fig. 1. Relation between gains of the first harmonic responses of vestibular nuclear neurons (A) and medullary reticular neurons (B) to macular and neck inputs evaluated at standard parameters of stimulation. In both diagrams the gain of the macular response (ordinate) is compared to that of the neck response (abscissa) for each unit. The line corresponding to slope 1 would apply if both response gains were equal. Among the convergent units, 52 out of 58 vestibular nuclear neurons and 45 out of 71 medullary reticular neurons were antidromically identified as projecting to the lumbosacral cord (●); the remaining neurons were not driven antidromically (○). (From [29, 39]).

sponses ($n = 53$) and $+51.4 \pm 16.9°$ for the neck responses ($n = 56$). Moreover, most of the responsive units were excited by side-down tilt of the whole animal (42/58 units, i.e. 72.4%) and by side-up neck rotation (48/58 units, i.e. 82.8%).

The units receiving convergent inputs from labyrinth and neck receptors were subdivided according to the absolute difference in the phase angle of re-

sponses to the individual macular and neck inputs elicited by standard parameters of stimulation ($\Delta\varphi$). Specifically, 53 out of 58 convergent units (i.e. 91.4%) were characterized by reciprocal ('out of phase') responses, i.e. $\Delta\varphi > 90°$, while only 5 out of 58 units (i.e. 8.6%) were characterized by parallel ('in phase') responses, i.e. $\Delta\varphi < 90°$ to both inputs. Moreover, the majority of the 53 units showing a

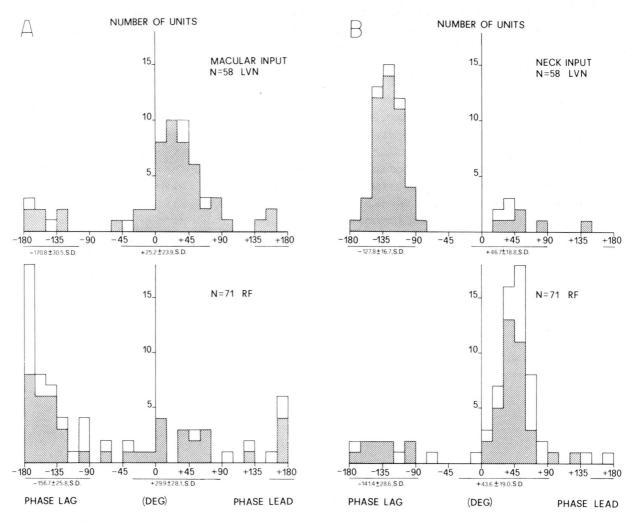

Fig. 2. Comparison of the phase angle of the first harmonic responses of vestibular nuclear neurons and medullary reticular neurons to sinusoidal stimulation of macular receptors (A) and neck receptors (B) at standard parameters. Among the 58 vestibular neurons and the 71 medullary reticular neurons receiving convergence from the macular and neck inputs, 52 were lVS and 45 were lRS neurons (shaded columns), the remaining units being not antidromically activated (open columns). Positive and negative numbers in the abscissa indicate in degrees the phase lead and lag, respectively, of the responses with respect to the extreme side-down displacement of the animal (A) or of the neck (B) as indicated by 0°. Mean value and standard deviation (S.D.) of the phase angle of responses are underlined below each histogram. (From [29, 39]).

$\Delta\varphi$ of the responses higher than 90° (i.e. 38 units, 71.7%) were excited by side-down tilt of the whole animal and side-up neck rotation, while most of the 5 units showing a $\Delta\varphi$ of the responses lower than 90° (i.e. 3 units, 60%) were excited during side-up animal tilt and neck rotation.

It is of interest that in the group of 53 units displaying reciprocal responses, the gains of the macular (0.55 ± 0.50 imp./s/deg, mean ± S.D.) and the neck responses (0.61 ± 0.46 imp./s/deg) were slightly higher than those obtained from the whole population of responsive units, the average ratio of the gains (G_N/G_M) corresponding to 1.67 ± 1.62 (mean ± S.D.).

Contrary of the units displaying reciprocal responses, the 5 units that showed parallel responses had gains of the macular (0.24 ± 0.19 imp./s/deg, mean ± S.D.) and the neck responses (0.29 ± 0.11 imp./s/deg) that were on average lower than those obtained from the whole population of responsive units; in this instance the ratio of the gains was 1.54 ± 0.54 (mean ± S.D.).

Convergence of macular and neck inputs on medullary reticulospinal neurons

Pompeiano et al. [29] have recorded the responses of 127 units histologically identified as being located in the inhibitory area of the medullary RF during independent stimulation of macular and neck receptors. Among the tested neurons, 77 units were activated by electrical stimulation of the spinal cord between Th12 and L1 (lRS neurons; conduction velocity of the corresponding axons 67.6 ± 27.5 m/s, mean ± S.D.). Of the 127 medullary reticular neurons, 84 (66.1%) displayed a periodic modulation of their firing rate during roll tilt of the animal at the standard parameters; moreover, 50 out of these 84 units were antidromically activated by spinal cord stimulation. Among the same population of 127 neurons, 93 units (73.2%) responded to neck rotation at the same parameters reported above; moreover 59 out of these 93 units projected to the lumbosacral cord.

Among the 127 units submitted to sinusoidal stimulation of macular and neck receptors, 71 units (55.9%) received convergent input from both types of receptors. Histological controls indicated that these convergent units were distributed throughout the nucleus reticularis gigantocellularis, magnocellularis and ventralis. Moreover, 45 out of 71 convergent units were lRS neurons.

The firing rate of all the medullary reticular neurons receiving convergent inputs from both macular and neck receptors was 11.9 ± 8.9 imp./s (mean ± S.D., $n = 71$). The gain of these units was higher for the neck responses (0.49 ± 0.41 imp./s/deg, mean ± S.D.) than for the macular responses (0.40 ± 0.39 imp./s/deg) (paired t-test, $p < 0.001$). Fig. 1B relates the gain of the neck response to that of the macular response for each reticular unit receiving convergent input from both types of receptors. In this instance the ratio between the response gains to the neck input and the macular input (G_N/G_M) averaged 1.80 ± 1.55 (mean ± S.D.) for all the 71 units tested, corresponding to 1.90 ± 1.50 (mean ± S.D.) for the 45 lRS neurons.

The distribution of the phase angle of the macular and the neck responses for the convergent reticular neurons is illustrated in the lower histograms of Fig. 2A and B, respectively. Most units responded preferentially to the direction of stimulus orientation and showed a phase lead with respect to the extreme side-down (0°) or side-up (180°) displacement of + 24.9 ± 26.3° (mean ± S.D.) for the macular responses ($n = 64$) and + 42.7 ± 20.9° for the neck responses ($n = 67$). Moreover, the majority of the responsive units were excited by side-up tilt of the whole animal (49/71 units, i.e. 69.0%) and by side-down neck rotation (55/71 units, i.e. 77.5%).

Following the criteria reported in the previous section, the convergent units were subdivided according to the difference in the phase angle of responses to the individual macular and neck inputs ($\Delta\varphi$). Specifically, 58 out of 71 convergent units (i.e. 81.7%) were characterized by reciprocal responses, i.e. $\Delta\varphi > 90°$, while only 13 out of 71 units (i.e. 18.3%) showed parallel responses, i.e. $\Delta\varphi < 90°$. Moreover, the majority of the 58 units showing 'out of phase' responses (i.e. 44 units, 75.9%) were excited by side-up tilt of the whole animal and side-down neck rotation, while most of the 13 units showing 'in phase' responses (i.e. 7 units, 53.8%) were excited during side-down animal tilt and neck rotation.

It is worth mentioning that among the group of 58 units displaying reciprocal responses, the gains of the macular responses (0.39 $\pm$ 0.36 imp./s/deg, mean $\pm$ S.D.) and the neck responses (0.52 $\pm$ 0.41 imp./s/deg) did not greatly differ from those obtained from the whole population of responsive units (t-test between the means, $p > 0.05$), the ratio of the gains (G_N/G_M) corresponding to 1.68 $\pm$ 1.18 (mean $\pm$ S.D.). Similarly, the 13 units that showed parallel responses had gains of the macular (0.41 $\pm$ 0.52, S.D. imp./s/deg, mean $\pm$ S.D.) and the neck responses (0.39 $\pm$ 0.41 imp./s/deg) comparable to the values obtained from the whole population of responsive units; moreover, the ratio of the gains was 2.44 $\pm$ 2.61 (mean $\pm$ S.D.).

Interaction between macular and neck responses during head rotation

The responses of vestibular nuclear neurons [5] as well as of medullary reticular neurons [29] receiving convergent neck and macular vestibular inputs were evaluated in detail during combined receptors activation elicited by head rotation at the standard parameters. Each of the units examined during head rotation responded in a fashion predicted from the vectorial summation of responses obtained from the separate macular and neck stimulations. This finding was observed irrespective of the gain and phase relation between the two responses.

In particular, a cancellation of the labyrinth and neck responses during head rotation occurred only when the individual responses had the same gain and were exactly 180° out of phase. When, most frequently, the response gains of the neck and macular inputs were slightly different, the phase angle of response to head rotation approached an intermediate value (about 90°) in those instances in which the responses were almost in opposition of phase; this value decreased progressively below 90°

when the peaks of the two individual responses became more and more in phase. In these instances, the more prominent the gain of the unit response to one input with respect to the other, the smaller the difference between the phase angle of the response to head rotation and that to the prominent input. This is actually what one would expect on the basis of vectorial summation of the responses. In all instances, the experimental values of the gain and phase angle of response obtained during head rotation corresponded closely to the component values of the vector predicted by a linear summation of the separate macular and neck responses.

Discussion

Responses of VS and medullary RS neurons to macular and neck inputs

Previous experiments had shown that lVS neurons [22, 30] as well as medullary lRS neurons projecting to the lumbosacral cord [21, 38] responded to roll tilt of the animal and neck rotation at 0.026 Hz, $\pm$ 10°. The unit responses to animal tilt were obtained with stimuli that were subthreshold for vestibular nuclear responses to the angular input (cf. [31, 36]), thus being attributed to stimulation of macular vestibular receptors. On the other hand, the responses to neck rotation were attributed to stimulation of deep neck receptors, i.e. joint and/or muscle spindle receptors, that are in part at least related to the atlanto-occipital and the atlanto-axial joints and membranes [1, 23] and are innervated by the dorsal root ganglia C1–C2 [12, 13].

Experiments reviewed in this chapter [29, 39] have shown that a large proportion of LVN neurons (48.7%) as well as of medullary reticular neurons (55.9%), most of which were identified antidromically as projecting to the lumbosacral segments of the spinal cord, responded with a periodic modulation of the firing rate to individual stimulation of both macular vestibular and neck receptors, while 35.3% of the LVN neurons and 27.6% of the medullary reticular units responded to the macular input or to the neck input only. Moreover, the convergent units – particularly those located in LVN – showed a higher gain than that of the units responding only to animal tilt or neck rotation.

If we compare the response characteristics of the convergent vestibular and reticular neurons, namely of the lVS and the lRS neurons, to the neck and the macular inputs, some differences are observed. In particular, the gain of the neck responses was on average higher than that of the macular responses at the standard parameters of stimulation. Moreover, the neck responses showed on average a larger phase lead with respect to position than the responses of the same neurons to the macular input. This finding can be of great importance in the free-moving animal where, during the vestibulospinal reflexes acting on the limb musculature, an activation of neck receptors may occur as a result of the reflex contraction of the neck musculature following labyrinth stimulation (for references see [42]). In this instance the prominent phase lead of responses of the lVS and the lRS neurons to neck rotation might anticipate the arrival of the corresponding volleys on limb extensor motoneurons, thus compensating for the later recruitment of the neck receptors with respect to the labyrinth receptors when head position is changed in space.

Patterns of convergence of macular and neck inputs on VS and medullary RS neurons projecting to the lumbosacral cord

Among the LVN neurons, namely the lVS neurons projecting to the lumbosacral segments of the spinal cord, two populations of convergent neurons were found [39]. In the first and most prominent group (53/58, i.e. 91.4%), the responses to the macular and neck inputs were organized reciprocally, i.e. 'out of phase', and were mainly characterized by excitation during side-down tilt of the whole animal and side-up neck rotation. In the other group (5/58, i.e. 8.6%), the units showed parallel responses to the individual macular and neck inputs, i.e. 'in phase', being mainly characterized by excitation during side-up animal tilt and neck rotation. The smaller proportion of convergent LVN neurons showing

reciprocal responses (45/75, i.e. 60%) and the higher proportion of convergent LVN neurons showing parallel responses (30/75, i.e. 40%) to the two inputs, as reported in a previous study [5], can be attributed to the fact that the whole extent of Deiters' nucleus was explored in these experiments, thus including neurons projecting not only to the limbs but also to the neck extensor motoneurons.

Patterns of convergence similar to those described for the lVS neurons were also found among the medullary lRS neurons projecting to the same segments of the spinal cord [29]. Even in this instance most of the convergent units (58/71, i.e. 81.7%) showed reciprocal responses to the macular and neck inputs, while the remaining units (13/71, i.e. 18.3%) showed parallel responses. However, the majority of the medullary reticular neurons showing reciprocal responses to the individual macular and neck inputs were characterized by excitation during side-up tilt of the whole animal and side-down neck rotation. On the other hand, the majority of the medullary reticular units showing parallel responses to the two inputs were characterized by excitation during both side-down animal tilt and neck rotation. These responses were just opposite to those of the vestibulospinal neurons projecting to the lumbosacral segments of the spinal cord. The pathways and the mechanisms by which the macular and the neck inputs produce opposite response patterns at the level of the homogeneous populations of lVS and medullary lRS neurons have been discussed in detail in previous studies [6, 11, 27].

The vestibulospinal as well as the reticulospinal neurons receiving convergent labyrinth and neck inputs are probably involved in the postural changes of the limb muscles during the tonic labyrinth and neck reflexes (see [28]). However, while the LVN exerts an excitatory influence on ipsilateral extensor motoneurons ([16]; for references see [26, 42]), the medullary reticular neurons are probably inhibitory in function. This conclusion is supported by the fact that the latter neurons were recorded from the medullary inhibitory area of Magoun and Rhines [19], i.e. from that region which, upon stimulation, produces postsynaptic inhibition in hindlimb motoneurons [10, 15, 25]; further arguments supporting this hypothesis have been reported in a previous study [29]. Particularly relevant in this connection is the demonstration that a progressive increase in resting discharge of these reticular neurons leads to a parallel decrease in postural activity [37].

If we consider the two populations of excitatory VS and inhibitory RS neurons showing *reciprocal* 'out of phase' responses to the labyrinth and neck inputs, we may explain why side-down tilt of the whole animal produces contraction of the ipsilateral and relaxation of contralateral limb extensors, whereas side-down neck rotation produces the opposite posture (see Introduction). In particular, the increased activity of ipsilateral limb extensor motoneurons during side-down tilt would be due to both an increased discharge of the excitatory lVS neurons and a reduced discharge of the inhibitory lRS neurons (disinhibition); on the other hand, the reduced activity of ipsilateral limb extensor motoneurons during side-down neck rotation would be due to both a reduced discharge of the excitatory lVS neurons (disfacilitation) and an increased activity of the inhibitory lRS neurons.

As to the two populations of vestibulospinal and reticulospinal neurons projecting to the lumbosacral segments of the spinal cord and showing *parallel* 'in phase' responses to macular and neck stimulations, it appears that the majority of the excitatory lVS neurons undergo a decrease in firing rate during side-down animal tilt and neck rotation, while the majority of the inhibitory lRS neurons undergo an increase in firing rate for the same direction of animal and neck orientation. In this instance, both macular and neck inputs might contribute to some synergistic influences on limited groups of motoneurons innervating hindlimb muscles. We cannot exclude, however, that some of these VS and RS neurons converge on motoneurons controlling axial muscles.

Independently upon the patterns of convergence of macular vestibular and neck inputs within the medullary structures, the responses of VS and RS neurons to head rotation leading to combined stimulation of both types of receptors closely corresponded to the values obtained by vectorial summation of the responses to the individual inputs, as originally shown by Boyle and Pompeiano [5] and Pompeiano et al. [29] (cf. [2]) for neck-canal interaction). It is of interest that when the lVS and the medullary inhibitory lRS neurons displayed a reciprocal pattern of neck–vestibular convergence, the labyrinth and neck responses neither showed an equal gain nor were they exactly 180° out of phase with respect to each other; in these instances residual responses of both the excitatory lVS and the inhibitory lRS neurons might occur during head rotation. In particular, the lVS neurons, which were mainly excited during side-down animal tilt and side-up neck rotation, would show small amplitude and large phase lag of the responses with respect to those obtained during animal tilt, while the medullary lRS neurons, which showed mainly the opposite response pattern, would display responses to head rotation of small amplitude and large phase lead with respect to those obtained during neck rotation. As to the inputs which showed a parallel pattern of neck–vestibular convergence, it is likely that the lVS neurons which were mainly excited during side-up animal tilt and neck rotation would show during head rotation large amplitude and small phase lead of the responses with respect to side-up head displacement; on the other hand, the majority of the medullary lRS neurons, which were mainly excited during side-down animal tilt and neck rotation, would display during head rotation large amplitude and small phase lead of the responses with respect to side-down head displacement.

These predicted patterns of unit responses to head rotation were originally documented at the level of unidentified LVN neurons [5], and the results obtained were also confirmed at the level of the medullary inhibitory lRS neurons [29].

The persistence of some unit responses of both excitatory lVS neurons and presumably inhibitory lRS neurons during combined macular and neck stimulations would be integrated at motoneuronal level, thus leading to some residual component of the EMG responses during costimulation of macular and neck receptors [9, 20].

The demonstration that in the frequency domain the gain and the phase angle of the responses of individual lVS [3, 4, 35] and lRS [21, 38] neurons to either macular vestibular or neck inputs may change, offers new possibilities of extending our observation by studying the modalities of interaction between the two inputs for a wide range of stimulus parameters.

Acknowledgements

This study was supported by the NIH grant NS 07685-19 and a grant from the Ministero della Pubblica Istruzione, Rome, Italy.

References

[1] Abrahams, V.C. and Richmond, F.J.R. (1988) Specialization of sensorimotor organization in the neck muscle system. In O. Pompeiano and J.H.J. Allum (Eds.), *Vestibulospinal Control of Posture and Locomotion, Progress in Brain Research, Vol. 76*, Elsevier, Amsterdam, pp. 125–135.

[2] Anastasopoulos, D. and Mergner, T. (1982) Canal–neck interaction in vestibular nuclear neurons of the cat. *Exp. Brain Res.*, 46: 269–280.

[3] Boyle, R. and Pompeiano, O. (1980) Reciprocal responses to sinusoidal tilt of neurons in Deiters' nucleus and their dynamic characteristics. *Arch. Ital. Biol.*, 118: 1–32.

[4] Boyle, R. and Pompeiano, O. (1980) Responses of vestibulospinal neurons to sinusoidal rotation of the neck. *J. Neurophysiol.*, 44: 633–649.

[5] Boyle, R. and Pompeiano, O. (1981) Convergence and interaction of neck and macular vestibular inputs on vestibulospinal neurons. *J. Neurophysiol.*, 45: 852–868.

[6] Coulter, J.D., Mergner, T. and Pompeiano, O. (1976) Effects of static tilt on cervical spinoreticular tract neurons. *J. Neurophysiol.*, 39: 45–62.

[7] De Kleijn, A. (1920) Tonische Labyrinth- und Halsreflexe auf die Augen. *Pflügers Arch.*, 186: 82–97.

[8] Ezure, K. and Wilson, V.J. (1983) Dynamics of neck-to-forelimb reflexes in the decerebrate cat. *J. Neurophysiol.*, 50: 688–695.

[9] Ezure, K. and Wilson, V.J. (1984) Interaction of tonic neck and vestibular reflexes in the forelimb of the decerebrate cat. *Exp. Brain Res.*, 54: 289–292.

[10] Jankowska, E., Lund, S., Lundberg, A. and Pompeiano, O. (1968) Inhibitory effects evoked through ventral reticulospinal pathways. *Arch. Ital. Biol.*, 106: 124–140.

[11] Kubin, L., Magherini, P.C., Manzoni, D. and Pompeiano, O. (1980) Responses of lateral reticular neurons to sinusoidal stimulation of labyrinth receptors in decerebrate cat. *J. Neurophysiol.*, 44: 922–936.

[12] Kubin, L., Magherini, P.C., Manzoni, D. and Pompeiano, O. (1981) Responses of lateral reticular neurons to sinusoidal rotation of neck in decerebrate cat. *Neuroscience*, 6: 1277–1290.

[13] Kubin, L., Manzoni, D. and Pompeiano, O. (1981) Responses of lateral reticular neurons to convergent neck and macular vestibular inputs. *J. Neurophysiol.*, 46: 48–64.

[14] Lindsay, K.W., Roberts, T.D.M. and Rosenberg, J.R. (1976) Asymmetric tonic labyrinth reflexes and their interaction with neck reflexes in the decerebrate cat. *J. Physiol. London*, 261: 583–601.

[15] Llinás, R. and Terzuolo, C.A. (1964) Mechanisms of supraspinal actions upon spinal cord activities. Reticular inhibitory mechanisms on alpha extensor motoneurons. *J. Neurophysiol.*, 27: 579–591.

[16] Lund, S. and Pompeiano, O. (1968) Monosynaptic excitation of alpha-motoneurons from supraspinal structures in the cat. *Acta Physiol. Scand.*, 73: 1–21.

[17] Magnus, R. (1924) *Körperstellung*. Springer, Berlin, 740 pp.

[18] Magnus, R. and De Kleijn, A. (1912) Die Abhängigkeit des Tonus der Extremitätenmuskeln von der Kopfstellung. *Pflügers Arch.*, 145: 455–548.

[19] Magoun, H.W. and Rhines R. (1946) An inhibitory mechanism in the bulbar reticular formation. *J. Neurophysiol.*, 9: 165–171.

[20] Manzoni, D., Pompeiano, O., Srivastava, U.C. and Stampacchia, G. (1983) Responses of forelimb extensors to sinusoidal stimulation of macular labyrinth and neck receptors. *Arch. Ital. Biol.*, 121: 205–214.

[21] Manzoni, D., Pompeiano, O., Stampacchia, G. and Srivastava, U.C. (1983) Responses of medullary reticulospinal neurons to sinusoidal stimulation of labyrinth receptors in decerebrate cat. *J. Neurophysiol.*, 50: 1059–1079.

[22] Marchand, A.R., Manzoni, D., Pompeiano, O. and Stampacchia, G. (1987) Effects of stimulation of vestibular and neck receptors on Deiters neurons projecting to the lumbosacral cord. *Pflügers Arch.*, 409: 13–23.

[23] McCouch, G.P., Deering, I.D. and Ling, T.H. (1951) Location of receptors for tonic neck reflexes. *J. Neurophysiol.*, 14: 191–195.

[24] Mittelstaedt, H. (1964) Basic control patterns of orientational homeostasis. *Symp. Soc. Exp. Biol.*, 18: 365–385.

[25] Peterson, B.W., Pitts, N.G. and Fukushima, K. (1979) Reticulospinal connections with limb and axial motoneurons. *Exp. Brain Res.*, 36: 1–20.

[26] Pompeiano, O. (1975) Vestibulo-spinal relationships. In R.F. Naunton (Ed.), *The Vestibular System*, Academic Press, New York, pp. 147–180.

[27] Pompeiano, O. (1979) Neck and macular labyrinthine influences on the cervical spinoreticulocerebellar pathway. In R.

154

Granit and O. Pompeiano (Eds.) *Reflex Control of Posture and Movement, Progress in Brain Research, Vol. 50*, Elsevier Amsterdam, pp. 501–514.

[28] Pompeiano, O. (1984) A comparison of the response characteristics of vestibulospinal and medullary reticulospinal neurons to labyrinth and neck inputs. In. C.D. Barnes (Ed.), *Brainstem Control of Spinal Cord Function, Research Topics in Physiology, Vol. 6*, Academic Press, Orlando, pp. 87–140.

[29] Pompeiano, O., Manzoni, D., Srivastava, U.C. and Stampacchia, G. (1984) Convergence and interaction of neck and macular vestibular inputs on reticulospinal neurons. *Neuroscience*, 12: 111–128.

[30] Pompeiano, O., Manzoni, D., Marchand, A.R. and Stampacchia, G. (1987) Effect of roll tilt of the animal and neck rotation on different size vestibulospinal neurons in decerebrate cats with the cerebellum intact. *Pflügers Arch.*, 409: 24–38.

[31] Precht W. (1974) The physiology of the vestibular nuclei. In H.H. Kornhuber (Ed.), *Handbook of Sensory Physiology, Vol. 6 (1)*, Springer, Berlin, pp. 353–416.

[32] Roberts, T.D.M. (1973) Reflex balance. *Nature*, 244: 156–158.

[33] Roberts, T.D.M. (1978) *Neurophysiology of Postural Mechanisms.* (2nd Edn.), Butterworths, London, 415 pp.

[34] Schor, R.H. and Miller, A.D. (1981) Vestibular reflexes in neck and forelimb muscles evoked by roll tilt. *J. Neurophysiol.*, 46: 167–178.

[35] Schor, R.H. and Miller, A.D. (1982) Relationship of cat vestibular neurons to otolith-spinal reflexes. *Exp. Brain Res.*, 47: 137–144.

[36] Shimazu, H. and Precht, W. (1965) Tonic and kinetic responses of cat's vestibular neurons to horizontal angular acceleration. *J. Neurophysiol.*, 28: 991–1013.

[37] Srivastava, U.C., Manzoni, D., Pompeiano, O. and Stampacchia, G. (1982) State-dependent properties of medullary reticular neurons involved during the labyrinth and neck reflexes. *Neurosci. Lett. Suppl.* 10: S461.

[38] Srivastava, U.C., Manzoni, D., Pompeiano, O. and Stampacchia, G. (1984) Responses of medullary reticulospinal neurons to sinusoidal rotation of neck in the decerebrate cat. *Neuroscience*, 11: 473–486.

[39] Stampacchia, G., Manzoni, D., Marchand, A.R. and Pompeiano, O. (1987) Convergence of neck and macular vestibular inputs on vestibulospinal neurons projecting to the lumbosacral segments of the spinal cord. *Arch. Ital. Biol.*, 125: 201–224.

[40] Von Holst E. and Mittelstaedt H. (1950) Das Reafferenzprinzip. Wechselwirkungen zwischen Zentralnervensystem und Peripherie. *Naturwissenschaften*, 37: 464–476.

[41] Wilson, V.J. (1988) Convergence of neck and vestibular signals on spinal interneurons. In O. Pompeiano and J.H.J. Allum (Eds.), *Vestibulospinal Control of Posture and Locomotion, Progress in Brain Research, Vol. 76*, Elsevier, Amsterdam, pp. 137–143.

[42] Wilson, V.J. and Melvill Jones, G. (1979) *Mammalian Vestibular Physiology*, Plenum Press, New York, 365 pp.

O. Pompeiano and J.H.J. Allum (Eds.)
Progress in Brain Research, Vol. 76
© 1988 Elsevier Science Publishers B.V. (Biomedical Division)

CHAPTER 13

Integration of vestibular and neck afferent signals in the central cervical nucleus

T. Hongo[2], T. Kitama[1] and K. Yoshida[1]

[1]Department of Physiology, Institute of Basic Medical Sciences, University of Tsukuba, Tsukuba, Ibaraki-ken 305, and [2]Department of Neurophysiology, Institute of Brain Research, School of Medicine, University of Tokyo, Hongo 7-3-1, Bunkyo-ku, Tokyo 113, Japan

The responses of spinocerebellar tract neurons in the CCN to natural stimulation of vestibular and neck muscle receptors were investigated in decerebrate cats. The spike activity of single CCN neurons was recorded extracellularly with a floating microelectrode in the C2 segment of the spinal cord. CCN neurons exhibited clear modulation of firing activity in response to sinusoidal rotation of the head in the vertical planes but not to rotation in the horizontal semicircular canal plane. The response to vertical rotation was attributed to stimulation of the vertical semicircular canals, since selective stimulation of otolith organs by static tilt of the head in the same plane had no effect. The response was approximately in phase with the head angular velocity at 0.05–2.0 Hz. Vector analysis suggested that the optimal orientation of vertical rotation varied considerably among neurons. The CCN neurons increased or decreased their firing rate in response to stretch of dorsal neck muscles. The time course of the responses suggested that muscle spindle primaries were most likely to be the receptors responsible for both excitatory and inhibitory responses. The input was highly muscle specific in that most CCN neurons received excitation from one muscle or two synergists, and that a group of neurons was specifically inhibited from biventer cervicis and complexus. The vestibular and neck muscle afferent signals converged with specific patterns of combination on individual CCN neurons. It is suggested that each CCN neuron integrates signals from the labyrinth and the neck and provides the cerebellum with information concerning the head movement in a certain vertical direction.

Introduction

The CCN existing in the C1–C4 segments [23] is now known to receive inputs from the neck and the labyrinth, and to project to the cerebellum as a major spinocerebellar tract of the upper cervical cord. Since Matsushita and Ikeda [16] and Wiksten [29] first demonstrated its spinocerebellar nature using the technique of retrograde transport of HRP, the knowledge of the input and output organizations of the CCN neurons has accumulated in the last decade. The mode of projection of CCN neurons to the cerebellum, including the main termination in labules I–II, has been well documented anatomically [14–18, 30, 31, 35] and electrophysiologically [10] in the cat. Dense projection to the CCN of cervical dorsal root fibres has long been recognized [13, 22, 27, 32]. Subsequent anatomical [3, 12, 28] and physiological [1, 12] studies demonstrated that the CCN receives afferent input from the dorsal neck muscles. Another major source of sensory input to the CCN has been shown to originate from the vestibular labyrinth. In a previous study we have shown that CCN neurons are excited by electrical stimulation of the contralateral vestibular nerve and inhibited from the ipsilateral vestibular nerve [11]. Stimulation of individual ampullary nerves further indicated that the semicircular canals

---

Abbreviations: BCC, biventer cervicis and complex; CCN, central cervical nucleus; HRP, horseradish peroxidase; OCC, obliques capitis caudalis; RCD, rectus capitis dorsalis; Spl, splenius.

constitute a source from which the vestibular effect is evoked.

In the present study we have attempted to investigate the dynamic properties of the responses of CCN neurons to natural stimulation of vestibular and neck muscle receptors in order to elucidate the functional role of the CCN spinocerebellar tract. We will describe the responses of single CCN neurons to sinusoidal rotation and static tilt of the head and also to muscle stretch. In addition, some preliminary data, suggesting a highly specific pattern of convergence from vestibular and neck muscle afferents, will be presented.

Experiments were performed on decerebrate cats prepared under halothane anaesthesia. The animal was immobilized with pancuronium bromide and maintained under artificial respiration. Blood pressure in the femoral artery was monitored and maintained above 100 mmHg, and rectal temperature was kept at 37–38°C throughout the experiment. Bipolar silver-ball electrodes were placed on the round and oval windows for electrical stimulation of the vestibular nerves. Ensembles of needle electrodes were inserted into the white matter of the cerebellar anterior lobe for stimulation of spinocerebellar axons. Various neck muscles were dissected with the innervation kept intact and prepared for natural stimulation. After laminectomy from C1 to C4, the spinal cord was transected between the C3 and C4 segments. This was done to eliminate a possible sensory inflow from the body and limbs during rotation and tilt for vestibular stimulation.

The spike activity of single CCN neurons was recorded extracellularly with a floating microelectrode in the C2 segment of the left side. CCN neurons were identified by antidromic activation from the anterior lobe vermis, and only those which were activated orthodromically following electrical stimulation of the contralateral (right) vestibular nerve were selected for further analysis.

Responses to input from the vestibular labyrinth

Responses of single CCN neurons to whole-body rotation were examined. With the head tilted nose-down by 27° the animal was rotated sinusoidally in three orthogonal planes which were approximately coplanar with canal planes. For stimulation of the horizontal canal pair, the animal was rotated in the earth-horizontal plane (HC mode). For stimulation of the right anterior–left posterior canal pair (r-AC mode) and the right posterior–left anterior canal pair (r-PC mode), the animal was rotated in the vertical plane orienting 45° and 135° from the sagittal plane (clockwise as viewed from above), respectively. Thus the r-AC and the r-PC mode rotations should stimulate both vertical canals and otolith organs. To evaluate the contribution of otolith inputs, responses to static tilts which should provide pure otolith stimuli were also examined.

Fig. 1A exemplifies responses of a left CCN neuron to sinusoidal rotation in the r-AC plane at 0.5 Hz with an amplitude of $\pm 13.5°$/s. The firing rate was modulated in an approximately sinusoidal manner around the resting level (45 spikes/s, see record in Fig. 1B, middle traces). Fig. 1B shows the steady-state activity of the same neuron at the standard position (middle traces) and during 10° static tilt in the same r-AC plane in both directions (left and right traces). Although the angular displacement during the tilt was more than twice as large as the positional change that occurred during sinusoidal stimulus, the tilt stimuli elicited no appreciable change in the firing rate. Thus the clear modulation of firing rate during rotation shown in Fig. 1A was attributable to stimulation of vertical canals.

The vast majority of CCN neurons exhibited clear modulations of firing rate in response to rotation in the vertical plane of either r-AC or r-PC mode or both, but not to HC mode rotation. In contrast, static tilts in these planes had no effect in any of the CCN cells examined. In a few cells, weak modulations were observed during HC mode rotation. Such weak modulations could, however, be well accounted for as caused by stimulation of the vertical canals, because the vertical canals cannot be exactly perpendicular to the plane of rotation due to variations of the canal orientations [5]. In fact, stimulation of the vertical canals evoked

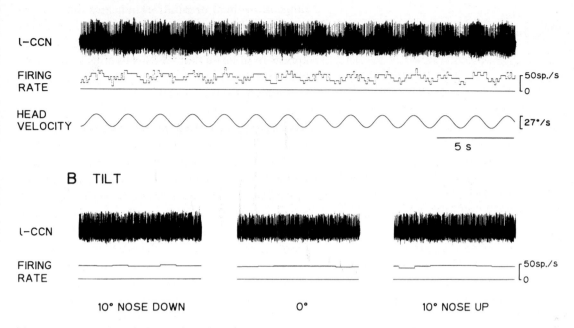

Fig. 1. Responses of a left CCN cell to sinusoidal rotation at 0.5 Hz (A) and to static tilt (B) in r-AC plane. In the head velocity curve in A, upward deflexion indicates right side-nose down direction. See text for further explanations.

strong effects on these cells, and when the head position was changed by 10° from the standard 27° pitch to 17° pitch, the modulation due to horizontal rotation changed just as expected if the vertical canals were responsible. In regard to the receptor origin of the vestibular input, therefore, it can be concluded that the CCN cells so far analysed received input only from the vertical canals.

The gain and phase with respect to the head velocity were computed from the average of responses to 10–100 successive stimulus cycles. Within the range of stimulus amplitudes employed (2.3 to 13.5°/s, at 0.5 Hz), the response amplitudes varied with the stimulus amplitudes in an approximately linear manner, i.e. the gain was constant. The phase of response was essentially independent of the stimulus amplitude. For example, the cell shown in Fig. 2 exhibited response amplitudes of 4.3, 8.6, and 11.7 (spikes/s/(°/s) for stimulus velocities of 4.5, 9.0 and 13.5°/s, respectively. The phase was about 0°, and varied by no more than 4° for these three stimulus amplitudes.

In most CCN cells tested, the phase of response was approximately in phase with the head velocity that should excite the contralateral canal, ranging from + 30° (lead) to − 30° (lag) at 0.5 Hz. The phase was roughly constant over frequencies from 0.05 to 2.0 Hz. These phase properties were similar to those of vestibular nucleus neurons [21, 26]. In some cells, the response to r-PC mode rotation was about 180° out of phase, i.e. firing rate decreased during contralateral posterior canal activation. Since no excitatory effects on CCN cells were found after electrical stimulation of the ipsilateral vestibular nerve [11], these cells were considered to be inhibited from the contralateral (right) posterior canal.

Gain of responses to r-AC mode and r-PC mode rotations varied considerably from neuron to neuron. While some neurons responded almost exclusively to either r-AC or r-PC mode rotation, others were responsive to both (Fig. 2A). To obtain a quantitative measure of the total canal input to each cell, the orientation of the vertical plane at which rotation would evoke a maximum response

A   B

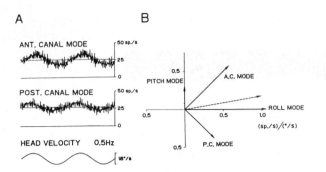

Fig. 2. Responses of a left CCN cell to sinusoidal rotation in different vertical planes. (A) Modulation of firing rate to r-AC mode (top) and r-PC mode (middle) rotations at 0.5 Hz. Averaged from 30 cycles. (B) Solid vectors represent the gain of the response to r-AC mode, r-PC mode, pitch mode and roll mode rotations. The dotted vector indicates the predicted response in the optimal plane. See text for further explanations.

(optimal plane), and the gain in the optimal plane were calculated in individual cells. These were obtained from the gain and phase of r-AC and r-PC mode responses at 0.5 Hz, assuming a linear summation of effects from different canals. Fig. 2 illustrates for one cell the actual r-AC and r-PC mode responses and the predicted response at the optimal plane. This cell exhibited clear modulations in response to both r-AC and r-PC mode rotations (Fig. 2A). The gain and phase of the r-AC mode response were 0.82 (spikes/s)/(°/s) and − 20.1°, and those of the r-PC mode response were 0.63 (spikes/s)/(°/s) and + 12.6°, respectively. In Fig. 2B each response is represented in vector form where the vector length is proportional to the gain and the polar angle shows the orientation of the rotation plane. Vectorial summation of the r-AC and r-PC mode responses predicted the optimal plane at 81° (clockwise from the sagittal plane) and the maximum gain of 0.99 (spikes/s)/(°/s) (dotted vector). The actual responses to pitch and roll mode rotations were in good agreement with the prediction (Fig. 2B), indicating the validity of the assumption of linear summation.

Similar analyses in 10 CCN cells so far studied showed that the gain of the optimal response ranged from 0.32 to 2.18 (spikes/s)/(°/s) and the op-

timal orientation varied from 9° to 157°. The wide range of optimal orientation indicates that a given rotation influences the activity of individual cells differentially. The available data, though limited, appear to indicate that CCN cells consist of subpopulations having different directional sensitivities for vertical rotations (see Fig. 5).

Responses to input from the neck muscles

The responses of CCN neurons to electrical stimulation of the dorsal root of cervical segments and of various peripheral nerves in the neck and the forelimb have been studied by Hirai et al. [9, 12] and Abrahams et al. [1]. These studies have shown that monosynaptic excitatory effects are exerted by afferents from neck muscles and are conveyed via the dorsal roots of the upper cervical segments. No detectable excitation with a monosynaptic latency was elicited from the forelimb nerves, though nerves from shoulder muscles were not tested. We were unsuccessful in finding effects clearly ascribable to afferents from vertebral joints or ligaments, which have been reported to cause neck–limb [20] or neck–ocular reflex actions [8]. Detailed analyses were therefore focused on the effects from the neck muscle afferents in the previous study [12].

The main findings obtained by using electrical stimulation of the neck muscle nerves were as follows.

(1) Monosynaptic excitation was evoked in CCN neurons after stimulation of nerves to dorsal neck muscles such as Spl, BCC, OCC and RCD.

(2) Thresholds for the monosynaptic excitation were near the threshold of the nerve, suggesting that it was caused by group I afferents.

(3) The excitatory input was muscle specific in that individual neurons received excitation from one muscle, or from synergists (e.g. BCC–RCD, Spl–OCC). There were some cells in which convergence from BCC and Spl occurred, but then the excitatory effect from one muscle overwhelmed that from the other.

(4) Inhibition could also be evoked at short latencies after stimulation of BCC but not Spl.

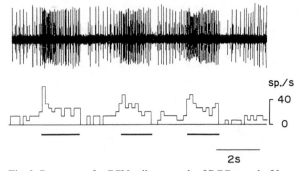

Fig. 3. Response of a CCN cell to stretch of BCC muscle. Upper trace: extracellular spikes of single CCN cells recorded through a high-pass filter. Lower trace: firing frequency of the larger unit in the upper trace. The solid lines in the bottom indicate the periods of muscle stretch.

Based on these results, we attempted to investigate effects of natural stimulation of the muscle (stretch or local pressure) on the firing activity of single CCN neurons recorded extracellularly. A floating microelectrode was useful for this test. Fig.

3 shows an example of responses of a single CCN neuron to stretching the BCC muscle. Note that the firing rate greatly increased transiently at the early phase of stretch, maintained an elevated level during stretch, and abruptly decreased even to pause when the muscle was released. The firing pattern was very similar to that of muscle spindle primaries in possessing both dynamic and static responses [19, 24], suggesting that the excitatory effect was of group Ia fibre origin. The interpretation is in good agreement with the observation that fibres identified to originate from spindle primaries distribute terminals in the CCN as revealed by their intra-axonal staining with HRP (Fig. 4 [12]). The excitatory responses of CCN neurons to muscle stretch were usually as in Fig. 3, and were seen in about 70% of CCN neurons examined.

Decrease of the firing rate was also produced by muscle stretch in some CCN cells. Since electrical stimulation of the nerve to the muscle stretched also

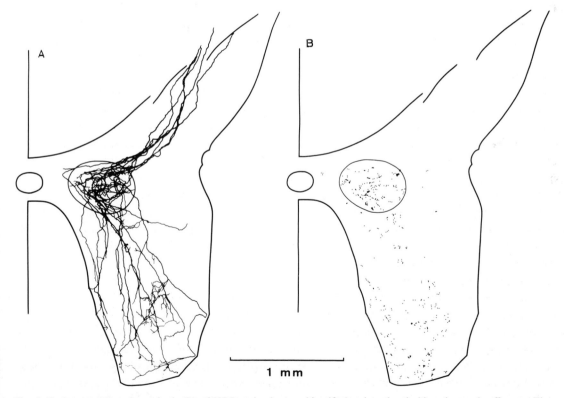

Fig. 4. Trajectory (A) and terminals (B) of HRP-stained axons identified as low-threshold neck muscle afferents. Five collaterals are superimposed at the C2 segment. (From [12]).

caused suppression, the effect was interpreted as due to inhibition caused by stretch-evoked impulses in the nerve from that muscle and not due to unloading of other muscles that supplied excitatory input to the CCN cell. The inhibition was probably also of group Ia fibre origin, since it occurred with a small stretch and persisted throughout the period of stretch.

The receptive field for the excitation and inhibition caused by muscle stretch was explored in individual CCN neurons. The input was found to be muscle specific, in general agreement with the results obtained by electrical stimulation of the muscle nerves [12]. The excitatory input, when present, originated from single or synergic muscles of either the BCC–RCD group or the Spl–OCC group, while inhibition came from BCC and not from any other muscles examined. These results indicated that CCN neurons consist of subgroups, each of which receive specific spatial pattern of excitatory and/or inhibitory inputs from muscle spindle afferents of different neck muscles. According to the patterns of muscle input, the following four subgroups of CCN neurons have so far been observed: (1) those excited from BCC; (2) those inhibited from BCC; (3) those excited from Spl–OCC; (4) those excited from Spl–OCC and inhibited from BCC.

Convergence of inputs from the semicircular canal and the neck muscles

The majority of CCN cells examined received inputs from both the labyrinth and the neck muscles, in agreement with the previous results obtained by electrical stimulation [9, 11]. We therefore attempted to disclose the pattern of convergence from the two sources onto the same CCN neurons. Despite technical difficulties we could complete, in a limited number of cells, most of the necessary tests using rotation and muscle stretch without losing the cell recorded from. The results obtained in 6 cells are shown in Fig. 5, where the origin of muscle for excitation and inhibition by stretch (A) and the vector (gain and direction) of the response at the optimal plane as defined above (B) are given for each

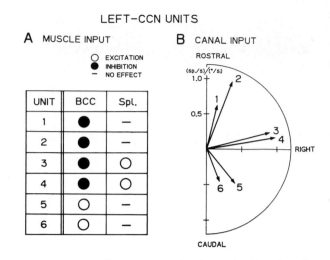

Fig. 5. Patterns of convergence of neck muscle (A) and vestibular (B) inputs to 6 CCN neurons. In B the response gain and orientation of optimal plane are shown in vector form, as in Fig. 2. The number attached to each vector refers to the unit in A. See text for further explanations.

cell. The diagram in B shows that the directions of the optimal plane are anterior in units 1 and 2, lateral in units 3 and 4, and posterior in units 5 and 6. It is interesting to note that the differences in the canal input are well correlated with the pattern of input from neck muscles. Cells with anterior vectors were inhibited from BCC without effects from Spl; cells with lateral vectors were excited from Spl and inhibited from BCC; and cells with posterior vectors were excited from BCC with no effects from Spl. Such highly specific patterns of convergence suggest that each CCN neuron integrates sensory signals related to the head movement in a particular direction, with respect to both body and space.

Discussion

Our results demonstrate that the CCN neurons receive afferent signals arising from both the vestibular and neck muscle receptors and provide the cerebellum with integrated information about the head movement with respect to the trunk and space. One of the striking features of the vestibular input is that CCN neurons receive input only from the vertical canals. The absence of the horizontal canal input is in agreement with the previous results obtained by electrical stimulation of the individual ampullary nerves [11]. The previous study [11] has also revealed various patterns of convergence from different vertical canals on single CCN neurons. The present results extend this previous finding by showing that each cell has its own optimal orientation of vertical rotation which varied widely among neurons. Similar convergence from different canal pairs has been observed in some second-order vestibular neurons [2]. It remains to be studied whether the convergence takes place at the vestibular nuclei or at the CCN. As for the contribution of the otolith input, selective stimulation of the otolith organs by static tilt was shown to have negligible effect. In this regard it should be pointed out that the functional organization of vestibular inputs to CCN neurons is quite different from that to dorsal neck motoneurons, in which both the horizontal canal and the otolith organs also make a substantial contribution to the vestibular induced activity [2, 4, 6, 7, 25, 34].

The properties of the response of CCN neurons to muscle stretch are in general accordance with the previous electrophysiological and anatomical findings [12], in showing that the input is of muscle spindle origin and the receptive field of each cell is limited to one muscle or close synergists.

A close correlation was found between the optimal direction of the head rotation for vestibular stimulation and the pattern of muscle input in each cell (see Fig. 5). Given the complex geometry of neck muscles and their actions, it is difficult to give a simple explanation for the highly specific pattern of convergence of the two inputs. Nevertheless it would be of interest to consider the manner of interaction of the two signals when the head is passively rotated with respect to a stationary trunk. The result in Fig. 5 suggests that if a CCN neuron is excited from the labyrinth by a passive head rotation toward its preferred direction, effects from neck muscles are either inhibition from stretched muscles or disfacilitation from released muscles. If the head is moved to the opposite direction, the canal input would be inhibitory while changes in muscle length would produce either disinhibition or facilitation. It therefore appears that effects from the vestibular and neck receptors are of opposite polarity and may more or less cancel each other. It is interesting to note that similar opposite effects of vestibular and neck afferent actions have been shown in interneurons of the lower cervical cord, though mainly otolith inputs appear to contribute in these neurons [33].

References

[1] Abrahams, V.C., Anstee, G. and Richmond, F.J.R. (1979) Neck muscle and trigeminal input to the upper cervical cord and lower medulla of the cat. Can. J. Physiol. Pharmacol., 57: 642–651.

[2] Baker, J., Goldberg, J. and Peterson, B. (1985) Spatial and temporal properties of the vestibulocollic reflex in decerebrate cats. J. Neurophysiol., 54: 735–756.

[3] Bakker, D.A., Richmond, F.J.R. and Abrahams, V.C. (1984) Central projections from cat suboccipital muscles: A study using transganglionic transport of horseradish peroxidase. J. Comp. Neurol., 288: 409–421.

[4] Berthoz, A. and Anderson, J.H. (1971) Frequency analysis of vestibular influence on extensor motoneurons. II. Relationship between neck and forelimb extensors. Brain Res., 34: 376–380.

[5] Estes, M.S., Blanks, R.H.I. and Markham, C.H. (1975) Physiologic characteristics of vestibular first-order canal neurons in the cat. I. Response plane determination and resting discharge characteristics. J. Neurophysiol., 38: 1232–1249.

[6] Ezure, K. and Sasaki, S. (1978) Frequency-response analysis of vestibular induced neck reflex in cat. I. Characteristics of neural transmission from horizontal semicircular canal to neck motoneurons. J. Neurophysiol., 41: 445–458.

[7] Ezure, K., Sasaki, S., Uchino, Y. and Wilson, V.J. (1978) Frequency-response analysis of vestibular-induced neck reflex in cat. II. Functional significance of cervical afferents and polysynaptic descending pathways. J. Neurophysiol., 41: 459–471.

[8] Hikosaka, O. and Maeda, M. (1973) Cervical effects on abducens motoneurons and their interaction with vestibulo-ocular reflex. Exp. Brain Res., 18: 512–530.

[9] Hirai, N., Hongo, T. and Sasaki, S. (1978) Cerebellar projection and input organizations of the spinocerebellar tract arising from the central cervical nucleus in the cat. Brain Res., 157: 341–345.

[10] Hirai, N., Hongo, T. and Sasaki, S. (1984) A physiological study of identification, axonal course and cerebellar projec-

162

tion of spinocerebellar tract cells in the central cervical nucleus of the cat. *Exp. Brain Res.*, 55: 272–285.

[11] Hirai, N., Hongo, T., Sasaki, S. and Yoshida, K. (1979) The neck and labyrinthine influences on cervical spinocerebellar tract neurons of the central cervical nucleus in the cat. In: R. Granit and O. Pompeiano (Eds.), *Reflex Control of Posture and Movement, Progress in Brain Research, Vol. 50*, Elsevier, Amsterdam, pp. 529–536.

[12] Hirai, N., Hongo, T., Sasaki, S., Yamashita, M. and Yoshida, K. (1984) Neck muscle afferent input to spinocerebellar tract cells of the central cervical nucleus in the cat. *Exp. Brain Res.*, 55: 286–300.

[13] Imai, Y. and Kusama, T. (1969) Distribution of the dorsal root fibers in the cat. An experimental study with the Nauta method. *Brain Res.*, 13: 338–359.

[14] Matsushita, M. and Hosoya, Y. (1982) Spinocerebellar projections to lobules III to V of the anterior lobe in the cat, as studied by retrograde transport of horseradish peroxidase. *J. Comp. Neurol.*, 208: 127–143.

[15] Matsushita, M., Hosoya, Y. and Ikeda, M. (1979) Anatomical organization of the spinocerebellar system in the cat, as studied by retrograde transport of horseradish peroxidase. *J. Comp. Neurol.*, 184: 81–106.

[16] Matsushita, M. and Ikeda, M. (1975) The central cervical nucleus as cell origin of a spinocerebellar tract arising from the cervical cord: a study in the cat using horseradish peroxidase. *Brain Res.*, 100: 412–417.

[17] Matsushita, M. and Okado, N. (1981) Spinocerebellar projections to lobules I and II of the anterior lobe in the cat, as studied by retrograde transport of horseradish peroxidase. *J. Comp. Neurol.*, 197: 411–424.

[18] Matsushita, M., Tanami, T. and Yaginuma, H. (1984) Differential distribution of spinocerebellar fiber terminals within the lobules of the cerebellar anterior lobe in the cat: an anterograde WGA–HRP study. *Brain Res.*, 305: 157–161.

[19] Matthews, P.B.C. (1972) *Mammalian Muscle Receptors and their Central Actions*, Arnold, London, pp. 20–194.

[20] McCouch, G.P., Deering, I.D. and Ling, T.H. (1951) Location of receptors for tonic neck reflexes. *J. Neurophysiol.*, 14: 191–195.

[21] Melvill Jones, G. and Milsum, J.H. (1970) Characteristics of neural transmission from the semicircular canal to the vestibular nuclei of cats. *J. Physiol. London*, 209: 295–316.

[22] Ranson, S.W., Davenport, H.K. and Doles, E.A. (1932) Intramedullary course of the dorsal root fibers of the first three cervical nerves. *J. Comp. Neurol.*, 54: 1–12.

[23] Rexed, B. (1954) A cytoarchitectonic atlas of the spinal cord of the cat. *J. Comp. Neurol.*, 100: 297–379.

[24] Richmond, F.J.R. and Abrahams, V.C. (1979) Physiological properties of muscle spindles in dorsal neck muscles of the cat. *J. Neurophysiol.*, 42: 604–617.

[25] Schor, R.H. and Miller, A.D. (1981) Vestibular reflexes in neck and forelimb muscles evoked by roll tilt. *J. Neurophysiol.*, 46: 167–178.

[26] Shinoda, Y. and Yoshida, K. (1974) Dynamic characteristics of responses to horizontal head angular acceleration in vestibuloocular pathway in the cat. *J. Neurophysiol.*, 37: 653–673.

[27] Shriver, M.E., Stein, B.M. and Carpenter, M.B. (1968) Central projections of spinal dorsal roots in the monkeys. I. Cervical and upper thoracic dorsal roots. *Am. J. Anat.*, 123: 27–74.

[28] Takahashi, O., Takeuchi, Y. and Matsushima, R. (1985) Direct connections of primary afferent fibers with central cervical nucleus neurons projecting to the cerebellum in the cat. *Brain Res.*, 328: 390–395.

[29] Wiksten, B. (1975) The central cervical nucleus – a source of spinocerebellar fibres, demonstrated by retrograde transport of horseradish peroxidase. *Neurosci. Lett.*, 1: 81–84.

[30] Wiksten, B. (1979) The central cervical nucleus in the cat. II. The cerebellar connections studied with retrograde transport of horseradish peroxidase. *Exp. Brain Res.*, 36: 155–173.

[31] Wiksten, B. (1979) The central cervical nucleus in the cat. III. The cerebellar connections studied with anterograde transport of ^{3}H-leucine. *Exp. Brain Res.*, 36: 175–189.

[32] Wiksten, B. and Grant, G. (1983) The central cervical nucleus in the cat. IV. Afferent fiber connections. An experimental anatomical study. *Exp. Brain Res.*, 51: 405–412.

[33] Wilson, V.J., Ezure, K. and Timerick, S.J.B. (1984) Tonic neck reflex of the decerebrate cat: Response of spinal interneurons to natural stimulation of neck and vestibular receptors. *J. Neurophysiol.*, 51: 567–577.

[34] Wilson, V.J. and Maeda, M. (1974) Connections between semicircular canals and neck motoneurones in the cat. *J. Neurophysiol.*, 37: 346–357.

[35] Yaginuma, H. and Matsushita, M. (1986) Spinocerebellar projection fields in the horizontal plane of lobules of the cerebellar anterior lobe in the cat: an anterograde wheat germ agglutinin–horseradish peroxidase study. *Brain Res.*, 365: 345–349.

O. Pompeiano and J.H.J. Allum (Eds.)
Progress in Brain Research, Vol. 76
© 1988 Elsevier Science Publishers B.V. (Biomedical Division)

CHAPTER 14

Dynamic and kinematic properties of the vestibulocollic and cervicocollic reflexes in the cat

B.W. Peterson, J.F. Baker, J. Goldberg and J. Banovetz

Department of Physiology, Northwestern University Medical School, 303 East Chicago Avenue, Chicago, IL 60611, U.S.A.

In situations where the body and head can move independently, the VCR and CCR must work together to stabilize the head with respect to space and with respect to the body. The dynamic and kinematic properties of these two reflexes appear to be organized to promote relatively simple, linear interactions between them over a wide range of head movement frequencies. Neck EMG outputs produced by both reflexes exhibit nearly identical second-order lead characteristics as stimulus frequencies increase from 0.5 to 5.0 Hz. Their input/output curves are matched so that the threshold of the VCR is offset by the high sensitivity of the CCR at low stimulus amplitudes. In addition, the patterns of muscle activation produced by the two reflexes in the decerebrate cat are quite similar. Direct evidence of linear summation of the VCR and CCR has been obtained in situations where the head rotates with respect to a stationary trunk [16, 22] and where animals make head motions to compensate for rotation of the trunk [3, 22]. In the latter situation, the two reflexes appear to play an important role in stabilizing the head of the cat at frequencies below about 3 Hz [3]. In primates, however, voluntary head movements may override this reflex stabilization [1, 25].

Introduction

This chapter will examine the properties of two reflexes that contribute to head stabilization: the vestibulocollic and cervicocollic reflexes. The VCR arises when receptors of the vestibular labyrinth are activated by motion of the head with respect to space and elicit reflex contractions of muscles that would act to oppose that motion. The CCR is a stretch reflex of the neck muscles that acts to oppose movement of the head with respect to the trunk. As in other somatomotor systems, a central problem in neck motor control is how neck motor signals and the muscle forces that they produce are matched to the dynamic and kinematic properties of the musculoskeletal system that they control. Recent advances in defining the mechanics of the head–neck system have opened the way for attempts to understand the functional significance of dynamic and kinematic properties of the VCR and CCR.

Initial attempts to model the neck musculoskeletal system examined its properties in a single plane of motion. Bizzi et al. [1] developed a lumped-parameter second-order model of horizontal (yaw) head movements based on measurements of the head and neck in the Rhesus monkey. Schor et al. [2] have recently shown that a similar model can account for both the frequency response and step response of the human VCR when appropriate delays are added within the reflex pathways. Both models indicated that dynamic properties of the passive head–neck system could be reasonably approximated by a model containing three parameters: head in-

---

Abbreviations: CCR, cervicocollic reflex; CNS, central nervous system; EMG, electromyograph; ODD, orientation-dependent dynamics; SCC, semicircular canal; VCR, vestibulocollic reflex.

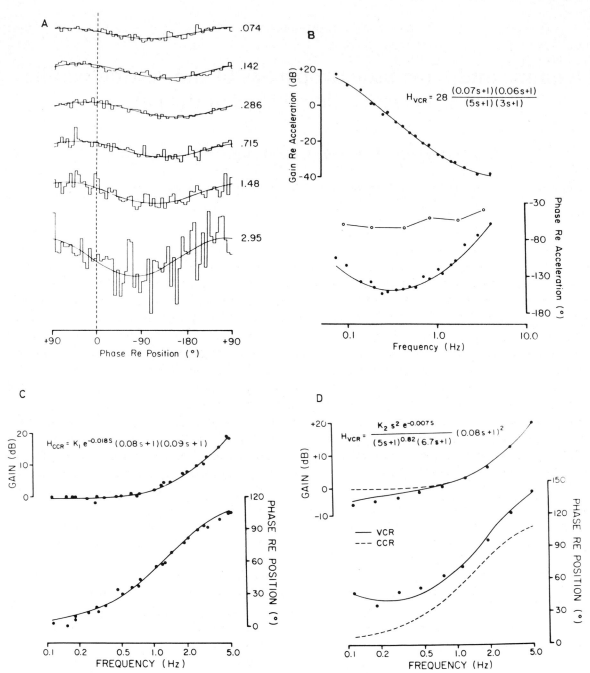

Fig. 1. (A,B) Dynamics of the VCR (adapted from [11]). The EMG of the left complexus muscle was recorded during whole-body rotation where the angular position of the platform holding the animal was modulated by a wave equal to the sum of 10 sinusoids in the 0.074–1.648 and 0.185–4.117 frequency ranges. (A) Modulation of the rectified, averaged EMG together with the best-fitting sinusoid at six representative frequencies. Phase and gain are referenced to the peak rightward deviation of the turntable. (B) The gains and phases of EMG modulation (●) together with the best-fitting transfer function (continuous line). In this Bode diagram gains and phases of EMG modulation are plotted with respect to angular acceleration in the on direction of the muscle. 0 dB equals 1% EMG modulation/deg/s². The open circles and broken line show the phase behaviour of an irregular canal afferent for comparison. (C,D) Comparison of the dynamics of the CCR and VCR (from [23]). The Bode diagram in C illustrates the behaviour of CCR evoked

ertia (*I*), neck viscosity (*B*) and neck elasticity (*K*). Fig. 4. shows a similar three-parameter model of the cat's head–neck system including the VCR and CCR developed by Goldberg and Peterson [3]. Although this chapter will concentrate on relatively simple lumped-parameter models of the type described above, the reader should be aware of attempts to develop more realistic models in which agonist and antagonist muscles are represented by both series and parallel visco-elastic elements [4].

Viviani and Berthoz [5] used the lumped-parameter approach to analyse head movements in the pitch plane. They found that it was necessary to consider at least two axes of rotation to model these movements adequately. Adding additional degrees of freedom in the motion of the head–neck system greatly increases the complexity of the model. It is therefore important to determine precisely which of the neck joints exhibit significant rotation during normal behaviour. Vidal and coworkers [6, 7] have examined this problem by making fluoroscopic observations of head movement behaviour in a number of species. They found that yaw rotations occur primarily about the C1–C2 joint, pitch rotations about either C1–skull or C7–Th1 and roll rotations about joints between C2 and C5. Thus head movements in 3 dimensions involve approximately six rotational degrees of freedom out of the many that are possible for a linkage of seven vertebrae.

In early models restricted to yaw rotations, the 30 neck muscles that insert on the head were treated as two synergistic groups producing either rightward or leftward rotations (e.g. [4]). To understand the full range of 3-dimensional head movements, it is necessary to discard such simplifications and determine the precise action of each muscle. Baker and Wickland [8] report such an analysis based on stereotaxic measurements of the origins and inser-

tions of the 30 muscles in the cat. These observations, together with anatomical analyses described by Richmond and Vidal [6] provide the basis for understanding the observations of kinematic features of the VCR and CCR that are described below.

In the sections that follow, our goal is to try to understand the key features of neck motor programming by observing patterns of muscle activation during attempted head stabilization. In each case muscle activity was recorded with EMG electrodes implanted in a number of neck muscles while the animal was rotated in a number of different planes in order to activate the VCR or CCR either separately or in combination. The data allow us to examine the following questions: (1) Are the dynamic properties (timing, gain and phase as a function of rotation frequency) of the reflexes appropriate to overcome the second-order mechanical properties of the musculoskeletal system? (2) Can the spatial properties of the motor commands be related to the pulling actions of the neck muscles? (3) Do dynamic properties of motor signals vary with spatial orientation or are they independent? (4) How do the VCR and CCR interact? (5) What is the relation between movements produced by muscle activation and by passive properties of the head–neck system?

Properties of the VCR

Dynamics

The simplest situation for studying the dynamics of the VCR is during yaw rotations of the whole body where neck muscle activation is due solely to activation of the horizontal SCCs. As illustrated in Fig. 1A–C, the dynamics of the VCR can be quantified by measuring the gain and phase of the EMG re-

in the right complexus muscle by rotation of the animal's body with its head held fixed in space. The data are plotted with respect to platform angular position. Points were obtained from 3 multiple-frequency runs. The curves plot the best-fitting transfer function, determined by a least-squares fitting procedure, whose LaPlace transform is given above the data. The points in D plot the behaviour of the VCR evoked in the same muscle in the same cat by whole-body rotation. The solid line shows the behaviour of the best-fitting transfer function, which is given above the data. The dashed lines show the transfer function from C for comparison. Phase is relative to peak leftward head rotation for VCR or peak rightward body rotation for CCR.

sponse elicited by sinusoidal rotation at a number of different frequencies. Berthoz and Anderson [9] and Ezure and Sasaki [10] measured the frequency response of the horizontal VCR at frequencies of 0.01–1.0 Hz. Fig. 1A,B is from Bilotto et al. [11], who extended the frequency range to 5 Hz. As indicated by the transfer function in the figure, the VCR can be modelled as a second-order lag–lead system containing two poles and two zeros. Beginning with the angular acceleration stimulus sensed by the SCCs, the poles shift the EMG response at 0.1–1.0 Hz toward a signal resembling angular position. At frequencies above 1.0 Hz the two zeros shift the EMG response back towards a signal resembling angular acceleration. This form of motor output is appropriate for matching the mechanical loading of a second-order spring–pendulum system, which is dominated by position-related elasticity at low frequencies and by acceleration-related inertia at high frequencies. Thus question one can be answered in the affirmative for the VCR.

It is also of interest to consider how the proces-

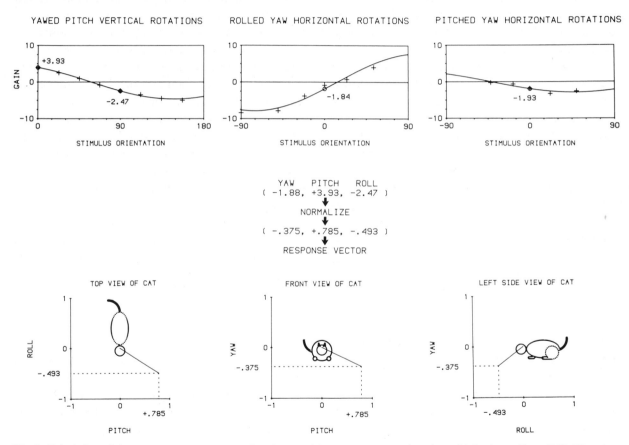

Fig. 2. Calculation of the response vector representing the muscle's response to rotations in multiple planes (from [15]). The upper plots show the gains of the EMG response as a function of the orientation of the plane of rotation in three rotation series. In the 'Yawed Pitch' series, rotations are in earth-vertical planes with 0° equal to pitch, 90° equal to roll. In the 'Rolled Yaw' series, rotations are about the earth-vertical axis with the animal's body either upright (0°) or rolled towards a side-lying position (+ 90° equals right ear down and − 90° left ear down). In the 'Pitched Yaw' series, rotations are about the earth-vertical axis with the animal's body either upright (0°) or pitched upwards (negative angles) or downwards (positive angles). Values for the pitch and roll response of the muscle are taken from the sinusoidal function (solid line) fitted to the 'Yawed Pitch' data. The yaw response is taken to be the average of values obtained from fits to 'Rolled Yaw' and 'Pitched Yaw' data. The length of the vector represented by these 3 values is then normalized to one and displayed as shown at the bottom of the figure.

sing represented by the two poles and two zeros occurs. The dashed line in the phase portion of Fig. 1B indicates the response of irregular vestibular afferents from the horizontal SCC, which are believed to be the afferents responsible for the VCR [11, 12]. The afferent response can be described by a transfer function with one pole and one zero. This leaves a second pole and second zero to be added by neural circuitry of the VCR, which agrees with observations of Wilson et al. [13], who observed VCR responses elicited by electrical stimuli that bypassed the dynamics of the SCCs. Thus the horizontal VCR can be viewed as two concatenated first-order lag–lead systems, one representing the horizontal SCCs, the other the CNS.

A different pattern of dynamic processing occurs when the VCR is elicited by rotation in vertical planes, which excites both SCCs and otolith organs. The latter are sensitive to the position of the head with respect to gravity and add a static component to the vertical VCR response at low frequencies [9, 14]. Otherwise the dynamics resemble those of the horizontal VCR [15, 16].

Kinematics

In studying the kinematics of the VCR, we are interested in how the 30 neck muscles in the cat are activated during rotations in different planes in space. If the VCR is viewed as stabilizing the same 6 degrees of freedom of rotation that cats employ during voluntary movements, there are more muscles than are needed. As a result the system is overcomplete and theoretically many different patterns of

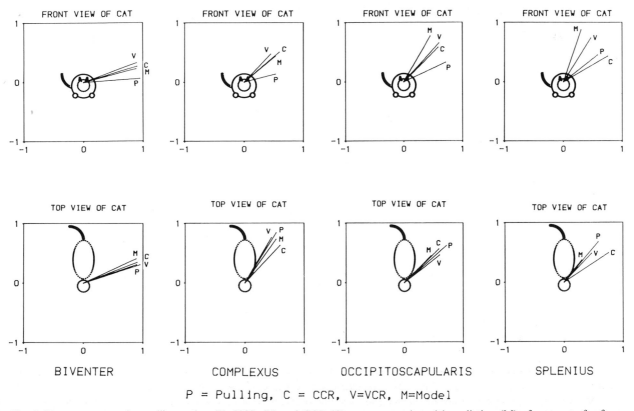

P = Pulling, C = CCR, V=VCR, M=Model

Fig. 3. Vectors representing pulling action (P), VCR (V) and CCR (C) responses and model prediction (M) of responses for four right-sided neck muscles. The VCR and CCR data are averaged from 4 and 2 animals respectively [19]. The model prediction is from the tensorial model of VCR [18]. The pulling direction is from anatomical measurements of neck muscle origins and insertions [8] and has been *reflected* for easy comparison with other vectors.

muscle activity could be used to counter a given rotation of the head and body in space [17, 18]. However, as illustrated in Fig. 2, Baker et al. [15] observed the spatial pattern of neck muscle activation produced by whole body rotation in 24 different planes and found that each muscle was maximally activated by rotation in a preferred plane that was consistent within and across animals. Responses to rotations in other planes fell off as the cosine of the angle between those planes and the preferred plane. Banovetz et al. [19] have recently extended these findings from the decerebrate to the alert cat.

How can the preferred directions of activation of neck muscles during the VCR be related to the pulling directions of those muscles? As shown by Pellionisz and Peterson [18], we should not expect activation and pulling directions to be aligned and, in fact, they are not (see Fig. 3). Since the system is overcomplete, any attempt to predict activation directions from pulling directions must assume some

optimality criterion that governs the selection of a single 'best' motor output pattern by the CNS. Pellionisz and Peterson [18] have constructed a tensorial model [20] of the VCR that uses as its criterion the Moore-Penrose Generalized Inverse [17, 21, 22], a solution that minimizes the sum-of-squares of muscle activity required to execute a movement. As illustrated in Fig. 3, the model gives reasonably close predictions of the observed activation directions. Thus the CNS may be selecting a criterion that generates movements with the minimum co-contraction or energy expenditure.

The kinematic observations described above were all made at higher frequencies of rotation where the VCR is dominated by SCC input. When responses are studied at frequencies close to 0.2 Hz, where otolith and canal signals are approximately equal in amplitude, another complexity arises, which we term orientation-dependent dynamics or ODD. As illustrated in Fig. 4, ODD manifests as

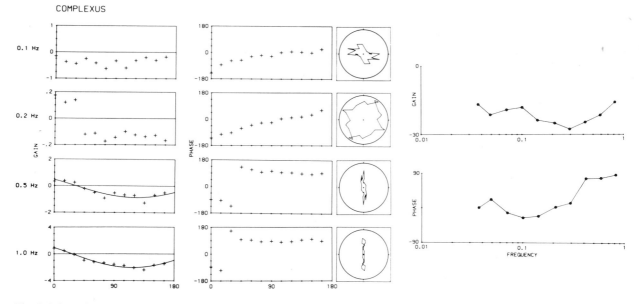

Fig. 4. Orientation-dependent dynamics of the complexus muscle response to rotations in 12 vertical planes (modified from [15]). The plots at left show the gain and phase of the EMG response in the 'Yawed Pitch' series where 0° equals pitch and 90° equals roll. At high frequencies the response has fixed phase ($\pm 90°$) and sinusoidally varying gain as in Fig. 2. At lower frequencies, however, gain is relatively constant (± 0.15 at 0.2 Hz) and the phase shifts with orientation of rotation plane. This behaviour is reflected in an open phase plane plot (third column) where gain is plotted as a function of rotation plane orientation in polar coordinates. The right column is a Bode diagram of the response in the roll (90°) plane as a function of frequency. The low gain at 0.2 Hz suggests competition of the canal and otolith components of the response at this frequency.

a VCR that is equally strong in many planes of rotation but has different dynamics in different planes [15]. It appears to arise when the otolith and canal components of the VCR have different preferred planes of activation so that muscles exhibit a strong position-related response in one plane, typically the roll plane, and a strong velocity-related response in another plane, typically the pitch plane. Functionally, ODD makes sense because the inertia of the head–neck system varies greatly with the axis of rotation.

Properties of the CCR

Dynamics

Peterson et al. [23] were the first to study the dynamics of the CCR. They also examined the linearity of both VCR and CCR by studying neck EMG responses in decerebrate cats exposed to graded whole-body rotations or graded rotations of the body about an earth-fixed head. While the VCR exhibited a threshold amplitude below which no response occurred, the CCR exhibited a complementary region of high sensitivity for rotations less than about 2° in amplitude. Peterson et al. [23] speculate that this region may arise because neck muscle spindles contributing to the CCR have a high sensitivity to small stretches like that observed in limb muscle spindles [24]. Functionally the complementary low-amplitude behaviour of the VCR and CCR means that the combined output of the two, which occurs during rotation of the head on a stationary trunk, will be more linear than the output of either alone.

The frequency response of the CCR also seems to be ideal for promoting simple interaction with the VCR. As illustrated in Fig. 1D, the CCR exhibits a static stretch response at low frequencies and a second-order lead at high frequencies that is closely matched to that of the VCR. In fact, Peterson et al. [23] found that the time constants of the two lead terms (zeros) of the CCR were closely correlated with those of the VCR in their animals. This suggests that the dynamics of the two reflexes are matched to allow them to interact in a simple fashion at all frequencies.

Kinematics

Banovetz et al. [19] have recently begun a multidimensional study of the CCR in both alert and decerebrate cats. Observations in the alert animal indicate that the amplitude of the CCR is under strong supraspinal control, which often suppresses it entirely. In the decerebrate state, however, the reflex is released and its spatial properties can be investigated. Preliminary observations, represented by the optimal response direction vectors in Fig. 3, suggest that the kinematic properties of the CCR are also quite close to those of the VCR. Once again this similarity would serve to promote simple interaction of the VCR and CCR in stabilizing the head.

Interaction of VCR, CCR and neck mechanics

Interaction of VCR and CCR

Peterson et al. [23] studied neck EMG output in two situations where the VCR and CCR are activated together. The simplest case is where the head is rotated on a fixed trunk, causing the VCR and CCR to work together to oppose the rotation. In all animals the EMG output in this case was found to be the vectorial sum of the EMG activation observed when the VCR and CCR were elicited by a rotation of the same amplitude and frequency. Dutia et al. [16] provide evidence for a similar summation of VCR and CCR during head rotations in the sagittal plane.

A more complex interaction of the VCR and CCR occurs when the animal's body is rotated with the head free to rotate on the trunk. This situation is referred to as 'closed loop' since head movements induced by the VCR and CCR alter the input to these two reflexes. As illustrated in Fig. 5A–E, the linearity of the VCR–CCR system in the closed-loop case can be estimated by predicting the EMG response with the head free from VCR and CCR responses measured with the head restrained. Two steps are required to arrive at the estimate. First the VCR response is corrected to reflect the actual movement of the head relative to space in the free-head condition (Fig. 5D). Then the CCR response that would be produced by the observed motion of the head relative to the trunk is added to the first estimate (Fig. 5E). As illustrated, this procedure gave good prediction of the observed data in all cases where stimuli were in the linear range for the VCR and CCR. Thus, the combined motor output produced by the VCR and CCR is simply the sum of the EMG activation produced by each alone.

Interaction of reflexes and head mechanics

The forces and torques responsible for head stabilization arise not only from closed-loop operation of the VCR and CCR but also from mechanical forces

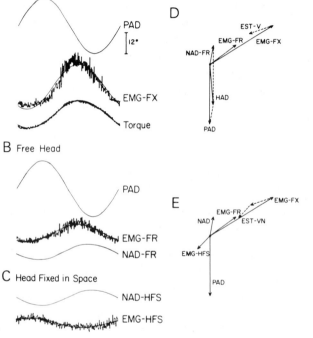

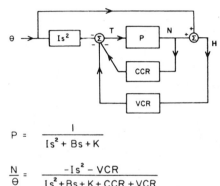

$$P = \frac{1}{Is^2 + Bs + K}$$

$$\frac{N}{\Theta} = \frac{-Is^2 - VCR}{Is^2 + Bs + K + CCR + VCR}$$

Fig. 5. (A–E) Vestibular and neck reflex contribution to the closed-loop VCR response. (A) The EMG activity in the right splenius muscle and head torque during 15°, 0.2 Hz whole-body rotation (PAD) with the head fixed to the turntable. (B) The activity of same muscle and angular counterrotation of the head (NAD-FR) during identical platform rotation with the head free to rotate. (C) The EMG activity of the same muscle during rotation of the body about the earth-fixed head with amplitude and phase of rotation set equal to NAD-FR. (D) A vector diagram in which stimuli and EMG responses are represented by solid vectors with lengths proportional to the amplitude and with polar angle equal to the phase of the stimulus or response measured with respect to the peak rightward deviation of the turntable. The dashed lines indicate the vector summation of PAD and NAD-FR to obtain the angular deviation of the head with respect to space (HAD) during closed-loop VCR. The dotted vector EST-V indicates the change in EMG response predicted as a result of the changed vestibular stimulus in the closed-loop situation. (E) A similar diagram to which the vector representing the neck reflex response (EMG-HFS) has been added. Addition of this vector to the EST-V vector produces EST-VN, the estimated closed-loop response after compensating for vestibular and neck reflex effects. Note the close agreement with the measured closed-loop response (EMG-FR). (F) Biomechanical model of the head-position-control system. The block diagram describes factors that determine head position during passive rotation of the body. The first equation below the diagram gives the transfer function of the neck motor plant. The second equation gives the overall transfer function relating rotation of the head on the body (N) to the applied rotation of the body (θ). Other symbols are: B, viscosity of neck musculature; head position in space; I, head inertia; K, spring constant of neck musculature; P, neck motor plant; s, LaPlace operator; T, torque applied to head.

produced by the head–neck musculoskeletal system. Goldberg and Peterson [3] used the head movement model shown in Fig. 5F and measurements of cat head stabilization at frequencies from 0.2 to 5 Hz to explore the interaction of reflex and mechanical contributions to stabilizing head movements. They began with observations of head movements in deeply anaesthetized cats where the VCR and CCR were absent. These showed that the neck mechanics behave like an underdamped second-order spring–pendulum system with a resonance at about 2 Hz. A key feature of such a system is that the movements it produces decline as the square of the frequency below the resonance point. Thus during rotation of the body at frequencies below 0.5 Hz, there was very little rotation of the head on the trunk while at frequencies above the resonance point, head inertia tended to hold the head fixed in space so that head rotation on the trunk was equal and opposite to the applied body rotation.

When they performed the same measurements on alert cats exposed to pseudo-random rotations in the dark, Goldberg and Peterson [3] found that the resonance point had shifted to about 4 Hz, probably because of the higher visco-elasticity of the active neck muscles. They also found that compensatory head movements did not decline as the square of frequency below this resonance point. Rather the animal produced compensatory movements with a constant gain of 0.5 at frequencies from 0.2 to 2.0 Hz. Since mechanically induced movements rapidly decline to negligible levels in this range, the compensatory movements must have been produced by the VCR and CCR. Referring to the equations in Fig. 5F, if the VCR and CCR were equal, the closed-loop transfer function would reduce to $H(s) = -VCR/VCR + CCR = -1/2$. Since the minus sign indicates movements in the compensatory direction, a simple summation of a VCR and CCR with equal gains and dynamic properties can account for the head stabilization seen in the alert cat at low frequencies of body rotation.

The simple head stabilization strategy observed by Goldberg and Peterson [3] may not always apply. As described earlier, Banovetz et al. [19] have found that cats can suppress the CCR under some circumstances. This would allow them to produce compensatory movements with a gain approaching −1.0. Bizzi et al. [1] also found very low CCR gains in the Rhesus monkey. It is also possible that the VCR may be suppressed, at least in humans, where Guitton et al. [25] found that compensatory head movements were present only when subjects generated them voluntarily. Nevertheless, Goldberg and Peterson's [3] findings demonstrate that the VCR and CCR can interact in a simple way to produce stabilizing head movements. This interaction is greatly facilitated by the simple features of these two reflexes that were described earlier: identical dynamics and kinematics, offsetting amplitude nonlinearities and additive interaction.

References

[1] Bizzi, E., Dev, P., Morasso, P. and Polit, A. (1978). Effect of load disturbances during central initiated movements. *J. Neurophysiol.*, 41: 542–556.

[2] Schor, R.H., Kearney, R.E. and Dieringer, N. (1988) Reflex stabilization of the head. In B.W. Peterson and F.J. Richmond, (Eds.), *Control of Head Movement*, Oxford University Press, New York, pp. 141–166.

[3] Goldberg, J. and Peterson, B.W. (1986) Reflex and mechanical contributions to head stabilization in alert cats. *J. Neurophysiol.*, 56: 857–875.

[4] Zangemeister, W.H., Lehman, S. and Stark, L. (1981) Simulation of head movement trajectories: model and fit to main sequence. *Biol. Cybern.*, 41: 19–32.

[5] Viviani, P. and Berthoz, A. (1975) Dynamics of the head–neck system in response to small perturbation: analysis and modeling in the frequency domain. *Biol. Cybern.*, 19: 19–37.

[6] Richmond, F.J.R. and Vidal, P.P. (1988) The motor system: joints and muscles of the neck. In B.W. Peterson and F.J. Richmond (Eds.), *Control of Head Movement*, Oxford University Press, New York, pp. 1–21.

[7] Vidal, P.P., Graf, W. and Berthoz, A. (1986) The orientation of the cervical vertebral column in unrestrained awake animals. I. Resting position. *Exp. Brain Res.*, 61: 549–559.

[8] Baker, J. and Wickland, C. (1988) Kinematic properties of the vestibulocollic reflex. In B.W. Peterson and F.J. Richmond (Eds.), *Control of Head Movement*, Oxford University Press, New York, pp. 167–177.

[9] Berthoz, A. and Anderson, J.H. (1971) Frequency analysis of vestibular influence on extensor motoneurons. II. Rela-

172

tionship between neck and forelimb extensors. *Brain Res.*, 34: 376–380.

[10] Ezure, K. and Sasaki, S. (1978) Frequency-response analysis of vestibular-induced neck reflex in cat. I. Characteristics of neural transmission from horizontal semicircular canal to neck motoneurons. *J. Neurophysiol.*, 41: 445–458.

[11] Bilotto, G., Goldberg, J., Peterson, B.W. and Wilson, V.J. (1982) Dynamic properties of vestibular reflexes in the decerebrate cat. *Exp. Brain Res.*, 47: 343–352.

[12] Moschovakis, A.K., Highstein, S.M. and Goldberg, J.M. (1985) Differential projections of regularly and irregularly discharging vestibular primary afferents in the barbiturate anesthetized squirrel monkey. *Soc. Neurosci. Abstr.*, 11: 321.

[13] Wilson, V.J., Peterson, B.W., Fukushima, K., Hirai, N. and Uchino, Y. (1979) Analysis of vestibulocollic reflexes by sinusoidal polarization of vestibular afferent fibers. *J. Neurophysiol.*, 42: 331–346.

[14] Schor, R.H. and Miller, A.D. (1981) Vestibular reflexes in neck and forelimb muscles evoked by roll tilt. *J. Neurophysiol.*, 46: 167–178.

[15] Baker, J., Goldberg, J. and Peterson, B.W. (1985) Spatial and temporal response properties of the vestibulocollic reflex in decerebrate cats. *J. Neurophysiol.*, 54: 735–756.

[16] Dutia, M.B. and Hunter, M.J. (1985) The sagittal vestibulocollic reflex and its interaction with neck proprioceptive afferents in the decerebrate cat. *J. Physiol. London*, 359: 17–29.

[17] Pellionisz, A. (1984) Coordination: a vector-matrix description of transformations of overcomplete CNS coordinates and a tensorial solution using the Moore-Penrose generalized inverse. *J. Theor. Biol.*, 110: 353–375.

[18] Pellionisz, A. and Peterson, B.W. (1988) A tensorial model of neck motor activation. In B.W. Peterson and F.J. Richmond (Eds.), *Control of Head Movement*, Oxford University Press, New York, pp. 178–186.

[19] Banovetz, J.M., Rude, S.A., Perlmutter, S.I., Peterson, B.W. and Baker, J.F. (1987) A comparison of neck reflexes in alert and decerebrate cats. *Soc. Neurosci. Abstr.*, in press.

[20] Pellionisz, A. and Llinás, R. (1980) Tensorial approach to the geometry of brain function. Cerebellar coordination via a metric tensor. *Neuroscience*, 5: 1761–1770.

[21] Albert, A. (1972) *Regression and the Moore-Penrose Pseudoinverse*, Academic Press, New York.

[22] Bickley, W.G. and Gibson, R.E. (1962) *Via Vector to Tensor*, John Wiley and Sons, New York.

[23] Peterson, B.W., Goldberg, J., Bilotto, G. and Fuller, J.H. (1985) Cervicocollic reflex: its dynamic properties and interaction with vestibular reflexes. *J. Neurophysiol.*, 54: 90–109.

[24] Hasan, Z. and Houk, J.C. (1975) Transition in sensitivity of spindle receptors that occurs when muscle is stretched more than a fraction of a millimeter. *J Neurophysiol.*, 38: 673–689.

[25] Guitton, D., Kearney, R.E., Wereley, N. and Peterson, B.W. (1986) Visual, vestibular and voluntary contributions to human head stabilization. *Exp. Brain Res.*, 64: 59–69.

O. Pompeiano and J.H.J. Allum (Eds.)
Progress in Brain Research, Vol. 76
© 1988 Elsevier Science Publishers B.V. (Biomedical Division)

CHAPTER 15

Interaction between vestibulocollic and cervicocollic reflexes: automatic compensation of reflex gain by muscle afferents

M.B. Dutia

Department of Physiology, University Medical School, Teviot Place, Edinburgh EH8 9AG, U.K.

Recent experiments on the sagittal VCR in the decerebrate cat have examined the possible contribution from otolith afferents to this reflex, and the interaction of the sagittal VCR with afferent inputs from muscle stretch receptors in the neck muscles. The role of otolith afferents has been investigated by comparing, during very slow sinusoidal movements of the head, the response of the sagittal VCR with that known for the horizontal (yaw) VCR. Unlike the horizontal VCR whose ability to follow low frequencies of head movement is limited by the time constant of integration of horizontal semicircular canal inputs, the sagittal VCR shows relatively constant gain and phase at frequencies between 0.015 and 0.1 Hz. This indicates a functionally significant role at low frequencies for an input signal related to actual head position, presumably from otolith afferents whose activity is modulated by head movement in the sagittal (pitch) plane but not by horizontal (yaw) movements. Separate experiments in which the biventer cervicis muscles were systematically stretched or shortened during 1 Hz vestibular stimulation have shown that the sagittal VCR interacts powerfully with afferent inputs from stretch receptors (presumably muscle spindles) in these muscles. The reflex response to a given head movement is amplified severalfold if the muscles are lengthening during vestibular stimulation, or attenuated and even abolished if they are shortening. The combined reflex response to head movement and muscle stretching is estimated reasonably well by a linear addition between the VCR and the CCR evoked by sinusoidal stretching alone.

Introduction

Vestibular reflexes in the neck muscles (VCRs) serve to stabilize the position of the head in relation to the trunk. They are in several ways analogous to the vestibulo-ocular reflexes, which stabilize the eyes within the head. These reflexes provide useful experimental models of mammalian motor control systems: particular motoneuron pools (neck or extra-ocular motoneurons) may be repetitively and reproducibly activated by natural vestibular stimulation, under controlled conditions. Vestibulo-ocular reflexes have been extensively studied in animals and man (cf. [6,11]). However, VCRs are perhaps the better model of typical *skeletomotor* systems. The neck muscles, like the muscles of the limbs, deal with an inertial load (the head) that continuously interacts with external forces including gravity.

This paper describes recent experiments in which we have used the VCR system as a model in which to study the functional role of muscle stretch receptor afferent feedback in regulating the force of contraction of the neck muscles [3,4]. The results suggest that muscle spindle afferents 'servo-assist' in the dynamic control of muscle contraction, amplifying or attenuating the reflex response to a given vestibular stimulus according to the instantaneous

---

Abbreviations: BC, biventer cervicis; CCR, cervicocollic reflex; VCR, vestibulocollic reflex.

operating conditions of the neck muscles themselves.

Methods

The experiments described here were carried out on the VCR evoked by sinusoidal nose-up, nose-down movements of the head of the precollicular decerebrate cat (the sagittal VCR). The experimental preparation, data recording and analysis methods have been described in detail elsewhere [3]. In brief, the decerebrate animal was supported in a metal frame and its head was fixed in a head-holder attached to the armature of a large printed-circuit motor. The motor was positioned so as to produce sinusoidal movements of the head in the sagittal (pitch) plane, about an axis passing transversely through the atlanto-occipital joint. Stimulation of neck proprioceptors during head movement was avoided by detaching the neck muscles from the skull.

The neck extensor muscles biventer cervicis (BC) of the left and right sides were exposed, detached from the lamboidal crest and separated down the midline. In most experiments both muscles were connected to an electromagnetic muscle stretcher by stout threads; in some experiments only one of the muscles was attached to the stretcher while the other was fixed to a rigid bar. The printed-circuit motor and the muscle stretcher could be driven by a sinusoidal waveform from a function generator. The driving signal to the muscle stretcher was routed through a programmable analogue-delay line. It was thus possible to evoke in the BC muscles the VCR (motor driven alone), CCR (stretcher driven alone), or both VCR and CCR with the stretch stimulus either in phase with head movement (analogue delay = 0°), or out of phase with it (analogue delay = 180°).

EMG activity in the left and right BC muscles was recorded by surface electrodes stitched to the muscles, and after amplification and rectification was cycle-averaged by a microcomputer triggered by the function generator (see [3] for details). To allow comparision between cycle-averages with different levels of mean EMG activity they were normalized with respect to the mean level [2,3]. The amplitude and phase of EMG modulation at the frequency of head movement was determined from the Fourier transform of the cycle-average (e.g. Fig. 1, solid lines drawn through averaged EMG records). The gain of the VCR was measured as the percent modulation of mean activity per degree of head movement and expressed in dB (0 dB = 1% modulation/degree). CCR gain was measured similarly as percent modulation of mean activity per millimetre stretch of the muscle. Phase was measured with respect to either the maximum nose-down position of the head or the maximum stretch of the muscle, as appropriate. When head movement and muscle stretching were applied together, the gain and phase of the resulting 'combined' reflex were measured with respect to head position as for the VCR (see [4] for details).

Results

The sagittal vestibulocollic reflex

Fig. 1 shows example cycle-averages of rectified EMG-activity in the neck extensor muscles (BC)

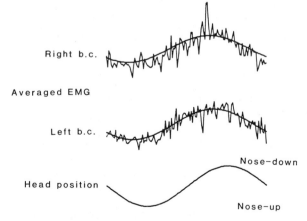

Fig. 1. Cycle-averages of rectified EMG activity in the right and left BC muscles (top and middle traces), during sagittal head movement at 0.1 Hz (bottom trace). The sinusoids drawn through the averaged records show the amplitude and phase of EMG modulation at the frequency of head movement obtained from the Fourier transform of the averaged record. Amplitude of head movement is 7.5° peak-to-peak.

during sinusoidal nose-up, nose-down head movement at 0.1 Hz. These averages were obtained with the muscles held at a fixed length close to their in vivo resting length. EMG activity in both left and right BC muscles increases with head movement in the nose-down direction, and declines as the head moves in the nose-up direction. This is the action of the sagittal VCR, which in the intact animal would resist downward displacements of the head. At this frequency of head movement EMG modulation leads actual head position by some 30°, so that peak EMG activity occurs before the head reaches its maximum nose-down position. At higher frequencies of head movement in the physiological range (1 to 5 Hz), peak EMG activity occurs progressively earlier in the cycle and EMG modulation amplitude increases severalfold (see, for example, Fig. 2). The phase advance and increase in gain

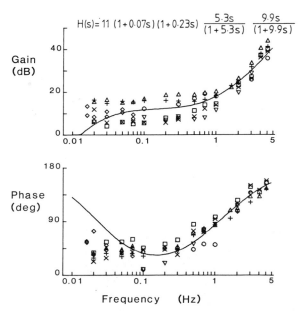

Fig. 2. Bode diagram of gain and phase (re head position) of the sagittal VCR in the frequency range 0.015–5 Hz. Each symbol represents a different experiment. The solid lines show the gain and phase predicted by the transfer function (top) which describes a second-order lead–lag system operating on the head angular velocity signals from the vertical semicircular canals. Note that the predicted values correspond well with actual values for higher frequencies of head movement, but deviate from them at low frequencies.

with frequency are modelled adequately by a second-order lead–lag system operating on head-velocity input signals from the semicircular canals [3].

The frequency response of the sagittal VCR in the range 0.1–5 Hz is very similar to that of the horizontal VCR evoked by head movements in the yaw plane [2,5]. Thus, while the maximum excitation vector of the BC muscles is close to the pitch (sagittal) plane [1], the same muscles would also assist in yaw movements of the head. However the synergistic, in-phase activation of the left and right BC muscles in the sagittal VCR is in contrast to the antagonistic, out-of-phase activation of the same muscle by head movements in the yaw plane. In combined pitching and yawing movements of the head, therefore, the degree to which the two BC muscles would be used as synergists or antagonists would presumably depend upon the relative intensity of vertical and horizontal canal afferent inputs and convergence between them [1,12]. In addition to this convergence between semicircular canal afferent inputs, a further likely contribution is from otolith afferents whose activity would be modulated by head movements in the sagittal (pitch) plane [1,9,10].

To investigate the extent to which otolith afferents contribute to the sagittal VCR, we have extended our earlier observations to include frequencies of head movement between 0.015 and 0.1 Hz (Fig. 2). At these low frequencies the afferent input related to head angular velocity from the semicircular canals is very small. If the sagittal VCR is driven solely by semicircular canal afferents, its performance at these low frequencies can be estimated using the second-order lead–lag model fitted to the data at higher frequencies (Fig. 2, solid lines). It would be expected that head movements at frequencies below 0.05 Hz would evoke progressively smaller reflex responses (decreasing gain), becoming more related to head velocity and acceleration rather than head position (advancing phase). The horizontal VCR evoked by yaw movements, in which the otolith afferents are not modulated, does behave as predicted by the solid lines in Fig. 2 [2,5]. However, as shown by the symbols in Fig. 2 (each of which represents a different experiment), the gain of the sagittal VCR does not decline, and phase remains on average about 30° in advance of head position, even at frequencies as low as 0.015–0.2 Hz.

This persistence of the sagittal reflex response during very slow movements of the head implies a significant role for an afferent input signal related to actual head position, presumably from the otolith receptors. It is interesting, however, that even at these low frequencies the sagittal VCR response maintains a phase lead of some 30–40° with respect to head position (Fig. 2). This is in contrast to the response of some forelimb and shoulder muscles to low-frequency vestibular stimulation [12].

The motor output of the sagittal VCR system appears therefore to be determined by systematic convergence between afferent inputs from the semicircular canals and the otolith afferents, the latter predominating at low frequencies of head movement. In addition, as described below, the VCR motor output also interacts powerfully with afferent feedback from muscle stretch receptors in the neck muscles themselves. This latter interaction presumably plays an important part in the behaving animal, where movements of the head on the neck would involve not only vestibular stimulation but also changes in length of the muscles of the neck.

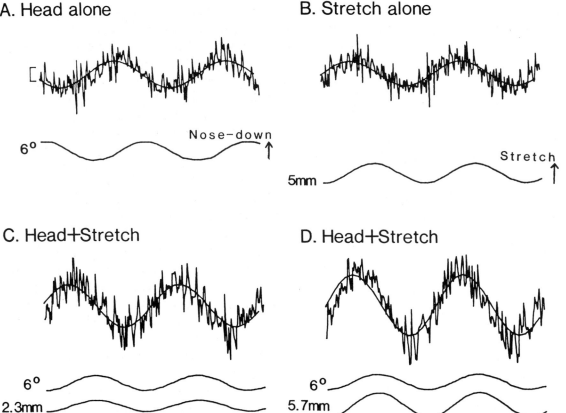

Fig. 3. Cycle-averages of EMG activity from a typical BC muscle showing interaction between the sagittal VCR and muscle stretching in phase with head movement. (A) EMG modulation evoked by head movement at 1 Hz (the sagittal VCR alone). The arrow indicates head movement in the nose-down direction. (B) EMG modulation evoked by sinusoidal stretching of the muscle also at 1 Hz (the CCR). The arrow indicates muscle stretch (increase in muscle length). (C,D) EMG modulation in response to muscle stretching of 2.3 and 5.7 mm amplitude respectively in phase with the vestibular stimulus.

Interaction of the sagittal vestibulocollic reflex and muscle stretching

For the remainder of the experiments described here, a 'standard' vestibular stimulus was employed of sinusoidal head movement of 6–8° amplitude at 1 Hz. Both BC muscles were attached by stout threads to a muscle stretcher and could thereby also be stretched sinusoidally at 1 Hz to evoke the CCR. The VCR evoked in the BC muscles by the 1 Hz vestibular stimulus was measured when the muscles were either held at a fixed length (VCR alone), or stretched sinusoidally in phase with head movement so that they were stretched as the head moved nose-downwards (VCR + CCR), or stretched out-of-phase with head movement so that they were shortened as the head moved nose-downwards (VCR − CCR).

Results from one BC muscle in a typical experiment are illustrated in Figs. 3 and 4. The reflex response to head movement with the muscles held at a constant length (VCR alone) is shown in Fig. 3A. Fig. 3B shows the EMG modulation evoked by a 5 mm peak-to-peak sinusoidal stretch of the muscle also at 1 Hz (the CCR). The effects of combining head movement and muscle stretching in phase (so that the muscle was stretched as the head moved downwards) are shown in Fig. 3C and D. EMG modulation evoked by combined head movement and muscle stretching is larger than either the VCR or the CCR alone, even for small stretch amplitudes (e.g. Fig. 3C). Larger stretch amplitudes evoked a proportionately larger combined reflex response (e.g. Fig. 3D). When the sinusoidal stretching was applied 180° out of phase with head movement, so that the muscles shortened as the head moved in the nose-down direction, the combined reflex response became smaller (Fig. 4B cf. 4A). The reduction in the amplitude of modulation of the EMG was also in proportion to the amplitude of stretch. In some experiments larger stretches (6-8 mm) reduced the amplitude of EMG modulation to below the noise level in the record, effectively abolishing it.

Fig. 5 shows the results from one experiment where the gain and phase of the combined reflex

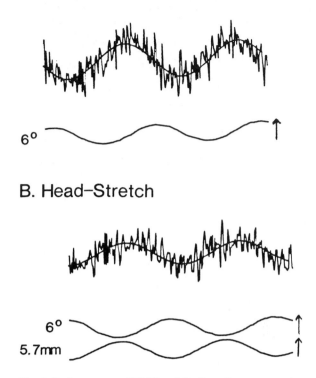

A. Head alone

B. Head–Stretch

Fig. 4. Cycle-averages of EMG activity from the same muscle as in Fig. 3, showing the effects of muscle stretching 180° out-of-phase with head movement: (A) the sagittal VCR alone; (B) head movement with muscle stretching out-of-phase with it.

were systematically measured over a range of stretch amplitudes applied either in phase or out of phase with head movement. The open circles in Fig. 5 show the gain and phase of the VCR alone measured at various times during the experiment. The measurements of gain and phase of the combined reflex obtained with muscle stretching in phase with head movement are plotted to the right (×), while those obtained with muscle stretching 180° out-of-phase with head movement are plotted to the left (+). The broken horizontal lines show the mean values of gain and phase of the VCR alone in this experiment.

The increase in gain of the combined reflex (G_C) with in-phase stretching, and the decrease with out-of-phase stretching, are predicted reasonably well by the vectorial sum of the VCR (G_V) and the CCR

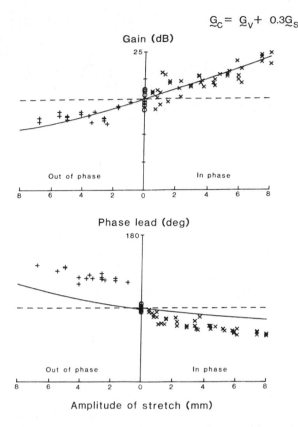

$$\underset{\sim}{G_C} = \underset{\sim}{G_V} + 0.3\underset{\sim}{G_S}$$

Gain (dB)

Out of phase   In phase

Phase lead (deg)

Out of phase   In phase

Amplitude of stretch (mm)

Fig. 5. Gain (upper) and phase (lower) of the combined reflex response to head movement and muscle stretching, plotted against the amplitude of stretch: O, gain and phase of the sagittal VCR alone measured at various times during the experiment; ×, gain and phase of the combined reflex response obtained with stretching in phase with head movement; +, those obtained with stretching 180° out-of-phase. Solid lines indicate the gain and phase of the combined reflex (G_C) predicted by a vectorial sum (top) of the VCR (G_V) and the CCR (G_S). (From [4].)

(G_S) for each amplitude of stretch (Fig. 5, top; solid lines), taking into account a proportionally constant K ($= 0.35$ in this experiment) by which the CCR is scaled. In addition, the dependence of the CCR upon the amplitude of stretching [4], which results in a decrease in CCR gain of some 8 dB as the peak-to-peak amplitude of stretching increases from 1 to 8 mm, is also taken into account in calculating the expected combined reflex response (solid lines in Fig. 5). While this linear vectorial addition predicts the gain of the combined reflex response

quite well, there is a small but consistent discrepancy between the predicted and measured values of phase (Fig. 5, lower plot). This may be due to nonlinearities either in the responses from the BC muscle spindles stimulated in the CCR, or in the recruitment and release of motoneurons during EMG modulation.

Thus, the amplitude of the BC reflex response to a constant vestibular stimulus is dynamically regulated by the simultaneous muscle stretch receptor afferent input from the muscles themselves. The reflex response is either amplified severalfold if the muscles are lengthening as the head moves in the nose-down direction (Fig. 5, ×), or attenuated and even abolished if the muscles are shortening as the head moves downward (Fig. 5, +).

In some experiments, we arranged to stretch only one of the BC muscles while the other was held at a fixed length, in order to determine if the two BC motoneuron pools were linked by excitatory or inhibitory influences during the VCR. The results of one such experiment are shown in Fig. 6. In this case the right BC muscle was attached to the stretcher while the left was fixed to a rigid bar. Head movement alone elicited the normal VCR response in both muscles (Fig. 6A). When the right BC muscle was stretched sinusoidally the CCR was evoked in this muscle, with no EMG modulation on the left side (Fig. 6B). When head movement and stretching were combined, the amplitude of EMG modulation in the right muscle approximately doubled while that in the left muscle was the same as with vestibular stimulation alone (Fig. 6C). This indication that the effects of muscle stretching were restricted to the stimulated muscle were confirmed when the result of stretching only the right muscle during the VCR was compared with that obtained earlier in the experiment when both muscles were stretched together. The increase in gain in the stimulated (right) muscle was as great as when both muscles were stretched together, indicating that muscle afferents from the contralateral muscle did not contribute significantly to the VCR–CCR interaction. It would appear therefore that the BC motoneuron pools are organized as essentially inde-

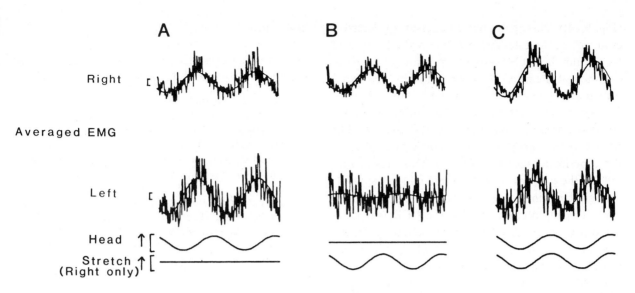

Fig. 6. Cycle-averages of EMG activity from the right and left BC muscles in one experiment to show the effects of stretching only one of the muscles. (A) VCR in both muscles evoked by head movement at 1 Hz. (B) CCR (stretch reflex) evoked in the right muscle by stretching at 1 Hz while the left muscle was held fixed. (C) Response to combined head movement and stretching of the right muscle. Note potentiation of reflex gain in the right muscle while response in the left muscle is the same as with head movement alone. (From [4].)

pendent entities free of mutual reflex linkages. This presumably allows flexibility in their separate recruitment and control either as synergists or antagonists in the context of a particular head trajectory.

Discussion

The experiments described here illustrate the convergence of afferent inputs from semicircular canal, otolith and muscle receptors in generating the reflex response of the neck extensor muscles to displacements of the head in the sagittal plane. The contribution of the otolith afferents to the sagittal VCR, as in the roll VCR and [8], extends its head-stabilizing action to low frequencies of head movement (0.015–0.02 Hz and presumably below). The role of muscle stretch receptor afferents (presumably from muscle spindles in the BC muscles) appears to be to 'servo-assist' in the reflex contraction of the BC muscles, amplifying or attenuating the motoneurons' response to the vestibular stimulus in the context of the operating conditions of the muscles themselves. Lengthening of the BC muscles marked-

ly potentiates the gain of the combined reflex, while shortening reduces the combined reflex gain and may even abolish it.

In the intact animal, such interactions between the VCR and CCR may be expected to occur frequently as a result of movements of the spinal column relative to the head during walking, running and jumping. Thus a given movement of the head may be accompanied under different circumstances by larger or smaller changes in length of the neck muscles. Effective head stabilization therefore requires that the force of contraction of the neck muscles is dynamically regulated, not just with respect to the vestibular stimulus but also in relation to the movement of the spinal column to which the neck muscles are attached. This integration of head and neck position is achieved by the additive interaction between the VCR and the CCR, and results in a sensitive and effective system for stabilizing the head on the neck.

The combined reflex response to head movement and muscle stretching is estimated reasonably well by a linear addition between the VCR and the CCR

(Fig. 5; [4]). This agrees with the results of Peterson et al. [7] on the interaction between the horizontal VCR and the CCR evoked by whole-body rotations about the neck. However, while in their experiments the gains of the VCR and the CCR (with respect to angular rotation of the body) were similar, in the present experiments the CCR gain had to be scaled by a proportionality constant K (0.35 in the experiment shown in Fig. 5). This presumably reflects the fact that in the present experiments, although the gain of the VCR was measured per degree of head rotation, that of the CCR was measured per millimetre of stretch of the muscle. In the simplest case the present results imply that in the intact animal, where the neck muscles are attached to the skull, a downward head movement of 1° would stretch the BC muscles by about 0.35 mm. The value of K might thus represent a factor by which the VCR–CCR interaction is 'calibrated' in each animal, related to the amount of muscle stretching that would normally occur with head movement [4]. Alternatively it is possible that K represents a factor by which the gain of the CCR may be modified (for example through the gamma fusimotor system acting on the muscle spindles in the BC muscles), to make the VCR–CCR interaction more or less sensitive to changes in length of the neck muscles. The value of K appeared to remain the same throughout a given experiment, however (e.g. Fig. 5), and this suggests that it may represent a fixed 'calibration' between the VCR and the CCR.

Acknowledgements

I am grateful to M.J. Hunter and R.F. Price for their help in much of this work, and the Medical Research Council for financial support.

References

[1] Baker, J., Goldberg, J. and Peterson, B.W. (1985) Spatial and temporal response properties of the vestibulo-collic reflex in decerebrate cats. *J. Neurophysiol.*, 54: 735–756.

[2] Bilotto, G., Goldberg, J., Peterson, B.W. and Wilson, V.J. (1982) Dynamic properties of vestibular reflexes in the decerebrate cat. *Exp. Brain. Res.*, 47: 343–352.

[3] Dutia, M.B. and Hunter, M.J. (1985) The sagittal vestibulo-collic reflex and its interaction with neck proprioceptive afferents in the decerebrate cat. *J. Physiol. London*, 359: 17–29.

[4] Dutia, M.B. and Price, R.F. (1987) Interaction between the vestibulo-collic reflex and the cervico-collic stretch reflex in the decerebrate cat. *J. Physiol. London*, 387: 19–30.

[5] Ezure, K. and Sasaki, S. (1978) Frequency-response analysis of vestibular-induced neck reflex in cat. I. Characteristics of neural transmission from the horizontal semicircular canal to neck motoneurones. *J. Neurophysiol.*, 41: 445–458.

[6] Ito, M. (1984) *The Cerebellum and Neural Control*, Raven, New York, pp. 406–424.

[7] Peterson, B.W., Goldberg, J., Bilotto, G. and Fuller, J.H. (1985) Cervico-collic reflex: its dynamic properties and interaction with vestibular reflexes. *J. Neurophysiol.*, 54: 90–109.

[8] Schor, R.H. and Miller, A.D. (1981) Vestibular reflexes in neck and forelimb muscles evoked by roll tilt. *J. Neurophysiol.*, 46: 167–178.

[9] Schor, R.H., Miller, A.D. and Tomko, D.L. (1984) Responses to head tilt in cat central vestibular neurons. I. Direction of maximal sensitivity. *J. Neurophysiol.*, 51: 136–146.

[10] Schor, R.H., Miller, A.D., Timerick, S.J.B. and Tomko, D.L. (1985) Responses to head tilt in cat central vestibular neurons. II. Frequency dependence of neural response vectors. *J. Neurophysiol.*, 53: 1444–1452.

[11] Wilson, V.J. and Melvill-Jones, G. (1979) *Mammalian Vestibular Physiology*, Plenum, New York, 365 pp.

[12] Wilson, V.J., Schor, R.H., Suzuki, I. and Park, B.R. (1986) Spatial organisation of neck and vestibular reflexes acting on the forelimbs of the decerebrate cat. *J. Neurophysiol.*, 55: 514–526.

O. Pompeiano and J.H.J. Allum (Eds.)
Progress in Brain Research, Vol. 76
© 1988 Elsevier Science Publishers B.V. (Biomedical Division)

CHAPTER 16

Neck influences on posturokinetic responses to cortical stimulation

Y. Gahery[1] and O. Pompeiano[2]

[1]Laboratoire de Neurosciences Fonctionelles, Unité de Neurosciences Intégratives, CNRS., 31 Chemin Joseph-Aiguier, 13402 Marseille, CEDEX 9, France and [2]Dipartimento di Fisiologia e Biochimica, Università di Pisa, Via S.Zeno 31, 56100 Pisa, Italy

Experiments were performed in cats in order to establish whether the postural adjustments which accompany limb movements induced by motor cortex stimulation share the same efferent pathways as the postural reflexes elicited by labyrinth and neck afferent volleys, which act on neurons of the lateral vestibulospinal pathway either directly or through the precerebellar LRN and the cerebellar loop. The limb movements induced by cortical stimulation are accompanied by postural adjustments occurring at the same time as or slightly before the movement itself and are therefore clearly different both from postural preparations (which cannot occur under these conditions) and from postural reactions (which are reflexly triggered). The postural responses were studied in unrestrained, unanaesthetized cats by analysing the vertical forces exerted under the limbs and were found to be characterized by a diagonal pattern, i.e. a decrease in the vertical force exerted under the limb diagonally opposite to the moving limb and an increase in the force under the other two limbs. Unilateral neck deafferentation and unilateral lesion of the LRN had very similar effects on both postural tonus and postural adjustments. In both instances a postural asymmetry occurred, which was characterized by ipsilateral hypertonia and contralateral hypotonia of the limb extensor musculature. The threshold values of cortical stimulation inducing limb flexion movements increased on the hypertonic side (ipsilateral to the lesions) and decreased on the hypotonic side. The force variations decreased in amplitude and speed when the performing limb was ipsilateral to the hypertonic side, while the opposite occurred when the other side of the motor cortex was stimulated. Finally, the slopes of the response curves (representing the absolute values of the force variations as a function of the stimulus strength expressed in multiples of the threshold) were analysed before and after the lesions. With both kinds of lesions, the slope of the response curve of all four limbs decreased when the performing limb was ipsilateral to the hypertonic side, but increased if it was ipsilateral to the hypotonic side. Besides these findings, several experimental results indicate that cortical influences may be exerted on the lateral vestibular nucleus of Deiters via the LRN, i.e. the same precerebellar structure which is involved in the postural reactions originating from labyrinth and neck receptors. Experiments of monitoring the unit activity of lateral vestibulospinal neurons during cortical movements are required to find out whether Deiters' nucleus is directly involved in the postural adjustments which accompany the limb flexion induced by motor cortex stimulation.

Introduction

Besides 'postural preparations' facilitating voluntary or deliberate movements and 'postural reactions' compensating for the perturbations or disequilibrium resulting from a given movement, there are 'postural adjustments' which occur at the same time as the movement itself. These postural responses have been recently analysed both in humans and in quadrupeds (for references see [24,49]).

Conditioned limb movements in the dog [27,34,52]

Abbreviations: LRN, lateral reticular nucleus; LVN, lateral vestibular nucleus; lVS, lateral vestibulospinal.

and placing reactions in the cat [16,27,50,51,57] are accompanied by vertical force variations under the three other limbs. These force variations exhibit a diagonal pattern: the force exerted by the limb diagonally opposite to the moving one decreases while the force exerted by the other two increases. The same pattern of diagonal variations of vertical force also occurs for limb flexion induced by stimulation of the motor cortex [25,26]. These changes in force do not result from a feedback elicited by peripheral modifications brought about by the movement, as shown by considering the latencies of these responses: in fact, the postural adjustments occur at the same time or even precede the movement itself [26]. Therefore, a central command is responsible for this kind of postural responses, in contrast to 'postural reactions' which are reflexly triggered from the periphery.

Two prominent sources of postural reflexes are the neck receptors and the labyrinth receptors. In particular, rotation about the longitudinal axis of the animal ([22,47,60]; cf. [18,45]) on the one hand, and rotation of the neck with a stationary head on the other ([21,22,47]; cf. [18,45]), leading to selective stimulation of labyrinth and neck receptors, produce asymmetric changes in posture, such as contraction of ipsilateral limb extensors during side-down animal tilt and relaxation during side-down neck rotation (cf. also [43]). These effects were attributed to an increased or a decreased neuronal discharge, respectively, of the LVN of Deiters [4-6,48,61,64], which exerts an excitatory influence on ipsilateral extensor motoneurons ([44]; cf. [53]). Just the opposite results were observed for the other direction of animal or neck orientation.

The labyrinth and neck inputs may affect the activity of the LVN neurons not only directly, but also by utilizing the LRN. This precerebellar structure receives both crossed and uncrossed spinoreticular fibres [14]. However, while the crossed spinoreticular neurons which have a bilateral receptive field are monosynaptically excited by the lVS tract [12,32,58], the uncrossed spinoreticular neurons which have an ipsilateral receptive field escape this monosynaptic control ([10]; cf. [17]).

If we consider now the vestibulospinal reflexes, it appears that the increased discharge of lVS neurons during side-down animal tilt activates not only the ipsilateral limb extensor motoneurons [53], thus increasing the postural activity on this side, but also neurons of the crossed spinoreticulocerebellar pathway [17] passing through the LRN ([36,38]; cf. [54]). The resulting excitation of Purkinje cells of the contralateral hemivermis [19] would then inhibit the underlying Deiters' nucleus, thus contributing to the reduced postural activity which affects the limbs contralateral to the side of the animal displacement.

As to the cervicospinal reflexes, the reduced discharge of lVS neurons, leading to a decreased postural activity in the ipsilateral limbs during side-down neck rotation [5,6,48,64], can in part at least be due to activation of neurons of the uncrossed spinoreticulocerebellar pathway passing through the LRN [37,38], as well as of Purkinje cells of the ipsilateral hemivermis [19,20], leading to inhibition of the underlying Deiters' nucleus. The reduced activity of the corresponding VS neurons would also decrease the neuronal discharge of the crossed spinoreticulocerebellar pathway passing through the LRN. In this instance, the resulting disfacilitation of Purkinje cells of the contralateral hemivermis would lead to disinhibition of the underlying Deiters' nucleus, thus contributing to the increased postural activity which affects the limbs contralateral to the side of the neck displacement.

As a result of these findings it appears that the postural reflexes of both labyrinth and neck origin borrow a common pathway represented by the precerebellar LRN, which acts on the lVS neurons through the cerebellar loop. Even if postural adjustments which accompany limb movements following motor cortex stimulation are different in nature with respect to postural reflexes, they may share the same efferent pathways described above.

The main aims of the studies reported here were to test this hypothesis in two ways. Firstly, by evaluating the postural adjustments induced by cortical stimulation after unilateral neck deafferentation, since the neck input converges with the labyrinth input on the precerebellar LRN. Secondly, by evaluating the postural adjustments induced by cortical stimulation after unilateral lesion of the LRN, which may influence the discharge of lVS neurons through the cerebellar loop.

Postural adjustments accompanying limb movements induced by cortical stimulation

As seen in the Introduction, three kinds of postural responses may be associated to a given movement: 'postural preparations', 'postural adjustments' and 'postural reactions'. These responses differ in their time of occurrence with regard to the onset of the movement itself. Most often, all three are associated with the same movement and may also overlap. Therefore, it is difficult to distinguish them; it is particularly difficult to separate postural preparation from postural adjustments. The experimental evidence indicates that limb movements induced by motor cortex stimulation in the cat are accompanied by postural adjustments occurring at the same time or slightly before the movement itself [25,26]. Thus, these postural responses are clearly different from both postural preparations (which cannot occur in these conditions) and postural reactions (which are reflexly triggered).

The postural responses were studied in unrestrained, unanaesthetized cats by analysing the vertical forces exerted under the limbs. For that purpose the cats were trained to freely stand (for about 45–60 minutes) on four platforms equipped with strain gauges, allowing the measurement of forces with a precision of 20 g. Cortical stimulations were delivered through nickel-chrome electrodes implanted in the motor cortex of both sides at a depth of 1.5 mm. These electrodes, having a diameter of 250 μm and a resistance of 50–80 KΩ, were cemented to the bone and wired to a connector fixed to the cranium. Electric impulses were applied between these electrodes and an indifferent silver-wire anode placed in the left frontal sinus. Stimulations used to induce limb flexions were delivered by a completely programmable stimulator [23] and consisted of 50–100 ms trains of 0.5 ms square waves at a frequency of 200/s and at 1–3 V.

The vertical force values exerted under the limbs were transduced as potential variations by the strain gauges and converted into digital values before being stored in the memory of a PDP 11/40 computer. In order to make valid comparisons between the responses obtained, it was necessary to deliver cortical stimulations in standard postural conditions. For this purpose, the computer constantly analysed the postural parameters and delivered the stimulus only when conditions of weight distribution (equal under each of the four limbs) and postural stability (rate of displacement of the resultant of forces below a predetermined value) had been fulfilled for 1 s.

All the cortical stimulation sites used in these experiments gave rise to localized movements affecting a single joint, eliciting a fore- or hindlimb flexion. In order to facilitate the measurement of the amplitude of flexion, the intensity of cortical stimuli was so chosen that the moving limb remained in contact with the supporting platform. The amplitude of flexion was then the variation of vertical force and was automatically determined by the computer, which calculated the difference between the extreme vertical force measured during the first 300 ms and the mean value of the first four points immediately preceding the force development. Threshold values of cortical stimulations were also automatically measured by the computer following a standard protocol [23], in order to verify the constancy of stimulation conditions and as an important parameter for comparison between different experimental conditions. These thresholds (the smallest voltage values eliciting a change in the force measured under the moving limb) were determined with an accuracy of 0.1 V, each value being tested twice and the mean of the two responses being retained.

In these conditions, postural responses accompanying a limb flexion were characterized by a diagonal pattern. Specifically, for a cortical stimulation eliciting flexion of the left forelimb, the force always decreased under the right hindlimb but increased under the right forelimb and the left hindlimb (Fig. 1). On the other hand, if the performing limb was

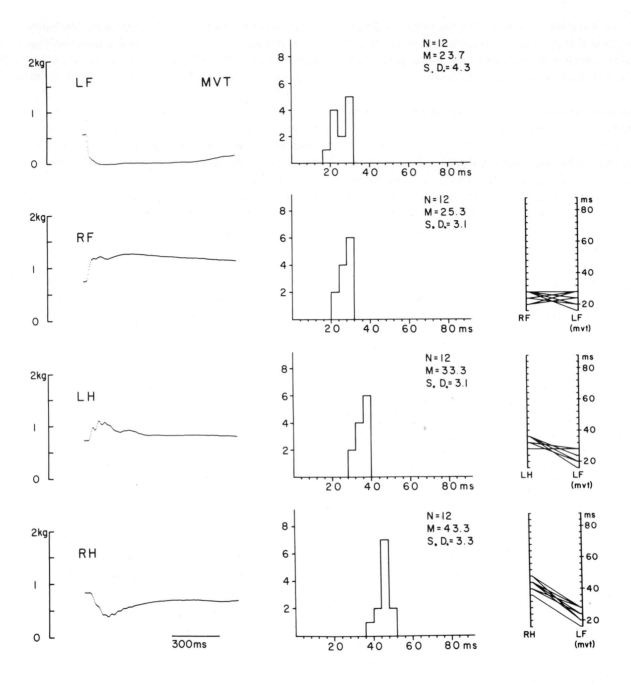

Fig.1. Force variations recorded under the four limbs following stimulation of the forelimb region of the right motor cortex leading to flexion of the left forelimb. On the left side, averaged curves representing the weight shifts for a series of 12 stimulations; MVT, movement limb (performing limb); LF, RF, left and right forelimb; LH, RH, left and right hindlimb. In the middle are represented the corresponding latency histograms for the 12 stimulations (N) with the mean (M) and standard deviation (S.D.). On the right side, the graphs of paired values between the limb in movement and each of the other limbs show that the force variations recorded under the postural forelimb (RF) have, for some stimulations, shorter latencies than those corresponding to the performing limb (LF). (From [26].)

the left hindlimb, the force increased under the left forelimb and the right hindlimb while a decrease was observed under the right forelimb.

The latencies of the force variations are very important as their evaluation leads to the conclusion that these postural responses cannot be reflexly triggered but result from a central command, thus being attributed to postural adjustments rather than to postural reactions. In all cases, the shortest latencies were those observed under the forelimbs. When forelimb flexions were elicited by cortical stimulation, the latencies were about the same for the two forelimbs and were in most cases in the range of 22 to 28 ms (time between the beginning of stimulus and the onset of force variation). Even though the mean latency was generally slightly smaller for the performing limb, the force variation recorded under the other forelimb could in some instances display the smallest latency of the two (Fig. 1). Postural responses under the hindlimbs occurred 10 to 20 ms later. In the case of flexion of the hindlimbs, the shortest latencies were still observed under one of the anterior, postural limbs. The fact that these postural responses occurred simultaneously with or before the movement indicates that they cannot result from perturbations brought about at the periphery by the movement, but are centrally triggered.

An interesting feature of these responses is the tied coupling between the movement and the associated postural responses. This was particularly evident when considering the curves relating the amplitudes of force variations with different supraliminal values of stimulation. These curves were automatically established by the computer, which calculated the mean of four responses for each stimulus strength and delivered five values of voltage from threshold (1T) to 1.25, 1.50, 1.75 and 2T. The responses curves were obtained for the performing limb as well as for the three other postural limbs. It was thus possible to observe that when the amplitude of the flexion induced by the stimulation increased, the amplitude of the postural responses increased as well. The threshold values were about the same, which means that the smallest stimulus

inducing flexion of one of the limbs also induced a postural response of the other limbs. Moreover, the slopes of the four curves evolved similarly: when the slope of the curve corresponding to the flexion limb increased, the slope of the other curves also increased.

The observation of both the latencies and amplitudes of the force variations leads to the establishment of another characteristic, i.e. that the sum of the decreasing forces evaluated in absolute value during the response does not always correspond to the sum of the increasing forces. These variations in the total apparent weight of the cat correspond to a vertical displacement of the centre of gravity, as reported recently [30].

Effects of unilateral neck deafferentation on posture and postural adjustments accompanying limb movements

Postural changes

Since the work of the De Kleijn [18] and Magnus [45] it has been known that the proprioceptive input arising from neck receptors plays an important role in the control of posture and movements. However, in spite of the numerous attempts made in the past, the postural and motor deficits resulting from unilateral neck deafferentation in the cat have been specified only recently [46].

In particular, unilateral section of the cervical dorsal roots C1–C3 produced a postural asymmetry, characterized by ipsilateral hypertonia and contralateral hypotonia of the limb extensor muscles, a syndrome which was opposite in sign with respect to that elicited following unilateral section of the VIII nerve. In addition, the head of the animal was generally turned to the contralateral side and rotated about the naso-occipital axis, with the contralateral side down. The postural asymmetry of the limb musculature induced by unilateral neck deafferentation was reversed by section of the ipsilateral VIIIth nerve or ablation of the contralateral vermal cortex of the cerebellar anterior lobe.

The placing reactions were also affected by the

cervical radicotomy, with a transient loss of the proprioceptive placing reaction and a persistent deficit of the tactile placing reflex in the limbs ipsilateral to the side of the neck deafferentation. These effects were not reversed by the additional lesions described above.

Effects on postural adjustments

In order to analyse the effects of unilateral neck deafferentation on postural adjustments, the forelimb region of the motor cortex was stimulated in chronically implanted cats under the conditions described above. Cortical stimulation still induced both limb movement and the associated diagonal postural responses (Fig. 2A). However, several response parameters were modified [28,29].

Thresholds

The response threshold for flexion of the performing limb increased on the hypertonic side (ipsilateral to the cervical rhizotomy) and decreased on the hypotonic side. The tied coupling between movement and postural adjustments was confirmed by the fact that the changes in threshold of the performing limb were accompanied by parallel changes in threshold of the limbs involved in the postural adjustments.

Amplitudes and latencies

Latencies of force variations increased when the performing limb was ipsilateral to the hypertonic side, while the force variations themselves decreased in amplitude and speed. The opposite occurred when the performing limb was ipsilateral to the hypotonic side. Once again, these modifications affected the responses of the performing limb as well as those of the other three postural limbs (Fig. 2B).

Slopes of the response curves

The response curves relating the force variations to the stimulus strength applied to the motor cortex were calculated before and after the lesions. It was shown that the slope of the response curve of the moving limb as well as of the limbs involved in the postural adjustments decreased following stimulation of the motor cortex at different stimulus intensities if the performing limb was ipsilateral to the hypertonic side, but increased if the performing limb was ipsilateral to the hypotonic side (Fig. 3).

Effects of unilateral lesion of the lateral reticular nucleus on posture and postural adjustments accompanying limb movements

Postural changes

Unilateral lesion of the LRN produced a postural asymmetry, due to ipsilateral hypertonia and contralateral hypotonia of the limb extensor muscles. The lesion also elicited, in the ipsilateral limbs, a transient loss of the proprioceptive placing reaction and a persistent deficit of the tactile placing reflex. These postural and reflex changes were similar to those induced by unilateral neck deafferentation and were observed both after electrolytic destruction [15] and after kainic acid lesion of the LRN [59]. The effects may thus be attributed to selective destruction of lateral reticular neurons and not to damage of neighbouring or passage fibres.

Marked motor deficits appeared after the lesion. During the first days, the cats were unable to stand or walk. Later, they often fell while walking and, during standing, the contralateral limbs often sag under the weight of the body. This behaviour was attributed to the postural changes described above. It is of interest that the postural asymmetry characterized by an increased tonic contraction of the extensor muscles of the ipsilateral limbs and a decrease of the extensor tonus of the contralateral limbs was reversed by section of the ipsilateral VIIIth nerve, lesion of the ipsilateral Deiters' nucleus or ablation of the contralateral vermal cortex of the cerebellar anterior lobe. In these cases, interruption of the crossed vestibulocerebellar loop at different levels fully reversed the postural asymmetry produced by unilateral lesion of the LRN. These additional lesions did not reverse the effects on the proprioceptive placing reaction or the tactile placing reflex [15].

187

Effects on postural adjustments

The experimental procedure chosen for studying the effects of unilateral neck deafferentation described above, was also used to study the effects of unilateral lesion of the LRN on postural adjustments induced by cortical stimulation. In these experiments, the LRN was destroyed either by electrolytic lesion or by local injection of kainic acid. As in the pre-

vious experiments submitted to dorsal radicotomy, cortical stimulation still induced both limb movement and the associated diagonal postural pattern, but with modification of several response characteristics.

Thresholds

Evaluation of thresholds for forelimb flexion was made before and up to 3–8 weeks after the lesion

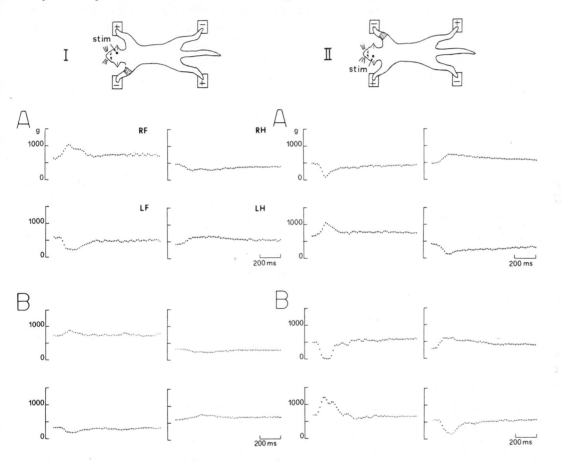

Fig.2. Averaged curves representing the weight shift occurring during movement of the left forelimb (I) or the right forelimb (II) elicited by stimulation of the corresponding region of the motor cortex before and after left-side neck deafferentation. On the ordinates the force is given in grams. LF, RF, left and right forelimb; LH, RH, left and right hindlimb. (A) Averaged samples of the force variations elicited by stimulating the forelimb region of the right (I) or left (II) motor cortex with 50 ms trains of 0.5 ms pulses at 200/s, 2.0 V or 1.2 V, respectively. The results were obtained 3 and 6 days, respectively, prior to the neck deafferentation. (B) Averaged samples of force variations elicited by stimulating the same regions of the motor cortex with the same parameters as above, but 7 and 8 days, respectively, after section of the left dorsal roots C1–C2. Note in I the great reduction in the weight change of the performing left forelimb made hypertonic by the unilateral neck deafferentation and the parallel decrease in force variations related to the postural adjustments in the remaining three limbs. On the other hand, in II there is a great increase in the weight change of the performing right forelimb made hypotonic by the unilateral neck deafferentation and a parallel increase in force variations accompanying the postural adjustments in the remaining three limbs. (Modified from [29].)

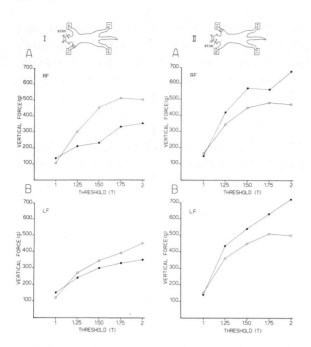

Fig.3. Slopes of the averaged curves showing the force variations in the forelimb elicited by stimulation of the forelimb region of the right (I) or left (II) motor cortex at increasing stimulus intensities, before and after left-side neck deafferentation. For experimental details see legend to Fig.2. The ordinates represent the absolute values of weight variations (increases or decreases) in grams, and the abscissae the stimulus intensities expressed in multiples of threshold for force variations (50 ms trains of 0.5 ms pulses at 200/s). Each point on the curve corresponds to the mean amplitude obtained by four stimuli applied at each of the four stimulus intensities used. LF, RF, left and right forelimb. (I) Response curves obtained 3 days before (○) and 7 days after (●) unilateral neck deafferentation. The slopes of the averaged response curves obtained by stimulating the forelimb region of the right motor cortex decreased to 76.0% and 68.0% of the control values in the left and the right forelimb, respectively, after section of the left dorsal roots C1–C2. (II) Response curves obtained 5 days before (○) and 8 days after (●) unilateral neck deafferentation. The slopes of the averaged curves obtained by stimulating the forelimb region of the left motor cortex increased to 127.0% and 144.0% of the control values in the left and right forelimb, respectively, after section of the left dorsal roots C1–C2. (Modified from [29].)

performed ipsilaterally to the side of cortical stimulation. In these instances, the threshold measurements involved the forelimb whose extensor tonus was reduced. There was a decrease in threshold of both limb flexion and associated postural responses

induced by motor cortex stimulation after the lesion, which corresponded on the average to 82% of the control value [55].

Slopes of the response curves

The response curves were calculated before and after lesion for cortical stimulations ipsilateral or contralateral to the lesioned side. By stimulating the right motor cortex, contralateral to the side of the LRN lesion, the slope decreased for the performing limb (left forelimb) as well as for the postural limbs. The opposite result was obtained when stimulating the left motor cortex; in this instance the slope of the response curve increased for the moving limb (right forelimb) as well as for the three other postural limbs.

Discussion

The experiments summarized in the present report have shown that the postural adjustments which accompany limb movements elicited by stimulation of the motor cortex can be affected either by unilateral section of dorsal cervical roots or by unilateral lesion of the LRN. In particular, the posturokinetic responses increased in amplitude when the performing limb was located on the hypotonic side, contralateral to either the neck deafferentation or the LRN lesion, but decreased in amplitude when the moving limb was located on the hypertonic side, i.e. ipsilateral to the lesions.

Since the LRN represents one of the main precerebellar structures which integrate both the labyrinth and neck inputs and, through the cerebellar vermis and Deiters' nucleus, intervene in the reflex control of posture during the vestibular and neck reflexes (see Introduction), we postulated that even the postural responses which accompany the limb movements induced by cortical stimulation utilize the same precerebellar and vestibular structures.

Let us examine first the evidence that the cortical influences on posture can be exerted through vestibulospinal neurons originating from Deiters' nucleus. It is known that stimulation of the motor cortex of the cat evokes responses from the cerebellar cortex which are somatotopically organized [1,33,62, 63]. These responses are at least in part mediated through mossy fibres [3,56]. Among the regions of the cerebellar cortex receiving these cortical projections there is also the zone B projecting to the LVN [13,65]. This finding may explain why a large proportion of LVN neurons, some of which are antidromically identified as vestibulospinal neurons, responded to electrical stimulation of the forelimb region of the contralateral motor cortex [42]; however, no response could be detected in Deiters' nucleus after partial cerebellectomy [31]. It therefore appears that motor cortical output is delivered to the LVN through a cerebellar loop (cf. [35]).

One of the precerebellar structures which can be influenced by cortical stimulation is the LRN, which receives descending fibres from the contralateral sensorimotor cortex, especially the anterior sigmoid gyrus [7,40,41,66], and projects mossy fibres to the cerebellum [11]. Cortical activation of LRN neurons has been attributed to collaterals of corticospinal fibres [8,67], but Alstermark and Lundberg [2] have shown that the LRN receives inputs from corticofugal neurons separate from corticospinal tract neurons. Independent of the modalities of this projection, it appears that the cortical fibres terminate in the magnocellular part of the LRN [7], i.e. in that area which induces postural deficits following lesion, thus being able to influence the ipsilateral vermal cortex of the cerebellar anterior lobe and then the Deiters' nucleus [15]. In addition to a direct projection to the LRN, the anterior sigmoid gyrus may also send an indirect projection to the LRN through the red nucleus (cf. [14]).

It is very likely that in our experiments stimulation of the forelimb region of the motor cortex increased the discharge of both the contralateral LRN and the Purkinje cells of the corresponding hemivermis, thus leading to inhibition of the underlying Deiters' nucleus. Since the latter structure exerts a direct excitatory influence on ipsilateral limb extensors, the postural activity in the corresponding limb would decrease, a finding which might facilitate the cortically induced flexion of the performing limb. The reduced discharge of this Deiters' nucleus would also decrease the neuronal activity of the crossed spinoreticulocerebellar pathway, thus decreasing the excitatory input to the contralateral hemivermis. The resulting disinhibition of the corresponding Deiters' nucleus would then lead to facilitation of the extensor motoneurons, which would increase the tonic contraction in the extensor muscle ipsilateral to the cortical stimulation. The main pathways involved in these mechanisms are schematically represented in Fig. 4.

The finding that the postural adjustments which occur in the hindlimbs following stimulation of the forelimb region of the motor cortex are opposite in sign with respect to those affecting the forelimbs can easily be understood if we consider the following:

(1) The cerebrocerebellar projections originating from the fore- and hindlimb area of the sensorimotor cortex are not sharply separate in the cerebellar vermis to occupy lobuli III, IV and V in a caudorostral orientation, but an organization can also be recognized in a laterolateral orientation. In particular, the fore- and hindlimb areas dominate in a medial and lateral longitudinal strip, respectively, extending in lobuli III, IV and V; moreover, prominent overlap exists between these narrow regions receiving projections from the fore- and hindlimb areas of the cerebral cortex [3,56]*.

(2) No clear correlation was seen within the LRN between the inputs from forelimb afferents and the forelimb sensorimotor cortex and from hindlimb afferents and the hindlimb sensorimotor cortex [58].

(3) Cortical stimulation may produce not only excitation but also inhibition in LRN neurons, a finding which does not necessarily depend on the pyramidal pathway [8,58].

(4) There are structural and functional bases for transforming an excitatory input to Purkinje cells

---

* A longitudinal pattern of projections from the LRN to the cerebellar cortex of the anterior lobe has been demonstrated autoradiographically [9,39].

190

of a given microzone into an inhibitory input on Purkinje cells of a neighbouring microzone [35].

It is likely that, in our experiments, unilateral neck deafferentation as well as unilateral lesion of the LRN produced a prominent unbalance in the

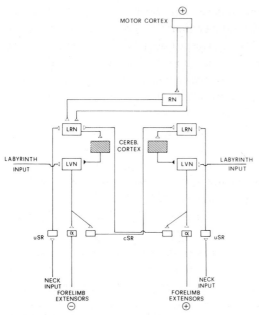

Fig.4. Anatomical pathways which are likely to be involved in posturokinetic responses after electrical stimulation of the forelimb region of the right motor cortex. Abbreviations: Cereb. cortex, vermal cortex of the cerebellum; LVN, lateral vestibular nucleus; LRN, lateral reticular nucleus; RN, red nucleus; cSR,uSR, crossed and uncrossed spinoreticular pathways; α, alpha motoneurons; △, excitatory synapses; ▲, inhibitory synapses. The decrease in vertical force elicited in the left forelimb (−) after stimulation of the forelimb region of the right motor cortex was probably due not only to activation of flexor motoneurons elicited by corticospinal and corticorubrospinal projections (not indicated in the figure) but also to activation of the forelimb region of the left LRN which, through a direct reticulocerebellar projection, inhibits the forelimb region of LVN, thus decreasing the extensor activity in the corresponding forelimb. On the other hand the increase in vertical force in the right forelimb (+) can be attributed to the reduced discharge of the left LVN, which produces disfacilitation not only of the ipsilateral forelimb extensor motoneurons but also of neurons of the cSR pathway, as well as of the forelimb region of the right LRN and the corresponding cerebellar cortex. The disinhibition of the right LVN would lead to an increase in vertical force in the corresponding forelimb. The reciprocal pattern of postural adjustments in the hindlimbs elicited by the same cortical stimulation can be attributed to several factors, as discussed in the text.

cerebellar and the vestibulospinal systems of both sides (cf. [15,46,59]), which was critically responsible not only for the postural asymmetry in the animal at rest, but also for the changes in amplitude of limb movements and of the accompanying postural adjustments induced by cortical stimulation.

In these instances a precise coordination was always observed between the limb movement occurring on the hypotonic or the hypertonic side and the accompanying postural responses: in particular an increase (or decrease) in amplitude of the performing limb flexion also induced an increase (or decrease) of the postural responses of the three other limbs. This tight coordination assumes a high level of integration and Deiters' nucleus represents a good candidate for such a role, due to both its connectivity and its involvement in several postural responses. It should be mentioned, however, that, in addition to the LRN, there are other precerebellar structures which can be involved not only in the postural reflex changes induced by labyrinth and neck stimulations, but also in the postural adjustments induced by cortical stimulation [55].

Further experiments are required in order to evaluate the role that Deiters' nucleus plays in the postural adjustments which accompany the limb flexion produced by motor cortex stimulation. This evidence cannot be obtained from lesion experiments (since unilateral destruction of the LVN results in dramatic impairment of posture), but rather by experiments of unit recording in which the discharge of well-identified LVN neurons projecting to different segments of the spinal cord could be monitored during motor cortex stimulation.

Acknowledgements

This study was supported by the NIH grant NS 07685-19 and a grant from the Ministero della Pubblica Istruzione, Roma, Italy.

References

[1] Adrian, E.D. (1943) Afferent areas in the cerebellum connected with the limbs. *Brain*, 66: 289–315.

[2] Alstermark, B. and Lundberg, A. (1982) Electrophysiological evidence against the hypothesis that corticospinal fibres

send collaterals to the lateral reticular nucleus. *Exp. Brain Res.*, 47: 148–150.

[3] Allen, G.I., Azzena, G.B. and Ohno, T. (1974) Somatotopically organized inputs from fore- and hindlimb areas of sensorimotor cortex to cerebellar Purkinje cells. *Exp. Brain Res.*, 20: 255–272.

[4] Boyle, R. and Pompeiano, O. (1980) Reciprocal responses to sinusoidal tilt of neurons in Deiters' nucleus and their dynamic characteristics. *Arch. Ital. Biol.*, 118: 1–32.

[5] Boyle, R. and Pompeiano, O. (1980) Responses of vestibulospinal neurons to sinusoidal rotation of neck. *J. Neurophysiol.*, 44: 633–649.

[6] Boyle, R. and Pompeiano, O. (1981) Convergence and interaction of neck and macular vestibular inputs on vestibulospinal neurons. *J. Neurophysiol.*, 45: 852–868.

[7] Brodal, P., Maršala, J. and Brodal, A. (1967) The cerebral cortical projection to the lateral reticular nucleus in the cat, with special reference to the sensorimotor cortical areas. *Brain Res.*, 6: 252–274.

[8] Bruckmoser, P., Hepp-Reymond, M.-C. and Wiesendanger, M. (1970) Cortical influence on single neurons of the lateral reticular nucleus of the cat. *Exp. Neurol.*, 26: 239–252.

[9] Chan-Palay, V., Palay, S.L., Brown, J.T. and Van Itallie, C. (1977) Sagittal organization of olivocerebellar and reticulocerebellar projections: autoradiographic studies with ^{35}S-methionine. *Exp. Brain Res.*, 30: 561–576.

[10] Clendenin, M., Ekerot, C.-F. and Oscarsson, O. (1974) The lateral reticular nucleus in the cat. III. Organization of component activated from ipsilateral forelimb tract. *Exp. Brain Res.*, 21: 501–513.

[11] Clendenin, M., Ekerot, C.-F., Oscarsson, O. and Rosén, I. (1974) The lateral reticular nucleus in the cat. I. Mossy fiber distribution in cerebellar cortex. *Exp. Brain Res.*, 21: 473–486.

[12] Clendenin, M., Ekerot, C.-F., Oscarsson, O. and Rosén, I. (1974) The lateral reticular nucleus in the cat. II. Organization of component activated from bilateral ventral flexor reflex tract (b VFRT). *Exp. Brain Res.*, 21: 487–500.

[13] Corvaja, N. and Pompeiano, O. (1979) Identification of cerebellar corticovestibular neurons retrogradely labeled with horseradish peroxidase. *Neuroscience*, 4: 507–515.

[14] Corvaja, N., Grofová, I., Pompeiano, O. and Walberg, F. (1977) The lateral reticular nucleus in the cat. I. An experimental anatomical study of its spinal and supraspinal afferent connections. *Neuroscience*, 2: 537–553.

[15] Corvaja, N., Grofová, I., Pompeiano, O. and Walberg, F. (1977) The lateral reticular nucleus in the cat. II. Effects of lateral reticular lesions on posture and reflex movements. *Neuroscience*, 2: 929–943.

[16] Coulmance, M., Gahery, Y., Massion, J. and Swett, J.E. (1979) The placing reaction in the standing cat: a model for the study of posture and movement. *Exp. Brain Res.*, 37: 265–281.

[17] Coulter, J.D., Mergner, T. and Pompeiano, O. (1976) Effects of static tilt on cervical spinoreticular tract neurons. *J. Neurophysiol.*, 39: 45–62.

[18] De Kleijn, A. (1920) Tonische Labyrinth-/und Halsreflexe auf die Augen. *Pflügers Arch.*, 186: 82–97.

[19] Denoth, F., Magherini, P.C., Pompeiano, O. and Stanojević, M. (1979) Responses of Purkinje cells of the cerebellar vermis to neck and macular vestibular inputs. *Pflügers Arch.*, 381: 87–98.

[20] Denoth, F., Magherini, P.C., Pompeiano, O. and Stanojević, M. (1980) Responses of Purkinje cells of cerebellar vermis to sinusoidal rotation of neck. *J. Neurophysiol.*, 43: 46–59.

[21] Ezure, K. and Wilson, V.J. (1983) Dynamics of neck-to-forelimb reflexes in the decerebrate cat. *J. Neurophysiol.*, 50: 688–695.

[22] Ezure, K. and Wilson, V.J. (1984) Interaction of tonic neck and vestibular reflexes in the forelimb of the decerebrate cat. *Exp. Brain Res.*, 54: 289–292.

[23] Gahery, Y. and Haour, R. (1981) Description and applications of a programmable stimulation system for electrophysiology, used as a computer peripheral. *Int. J. Bio-Med. Comput.*, 12: 109–123.

[24] Gahery, Y. and Massion, J. (1981) Co-ordination between posture and movement. *Trends Neurosci.*, 41: 199–202.

[25] Gahery, Y. and Nieoullon, A. (1974) Étude des reactions posturales accompagnant des mouvements provoquès par des stimulations corticales chez le chat. *J. Physiol., Paris*, 69: 250 A.

[26] Gahery, Y. and Nieoullon, A. (1978) Postural and kinetic co-ordination following cortical stimuli which induce flexion movements in the cat's limbs. *Brain Res.*, 149: 25–37.

[27] Gahery, Y., Ioffe, M.E., Massion, J. and Polit, A. (1980) The postural support of movement in cat and dog. *Acta Neurobiol. Exp.*, 40: 741–756.

[28] Gahery, Y., Pompeiano, O. and Coulmance, M. (1983) Effects of unilateral neck deafferentation on the posturo-kinetic limb responses following cortical stimulation in the cat. *Behav. Brain Res.*, 8: 247–248.

[29] Gahery, Y., Pompeiano, O. and Coulmance, M. (1984) Changes in posturo-kinetic limb responses to cortical stimulation following unilateral neck deafferentation in the cat. *Arch. Ital. Biol.*, 122: 129–154.

[30] Gahery, Y., Ioffe, M.E., Frolov, A.A. and Coulmance, M. (1985) Analysis of vertical displacements of the center of gravity in the cat during limb flexion induced by cortical stimulation. *J. Mot. Behav.*, 17: 463–479.

[31] Gildenberg, P.L. and Hassler, R. (1971) Influence of stimulation of the cerebral cortex on vestibular nuclei units in the cat. *Exp. Brain Res.*, 14: 77–94.

[32] Grillner, S., Hongo, T. and Lund, S. (1968) The origin of descending fibres monosynaptically activating spinoreticular neurones. *Brain Res.*, 10: 259–262.

[33] Hampson, J.L. (1949) Relationship between cat cerebral and cerebellar cortices. *J. Neurophysiol.*, 12: 37–50.

[34] Ioffe, M.E. and Andreyev, A.E. (1969) Inter-extremities co-

ordination in local motor conditioned reactions of dogs. *Zh. Vyssh. Nerv. Deyat. Pavlova*, 19: 557–565.

[35] Ito, M. (1984) *The Cerebellum and Neural Control*, Raven Press, New York, 580 pp.

[36] Kubin, L., Magherini, P.C., Manzoni, D. and Pompeiano, O. (1980) Responses of lateral reticular neurons to sinusoidal stimulation of labyrinth receptors in decerebrate cat. *J. Neurophysiol.*, 44: 922–936.

[37] Kubin, L., Magherini, P.C., Manzoni, D. and Pompeiano, O. (1981) Responses of lateral reticular neurons to sinusoidal rotation of neck in the decerebrate cat. *Neuroscience*, 6: 1277–1290.

[38] Kubin, L., Manzoni, D. and Pompeiano, O. (1981) Responses of lateral reticular neurons to convergent neck and macular vestibular inputs. *J. Neurophysiol.*, 46: 48–64.

[39] Künzle, H. (1975) Autoradiographic tracing of the cerebellar projections from the lateral reticular nucleus in the cat. *Exp. Brain Res.*, 22: 255–266.

[40] Künzle, H. and Wiesendanger, M. (1974) Pyramidal connections to the lateral reticular nucleus in the cat: a degeneration study. *Acta Anat.*, 88: 105–114.

[41] Kuypers, H.G.J.M. (1958) Anatomical analysis of corticobulbar connexions to the pons and lower brain stem in the cat. *J. Anat.*, 92: 198–218.

[42] Licata, F., Li Volsi, G., Maugeri, G. and Santangelo, F. (1986) Unitary responses to bilateral muscles and motor cortex stimulation in the lateral vestibular nucleus of the rat. *Neurosci. Lett. Suppl.*, 26: S548.

[43] Lindsay, K.W., Roberts, T.D.M. and Rosenberg, J.R. (1976) Asymmetric tonic labyrinth reflexes and their interaction with neck reflexes in the decerebrate cat. *J. Physiol. London*, 261: 583–601.

[44] Lund, S. and Pompeiano, O. (1968) Monosynaptic excitation of alpha-motoneurons from supraspinal structures in the cat. *Acta Physiol. Scand.*, 73: 1–21.

[45] Magnus, R. (1924) *Körperstellung*, Springer, Berlin, 740 pp.

[46] Manzoni, D., Pompeiano, O. and Stampacchia, G. (1979) Tonic cervical influences on posture and reflex movements. *Arch. Ital. Biol.*, 117: 81–110.

[47] Manzoni, D., Pompeiano, O., Srivastava, U.C. and Stampacchia, G. (1983) Responses of forelimb extensors to sinusoidal stimulation of macular labyrinth and neck receptors. *Arch. Ital. Biol.*, 121: 205–214.

[48] Marchand, A.R., Manzoni, D., Pompeiano, O. and Stampacchia, G. (1987) Effects of stimulation of vestibular and neck receptors on Deiters neurons projecting to the lumbosacral cord. *Pflügers Arch.*, 409: 13–23.

[49] Massion, J. and Gahery, Y. (1979) Diagonal stance in quadrupeds: a postural support for movement. In R. Granit and O. Pompeiano (Eds.), *Reflex Control of Posture and Movements, Progress in Brain Research, Vol.50*, Elsevier, Amsterdam, pp. 219–226.

[50] Massion, J. and Smith, A.M. (1974) Ventrolateral thalamic neurons related to posture during a modified placing reaction. *Brain Res.*, 71: 353–359.

[51] Massion, J., Swett, J.E., Coulmance, M. and Gahery, Y.

(1975) Postural adjustment associated with a placing movement. *Exp. Brain Res. Suppl.*, 23: 137.

[52] Polit, A. and Massion, J. (1979) Patterns of postural support during limb movement. *Soc. Neurosci. Abstr.*, 5: 382.

[53] Pompeiano, O. (1975) Vestibulo-spinal relationships. In R.F. Naunton (Ed.), *The Vestibular System*, Academic Press, New York, pp. 147–184.

[54] Pompeiano, O. (1981) Neck and macular labyrinth inputs on lateral reticular nucleus and their influences on posture. In O. Pompeiano and C.A. Marsan (Eds.), *Brain Mechanisms of Perceptual Awareness and Purposeful Behavior, IBRO Monograph Series, Vol. 8*, Raven Press, New York, pp. 233–260.

[55] Pompeiano, O., Gahery, Y. and d'Ascanio, P. (1983) Contribution of mossy fiber and climbing fiber pathways to the posturo-kinetic limb responses following cortical stimulation in the cat. *Behav. Brain Res.*, 8: 265–266.

[56] Provini, L., Redman, S. and Strata, P. (1968) Mossy and climbing fibre organization on the anterior lobe of the cerebellum activated by forelimb and hindlimb areas of the sensorimotor cortex. *Exp. Brain Res.*, 6: 216–233.

[57] Regis, H. and Trouche, E. (1974) Effet des ablations corticales et cérébelleuses sur la reaction de placement et l'ajustement postural. *J. Physiol. Paris*, 69: 289A–290A.

[58] Rosén, I. and Scheid, P. (1973) Responses to nerve stimulation in the bilateral ventral flexor reflex tract (bVFRT) of the cat. *Exp. Brain Res.*, 18: 256–267.

[59] Santarcangelo, E., Pompeiano, O. and Stampacchia, G. (1981) Effects of kainic acid lesions of lateral reticular nucleus in posture and reflex movements. *Arch. Ital. Biol.*, 119: 324–340.

[60] Schor, R.H. and Miller, A.D. (1981) Vestibular reflexes in neck and forelimb muscles evoked by roll tilt. *J. Neurophysiol.*, 46: 167–178.

[61] Schor, R.H. and Miller, A.D. (1982) Relationship of cat vestibular neurons to otolith-spinal reflexes. *Exp. Brain Res.*, 47: 137–144.

[62] Snider, R.S. and Eldred, E. (1948) Cerebral projections to the tactile, auditory and visual areas of the cerebellum. *Anat. Rec.*, 100: 714.

[63] Snider, R.S. and Eldred, E. (1951) Electro-anatomical studies on the cerebro-cerebellar connections in the cat. *J. Comp. Neurol.*, 95: 1–16.

[64] Stampacchia, G., Manzoni, D., Marchand, A.R. and Pompeiano, O. (1987) Convergence of neck and macular vestibular inputs on vestibulospinal neurons projecting to the lumbosacral segments of the spinal cord. *Arch. Ital. Biol.*, 125: 201–224.

[65] Voogd, J. (1964) *The Cerebellum of the Cat. Structure and Fibre Connections*, Van Gorcum, Assen, 215 pp.

[66] Walberg, F. (1958) Descending connections to the lateral reticular nucleus: an experimental study in the cat. *J. Comp. Neurol.*, 109: 363–389.

[67] Zangger, P. and Wiesendanger, M. (1973) Excitation of lateral reticular nucleus neurones by collaterals of the pyramidal tract. *Exp. Brain Res.*, 17: 144–151.

O. Pompeiano and J.H.J. Allum (Eds.)
Progress in Brain Research, Vol. 76
© 1988 Elsevier Science Publishers B.V. (Biomedical Division)

CHAPTER 17

Synergistic interactions and functional working range of the visual and vestibular systems in postural control: neuronal correlates

C. Xerri, L. Borel, J. Barthélémy and M. Lacour

Laboratoire de Psychophysiologie, Université de Provence, Centre de Saint-Jérôme, Rue H. Poincaré, 13397 Marseille CEDEX 13, France

Comparisons between experimental data on visual-vestibular convergences at the neural, motor and perceptual levels yield the following conclusions: (1) synergistic interactions between congruent visual and vestibular signals improve velocity coding during low-frequency and steady-state body motion; (2) visual signals generally predominate over vestibular signals in the low frequency range, while the contrary applies in the higher frequency range of movement; (3) visual and vestibular inputs might be weighted depending on their internal relevance. These common interaction characteristics suggest that visual and vestibular modulation of activity in vestibular neurons might constitute at least part of the neurophysiological substrate for visual-vestibular cooperation in postural regulation and self-motion perception. In fact, it is well known that the vestibular nuclei are involved in motor control through vestibulospinal influences [22,26,34]. Nevertheless visual-vestibular convergences have been found to occur in numerous nervous structures such as the superior colliculus [8], the cerebellum [21,33], and the primary visual cortex [24,29] as well as in the vestibular cortical area [12]. Systematic investigations on the way the two modalities interact in these structures would help to determine whether the complex interactions described in this review actually take place within the vestibular nuclei or are simply reflected there after being integrated in other nervous structures.

Introduction

Integration of plurimodal information within the CNS results in multiloop control of sensory-motor activities. A tight functional coupling has long been known to exist between the visual and vestibular systems which contribute to motion perception, oculomotor and postural control.

The apparent redundance of visual and vestibular signals co-activating the two sensory-motor systems enables the CNS to remove the ambiguity inherent to each modality. In fact, the vestibular receptors lack sustained information about constant velocity and provide the same neural message whether acceleration or deceleration occur in one direction or the opposite direction, and visual cues are equivocal as to whether self or object motion is taking place.

Visual and vestibular information converge onto central nervous structures where they are integrated. This integration might be used to build up internal reference systems for spatial orientation and postural balance. These structures therefore constitute favourable neuronal networks for studying the mechanisms underlying functional cooperations between the visual and vestibular systems.

Abbreviations: CNS, central nervous system; EMG, electromyograph; NPH, nucleus prepositus hypoglossi; NRTP, nucleus reticularis tegmenti ponti; Pt, pretectum; VN, vestibular nucleus.

The purpose of this report is to review some findings on visual–vestibular integration at the neuronal level. We shall consider here only unit activity recorded within the vestibular nuclei, which are a major site of visual–vestibular convergence. Some results of our recent investigations on visual-otolith interactions in the vestibular nuclei of the alert cat will be presented together with relevant data on EMG responses developed in extensor muscles. The main current hypothesis based on single unit studies will be discussed within the general frame of visual–vestibular functional cooperation in motion perception and postural control. The nature (retinal or extraretinal) of the visual signals activating vestibular neurons will not be discussed in the present report. This matter has been dealt with elsewhere in a recent paper [4].

Synergistic interactions between visual and vestibular motion cues

Visual–vestibular interactions within the vestibular nuclei have been described in many species: the goldfish [1,19], the rat [13,25], the rabbit [30], the cat [5,17], and the monkey [23,47]. These studies have shown that a direction-specific modulation of unit resting discharge is evoked by the movement of a large visual field. Another common finding was that most vestibular neurons respond synergistically to motion of the head and surround in opposite directions, i.e. to vestibular and visual inputs. Moreover, vestibular neurons have been found to respond with a sustained discharge to constant-velocity head rotation in the presence of a stationary visual surround. This noteworthy result supports the assumption that visual information enables the vestibular system to monitor constant velocity. It has also been demonstrated that visual input abolishes the phase lead (with respect to head velocity) characteristic of vestibular responses to low-frequency rotation [23,27].

It is somewhat surprising that visual–vestibular interactions in central neurons have been analysed almost exclusively during rotations which activate the semicircular canals. Since canal inputs are mainly used to regulate high-frequency body movement while otolith and visual inputs have a stronger stabilizing effect in the low frequency range [40,42], one realizes at this stage that important data on visual–vestibular interactions are lacking. However, some experiments performed on the paralysed cat [17] and rat [25] have shown that otolith-dependent units within the vestibular nuclei are also activated by linear acceleration of the animal and a large visual stimuli in opposite directions.

An experimental paradigm was designed to record in the alert cat the extracellular activity of vestibular nuclei neurons during separate or combined visual and otolith stimulation (Fig. 1A). The results reported here concern sinusoidal movement of the animal and/or visual surround in the vertical plane. The great majority of neuronal responses were found to encode the velocity of the animal motion (71% of the units) or the velocity of the visual surround motion (89% of the units). Fig. 1B illustrates a typical unit exhibiting consistent responses, i.e. the neuron was excited by movement of the visual surround in the direction opposite to that which provided excitation during otolith stimulation. This synergistic interaction can be further specified by comparing the phase and sensitivity of vestibular neurons recorded during movement of the animal in the dark (otolith input) and in the light in front of a fixed visual pattern (visual + otolith inputs). As shown in Fig. 1C, the mean phase (Φ) of the unit response was much less scattered around the peak of motion velocity (0°) when both sensory modalities were available (otolith response: $\Phi = -0.7 \pm 40.1°$; visual + otolith response: $\Phi = -4.9 \pm 16.8°$): the dispersion of the phase angle distribution was significantly less during visual + otolith stimulation (t-test, $p < 0.01$). Moreover, in most units the response sensitivity (percentage increase in mean firing rate per cm/s) was strongly enhanced from $5.7 \pm 4\%$/cm/s to $10.8 \pm 7\%$/cm/s ($p < 0.001$) when visual input was combined with otolith input. It therefore emerges that the existence of synergistic interactions between visual and vestibular signals is now firmly established in the case of vestibular neurons excited during rotation as well as translation.

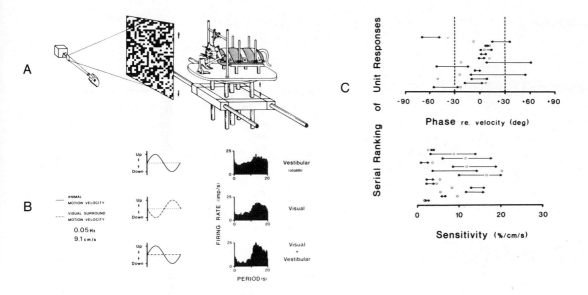

Fig. 1. Synergistic responses of vestibular nuclei neurons to visual and otolith motion cues. (A) Experimental set-up. Otolith receptors were stimulated by subjecting the animal to sinusoidal linear motion in the vertical plane, in total darkness. Visual (optokinetic) stimulation consisted of sinusoidally moving a black-and-white pseudorandom pattern in front of the stationary animal. Combined visual–otolith stimulation was obtained by moving the animal in front of the stationary visual surround. Visual stabilization was obtained by shifting the animal vertically together with the fixed visual surround. (B) Sequential histograms (average of 8 sweeps, 64 bins) illustrating synergistic integration of visual and otolith inputs in a typical neuron. Abscissa, period of the stimulus cycle (s); ordinate, firing rate (imp./s). The unit can be seen to have encoded velocity of the animal and visual surround. (C) Phase and sensitivity of response of 13 units to otolith (●), visual (○) and combined visual–otolith (▶) stimulation at 0.05 Hz. The magnitude of change in units response induced by a co-activation of visual and otolith receptors is given by the length of the horizontal bar. The unit response sensitivity was enhanced and the phase was shifted towards the peak of motion velocity (0°) when both inputs were combined. (Modified from [49].)

This basic feature of visual–vestibular convergences corroborates the findings reported by Thoden et al. [46], who observed an opposite direction-specific modulation of monosynaptic reflexes in cat limbs depending on whether optokinetic or vestibular stimuli (animal tilt) were used.

Our study on visual-otolith interactions confirms the results obtained during angular [1,19,47] as well as linear movement [17,25]: addition of a congruent visual input leads to an increase in the gain of unit response over that depending on purely vestibular stimulation, at least with low-frequency stimuli. Furthermore Daunton et al. [17] have also reported that in the cat visual input induces a phase shift of vestibular responses towards motion velocity. This indicates that a basic characteristic of vestibular nuclei neurons is their ability to process visual and

vestibular signals in order to yield more accurate velocity information. In another set of experiments we attempted to establish whether this notion also applies to the elaboration of motor responses. For this purpose, we examined the contribution of dynamic visual input to the EMG response of extensor neck muscle (splenius) stimulated under the same conditions as in the unit recordings. A modulation of the EMG responses during purely visual stimulation was sometimes observed below the 0.25 Hz stimulus frequency which did not lead to otolith-dependent muscle response. However, the influence of visual motion cues on neck muscle activity was clearly shown by comparing the responses evoked during otolith stimulation to those obtained during visual + otolith stimulation. The results shown in Fig. 2 indicate that muscle responses in-

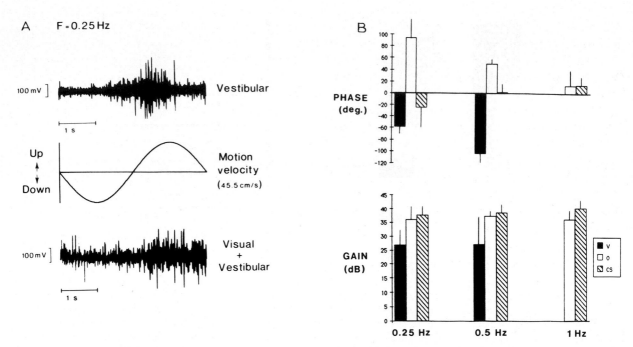

Fig. 2. Dynamic characteristics of neck muscle responses evoked during otolith and visual + otolith stimulation. (A) Modulation of EMG activity. Raw EMG response recorded from the splenius capitis muscle (single passage) during vestibular (animal movement in the dark) and visual + vestibular stimulation (animal movement in front of the stationary visual surround) at a frequency of 0.25 Hz. (B) Histograms showing the changes in the phase (degrees) and gain (dB) of EMG responses with respect to motion velocity at the 0.25, 0.50 and 1 Hz stimulus frequency. Values are the means of those recorded from left and right splenius muscles in 4 cats. The vertical lines represent the confidence intervals calculated at $p < 0.05$. Comparison between the phase values obtained during oto-lith (0) and visual + otolith stimulation (CS) shows that a phase shift towards motion velocity (0°) occurred when both inputs were available. (Modified from [9].)

duced by otolith stimulation were roughly in phase with downwards acceleration at 0.25 Hz, and displayed a phase lag of about −40° at 0.50 Hz and −80° at 1 Hz. The phase of responses evoked during costimulation was close to downward motion velocity over the whole frequency range studied. The phase shift from acceleration related to velocity related responses was the most prominent at 0.25 Hz (120° on the average). The amplitude of the oto-lith-dependent EMG modulation increased as a function of the input frequency, with a multiplying factor of about 5 through the frequency range tested. The gain of response was calculated with respect to velocity: the histograms show constant gain values from 0.25 Hz to 1 Hz. The gain evaluated during visual-otolith costimulation was comparable to that obtained during otolith stimulation,

indicating that the dynamic visual input did not significantly modify the amplitude of EMG responses, at least at motion frequencies higher than 0.25 Hz. The main influence of visual cues therefore seems to be confined to the splenius muscle response input-output phase relationship during vertical translation.

Interestingly, many studies support the idea that the velocity signal is the most significant kinematic parameter in the control of slow postural sway. For instance, body pitch can be induced by sinusoidal linear [32] or circular [38] movement of a visual scene. Both amplitude and phase of body pitch are related to the velocity of the visual surround up to 0.10 Hz. Furthermore, magnitude estimates of the subjective sensation of self-motion (vection) elicited by visual surrounds moving linearly are also related to stimulus velocity up to 0.10 Hz in the horizontal [6] as well as the vertical direction [7].

Functional working range of the visual and vestibular systems

One may consider that the conditions for optimal visual–vestibular cooperation are fulfilled, since each of the two sensory-motor systems has its own functional working range. The authors of all the studies dealing with visual–vestibular interactions at the neuronal level have used either trapezoidal- or sinusoidal-velocity stimuli; in the latter case a single stimulus frequency was tested, so that the opportunity of analysing the dynamic properties of these multisensory interactions in the frequency domain was missed. We therefore attempted to describe the frequency-dependent behaviour of vestibular nuclei neurons during separate and combined visual and otolith stimulation. Bode diagrams illustrating the dynamic unit responses within the 0.05–0.50 Hz decade (corresponding range of peak velocity: 0.09–0.91 m/s) are shown in Fig.3. The time course of discharge modulation is also presented so as to better visualize the magnitude of the changes in unit response. As a general rule, visual stimulation evoked significantly higher discharge modulation and response gain than otolith stimulation in the low frequency range ($\leqslant 0.25$ Hz), while the opposite was observed at frequences higher than 0.25 Hz (Fig. 3A,B). As far as phase was concerned, vestibular neurons encoded animal as well as visual-surround motion velocity and exhibited consistent responses in the 0.05–0.10 Hz frequency range. Above 0.10 Hz, otolith-dependent responses were characterized by a marked phase lead of about 100° at 0.25 Hz and 0.50 Hz, whereas visual-dependent responses displayed a phase lag above 0.25 Hz (about $-50°$ at 0.50 Hz) (Fig. 3C,D). Since the visual and otolith responses were out of phase from 0.10 Hz (about 130° at 0.25 Hz and 150° at 0.50 Hz), the two sensory systems did not encode the same kinematic parameters of motion in the higher frequency range.

Interestingly, the unit response parameters measured during combined visual-otolith stimulation were comparable to those obtained during visual stimulation, but differed significantly from the values recorded during otolith stimulation in the 0.05–0.25 Hz frequency range. On the contrary, the unit responses recorded during visual + otolith stimulation reached similar values to the 'vestibular curves' above the critical 0.25 Hz frequency. In a few cells we were able to study the effect of visual stabilization (animal and visual surround moving in phase, at the same velocity) as a function of the stimulus frequency. In this experiment, the otolith system was assumed to signal that the animal was moving while the visual system was assumed to indicate that the animal was stationary. As a rule, exclusion of visual motion cues induced a strong reduction in the amplitude of unit response: the lower the motion frequency, the more pronounced the attenuation. On comparing unit sensitivity in visual + otolith and visual stabilization conditions, the mean reduction was found to be about 80% at 0.05 Hz and 35% at 0.50 Hz (Fig.4).

It was proposed to correlate the neuronal events reported above with some characteristics of functional motor responses previously described in neck (splenius) and leg (soleus) extensor muscles in monkeys subjected to free fall [31]. The animal was unexpectedly dropped in front of a stationary (visual + otolith stimulation) or stabilized visual surround (suppression of visual motion cues) at various maximum accelerations (2.2 m/s² to 8.8 m/s²). As a rule, total exclusion of visual motion cues induced a powerful reduction in the muscular energy developed in both splenius and soleus muscles during the free fall. It is worth noting that the lower the fall acceleration, the stronger the reduction (Fig. 5). Moreover, the latency of muscle responses was increased during visual stabilization, and this effect was more pronounced at the lowest acceleration (2.2 m/s²). These results indicate that the dynamic contribution of visual motion cues to muscular responses is greater with slow falls than with rapid falls.

Neuronal as well as EMG data indicate that the visual and vestibular information can be combined

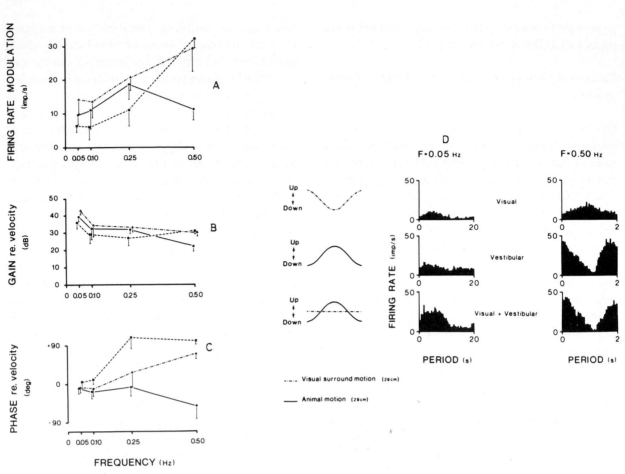

Fig. 3. Frequency-response curves of vestibular nuclei neurons to visual (●), otolith (■) and combined visual–otolith (▲) inputs. Amplitude of unit discharge modulation (A), gain (B) and phase (C) with respect to motion velocity (ordinates) in 13 units in the 0.05–0.50 Hz decade (abscissa) at a fixed 290 mm peak to peak amplitude (corresponding range of peak velocity: 0.09 to 0.91 m/s). Mean values and corresponding confidence limits at $p < 0.05$ (verticals bars) are given. Of the 13 units averaged, 9 were excited during downward visual and upward animal movement while 4 units were excited during upward visual and downward animal movement in the low frequency range. The phase angle of the response is expressed in degrees of phase lead (positive values) or lag (negative values) with respect to the peak velocity (0°) of the excitatory direction of motion at 0.05 Hz. Note that visual- and otolith-dependent responses were consistent up to 0.10 Hz but 120–150° out of phase above 0.10 Hz. During visual + otolith stimulation, the visual input predominated over the otolith input up to 0.25 Hz, while the opposite was observed as from 0.25 Hz. (D) Sequential histograms illustrating the responses of an individual neuron under the three experimental conditions, at the 0.05 and 0.50 Hz stimulus frequencies. (Modified from [49].)

so that the working range of vestibular neurons is extended. We observed that the sensitivity of the neuronal response to visual input was greater than that of otolith input in the low frequency range of linear motion, while the opposite was the case in the higher frequency range. Moreover, during visual stabilization, both unit sensitivity and EMG modu-

lation were reduced: the lower the frequency, the more pronounced the effect. These findings are in agreement with the well-known functional separation into low-frequency visual and high-frequency vestibular dominance which characterizes postural control. For instance, low-frequency postural oscillations with the eyes open have been reported as oc-

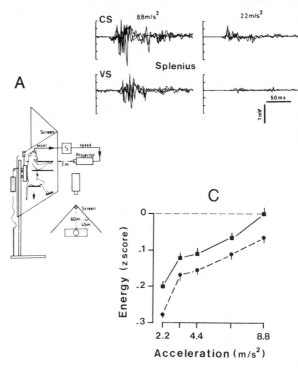

Fig. 4. Effect of the suppression of visual motion cues on the response of vestibular nuclei neurons. (A) Sequential histograms (64 bins) recorded at the frequencies of 0.05 and 0.50 Hz, showing that visual surround stabilization decreased the amplitude of unit response as compared to the normal visual–otolith interaction. (B) Mean response sensitivity of three units recorded during visual (V), otolith (O), combined visual + otolith (C) stimulation, and visual stabilization (VS). The values are expressed as a percentage of the sensivity measured during otolith stimulation. Note that the effect of VS was more pronounced at the lowest motion frequency (mean reduction of 80% and 35% at 0.05 Hz and 0.50 Hz, respectively). It is noteworthy that VS also decreased the otolith-dependent component of unit response. (Modified from [49].)

Fig. 5. Effect of the suppression of visual motion cues on muscle response to free fall. (A) Experimental set-up. A projector, the input of which consisted of the integral of vertical acceleration, and the output of which commanded the film motion, projected a black and white random pattern onto a V-shaped screen placed in front of the baboon. EMG activities were recorded during different accelerations of fall (8.8, 6.6, 4.4, 3.3, and 2.2 m/s^2) and with 2 visual surrounds: the visual scene either remained stationary on the screen (normal visual–vestibular costimulation: CS) or was moved downward at a velocity equal to that of the falling monkey (visual stabilization: VS). (B) EMG of the early response of splenius capitis muscle during falling at different accelerations under the two visual-surround conditions. Records consist of three superimposed raw EMG for three consecutive falls. (C) Energy of the early EMG responses to falling recorded from splenius muscle. Mean values obtained in three normal baboons are expressed as the Z score relative to the energy recorded at 8.8 m/s^2 with normal vision (values normalized to zero). Abscissa, amplitude of fall acceleration; ordinates, energy of the response in Z score; EMG activities are recorded during falls with normal vision (■), and with visual stabilization (●). Each point is given with its 1% confidence interval. Note the decrease in EMG responses as acceleration decreased and when the visual surround was stabilized. The lower the fall acceleration the greater the reduction in visual-stabilization condition. (Modified from [31].)

curring 50% less than with the eyes closed, in man [20] and dog [45]. The dynamic effect of vision on low-frequency perturbation of posture has also been demonstrated in subjects standing in front of a visual surround moving in a sinusoidal linear or circular manner. The postural instability was maximum in the 0.10 Hz to 0.30 Hz range of stimulus frequencies [32,39]. From experiments dealing with reflex responses to fore-aft platform displacement in normal and defective labyrinth subjects, Nashner [42] reached the conclusion that in the normal subject postural sway regulation is achieved by means of a combination of high-frequency (semicircular canals and somatosensory receptors) and low-frequency (otoliths and visual receptors) stabilization. We have shown that during low-frequency movements a distinction can still be made between the working range of otolith and visual channels. Nevertheless it would be an oversimplification to rule out the possibility that vision can intervene in transient postural adjustments [7,31] as well as high-frequency postural stabilization [2].

It is well known that vestibular nuclei are responsible for reflexes operating through vestibulospinal pathways [22,26,34]. Therefore, visual modulation of activity in vestibular nuclei neurons might form part of the neurophysiological substrate for visual and vestibular influences on postural regulation. In this respect, it seems likely that the neuronal population investigated in our study contributes to dynamic postural control rather than to gaze stabilization during linear motion by means of the vestibulo-ocular reflex. Indeed, no compensatory eye movement was elicited during vertical linear motion in the dark, at least within the frequency range studied, whereas this motion clearly induced a modulation of vestibular unit activity. Moreover, most of the neurons investigated were located in the lateral vestibular nucleus, which mainly projects to the spinal cord [10].

Modes of visual–vestibular integration in central vestibular neurons

Several attempts have been made to provide heuristic models of how visual and vestibular inputs interact. The mathematical analysis and modelling of these interactions has not yet been completed. The results of earlier investigations suggested that a nonlinear transformation of visual and vestibular signals may take place in the goldfish [19] and monkey [23]. However, according to Allum et al. [1], in the goldfish vestibular unit responses during rotation in the light can be described as an approximately linear combination of vestibular and optokinetic signals. Waespe and Henn [47], have shown in the monkey that the firing rate modulation of canal-related neurons was entirely dominated by the vestibular input during transient rotation whereas the response was entirely determined by the visual input during the period of constant velocity. They concluded that visual and vestibular signals were combined in a nonlinear fashion and proposed that a switching mechanism of interaction might be involved. Assuming a positive eye velocity feedback, Robinson [44] postulated that the activity in vestibular nuclei units during rotation in the dark is not identical to the activity which summates with the visual signal during rotation in the light. This author, without excluding some minor nonlinearity, has elaborated a theoretical model of interaction showing that a linear addition of vestibular and optokinetic signals might account for the responses obtained by Waespe and Henn. Contradictory conclusions seem to emerge from the studies cited above, but one cannot rule out the possibility that different modes of interaction may in fact co-exist in the same central nervous structure.

In our own study, we have provided the first description of visual-otolith interactions in a wide range of motion frequencies. This analysis enables us to better understand how visual and vestibular inputs converge, and how these signals are transformed into individual units. We found that both the gain and phase of unit responses recorded during combined stimulation were close, although not strictly equal (as suggested in the switching hypothesis), to the values determined by the dominant input (visual below 0.25 Hz, otolith above 0.25 Hz). These results point to the existence of a hierarchical type of convergence and support the hypothesis that a weighted summation of visual and vestibular inputs occurs. Besides this mode of interaction, a linear mode, i.e. an algebraic summation of the visual and otolith inputs, was encountered in some units [49]. Furthermore, when the visual system detected no relative movement between the animal and the environment (visual stabilization), the vestibular activity was much more attenuated than was to be expected on the basis of the otolith-dependent response (cf. Fig.4). This finding, which is comparable to that obtained by Waespe and Henn [48], suggests that the weighting process takes into account the degree of congruence between converging inputs. Visual stabilization was found to have stronger effects within the low frequency range of the movement. This can be explained by assuming that the CNS relies on the dominant, heavily weighted information, i.e. visual cues at low velocity and vestibular cues at high movement velocity. Interestingly, our study provides a neurophysiological counterpart to the nonlinear conflict model of motion perception elaborated by Young [50] and perfected by Zacharias and Young [51]. According to this mathematical model of visual-vestibular conflict, the weighting of the inputs is a function of the degree of consistency among the motion cues. The way in which visual and vestibular cues are combined more generally suggests that each source of information is evaluated in the CNS on the basis of the internal relevance of various covariant inputs to the environmental context.

Anatomical pathways relaying visual information to vestibular nuclei

Several pathways along which visual information reaches the VN have been identified. These pathways seem to be polysynaptic in view of the long latencies in the neuronal discharge modulation as well as in the induction of self-motion perception. Maekawa and Simpson [35,36] discovered a retino–pretecto–olivo–cerebello–vestibular circuit which is thought to be probably involved in the transmission of visual signals to the VN. The existence of other retinocerebellar pathways has been demonstrated [10,41]. Since the integrity of the cerebellum is not a prerequisite for the visually induced modulation of VN activity [28], other pathways and relays must be involved. Cazin et al. [14] and Precht and Strata [43] have shown, in the cat, that the

NRTP, which receives afferents from the Pt, conveys visual information to the VN. In fact, the integrity of the Pt, which receives direct retinal projections, is a prerequisite for optokinetic responses to be obtained in the VN; lesions of the NRTP also abolish these responses in the rat and cat. Furthermore, the response properties of these two structures are practically identical to those described in the VN. Cazin et al. [15], Magnin et al. [37], and Cazin et al. [16] have shown, using both autoradiographic and electrophysiological techniques, that the Pt→NPH→VN and/or Pt→NRTP→NPH→VN pathways are probably responsible for the optokinetic modulation of vestibular neurons.

Acknowledgements

This study was supported by U.A. C.N.R.S. 372, and grants from INSERM (No. 866011) and Ministère de la Recherche et de la Technologie (84.C.1311). The authors wish to thank Mrs M.R. Ibrahim for typing the manuscript, L. Agate for preparing the illustrations, and L. Bakalian and J.P. Roman for their technical assistance.

References

[1] Allum, J.H.J., Graf, W., Dichgans, J. and Schmidt, C.L. (1976) Visual-vestibular interactions in the vestibular nuclei of the goldfish. *Exp. Brain Res.*, 26: 463–485.

[2] Amblard, B. and Cremieux, J. (1976) Role of visual motion information in the maintenance of postural equilibrium in man. *Agressologie*, 17C: 25–36.

[3] Ansorge, K. and Grüsser-Cornehls, U. (1977) Visual and visual–vestibular responses of frog cerebellar neurons. *Exp. Brain Res.*, 29: 445–465.

[4] Barthélémy, J., Xerri, C., Borel, L. and Lacour, M. (1988) Neuronal coding of linear motion in the vestibular nuclei of the alert cat. II. Response characteristics to vertical visual stimulation. *Exp. Brain Res.*, in press.

[5] Bauer, R. and Hoffman, K.P. (1980) Responses of vestibular nucleus neurons in the visually deprived cat to optokinetic stimulation of central parts of the visual field. *Neurosci. Lett.*, 17: 237–241.

[6] Berthoz, A., Pavard, B. and Young, L.R. (1975) Perception of linear horizontal self motion induced by peripheral vision (linear-vection). Basic characteristics and visual–vestibular interactions. *Exp. Brain Res.*, 23: 471–489.

[7] Berthoz, A., Lacour, M., Soechting, J.F. and Vidal, P.P. (1979) The role of vision in the control of posture during linear motion. In R. Granit and O. Pompeiano (Eds.), *Re-*

flex Control of Posture and Movement, Progress in Brain Research, Vol. 50, Elsevier, Amsterdam, pp. 197–209.

[8] Bisti, S., Maffei, I. and Piccolino, L. (1974) Visuo-vestibular interactions in the cat superior colliculus. *J. Neurophysiol.,* 22: 146–155.

[9] Borel, L., Lacour, M. and Xerri, C. (1988) Response dynamics of the splenius neck muscle during vertical visual–otolith interactions. *Exp. Brain Res.,* in press.

[10] Brecha, N., Karten, H.J. and Hunt, S.P. (1980) Projections of the nucleus of the basal optic root in the pigeon: an autoradiographic and horseradish peroxidase study. *J. Comp. Neurol.,* 189: 615–670.

[11] Brodal, A., Pompeiano, O. and Walberg, F. (1962) *The Vestibular Nuclei and their Connections. Anatomical and Functional Correlations,* Oliver and Boyd, London, 193 pp.

[12] Büttner, U. and Büttner, U.W. (1978) Parietal cortex (2v) neuronal activity in the alert monkey during natural vestibular and optokinetic stimulation. *Brain Res.,* 153: 392–397.

[13] Cazin, L., Precht, W. and Lannou, J. (1980) Optokinetic responses of vestibular nucleus neurons in the rat. *Pflüger's Arch.,* 384: 31–38.

[14] Cazin, L., Precht, W. and Lannou, J. (1980) Firing characteristics of neurons mediating optokinetic responses to rat's vestibular neurons. *Pflüger's Arch.,* 386: 221–230.

[15] Cazin, L., Magnin, M. and Lannou, J. (1982) Non-cerebellar visual afferents to the vestibular nuclei involving the prepositus hypoglossal complex: an autoradiographic study in the rat. *Exp. Brain Res.,* 48: 309–313.

[16] Cazin, L., Lannou, J. and Precht, W. (1984) An electrophysiological study of pathways mediating optokinetic responses to the vestibular nucleus in the rat. *Exp. Brain Res.,* 54: 337–348.

[17] Daunton, N. and Thomsen, D. (1979) Visual modulation of otolith-dependent units in cat vestibular nuclei. *Exp. Brain Res.,* 37: 173–176.

[18] Daunton, N., Christensen, C. and Thomsen, D. (1981) Visual modulation of otolith responses: a paradigm for the study of self-motion perception and its neural substrate. In T. Gualtierotti (Ed.), *The Vestibular System: Function and Morphology,* Springer-Verlag, New York/Heidelberg/Berlin, pp. 452–462.

[19] Dichgans, J., Schmidt, C.L. and Graf, W. (1973) Visual input improves the speedometer function of the vestibular nuclei in the goldfish. *Exp. Brain Res.,* 18: 319–322.

[20] Edwards, A.S. (1946) Body sway and vision. *J. Exp. Psychol.,* 36: 526–535.

[21] Ghelarducci, B., Ito, M. and Yagi, N. (1975) Impulse discharges from flocculus cells of alert rabbits during visual stimulation combined with horizontal head rotation. *Brain Res.,* 87: 66–72.

[22] Grillner, S., Hongo, T. and Hund, S. (1970) The vestibulospinal tract. Effects on alpha motoneurons in the lumbosacral spinal cord in the cat. *Exp. Brain Res.,* 10: 94–120.

[23] Henn, V., Young, L.R. and Finley, C. (1974) Vestibular nucleus units in alert monkeys are also influenced by moving visual fields. *Brain Res.,* 71: 144–149.

[24] Horn, G. and Hill, R.M. (1969) Modifications of receptive fields of cells in the visual cortex occurring spontaneously and associated with body tilt. *Nature,* 221: 186–188.

[25] Horn, K.M., Miller, S.W. and Neilson, H.C. (1983) Visual modulation of neuronal activity within the rat vestibular nuclei. *Exp. Brain Res.,* 52: 311–313.

[26] Kato, M. and Tanji, J. (1971) The effects of electrical stimulation of Deiters' nucleus upon hindlimb γ-motoneurons in the cat. *Brain Res.,* 30: 385–395.

[27] Keller, E.L. and Daniels, P. (1975) Oculomotor related interaction of vestibular and visual stimulation in vestibular nucleus cells in alert monkey. *Exp. Neurol.,* 46: 187–198.

[28] Keller, E.L. and Precht, W. (1979) Visual-vestibular responses in vestibular nuclear neurons in the intact and cerebellectomized alert cat. *Neuroscience,* 4: 1599–1613.

[29] Kornhuber, H.H. and Da Fonseca, J.S. (1964) Optovestibular integration in the cat's cortex: a study of sensory convergence on cortical neurons. In B. Bender (Ed.), *The Oculomotor System,* Hoeber, New York, pp. 239–279.

[30] Kubo, T., Matsunaga, T. and Igarashi, M. (1979) Vestibular unitary responses to visual stimulation in the rabbit. *Acta Otolaryngol. Stockholm,* 88: 117–121.

[31] Lacour, M., Vidal, P.P. and Xerri, C. (1983) Dynamics of visual and vestibular control of rapid postural adjustments. In J.E. Desmedt (Ed.), *Motor Control Mechanisms in Man: Electrophysiological Methods and Clinical Applications,* Raven Press, New York, pp. 589–605.

[32] Lestienne, F., Soechting, J.F. and Berthoz, A. (1977) Postural readjustments induced by linear motion of visual scenes. *Exp. Brain Res.,* 28: 363–384.

[33] Lisberger, S.G. and Fuchs, A.F. (1974) Response of flocculus Purkinje cells to adequate vestibular stimulation in the alert monkey: fixation vs. compensatory eye movements. *Brain Res.,* 69: 347–353.

[34] Lund, S. and Pompeiano, O. (1968) Monosynaptic excitation of alpha motoneurons from supra-spinal structures in the cat. *Acta Physiol. Scand.,* 73: 1–21.

[35] Maekawa, K.E. and Simpson, J.I. (1972) Climbing fiber activation of Purkinje cells in the flocculus by impulses transferred through the visual pathways. *Brain Res.,* 39: 245–251.

[36] Maekawa, K.E. and Simpson, J.I. (1973) Climbing fiber responses evoked in the vestibulo-cerebellum of rabbit from visual system. *J. Neurophysiol.,* 36: 649–666.

[37] Magnin, M., Courjon, J.H. and Flandrin, J.M. (1983) Possible visual pathways to the cat vestibular nuclei involving the nucleus prepositus hypoglossi. *Exp. Brain Res.,* 51: 298–303.

[38] Mauritz, K.H., Dichgans, J. and Hufschmidt, A. (1977) The angle of visual roll motion determines displacement of subjective visual vertical. *Percept. Psychophysiol.,* 22: 557–562.

[39] Mauritz, K.H., Dichgans, J., Allum, J. and Brandt, Th. (1975) Frequency characteristics of postural sway in response to self induced and conflicting visual stimulation. *Pflügers Arch. Ges. Physiol.*, 335: Suppl. R 95.

[40] Money, K.E. and Scott, J.W. (1962) Functions of separate sensory receptors of non-auditory labyrinth of the cat. *Am. J. Physiol.*, 202: 1211–1220.

[41] Mower, G., Gibson, A., Robinson, F., Stein, J. and Glickstein, M. (1980) Visual ponto-cerebellar projections in the cat. *J. Neurophysiol.*, 43: 355–366.

[42] Nashner, L.M. (1970) *Sensory Feedback in Human Posture Control*, Sc.D. Thesis, MVT 70–3, Cambridge MA, Man Vehicle Laboratory, M.I.T., 198 pp.

[43] Precht, W. and Strata, P. (1980) On the pathway mediating optokinetic responses in vestibular nuclear neurons. *Neuroscience*, 6: 777–789.

[44] Robinson, D.A. (1977) Linear addition of optokinetic and vestibular signals in the vestibular nucleus. *Exp. Brain Res.*, 30: 447–450.

[45] Talbott, R.E. (1974) Modification of postural response of the normal dog by blind folding. *J. Physiol. London*, 243: 309–320.

[46] Thoden, U., Dichgans, J. and Savidis, Th. (1977) Direction-specific optokinetic modulation of monosynaptic hind limb reflexes in cats. *Exp. Brain Res.*, 30: 155–160.

[47] Waespe, W. and Henn, V. (1977) Neuronal activity in the vestibular nuclei of the alert monkey during vestibular and optokinetic stimulation. *Exp. Brain Res.*, 27: 523–538.

[48] Waespe, W. and Henn, V. (1978) Conflicting visual–vestibular stimulation and vestibular nucleus activity in alert monkeys. *Exp. Brain Res.*, 33: 203–211.

[49] Xerri, C., Barthélémy, J., Borel, L. and Lacour, M. (1988) Neuronal coding of linear motion in the vestibular nuclei of the alert cat. III. Dynamic characteristics of visual–otolith interactions. *Exp. Brain Res.*, in press.

[50] Young, L.R. (1970) On visual–vestibular interactions. In D.F. Proctor (Ed.), *Proceedings of the Fifth Symposium on the Role of the Vestibular Organs in Space*, NASA SP-314, pp. 205–210.

[51] Zacharias, G.L. and Young, L.R. (1981) Influence of combined visual and vestibular cues on human perception and control of horizontal rotation. *Exp. Brain Res.*, 41: 159–171.

SECTION IV

Vestibular Control of Locomotion

O. Pompeiano and J.H.J. Allum (Eds.)
Progress in Brain Research, Vol. 76
© 1988 Elsevier Science Publishers B.V. (Biomedical Division)

Overview

H. Forssberg

Departments of Neurophysiology, Physiology III and Pediatrics, Karolinska Institute, Lidingövägen 1, S-114 33 Stockholm, Sweden

During locomotion an animal has to deal with at least three different tasks. (1) It must perform the actual locomotor movements of the different limbs to support the body against gravity and to propel it forward. (2) It must adapt these movements to external conditions and to the goal of the animal. (3) It must maintain equilibrium during the movements. The organization of the CNS to deal with the first task is fairly well known today. Spinal pattern generators create the basic locomotor pattern, which is modified by peripheral reflexes. Centres in the brainstem control the activity of the pattern generators (for reviews see [1,2]). Much less is known about the neural control of the two latter tasks. Certainly, the vestibulospinal system has an important role to play. Before discussing the papers presented a brief summary of what is known about the vestibulospinal neurons and their action during locomotion will be given.

The lateral vestibulospinal system has monosynaptic connections onto extensor motoneurons of the knee and ankle joint of the cat's hindlimb [3,4]. Consistent with this, stimulation of Deiters' nucleus evokes enhanced activity in the extensor muscles in walking mecencephalic cats during MLR stimulation [5]. The response is, however, only present during the support phase when the extensor muscles are activated by the locomotor generator. Stimulation during the swing phase evokes no response at all. The same stimulation during fictive locomotion (i.e. the locomotor generator is activated but the cat

is paralysed with curare injections), can prolong the extensor bursts or prematurely terminate flexor bursts and initiate extensor bursts in addition to the enhancement of extensor activity during the extensor periods [6]. This means that the VS neurons can modify the amplitude of the locomotor output by a strong influence directly on the extensor motoneurons but can also change the temporal pattern by influencing the pattern generator itself. The latter effect is weaker and in the experimental situation of MLR-walking cats counteracted by powerful peripheral reflex mechanisms from the hip and the ankle preserving the rhythm.

During MLR-induced walking, VS neurons discharge phasically during the support phase. Deiters' nucleus is an important efferent output of the cerebellum [7]. The phasic activity of the VS neurons is completely dependent on the cerebellum, as it disappears after cerebellectomy [8]. The cerebellum receives rhythmic input via the dorsal spinocerebellar tracts, which convey information from the moving limb, and from the ventral spinocerebellar tracts, which transmit information from the spinal pattern generator (efference copy) [9].

When the vestibular apparatus is perturbed by a lateral tilt of a standing cat, most VS neurons are activated by a tilt in the ipsilateral direction and inhibited by a contralateral tilt. In MLR-walking cats there is a clear reduction of the tilt-induced activity compared to standing cats [10]. In fictive preparations, the responses of the VS neurons are rhythmi-

---

Abbreviations: CNS, central nervous system; MLR, mesencephalic locomotor region; VS, vestibulospinal.

cally modulated to be active only during the extensor period when the ordinary discharge is enhanced during an ipsilateral tilt [9].

There are thus phasic gain controls exerted in at least two different levels of this system. First, the cerebellum seems to modify the sensitivity of the VS neurons on the basis of phasic information coming from the spinal cord, only allowing information from external perturbations or central signals to get through during the extensor period. There might also be a general decrease of this gain in walking cats as compared to standing conditions. Secondly, the signals from the VS tract activate extensor motoneurons only during the extensor period. In this case it is presumably the central pattern generator which controls the transmission at the spinal level, opening up the pathways during the support phase and closing them during the swing phase.

My contribution (Chapter 19) does not specifically deal with the VS system but rather with equilibrium control during human locomotion. Supposedly the VS system is involved in this task, although postural responses are activated prior to voluntary movement and equilibrium disturbance. These results are interesting since they demonstrate phase-dependent modulations of the postural pattern. Functionally, this is very important as it allows different biomechanical demands to be met during the various phases of the step cycle. It also shows, on a behavioural level, the phasic gain control of information transmitted by descending motor systems.

The following discussion was focused on the finding that the fixed postural activation patterns that exist during stationary conditions could be modified both spatially and temporally during locomotion. The question was asked whether the term 'synergy' could still be used to describe a pattern which could be so dramatically changed. The synergy concept was defended by some, who argued there could be one or two original patterns that could be blended and that there could also be other motor activities that might influence and modify the original pattern.

One of the major parameters of postural control

is adjustment of muscle force during support phase. In previous studies, Mori has demonstrated that areas within the caudal pontine tegmentum reset the postural muscle tone during locomotion. The level of postural muscle tone greatly affects locomotor movements induced by stimulation of the MLR [11]. In his present contribution (Chapter 18), Dr. Mori demonstrated increased phasic and tonic activity in some VS neurons when the speed of locomotion is increased. He suggests that one task of the VS system could be to mediate the level of postural muscle tone during locomotion, e.g. enhancing amplitudes of locomotor bursts of the extensor muscles during fast locomotion. In the discussion, Mori states that he could not decide whether the increased discharge of the VS neurons was secondary to an increased stimulus strength in the MLR or due to changed peripheral input from the moving limbs.

Amblard et al. (Chapter 20) demonstrated the functional role of the vestibular system by studying the walking of vestibuloectomized cats in darkness. As already discussed, the cats had no problems solving the first task of locomotion, i.e. producing the basic locomotor synergy. They also had no problems controlling speed. As expected, they had great difficulty walking straight and in balancing. Remarkably, most of these deficits recovered when the cats were allowed to use their visual system.

References

[1] Grillner, S. (1981) Control of locomotion in bipeds, tetrapods, and fish. In V.B. Brooks (Ed.), *Handbook of Physiology, Section 1, The Nervous System, Vol. 2, Motor Control, Part 2*, American Physiology Society, Bethesda, pp. 1179–1236.

[2] Grillner, S., Stein, P.S.G., Stuart, D.G., Forssberg, H., and Herman, R.M. (1986) *Neurobiology of Vertebrate Locomotion* Wenner-Gren International Symposium, Series No. 45, McMillan, London.

[3] Lund, S. and Pompeiano, O. (1968) Monosynaptic excitation of alpha motorneurones from supra-spinal structures in the cat. *Acta Physiol. Scand.*, 73: 1–21.

[4] Grillner, S., Hongo, T. and Lund, S. (1970) The vestibulospinal tract. Effects on alpha-motoneurones in the lumbosacral spinal cord in the cat. *Exp. Brain Res.*, 10: 94–120.

[5] Orlovsky, G.N. (1972) The effect of different descending systems on flexor and extensor activity during locomotion. *Brain Res.*, 40: 359–371.

[6] Russel, D.S. and Zajac, F.E. (1979) Effects of stimulation of Deiters' nucleus and medial longitudinal fasciculus on the timing of the fictive locomotor rhythm induced in cats by dopa. *Brain Res.*, 177: 588–592.

[7] Pompeiano, O. (1967) Functional organization of the cerebellar projections to the spinal cord. In C.A. Fox and R.S. Snider (Eds.), *The Cerebellum, Progress in Brain Research, Vol. 25*, Elsevier, Amsterdam, pp. 282–321.

[8] Orlovsky, G.N. (1973) Activity of vestibulospinal neurons during locomotion. *Brain Res.*, 46: 85–98.

[9] Arshavsky, Y.I. and Orlovsky, G.N. (1986) Role of cerebellum in the control of rhythmic movements. In S. Grillner, P.S.G. Stein, D.G. Stuart, H. Forssberg and R.M. Herman (Eds.), *Neurobiology of Vertebrate Locomotion*. Wenner-Gren International Symposium Series No. 45. MacMillan, London, pp. 677–689.

[10] Orlovsky, G.N. and Pavlova, G.A. (1972) Response of Deiters' neurons during locomotion. *Brain Res.*, 42: 212–214.

[11] Mori, S., Kawahara, K., Sakamoto, T., Aoki, M. and Tomiyama, T. (1982) Setting and resetting of postural muscle tone in the decerebrate cat by stimulation of the brain stem. *J. Neurophysiol.*, 48: 737–748.

O. Pompeiano and J.H.J. Allum (Eds.)
Progress in Brain Research, Vol. 76
© 1988 Elsevier Science Publishers B.V. (Biomedical Division)

CHAPTER 18

The behaviour of lateral vestibular neurons during walk, trot and gallop in acute precollicular decerebrate cats

S. Mori[1], K. Matsuyama[1], K. Takakusaki[1] and T. Kanaya[2]

[1]Department of Physiology and [2]Department of Otolaryngology, Asahikawa Medical College, 4-5 Nishikagura, Asahikawa 078-11, Japan

During controlled locomotion in acute decerebrate cats, discharge characteristics of 90 Deiters' neurons were analysed. Representative Deiters' neurons changed their discharge from a tonic pattern (locomotor-unrelated) during slow walk to a phasic pattern (locomotor-related) during fast walk. Bursting discharge of these units was phase-locked with the bursting EMG activity of either the left or the right hindlimb extensor muscle. During trot, the same Deiters' neurons discharged twice in a single step cycle, and each bursting discharge was phase-locked with the bursting EMG activity of the left and the right hindlimb extensor muscles. During gallop, in which bursting EMG activities of bilateral hindlimb muscles appeared more or less in phase, such bursting discharges of the Deiters' neurons fused each other, thus being phase-locked with the bursting EMG activity. There were also activities of Deiters' neurons recruited at each transitional phase of locomotion from slow walk to fast walk, fast walk to trot and trot to gallop. These recruited Deiters' neurons either changed their discharge patterns in a sequence as described above or maintained a tonic pattern with an increase in the firing frequency in relation to the changes in the pattern of locomotion.

Introduction

For locomotion, functional integration of neuronal structures involved in postural control and locomotor control is essential [12,22]. Sherrington [30,31] described integration of posture and locomotion as 'posture follows movement like a shadow'. Acute precollicular–postmammillary decerebrate cats (locomotor preparation) provide us an unique model with which we can study the neuronal mechanisms involved in locomotion, because they are mainly equipped with automatic control mechanisms for the regulation of both posture and locomotion. In such preparations, it is not only possible to evoke locomotion but also to control locomotor patterns from slow walk to fast walk, and then to trot and even to gallop by changing the speed of a moving belt and the stimulus strength delivered to the MLR [26,32,33]. In each of the induced locomotor movements, a sequence of forelimb and hindlimb motion differs considerably; in the walk the limbs strike the supporting surface in the order left hindlimb–left forelimb–right hindlimb–right forelimb, in the trot two diagonal limbs work simultaneously while in the gallop the two limbs of one girdle are more or less in phase [9,36].

As one of the attempts to understand the neuronal mechanisms involved in automatic postural and locomotor control, we have recently proposed a working hypothesis that this system consists of the following three major subsystems [20]: (1) the

---

Abbreviations: EMG, electromyograph; GS, gastrocnemius–soleus; MLR, mesencephalic locomotor region; SLR, subthalamic locomotor region; TA, tibialis anterior.

locomotor-rhythm releasing or generating system; (2) the postural tonus regulating or power-control system, and (3) the locomotor phase-control system. Each of them constitutes a necessary condition for the satisfactory expression of well-coordinated four-legged locomotion. Some of the neuronal structures and pathways contributing to each system have already been identified and discussed in detail [17–19]. The locomotor phase-control system is composed of a spinocerebellar loop [4], and the activity of neuronal elements has been extensively studied both in mesencephalic cats and thalamic cats [2,3,23–25]. The vestibulospinal system is one of the descending pathways involved in this loop, and Deiters' neurons are an 'output' of the vestibular system [6].

As to the function of Deiters' neurons, Orlovsky suggested that the 'flow' of impulses descending in the vestibulospinal tract may adjust the level of extensor activity precisely in accordance with the phase of step, thereby controlling equilibrium during locomotion. Our recent study of the discharge characteristics of Deiters' neurons in the locomotor preparation demonstrated that, during slow walk, most Deiters' neurons regulate the overall excitability of extensor muscle tone of the hindlimbs so as to maintain static equilibrium of posture, and that, during fast walk, the same group of Deiters' neurons control the stance phase of the bilateral hindlimbs so as to maintain the left-right dynamic locomotor equilibrium [14]. In this article, we will show that Deiters' neurons change their discharge characteristics depending on the requirements for the execution of a given locomotor movement. We will further discuss, at the neuronal level of the brainstem, an adaptive control capability of the decerebrate cats in relation to the changes in the locomotor patterns.

Methods

Experimental procedures were similar to those described previously [17,19,21]. Under halothane anaesthesia, the animals were decerebrated at the precollicular–postmammillary level. The head of the animal and the dorsal spinal processes of the first three thoracic vertebrae were fixed in a stereotaxic frame. The body of the animal was supported by a rubber hammock at the abdominal level, and the limbs placed on a resting treadmill. The vertical distance between the hip and the surface of the treadmill was set so that locomotor movements were not hampered. EMGs were recorded by implanting bipolar electrodes made of thin (50 μm) stainless steel wires into bilateral GS and TA muscles. For eliciting locomotion on a moving belt, the MLR was stimulated with 20 to 60 μA pulses of 0.2 ms duration at 50 pulses/s. For inducing slow walk and fast walk, the stimulus strength to the MLR was kept constant while the speed of the moving belt was increased [14]. For inducing trot and gallop, stimulus strength to the MLR and the speed of the moving belt were increased independently or simultaneously according to the induced animal behaviour observed.

Discharge characteristics of Deiters' neurons were analysed during a variety of locomotor movements. The pattern of locomotor movements was determined from the observation on the animal behaviour and from the EMGs. For antidromic identification of Deiters' neurons projecting to the lumbosacral spinal cord, a pair of silver wires was placed under the spinal cord at L1. The spinal stimulation consisted of a pulse of 0.2 ms duration at 1 pulse/s [15]. The discharges of Deiters' neurons were recorded extracellularly by means of glass microelectrodes filled with Woods metal and a carbon fibre of 7 μm diameter (resistance 200–300 kΩ).

The spikes of Deiters' neurons were processed by means of a window discriminator when possible. In this study, 90 Deiters' neurons were studied during a variety of locomotor movements. The mean conduction velocity of these neurons was 88.5 $\pm$ 20.3 m/s, and their spontaneous firing frequency before locomotion was 13.9 $\pm$ 11.3 imp./s. At the end of each experiments, electrolytic lesions were made by passing a DC current of 30 μA for 30 s through the stimulating and recording microelectrodes. The brain was fixed in 10% formalin and stained with cresyl violet. The locations of electrode tips were determined with reference to the stereotaxic atlas of Berman [5].

Results and discussion

Adaptive capability of the locomotor preparation to the speed of the moving belt

Representation EMGs recorded from the left and the right GS muscles during walk, trot and gallop are illustrated in Fig. 1. All these EMGs were recorded from a single cat. The cycle time of locomotion was measured from the interstep interval. During walk with cycle time of about 1.0 s (A), termination of the left GS activity was immediately followed by a bursting discharge of the right GS muscles and vice versa. During a fast walk with a cycle time of about 0.55 s (B), the periods of bursting discharges in the left and the right GS muscles partly overlapped. During trot, the cycle time

shortened to about 0.45 s (C) and with this cycle time, the cat exhibited a diagonal pattern of locomotion. During gallop with cycle time of about 0.40 s (D), the periods of the bursting discharges in the bilateral GS muscles more or less overlapped. During this period of gallop, fore- and hindlimbs struck the moving belt in opposite order. This type of gallop was, therefore, considered to be the rotatory gallop, which was the preferred gait in intact cats [36]. It should be noted that the cat changed its locomotor movements from a given pattern to another pattern in a sequence without any difficulty.

The active periods of the left and the right GS muscles during walk, trot and gallop are summarized in Fig. 2 in a different form. In each locomo-

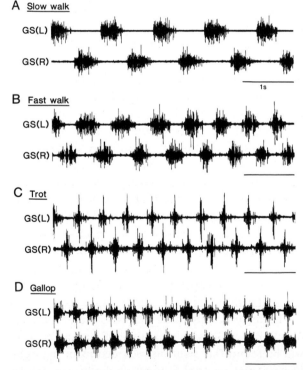

Fig. 1. EMGs recorded from the left (L) and the right (R) gastrocnemius–soleus (GA) muscles during slow walk (A), fast walk (B), trot (C) and gallop (D).

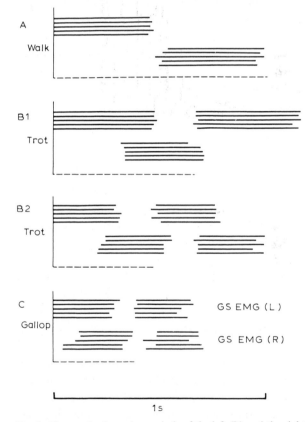

Fig. 2. Changes in the active periods of the left (L) and the right (R) gastrocnemius–soleus (GS) muscles during fast walk (A), trot (B1, 2) and gallop (C). The active period was measured from such EMG records in Fig. 1 and was represented by a bar. See text for details.

tor movement, the periods of bursting discharges in 5 consecutive step cycles were plotted for the left and for the right GS muscles. Since it has been demonstrated in cats that GS muscles are active throughout the stance phase (supporting phase) during overground locomotion with peaks at the start and end [27], it seems possible to estimate the supporting phase of the hindlimbs from the active periods of the GS muscles. Based on such a notion, Kanaya et al. [14] divided the locomotor pattern into slow walk with the presence of double support phase and fast walk with the presence of single support phase. Although Stuart et al. [36] did not describe the periods of the hindlimb support, their figures showed that they were shorter than 0.20 and 0.15 s for trot and gallop, respectively. In our study, the active periods of the GS muscles during trot and gallop were about 0.30 and 0.20 s, respectively. Despite such a difference, we think that smooth shifting of the EMG overlapping periods with the shortening of cycle time reflects the adaptive capability of the neuronal structures involved in postural control and locomotor control.

Adaptive capability of Deiters' neurons in relation to the changes in the pattern of induced locomotion

In acute mesencephalic cats and thalamic cats with intact cerebellum, Orlovsky [23] first correlated the discharge patterns of Deiters' neurons with the activity of hindlimb extensor muscles during locomotion evoked either by MLR stimulation or by exteroceptive stimuli. Among 109 Deiters' neurons studied, 73 neurons (67%) exhibited bursting discharges in relation to the step of the ipsilateral hindlimb while 36 neurons (33%) did not exhibit any modulation in their discharges. Fifty-seven of 73 modulated neurons (52%) showed maximal activity at the end of the swing phase or at the beginning of the stance phase and minimal activity at the end of the stance phase. Other Deiters' neurons had their maximal activity in the middle of the stance phase (4%), or had two maxima, one in the stance phase and another in the swing phase (5%), and had their maximal activity right at the end of the stance

phase or at the beginning of the swing phase (6%). Such modulation of Deiters' neuron discharges usually disappeared when the movement of the ipsilateral hindlimb in relation to the recording site of the Deiters' neurons was stopped. It was also found in decerebellate cats that not one of 52 Deiters' neurons showed any sign of periodic modulation during locomotion. These results demonstrated that the cyclic modulation of Deiters' neurons was closely linked with the limb movement.

Kanaya et al. [14] also studied the discharge characteristics of Deiters' neurons during slow walk and fast walk, and tried to reveal how Deiters' neurons change their discharge patterns in relation to the changes in the locomotor pattern. They found that during slow walk, in which the cycle time was about 1.7–1.0 s, 73% of recorded neurons discharged tonically. As the cycle time was shortened, the proportion of Deiters' neurons exhibiting tonic discharges decreased. By further shortening the cycle time to about 0.6–0.5 s, 80% of Deiters' neurons started to discharge phasically with relation to the extensor phase of step cycles. During a transitional period from slow walk to fast walk, in which cycle time was about 0.9–0.7 s, the overall discharge patterns of Deiters' neurons were not significantly different from those reported by Orlovsky [23]. These results indicate that the functional role played by each one of the Deiters' neurons is not fixed but changes depending on the relative requirements of whether the static or dynamic equilibrium of posture should be controlled during locomotion. These results also seem to reflect, at the neuronal level of the brainstem, an adaptive control capability of the decerebrate cats in relation to the speed of induced locomotion. Therefore, as a next step of this study, we tried to confirm this suggestion by studying the discharge characteristics of Deiters' neurons during trot and gallop.

The records illustrated in Fig. 3 were obtained during fast walk with cycle time of about 0.55 s. It will be found that neurons recorded from the right Deiters' nucleus exhibit bursting discharges during such a fast walk. The largest amplitude unit (a) was found to increase its firing frequency in phase with

Fast walk

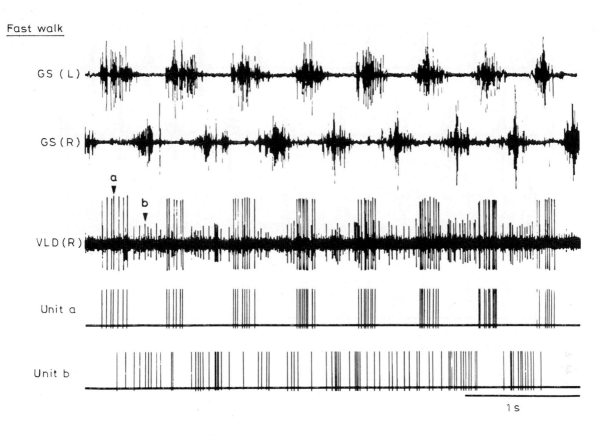

Fig. 3. Discharge pattern of representative Deiters' neurons (a and b) during fast walk. Note that unit 'a', recorded from the right Deiters' nucleus, fires in phase with the bursting discharge of the left (L) GS muscles.

the bursting discharge of the left GS muscles. From such a phase relation, unit 'a' was considered to belong to the contralateral type [14]. The visual examination of mass neuronal discharges in Fig. 3 indicates that there are activities of other neurons. The lower two traces are the representative spike trains of the Deiters' neurons obtained by processing actual records by means of a window discriminator. Unit 'a' showed clear cyclic modulation while unit 'b' tended to show tonic discharges with occasional increases in its firing frequency in phase with the bursting discharge of the right GS muscles. By shortening the cycle time to about 0.45 s, the locomotor pattern changed from fast walk to trot (Fig. 4). During such a period, the same Deiters' neuron (unit 'a' in Fig. 3) changed its discharge property from the contralateral type to the bilateral type;

each group of the bursting activities was phase-locked with the bursting discharges of the left and the right GS muscles, respectively. It was also found that the number of spikes within a burst discharge increased significantly during trot despite the shortening of the active period of the GS muscles. Unit 'b' also increased its tonic firing frequency from about 20 spikes/s during fast walk (Fig. 3) to about 40 spikes/s during trot (Fig. 4). Such Deiters' neurons could play an important role in maintaining the left–right dynamic locomotor equilibrium [13].

The neuronal activities of unit 'a' and unit 'b' were also analysed during gallop with the cycle time of about 0.40 s (Fig. 5). It will be seen from the EMGs illustrated in Fig. 5 that the active period of the left and the right GS muscles overlapped consid-

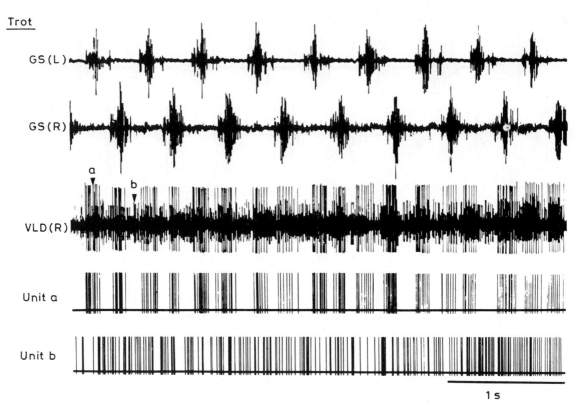

Fig. 4. Discharge pattern of Deiters' neurons during trot. See text for details.

erably, indicating in-phase movements of the bilateral hindlimbs. During such a period, unit 'a' further changed its discharge property, increasing its firing frequency significantly, corresponding to the overlapping period of the bilateral GS muscles while unit 'b' maintaining its tonic firing property. There were also quite a few newly recruited activities in other Deiters' neurons. From such results, it can be well understood that unit 'a', which was the representative Deiters' neuron, changed its firing property from tonic firing during slow walk to contralateral firing during fast walk, and sequentially to bilateral firing during trot and then to overlapping firing. Since gallop can be established by a gradual synchronization of the left and the right hindlimb movements as manifested in the increase in the overlapping periods of the bilateral GS muscles, it can be assumed that the periods of phasic neuronal activity associated with the bursting acti-

vities of the left and the right GS muscles gradually fused with each other, resulting in the significant increase in the firing frequency of a given Deiters' neuron. It should also be noted that such an increase in the firing frequency was observed even during the period in which activities of the bilateral GS muscles were absent.

Recruitment of Deiters' neurons in relation to the changes in the speed of locomotion

As the last step of this series of studies, the relative contribution of Deiters' neurons was studied in relation to the pattern of induced locomotion. For this, the number of Deiters' neurons was estimated from their spike height, although all of them were not antidromically identifiable. Three representative sets of records are illustrated in Fig. 6. During slow walk (A), the activities of two Deiters' neurons

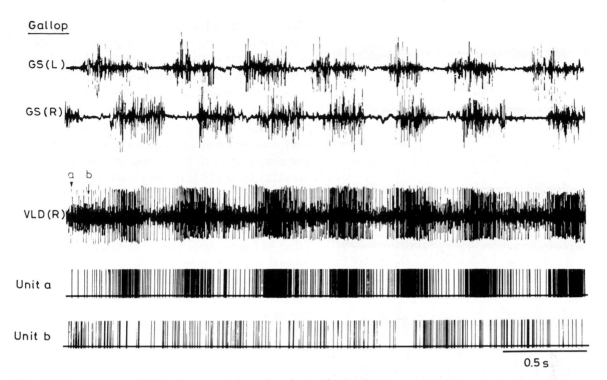

Fig. 5. Discharge pattern of Deiters' neurons during gallop. See text for details.

were clearly discernible, one of them firing in phase with the bursting discharge of the left GS muscles, while at least 4 neurons were identified during trot (B). During gallop (C), the number of recruited neurons significantly increased, each neuron also increasing its firing frequency significantly. In the record with a much faster sweep speed than that in Fig. 6C, it was possible to identify more than 10 active neurons (not illustrated). These results seem to emphasize the importance of recruitment of Deiters' neurons for switching the locomotor patterns from walk to trot, and then to gallop. Grillner [9] stated that, during rapid progression, the propulsive force must be 'injected' during a very brief period of time. Such 'injection' can be established by a significant and transient increase in the firing frequency of a 'command neuron'. At this stage of our study, we are not discussing whether or not Deiters' neurons are the command neurons for changing locomotor patterns. Our results clearly show that Deiters' neurons participate in such 'in-

jection' by increasing their firing frequencies significantly, and by recruiting a number of other Deiters' neurons, some of which may have been silent previously. It should be noted that most of the recruited Deiters' neurons tended to discharge tonically.

Of all brainstem neurons, the discharge patterns of Deiters' neurons and reticular neurons have been most extensively studied [7,23–25,34,35]. These neurons were conventionally classified as locomotor-related cells and unrelated cells. The former group of cells exhibited frequency modulation in relation to locomotor activity while the latter group of cells were clearly unrelated to the step-by-step control of locomotion. Obviously, locomotor-related Deiters' neurons participate in step-by-step control of locomotion. However, the function of locomotor-unrelated neurons has not been well studied and understood. With regard to the volitional control of locomotion, Armstrong [1] suggested that the production of general or 'global' changes such as initiation of or halting of locomotion, and

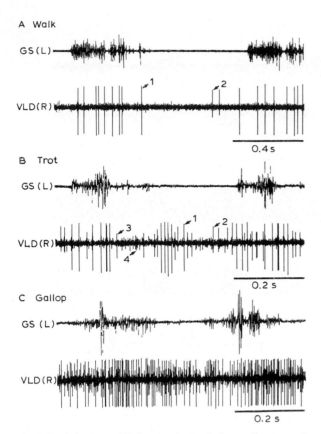

A Walk

GS (L)

VLD(R)

0.4 s

B Trot

GS (L)

VLD(R)

0.2 s

C Gallop

GS (L)

VLD(R)

0.2 s

Fig. 6. Recruitments of Deiters' neurons during walk, trot and gallop. See text for details.

even controlling the speed of locomotion, is commanded via variations in the levels of cortical drives to the SLR [11,38], the MLR or the pontomedullary reticular formation [16,24,29]. Such a notion seems to be applied to locomotor movements induced in the decerebrate locomotor preparation. It is a common observation that an increase in the stimulus intensity delivered to the MLR, increases the degree of extensor muscle tone in the hindlimbs, resulting in an increase in the speed of locomotion [20]. Garcia-Rill and Skinner [8] found that application of increasing amount of γ-aminobutyric acid antagonists into the MLR can differentially increase stepping frequency (walk–trot–gallop).

The possible role of the vestibulospinal system in the control of locomotion has also been studied by stimulating Deiters' nucleus during controlled locomotion or by ablation of the vestibular complex.

Orlovsky [23] found that stimulation of Deiters' nucleus enhanced the activity in extensor hindlimb muscles in cats walking on a moving belt. He also found that stimulation of these structures had no effect on the onset and cessation of muscular activity in a locomotor cycle. These results have led to the interpretation that the vestibulospinal system only acts on the output side and does not influence the neural network generating the locomotor pattern [28]. Orlovsky [24] also studied the acute effect of unilateral partial (Deiters' nucleus) vestibular complex lesions on controlled locomotion. He found ipsilateral abolition of hindlimb stepping, an effect which disappeared within 90 minutes. Yu and Eiderberg [37] studied the consequences of bilateral ablation of the vestibular complex. The cats were very severely ataxic and incapable of head support for nearly two weeks. They gradually regained the ability to stand and to walk on a moving belt, at first with a marked reduction of the extensor components of stepping. From these results, they suggested that the vestibulospinal system plays a major adjunctive role in the central control of the spinal stepping generators, selectively enhancing certain (extensor) elements of the step cycle. These results indicate that Deiters' neurons play a dual role, one controlling the power and the other rhythm of locomotion.

So far the inherent assumption has been that there is a standard 'posture' of the body during locomotion, but there are systematic modifications of posture in a number of situations [10]. These modifications need flexibility and modifiability in the neuronal structures involved in postural control and in locomotor control. Broadly speaking, both postural control and locomotor control can be regarded as a form of motor synergisms, and the synergisms must modify their activities to meet a variety of internal and external requirements. On this point, Arshavsky et al. [4] made a very interesting remark that the problem of interaction between different synergisms as well as between a given synergism and the environment could be solved much more easily if there was a special organ that selects only the essential part of the detailed information about the current state of the synergisms and the environment. They suggested that the cerebellum is such an organ. For the effective organization and recognition of the postural and locomotor synergisms, it is rather favourable for the postural and locomotor control systems to share common executing neuronal structures, and to have a common organizing structure i.e. the cerebellum. The selected information routed, through the cerebellum, would be able to activate these shared executing neuronal structures directly or indirectly with the intervention of complex problem solving [22]. Apparently, the vestibulospinal system is one such executing neuronal structure.

Our results and observations strongly indicate that the function of locomotor-unrelated Deiters' neurons should not be overlooked. As was shown in this study, the number of recruited Deiters' neurons was significantly greater during gallop than during walk and trot. Such an increase in the number of Deiters' neurons, regardless of whether they are tonic or phasic, along with an increase in the firing frequency of individual Deiters' neurons, will increase the power or postural muscle tonus required not only for shifting a locomotor pattern from trot to gallop but also for adequately setting the accompanying posture. The locomotor-related neurons will help to determine the locomotor phase of the left and the right hindlimbs by changing the pattern and the depth of firing frequency modulation. Conversely, the reverse shifting of the locomotor pattern from gallop to trot and even to walk can be established by a sequential derecruitment of Deiters' neurons and by a systematic change in the modulation pattern of locomotor-related neurons. In order to understand the adaptive capability of Deiters' neurons, we think that the populational activity of Deiters' nucleus must be considered. Our study seems to have suggested the possibility that Deiters' nucleus is one of the main constituents of the locomotor rhythm, power- and the phase-control systems [20], and that Deiters' nucleus itself changes the weight of the populational activity of cells participating in each subsystem so as to meet the internal and external requirements.

Acknowledgements

The authors express their sincere thanks to Dr. N. Shimoda for participating in a part of this study, to Dr. Y. Atsuta for his critical discussion, and to Miss. M. Nogami for typing. This study was supported by Ministry of Education and Culture of Japan Scientific Research Grant (B) 62480104 to S. Mori.

References

[1] Armstrong, D.M. (1986) Supraspinal contributions to the initiation and control of locomotion in the cat. *Prog. Neurobiol.*, 26: 273–361.

[2] Arshavsky, Yu.I., Berkinblit, M.B., Fukson, O.I., Gelfand, I.M. and Orlovsky, G.N. (1972) Activity of neurons of the DSCT during locomotion. *Biofizika*, 17: 487–494.

[3] Arshavsky, Yu.I., Berkinblit, M.B., Fukson, O.I., Felfand, I.M. and Orlovsky, G.N. (1972) Activity of neurons of the VSCT during locomotion. *Biofizika*, 17: 883–890.

[4] Arshavsky, Yu.I., Gelfand, I.M. and Orlovsky, G.N. (1983) The cerebellum and control of rhythmical movements. *Trends Neurosci.*, 6: 417–422.

[5] Berman, A.L. (1968) *The Brain Stem of the Cat. A Cytoarchitectonic Atlas with Stereotaxic Coordinates*, University of Wisconsin Press, Madison, 175 pp.

[6] Brodal, A., Pompeiano, O. and Walberg, F. (1962) *The Vestibular Nuclei and their Connections. Anatomy and Functional Correlations.* Oliver and Boyd, Edinburgh.

[7] Drew, T., Dubuc, R. and Rossignol, S. (1986) Discharge patterns of reticulospinal and other reticular neurons in chronic, unrestrained cats walking on a treadmill. *J. Neurophysiol.*, 55: 375–410.

[8] Garcia-Rill, E., Skinner, R.D. and Fitzgerald, J.A. (1985) Chemical activation of the mesencephalic locomotor region. *Brain Res.*, 330: 43–54.

[9] Grillner, S. (1975) Locomotion in vertebrates: central mechanisms and reflex interaction. *Physiol. Rev.*, 55: 247–304.

[10] Grillner, S. (1981) Control of locomotion in bipeds, tetrapods, and fish. In J.M. Brookhart and B.V. Mountcastle (Eds.), *Handbook of Physiology, Section 1, Vol.2, Motor Control, Part 2*, American Physiology Society, Bethesda, pp. 1179–1236.

[11] Grossman, R.G. (1958) Effects of stimulation of nonspecific thalamic system on locomotor movements in cat. *J. Neurophysiol.*, 21: 85–93.

[12] Gurfinkel, V.S. and Shik, M.L. (1973) The control of posture and locomotion. In A.A. Gydikov, N.T. Tankov and D.S. Kosarov (Eds.), *Motor Control*, Plenum Press, New York, pp. 217–234.

[13] Igarashi, M. and Alford, B.R. (1975) Animal behavioral studies of equilibrium. In D.B. Tower (Ed.), *The Nervous*

220

System, Human Communication and Its Disorders, Vol. 3, Raven Press, New York, pp. 125–135.

[14] Kanaya, T., Unno, T., Kawahara, K. and Mori, S. (1985) Functional roles played by Deiters' neurons during controlled locomotion in the mesencephalic cat. In M. Igarashi and F.O. Black (Eds.), *Vestibular and Visual Control on Posture and Locomotor Equilibrium*, Karger, Basel, pp. 193–199.

[15] Kawahara, K., Mori, S., Tomiyama, T. and Kanaya, T. (1985) Discharge of neurons in the midpontine dorsal tegmentum of mesencephalic cat during locomotion. *Brain Res.*, 341: 377–380.

[16] Mori, S., Shik, M.L. and Yagodnitsyn, A.S. (1977) Role of pontine tegmentum for locomotor control in mesencephalic cat. *J. Neurophysiol.*, 40: 284–295.

[17] Mori, S., Nishimura, H., Kurakami, C., Yamamura, T. and Aoki, M. (1978) Controlled locomotion in the mesencephalic cat: distribution of facilitatory and inhibitory regions within pontine tegmentum. *J. Neurophysiol.*, 41: 1580–1591.

[18] Mori, S., Nishimura, H. and Aoki, M. (1980) Brain stem activation of the spinal stepping generator. In J.A. Hobson and M.A.B. Brazier (Eds.), *Reticular Formation Revisited, IBRO Monograph Series, Vol. 6*, Raven Press, New York, pp. 241–259.

[19] Mori, S., Kawahara, K., Sakamoto, T., Aoki, M. and Tomiyama, T. (1982) Setting and resetting of postural muscle tone in the decerebrate cat by stimulation of the brain stem. *J. Neurophysiol.*, 48: 737–748.

[20] Mori, S., Kawahara, K. and Sakamoto, T. (1983) Supraspinal aspects of locomotion in the mesencephalic cat. In A. Roberts and B.L. Roberts (Eds.), *Neural Control*, Cambridge University Press, Cambridge, pp. 445–468.

[21] Mori, S., Sakamoto, T. and Ohta, Y. (1985) Neuronal mechanisms underlying 'plastic control changes' in the decerebrate, reflex standing cats. In C.D. Woody and D.L. Alkon (Eds.), *Neuronal Mechanisms of Conditioning*, Plenum Press, London, pp. 167–185.

[22] Mori, S. (1987) Integration of posture and locomotion in acute decerebrate cats and in awake, freely moving cats. *Prog. Neurobiol.*, 28: 161–195.

[23] Orlovsky, G.N. (1972) Activity of vestibulospinal neurones during locomotion. *Brain Res.*, 46: 85–98.

[24] Orlovsky, G.N. (1972) The effect of different descending systems on flexor and extensor activity during locomotion. *Brain Res.*, 40: 359–371.

[25] Orlovsky, G.N. (1972) Activity of rubrospinal neurons during locomotion. *Brain Res.*, 46: 91–112.

[26] Orlovsky, G.N. and Shik, M.L. (1976) Control of locomotion: a neurophysiological analysis of the cat locomotor system. In R. Porter (Ed.), *International Review of Physiology and Neurophysiology. Vol. 2*, University of Park Press, Baltimore, pp. 282–317.

[27] Prochazka, V.J., Tate, K., Westerman, R.A. and Ziccone, S.P. (1974) Remote monitoring of muscle length and EMG in unrestrained cats. *EEG Clin. Neurophysiol.*, 37: 649–653.

[28] Russel, D.F. and Zajac, F.E. (1979) Effects of stimulating Deiters' nucleus and medial longitudinal fasciculus on the timing of the fictive locomotor rhythm induced in cats by DOPA. *Brain Res.*, 177: 588–592.

[29] Shefchyk, S.J., Jell, R.M. and Jordan, L.M. (1984) Reversible cooling of the brainstem reveals area required for mesencephalic locomotion region evoked treadmill locomotion. *Exp. Brain Res.*, 56: 257–262.

[30] Sherrington, C.S. (1906) *The Integrative Action of the Nervous System*, Yale University Press, New Haven, 417 pp.

[31] Sherrington, C.S. (1910) Flexion reflex on the limb, crossed extension reflex and reflex stepping and standing. *J. Physiol. London*, 40: 28–121.

[32] Shik, M.L., Severin, F.V. and Orlovsky, G.N. (1966) Control of walking and running by means of electrical stimulation of the midbrain. *Biophysics*, 11: 756–765. (English translation of *Biofizika*, 11 (1966), 659–666.)

[33] Shik, M.L. and Orlovsky, G.N. (1976) Neurophysiology of locomotor automatism. *Physiol. Rev.*, 56: 465–501.

[34] Shimamura, M. and Kogure, I. (1983) Discharge patterns of rubrospinal neurons corresponding will quadripedal leg movements in thalamic cats. *Brain Res.*, 206: 27–34.

[35] Shimamura, M., Fuwa, T. and Kogure, I. (1985) Burst discharges of pontis reticular neurons in relation to forelimb stepping of thalamic and high spinal cats. *Brain Res.*, 346: 363–367.

[36] Stuart, D.G., Withey, T.P., Wetzel, M.C. and Goslow, G.E. Jr. (1973) The constraints for inter-limb coordination in the cat during unrestrained locomotion. In R.B. Stein, K.G. Smith and J.B. Redford (Eds.), *Control of Posture and Locomotion*, Plenum Press, London, pp. 537–560.

[37] Yu, J. and Eiderberg, E. (1981) Effects of vestibulospinal lesions upon locomotor function in cats. *Brain Res.*, 220: 179–183.

[38] Waller, W.H. (1940) Progression movements elicited by subthalamic stimulation. *J. Neurophysiol.*, 3: 300–307.

O. Pompeiano and J.H.J. Allum (Eds.)
Progress in Brain Research, Vol. 76
© 1988 Elsevier Science Publishers B.V. (Biomedical Division)

CHAPTER 19

Phasic modulation of postural activation patterns during human walking

H. Forssberg and H. Hirschfeld

Karolinska Institute, Departments of Neurophysiology, Physiology III and Pediatrics, Karolinska Institute, Lidingövägen 1, S-114 33 Stockholm, Sweden

In order to study postural control mechanisms during locomotion 8 subjects were instructed to walk on a treadmill and to pull a handle when given a signal that was triggered during different phases of the step cycle. Muscular activation patterns were studied by EMG recordings and movements by a photoelectric system (Selspot). Postural activity that preceded the voluntary arm contraction was superimposed on the ordinary locomotor bursts. During the different phases of the support phase there was considerable diversity in postural responses of the leg musculature. This included: the combination of muscles used, the temporal sequence and the spatial distribution of the relative magnitudes. The subtle and complex nature of these changes do not appear to be the result of stereotyped synergies. It is rather a practical example of phasic gain control in humans exerted at the spinal or supraspinal level.

Introduction

Bernstein [1] argued that it would be impossible for the brain to control each individual muscle during a movement. Instead, it was organized in a way that reduced the number of independent parameters that had to be controlled. This was achieved by a restricted number of synergies, which were programmed to activate appropriate muscles according to a fixed pattern.

Voluntary movements of the upper limbs are preceded by postural adjustments occurring in the trunk and lower limbs [2–4]. These movements are produced by consistent patterns of muscular contractions specific to the forthcoming voluntary movement in order to compensate for the equilibrium disturbance [5,6]. In agreement with Bernstein's hypothesis, the few recognized postural activation patterns were regarded as stereotyped synergies. The same synergies could be initiated either in advance of voluntary movements or evoked reflexively by somatosensory stimuli due to external perturbations causing the same disturbance of the equilibrium [7]. A continuum of postural movements could still be synthesized by combining two synergies in different magnitudes and temporal relations [8].

The pattern of muscular activation during the beginning of the support phase is similar to that during stationary standing and it was suggested that the same synergies are used [9]. During walking, the centre of mass (trunk) and the support surfaces (feet) are constantly moving in relation to each other. Different postural reactions are therefore needed at different phases of the step cycle to compensate for the same perturbation. In the experiments described in this report we have studied the postural activation pattern during different subphases of gait in order to see whether such a phasic change can be produced by mixing a few stereo-

---

Abbreviations: BIC, biceps; CNS, central nervous system; EMG, electromyograph; HAM, biceps femoris; LG, lateral gastrocnemius; RF, rectus femoris; TA, tibialis anterior; VL, vastus lateralis.

typed synergies. We found a gradual modulation of the activity in each muscle independent of the activity in synergistic or antagonistic muscles. These findings do not support the use of simple postural synergies during locomotion.

Methods

Eight subjects (19–39 years; 6 males, 2 females) were instructed to walk on a treadmill (2.5 × 0.8 m) at a comfortable walking speed (1–1.2 m/s) and to grip a handle with the left hand maintaining a preload of approximately 10 N. During randomly chosen step cycles a short tone burst was used to instruct the subjects to instantly perform a brisk pull on the handle. The tone bursts were triggered from left foot contact (pressure transducer) and timed to occur at 100 ms intervals during the whole step cycle.

Leg movements were recorded by a photoelectric system (Selspot; Selcom AB, Partille, Sweden) [10]. Six diodes were glued to the left leg to allow ankle, knee and hip-joint angles to be calculated from vectors drawn between adjacent diodes. EMG was recorded by surface electrodes from the left-arm BIC, and from the LG, TA, HAM and the VL and RF of the quadriceps group of the left leg. The signals were band-pass filtered (5th order Bessel, high pass 50 Hz, low pass 500 Hz) and full-wave rectified. Movement data from the Selspot and EMGs were multiplexed together with signals from footswitches on both feet, tone bursts and handle force, and fed into a minicomputer (HP 1000) for later analysis (for details see [10]).

EMG patterns during unperturbed treadmill walking and EMG signals associated with arm pulls respectively, were averaged ($n > 8$ stride cycles). The onset of associated postural activity in a given muscle was defined as the time when the EMG signal first deviated one standard deviation above the mean level of the unperturbed stride cycles. Temporal and spatial parameters for the associated postural activations followed the definitions of relative measurements as described earlier [9] in order to combine the results from all subjects.

(1) *Absolute latency* of a postural activation was the interval from tone command to the first increase of EMG.

(2) *Temporal organization* of an activation pattern was characterized by the delay of involved muscles from the absolute latency.

(3) *Spatial organization* of the activation patterns estimated the relative strength of the muscles involved. It was calculated as the area under the EMG envelope during the first 100 ms from the absolute latency and compared to maximal locomotor bursts, which were calculated in the same way.

Abbreviations

The support phases of the step cycles were divided in subphases. The postural responses were categorized to the subphase in which the first EMG response was detected: as follows

DS1 (double support 1), from left heel strike to right toe off.

SS1 (single support 1), from right toe off until the swing leg passes the support leg.

SS2 (single support 2), from the swing leg passing until right heel strike.

DS2 (double support 2), from right heel strike to left toe off.

TRST (transition to stance), 100 ms before left heel strike.

TRSW (transition to swing), 100 ms before left toe off.

Stride cycle events: LHS, left heel strike; LTO, left toe off; RHS, right heel strike; RTO, right toe off.

Results

Distribution of muscle activation

The hamstring and the gastrocnemius muscles were both activated during the early part of the support phase (i.e. TRST, DS1 and SS1) and preceded the voluntary activity of the biceps muscle (Fig. 1). These muscles were involved in the postural ankle synergy on the dorsal aspect of the leg, resisting a forward fall by ankle torque during stationary standing [7,8]. At the same time, however, the quadriceps group (VL and RF) on the ventral aspect was activated (Fig. 1). During SS1 the contribution of HAM and LG decreased while small EMG bursts were initiated in TA (Fig. 1). In later subphases (SS2 and DS2) the TA activity continued to increase while the activity of HAM and LG ceased. The contribution of the quadriceps muscles ceased during the middle of the support phase but reappeared again in the later parts, now in combination with the TA activity.

There was thus a clear change of postural activa-

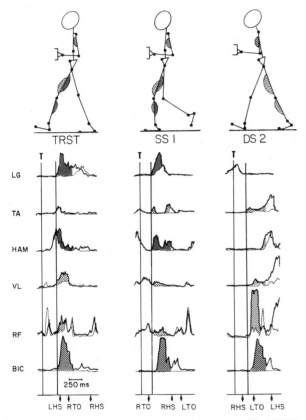

Fig. 1. The ensemble average of filtered and rectified EMGs from eight unperturbed step cycles (thin lines) of one subject are compared with eight step cycles of the same subject during handle pulls (thick lines) during TRST, SS1 and DS2. The vertical lines with T at the top indicate delivery of the tone signal and the subsequent lines denote the absolute latency to the first activated muscle of the postural response. The arrows show step cycle events. The stick figures at the top illustrate the distribution of muscle activity. Postural responses are indicated by different patterns on the ventral and dorsal aspects of the body.

tion patterns in distal parts of the leg. During early parts of the support phase when the body was behind the support leg and the whole foot was on the ground, muscles on the dorsal aspect of the leg contracted. Their action decelerated the forward rotation about the ankle and resisted an increased forward momentum of the body caused by the arm pull. In later parts of the support phase the body has passed the supporting foot and the heel has started to leave the floor. A similar activation pattern extending the ankle would in this position not rotate the body backwards but propell it upward and forward. The actual TA activation had the opposite effect, reducing the forward thrust generated by the locomotor burst of the gastrocnemius muscle. The early activation of VL and RF resisted knee flexion, which otherwise would have occurred because of the positioning of the body behind the foot. Such action was not needed when the body had moved forward. The RF contraction in late support phase had a decelerating effect on the forward movement of the body by resisting hip extension.

Spatial pattern

Both HAM and LG were maximally activated just prior to foot contact (TRST) and immediately afterwards (DS1). During this period there was no TA activation in any of the subjects (Figs. 1 and 2). This should be compared to the responses during the end of the support phase (DS2) when there was a maximal TA response in all subjects and only minimal activity in HAM and LG. From the beginning to the end of the support phase there was a smooth and gradual decrease of the HAM and LG responses concomitant to an increased intensity of the TA response. Thus, rather than a switch between two different response patterns, there was a gradual shift from one pattern to the other. In the middle of the support phase (SS1 and SS2) both responses were concomitantly activated with no or very small concordant delays (Figs. 1 and 2).

The relative contribution of HAM and LG varied extensively between consecutive steps of the same subject, although the phasic modulation of the two muscles followed each other for all subjects (Fig. 2). In one step the HAM response was largest, while LG was larger in the next trial. HAM and LG were thus not activated in one block with a fixed relation between EMG bursts and sudden cessation of activity by one muscle or the other. The strength of contraction of the two muscles appeared to be controlled separately.

Temporal pattern

The sequential order of initiation between the dorsal muscles HAM and LG was also dependent on the phase of the step cycle. In TRST, postural HAM activity always preceded the initiation of LG (44 ± 12 ms; $n = 8$ subjects; mean of means $\pm$ SD of means) (Figs. 1 and 3). HAM could be activated well in advance of foot contact if the signal was delivered during mid-swing. LG, on the other hand, was always delayed until a few ms before foot contact [9]. A proximal-to-distal order was also maintained during the beginning of the support phase (DS1) in all but one subject. Another subject had no HAM activity during this phase. The delay from the initiation of HAM to the initiation of LG decreased in DS1 (20 ± 18 ms; $n = 8$ subjects; mean of means $\pm$ SD of means) compared to TRST for all subjects and was significantly smaller ($p < 0.01$; *t*-test) for the whole group.

The sequential order was changed to a distal-to-proximal direction in five of eight subjects during SS1. The calculated mean of all subjects (Fig. 3) was also significantly reduced ($p < 0.02$; *t*-test) with activation of LG (30 ± 20 ms; $n = 8$ subjects; mean of means $\pm$ SD of means) before the HAM activity. During SS2 only two subjects activated LG in the postural response while most subjects only activated TA as the distal muscle. In both subjects LG was activated earlier than HAM.

Discussion

Are postural synergies used during locomotion?

Sudden arm movements perturbing the equilibrium during walking are preceded by postural responses

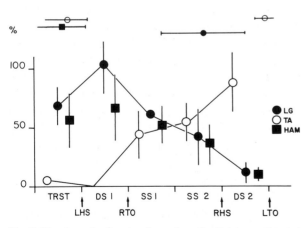

Fig. 2. The strength of postural muscle activation was estimated by calculation of the area during the first 100 ms between the EMGs of perturbed and unperturbed step cycles. The reference value (100%) was calculated in the same way under the EMG envelope of the maximal locomotor burst for each muscle. The horizontal bars at the top show the duration of normal locomotor activity.

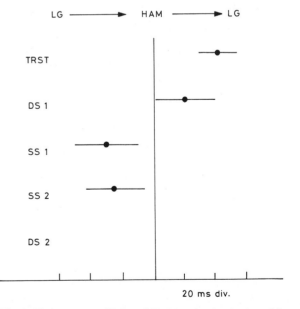

Fig. 3. The sequence of LG and HAM activation is plotted for the different subphases of support for all subjects ($n = 8$). The initiation of HAM is marked as a vertical midline; the circles to the left indicate the preceding LG activation and the circles to the right indicate subsequent LG activation. Note the time scale.

in leg and trunk muscles [9]. The present study demonstrates that different postural activation patterns are used during the support phase to resist the forward momentum of the upper part of the body due to an arm pull. In the early support phase, when the body is behind the supporting foot, muscles on the dorsal aspect of the leg are activated to resist an increased forward rotation about the ankle joint. This activity is accompanied with quadriceps activity resisting knee flexion. In the late support phase, when the body has passed the foot and the heel is lifted from the floor, a TA activation was again often accompanied by VL and RF activity, which reduced the forward thrust produced by the locomotor activity of the extensor muscles in the ankle and hip. There is not an abrupt switch from one pattern to another. Instead, there is a gradual shift of the activation of each individual muscle.

It has been argued that there is a limited number of postural synergies compensating for external or internal disturbances of equilibrium during static conditions [6,7,11]. The synergy concept implies a rigid structure of movement in which a certain number of muscles are activated in a fixed temporal and spatial pattern. Every time the synergy is elicited the sequencing between synergistic muscles should be the same, as should the relative intensity of the contractions [7]. A continuum of responses meeting changed configurations of the support surface could, however, be accomplished by sequential switches between two pure patterns or as hybrid blends [8,12].

There is not such a fixed structure of the postural activation patterns during walking. Muscles from different synergies are activated in different combinations. VL–RF are activated together with HAM–LG in the beginning of the support phase but concomitant with TA in later parts. During the middle of the support phase, when HAM–LG and TA are activated together, the contribution of VL–RF activity is smaller.

Secondly there is no fixed temporal pattern of muscle activation within a synergy. There is a proximal–distal sequence of HAM–LG initiation in the early support phase but a distal–proximal order in later parts. Thirdly, there is a change of the spatial relations of the contractions of the dorsal muscles seen in individual subjects.

The combination of different muscles and the modification of temporal and spatial relations suggest independent controllers of different muscles. The dynamically changing demands during the different phases of the step cycle can obviously not be met by the combination of a few stereotyped synergies which may be sufficient for different static conditions. If the synergy concept is to include responses seen during locomotion, it has to be broadened. For example, a synergy could indicate activation of a group of muscles from which temporal and spatial relations can be changed according to other mechanisms (e.g. locomotion).

Mechanisms of phasic modulation

Extensive studies on locomotor control during the last decades have uncovered complex locomotor patterns generated by neural networks in the spinal cord [13]. These circuits are controlled by cortical and subcortical systems via centres in the brainstem [14,15]. Reduced preparations (spinal or mesencephalic) may produce a complete basic locomotor rhythm but are not able to adapt the stereotyped pattern to the environment to any large extent [16]. To do so, supraspinal structures including the cerebellum and the vestibular system must be intact.

Several studies indicate that human locomotor control is organized in a similar hierarchic structure. Electrical stimulation of the analogue nuclei in the brainstem of nonhuman primates evokes locomotor activity that resembles normal locomotion [17]. Newborn human infants perform spontaneous locomotor-like steps when held erect [18] or supine [19]. Even human fetuses with severe malformations of the CNS only leaving the lumbar cord intact can carry out frequent stepping movements (H. Prechtl, personal communication). We think, therefore, that it may be justified to discuss the mechanisms of phasic modulation in man from the model of locomotor control in quadrupeds.

It is not known at which level in the motor hierarchy postural activation patterns are originating. The latency after external perturbations is about 90–100 ms [7], which could indicate supraspinal organization. Reflexes with corresponding latencies have, on the other hand, been described in spinal animals [20]. In either case, information to execute the postural reactions prior to the voluntary movements has to be transmitted through the spinal cord either as patterned information directly to the motoneurons or as simpler signals to spinal circuits producing the more specific activation pattern. Locomotor activity and environmental changes can interact and influence the outcome of the pattern on at least two different levels in the motor hierarchy.

Supraspinal level

Rhythmic signals related to hindlimb movements reach the cerebellum via spinocerebellar tracts. The dorsal tracts transmit detailed information from the moving limb while the ventral tracts convey information about the activity of the spinal pattern generator [21]. The ascending activity modulates the rhythm of cerebellar neurons inducing rhythmic discharge in vestibulospinal, reticulospinal and rubrospinal tracts. Detailed afferent information from the limb as well as which muscles will be activated next by the pattern generator is thus constantly available. The planning and programming of voluntary movement involve the construction of preceding postural adjustments according to the postural condition. With the information of limb dynamics and efference copy of the forthcoming locomotor activity such programming of the postural activity could be exerted at the supraspinal level.

Spinal level

In walking cats there is a phasic modulation of cutaneous reflexes evoked from the paw causing purposeful corrections of the limb movement at every moment of the step cycle [22]. The same mechanisms remain in walking cats after spinal cord transection as well as during fictive locomotion in spinal cats paralysed with curare injections [23,24]. As there is no phasic afferent inflow from the limbs in the paralysed cat; the phasic modula-tion of the cutaneous reflexes has to be exerted by the spinal pattern generator itself. A similar central modulation also occurs in descending vestibulospinal and reticulospinal tracts [25,26]. The continuous phasic modulation of the anticipatory postural reactions could thus be explained by the spinal pattern generator modulating the transmission in the pathways to the different muscle groups.

Acknowledgements

The study was supported by the Swedish Medical Research Council (4X-5925), Norrbacka-Eugenia Stiftelsen, Stiftelsen Solstickan and Omsorgsnämnden in Stockholm. The valuable comments of Dr. Leonard are gratefully acknowledged.

References

[1] Bernstein, N.A. (1967) *The Coordination and Regulation of Movements.* Pergamon Press, Oxford.

[2] Gelfand, I.M., Gurfinkel, V.S., Tsetlin, M.L. and Shik, M.L. (1971) Some problems in the analysis of movements. In I.M. Gelfand, V.S. Gurfinkel, S.V. Fomin and M.L. Tsetlin (Eds.), *Models of the Structural-Functional Organization of Certain Biological Systems,* MIT Press, Cambridge, pp. 229–345.

[3] Belen'kii, V.Y., Gurfinkel, V.S. and Pal'tsev, Y.I. (1967) On the elements of voluntary movement control. *Biofizika,* 12: 135–141.

[4] Pal'tsev, Y.I. and Elner, A.M. (1967) Preparatory and compensatory period during voluntary movement in patients with involvement of the brain of different localization, *Biofizika,* 12: 142–147.

[5] Bouisset S. and Zattara, M. (1981) A sequence of postural movements precedes voluntary movement. *Neurosci. Lett.,* 22: 263–270.

[6] Cordo, P.J. and Nashner, L.M. (1982) Properties of postural adjustments associated with rapid arm movements. *J. Neurophysiol.,* 47: 287–302.

[7] Nashner, L.M. (1977) Fixed patterns of rapid postural responses among leg muscles during stance. *Exp. Brain Res.,* 30: 13–24.

[8] Horak, F.B. and Nashner, L.M. (1986) Central programming of postural movements: adaption to altered support-surface configurations. *J. Neurophysiol.,* 55: 1369–1381.

[9] Nashner, L.M. and Forssberg, H. (1986) Phase-dependent organization of postural adjustments associated with arm movements while walking. *J. Neurophysiol.,* 55: 538–548.

[10] Halbertsma, J. (1983) The stride cycle of the cat: the modeling of locomotion by computerized analysis of automatic recordings. *Acta Physiol. Scand. Suppl.,* 521: 1–75.

[11] Nashner, L.M. and McCollum, G. (1985) The organization of human postural movements: a formal basis and experimental synthesis. *Behav. Brain Sci.*, 8: 135–172.

[12] Robertsson, G.A., Mortin, L.I., Keifer, J. and Stein, P.S.G. (1985) Three forms of scratch reflex in the spinal turtle: central generation of motor patterns. *J. Neurophysiol.*, 53: 1517–1534.

[13] Grillner, S. (1981) Control of locomotion in bipeds, tetrapods, and fish. In V.B. Brooks (Ed.), *Handbook of Physiology, Section 1, The Nervous System, Vol. 2, Motor Control*, American Physiology Society, Bethesda, pp. 1179–1236.

[14] Shik, M.L., Severin, F.V. and Orlovsky, G.N. (1966) Control of walking and running by means of electrical stimulation of the midbrain. *Biofizika*, 11: 659–666.

[15] Garcia-Rill, E. (1986) The basal ganglia and the locomotor regions. *Brain Res. Rev.*, 11: 47–63.

[16] Forssberg, H. (1979) On integrative motor functions in the cat's spinal cord. *Acta Physiol. Scand. Suppl.*, 474: 1–56.

[17] Eidelberg, E., Walden, J.G. and Nguygen, L.H. (1981) Locomotor control in macaque monkeys. *Brain*, 104: 647–663.

[18] Forssberg, H. (1985) Ontogeny of human locomotor control. I. Infant stepping, supported locomotion and transition to independent locomotion. *Exp. Brain Res.*, 57: 480–493.

[19] Thelen, E., Bradshaw, G. and Ward, J.A. (1981) Spontaneous kicking in month-old infants: manifestation of human central locomotor program. *Behav. Neurol. Biol.*, 32: 45–53.

[20] Ghez, C. and Shinoda, Y. (1978) Spinal mechanisms of the functional stretch reflex. *Exp. Brain Res.*, 32: 55–68.

[21] Arshavsky, Y.I. and Orlovsky, G.N. (1986) Role of cerebellum in the control of rhythmic movements. In S. Grillner (Ed.), *Neurobiology of Vertebrate Locomotion*, Vol. 45, Wenner-Gren International Series, Stockholm, pp. 677–689.

[22] Forssberg, H. (1979) Stumbling corrective reaction: a phase-dependent compensatory reaction during locomotion. *J. Neurophysiol.*, 42: 936–953.

[23] Forssberg, H., Grillner, S. and Rossignol, S. (1977) Phasic gain control of reflexes from the dorsum of the paw during spinal locomotion. *Brain Res.*, 132: 121–139.

[24] Andersson, O., Forssberg, H., Grillner, S. and Lindquist, M. (1978) Phasic gain control of the transmission in cutaneous reflex pathways to motoneurones during 'fictive' locomotion. *Brain Res.*, 149: 503–507.

[25] Russel, D.S. and Zajac, F.E. (1979) Effects of stimulation of Deiters nucleus and medial longitudinal fasciculus on the timing of the fictive locomotor rhythm induced in cats by dopa. *Brain Res.*, 177: 588–592.

[26] Drew, T. and Rossignol, S. (1984) Phase-dependent responses evoked in limb muscles by stimulation of medullary reticular formation during locomotion in thalamic cats. *J. Neurophysiol.*, 52: 653–675.

O. Pompeiano and J.H.J. Allum (Eds.)
Progress in Brain Research, Vol. 76
© 1988 Elsevier Science Publishers B.V. (Biomedical Division)

CHAPTER 20

Visual and vestibular control of locomotion in early and late sensory-deprived cats

A.R. Marchand, B. Amblard and J. Cremieux

Laboratoire de Neurosciences Fonctionnelles, Unité de Neurosciences du Comportement, 31 Chemin J. Aiguier F-13402 Marseille CEDEX 9, France CNRS

This study focuses on how the vestibular system intervenes in the control of locomotion in the cat, and evaluates the impact of the visual environment on the development and recovery of vestibular functions. Bilateral destruction of the vestibular receptors was therefore combined with selective visual deprivation, both neonatally and in adult animals. The task was specially designed to investigate specific components of goal-directed locomotion, such as dynamic balance, keeping a straight course, and paw guidance during walking, depending on the characteristics of the walking surface. The main criterion of performance was the average walking speed of the animal when subjected to various visual conditions, including stroboscopic illumination. The effects of vestibular deprivation at an early age on locomotion control were found to be no more severe than those of later lesions, which indicates that early developmental processes involving vestibular information do not impinge on nonvestibular functions. As to the vestibular-related functions, they seem to partly develop in conjunction with kinetic visual cues. For instance, navigation in darkness is impaired in strobe-reared subjects. Furthermore, in adult cats, vestibular signals may be used in conjunction with visual reafferent information, since visual paw guidance is impaired in labyrinthectomized cats during walking. However, vestibular control is both necessary and sufficient for dynamic balance, in that it does not depend upon visual experience, and cannot be properly handled by the visual channel in either early or late vestibular-deprived cats. Impairment of this dynamic balance function may partly explain the deficits observed in other components of locomotor control, namely zigzaging or difficulties over irregular ground after labyrinthectomy. The main effect of age in labyrinthectomized cats is visual: in early vestibular-deprived animals, enhanced use is made of positional visual cues to control the direction of locomotion.

Introduction

Walking adult cats can be fascinating to watch because of the sureness and smoothness of their gait. There is general agreement among physiologists that the vestibular system plays an essential role in this skilful performance. A distribution of functions seems to take place, however, across the various sensory systems involved, so that the visual system, for instance, may also participate in the control of locomotion, and, in some cases, partly compensate for any vestibular deficits [24, 40, 41]. It is also noteworthy that although the vestibular system matures very early [44], very young kittens are very clumsy and hesitant. Obviously, locomotion in the kitten has to be developed. Until now, however, it has not been clearly established whether or not normal development depends on sensory experience of a vestibular or visual kind, for instance in which case it would be affected by early sensory deprivation.

The acquisition of various postural reactions in the kitten has already been described in relation with the maturation of the vestibular system [43]. Very little is known, however, about the postural and locomotor development of cats with vestibular lesions: Blakemore and Papaioannou [5] have reported the existence in labyrinthectomized kittens of deficient tonic labyrinthine reflexes and righting reflexes during free fall. Early vestibular deprivation drastically deteriorates neither obstacle avoidance nor visually guided placing in kittens [17]. Adult cats which were neonatally labyrinthectomized showed no noticeable impairment of their ability to control their *static* equilibrium on a wide support [29]. Much more is known about the effects of vestibular deprivation in adult animals [1, 27, 41] and humans [35, 41]. Bilateral labyrinthectomy seems to have no or little effect on static equilibrium in the dog [34], whereas in humans [15] as well as in the monkey [12, 20], dynamic equilibrium performance on a narrow support is particularly severely affected after bilateral labyrinthectomy. On a wide surface, André-Thomas [1] reported that adult bilabyrinthectomized cats tended to zigzag.

Tasks of this kind also involve some visual control. Vision has often been shown to participate in the control of either static [3] or dynamic [11, 42] equilibrium in man, as well as playing a fast directional role in postural control in the normal falling baboon [24]. Postural responses of the cat to visual stimuli have also been described [6]. But as regards the possible role of vision in the control of locomotion, particularly in the cat, previous studies have been sparse [8].

Classically, vestibular deprivation, whether unilateral or bilateral, has been obtained by irreversible labyrinthectomy [27, 41] or canal-plugging [33]. These methods deprive the subject of sensory input, but they can lead to neuronal reorganization and/ or functional recovery. In the same way, although visual deprivation is reversible in the adult cat, it has not been established whether this is also true of long-term deprivation during development. Although people who have been blind from birth have been reported to exhibit some abnormal locomotion [32], total visual deprivation from birth does not seem to greatly disturb the goal-directed locomotion of adult cats [8] but does disturb the equilibrium of rats [13]. The selective visual deprivation obtained by stroboscopic illumination during development which is described here is known to

cause considerable changes in the visual system of the cat [7, 9, 14, 22, 23, 36].

Besides, a sensorimotor task is not a single unit from the sensory control point of view. We would like to suggest that there are at least four components in the visuovestibular control of locomotion in cats:

Visual definition of the goal. This visual function is probably subject to development.

Keeping a straight course. Vestibular lesions do deteriorate this function [1]; it does not seem to require a permanent visual control in the intact animal.

Dynamic equilibrium. Vestibular lesions do deteriorate this function [20].

Visual paw guidance. This function is known to be subject to development [17].

These components can be experimentally dissociated by manipulating the task and the sensory inputs. We propose to investigate how vestibular inputs are involved in the control of each component and to what extent each of these two types of input is both necessary and sufficient. Necessary means that no other input can play the same role, while sufficient means that no other inputs are involved simultaneously. This leads to the following questions: What is the specific contribution of the vestibular apparatus to the control of each component of goal-directed locomotion in adults? Does the vestibular apparatus make any specific contribution to the development of these components? How does the visual system contribute to these functions during development and in adults?

The results which are presented here have been partly published in Marchand and Amblard [30], and will be further developed in Marchand et al. (in preparation).

Methods

The method selected here was designed to assess deficits in cats deprived bilaterally of their vestibular receptors [30] by manipulating the task and the animals' early sensory experience. The first group of 3 cats was neonatally deprived of the peripheral vestibular apparatus and tested in adulthood, along with 3 control cats. The second group of 3 subjects, reared under normal conditions, was tested in adulthood both before and after chronic bilateral labyrinthectomy. The third group of 4 cats, reared from birth under pseudo-random stroboscopic illumination (frequency from 0.5 to 3.5 flashes/s [2]), was also tested before lesion and 8 months after recovery under normal visual conditions.

The single index of locomotor performance used was the average speed of locomotion over a distance of 2 meters, on various support surfaces (Fig. 1) and under various visual conditions, which were chosen so as to be able to differentiate between positional and kinetic visual information. The two can be effectively dissociated by using stroboscopic illumination so that, for instance, stroboscopic illumination at 4 flashes/s provides only positional cues when compared to darkness, while normal illumination provides both positional and kinetic cues. This distinction seems to have functional implications [37]. Trials in darkness were preceded by an initial visual orientation cue, since a dim light remained on as long as the cat was on the starting platform. Three groups of supports were chosen to reflect the three main components of locomotion. A wide support was used to test the ability to keep a straight course, particularly in darkness; whereas a narrow support was used to set the direction and test the dynamic equilibrium; locomotion over an irregular support (horizontal ladder) was used in particular to investigate visual and visuovestibular paw guidance. Lastly, the double rail was used as a reference situation, in which neither orientation, nor dynamic equilibrium, nor visual guidance requirements were especially dominant. Within 12 experimental sessions, the various supports and visual conditions (darkness; stroboscopic illumination with 2, 4 or 8 flashes/s; and normal illumination) were randomly assigned in order to avoid any bias due to motivational changes.

Results

Extent of visual recovery from early and late vestibular deprivation

Igarashi and his colleagues [20] have reported recovery from unilateral but not from bilateral lesions of the labyrinth in adult squirrel monkeys. Similar results were found after unilateral labyrinthectomy in the adult cat [45]. Here we investigated whether, in the cat, any recovery occurs after a neonatal bilateral lesion. Likewise, we wondered whether an ability to keep course might be developed after an early lesion, for instance on the basis of visual cues. Lastly, a labyrinthectomized cat might have some postural difficulties when supported by only three paws when walking and guiding the fourth.

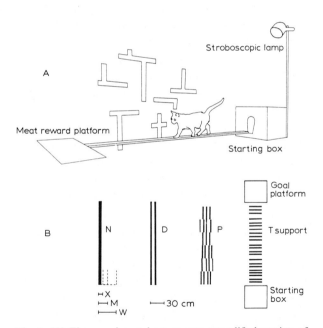

Fig. 1. (A) The experimental set-up was a modified version of that devised by Igarashi [18]. The cat had to walk from the starting box (right) to the meat-reward platform at the other end (left), over various supports. Time was measured by means of microswitches under each platform. Normal and flashlight bulbs were placed above the apparatus. (B) The crossing supports were either continuous supports of various widths (W, 40 cm; M, 20 cm; X, 9 cm; N, 6 cm), or a double rail (D, longitudinal rails 3 cm wide, 6 cm apart), or horizontal ladders (with flat transverse (T) rungs, 30 cm wide, irregularly spaced; or with the same rungs, 30 cm long, arranged parasagittally (P) in an irregular pattern).

Vestibular deficit

The vestibular deficit is shown in Fig. 2. In the absence of visual cues, as attested by the identical speeds of locomotion, keeping a straight course (wide support) appears to be equally (moderately) difficult for cats with lesions whether these were sustained neonatally or as adults. The same can be said of the control of dynamic balance, which is extremely deficient (as can be seen on the narrow supports), yet equally so in both groups.

Some supports (ladders, double rail, tilted platform) provided us with a test of tactile locomotion guidance (with the tilted W* support, the cats with

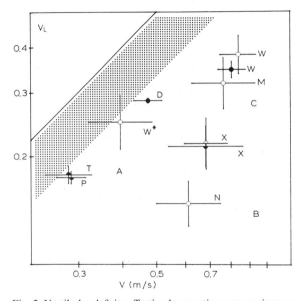

Fig. 2. Vestibular deficits affecting locomotion over various supports. Abscissae: average speed of locomotion in darkness of normal adult cats (with standard error bars). Ordinates: corresponding average speed in darkness of cats in which lesions were performed either at an early age or as adults. The diagonal line represents no deficit at all (same speed in both groups). The scale is logarithmic. The vertical distance to the diagonal of the point representing each support indicates the vestibular deficit, i.e. the speed ratio of cats with lesions to normal cats. Symbols represent cats in which lesions were performed at an early age (○) and as adults (●), respectively. Results are labelled according to paw adjustment requirements (group A: supports T, P, W*, and D: small, constant deficit), balance requirements (group B: narrow supports N and X; the greatest deficit), and straight-course requirements (group C: wide supports M and W; moderate deficit). W* means tilted wide support W (25° from horizontal). (From [30].)

lesions grappled on to the superior edge). These supports were crossed slowly by all the cats, but they differed from those requiring balance in that they revealed only a slight deficit in cats with lesions versus normal cats. This deficit (dotted area) was remarkably constant (speed about one third lower than normal) within this category of supports, regardless of the date of the lesion. This residual deficit on supports with few orientation or balance requirements may simply reflect a general slowing of motor activity as an adaptation to the lack of vestibular input. It does not seem to be reducible in cats which underwent lesions at an early age. In view of the lack of fully comparable situations, care should be taken here, however, in drawing conclusions.

Visual recovery

Fig. 3 shows the vestibular deficit under various visual conditions. For instance, the horizontal curve corresponding to the reference support D indicates that no increase at all occurred in the use of vision (with either static or kinetic cues) after labyrinthectomy.

In Fig. 3A, the traces coresponding to the cats with early lesions, on both wide and narrow supports, have a steeper slope than the traces corresponding to the cats which received lesions as adults. A better use of vision is therefore the main feature of the fuller recovery observed in labyrinthectomized cats when the lesion was performed at an early age. Their recovery included the ability to keep a straight course as well as to control balance, whereas after a lesion in adulthood, only the ability to keep a straight course can be recovered. The question thus arises as to whether visual recovery mainly involves information about velocity in the optical array or information about position and/or orientation.

It was observed, for example, in normal subjects (Fig. 4) that locomotion over wide supports was associated with greater use of positional cues (W support, upper trace, below 4 Hz), whereas locomotion over narrow supports seemed to involve mainly kinetic cues (N support, upper trace, above 4 Hz). In cats labyrinthectomized as adults, it can be seen

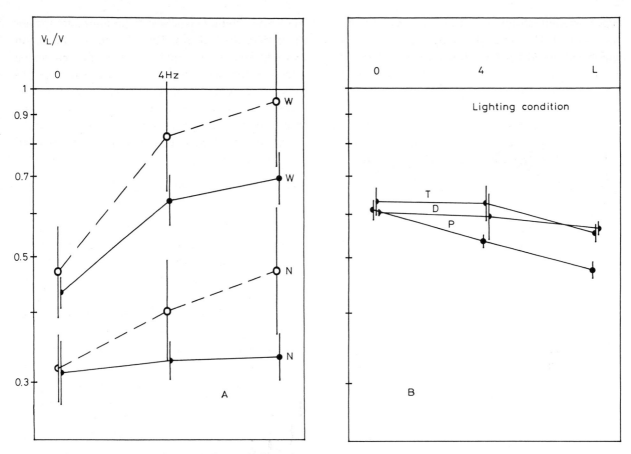

Fig. 3. Vestibular deficit (ratio of speeds before and after lesion) under various visual conditions, with standard error bars in control cats (normal rearing conditions) labyrinthectomized as adults (●), and ratio of speeds of cats labyrinthectomized at an early age versus control cats (○). Abscissae: visual conditions during testing; 0, darkness; 4, stroboscopic illumination frequency; L, continuous light. (A) Wide support (W) and narrow support (N). (B) Double support (D) and horizontal ladders (T and P).

(Fig. 3A) that recovery was mediated mainly by positional visual cues (0 to 4 Hz range), as far as locomotion over both wide and narrow supports was concerned. On the contrary, the use of kinetic visual cues remained approximately the same after as before the vestibular lesion (flat curves above 4 Hz), except over wide supports, where it increased, possibly indicating balance difficulties.

In addition, the fuller recovery observed in cats labyrinthectomized at an early age can be attributed primarily to the fact that they derived greater benefit from the positional cues, whereas they made only slightly better use of the kinetic cues. These cats used positional cues to reach a speed which was

nearly that of normal cats on wide supports, whereas on narrow supports they were still much slower than normal ones.

These results support the idea that in order to keep a straight course as well as to control dynamic balance, both early and late labyrinthectomized cats mainly compensate for the impairment by relying more than normal cats upon positional visual cues.

As regards paw guidance while walking over ladders, besides a possible tactile component, the main contribution seems to have been provided by positional cues (Fig. 4, supports P and T, NOR cats, PRE- and POST-OP, below 4 Hz), whereas kinetic cues contributed only to a lesser extent (same curves, above 8 Hz). Irregular supports of this kind, which require visual paw guidance, reveal the ex-

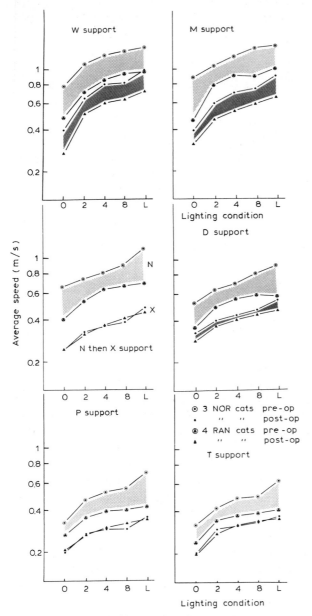

Fig. 4. Average speed of locomotion of normal (NOR) and strobe-reared (pseudo-random frequency, RAN) cats before (PRE-OP) and after (POST-OP) labyrinthectomy in adulthood. Abscissae: visual conditions during testing; 0, darkness; 2, 4, 8, stroboscopic illumination frequency; L, continuous light. Performances over each support are presented separately to allow comparison between groups.

istence of different visuovestibular interactions than those described above. Indeed, the use of vision seems to have been impaired rather than enhanced after the vestibular lesion (Fig. 3B). More specifically, on ladder P, which required lateral adjustments, the use of positional cues was found to decrease after the lesion, while on ladder T, which mainly involved distance adjustments, it remained constant.

Vestibular control of locomotion depends upon early visual experience

Visual deficits after strobe rearing

In Fig. 4, a comparison is made between the performance of strobe-reared and normal cats. The most striking feature of the strobe-reared cats' performances before the vestibular lesion was the fact that they were one fourth to one third lower than normal, regardless of the support and the visual conditions during the task (dotted areas). No selective impairment of balance was observed in the PRE-OP RAN cats. Paradoxially, this deficit, which must have been due to the visual rearing conditions, was found to exist even in darkness. Which nonvisual mechanism was impaired cannot be specified at this point. The deficit may however also have been associated with the visual definition of the goal, assuming that this visual component could precede the departure of the cat from the starting platform and the switching-off of the light. It should be noted that our strobe-reared cats exhibited pronounced myopia (− 5.70 ± 1.71), which may have interfered with their ability to locate a distant goal.

The main point of this type of early visual deprivation is obviously to suppress the mechanisms dealing with kinetic visual cues. It can be seen that this goal was achieved, since with supports (narrow support and ladders) on which these cues are particularly helpful for normal cats, strobe cats did not benefit from continuous illumination as compared with 8 Hz. Even in the POST-OP RAN group, which was exposed for eight months to normal illumination, no recovery of the use of kinetic visual cues was observed.

With increasing availability of positional visual information, the strobe cats improved their performances in the same proportion as normal cats, at least up to 8 Hz. This indicates that the use of positional information during locomotion is not particularly impaired by strobe-rearing, i.e. that a selective loss of kinetic cues has indeed occurred. This is further evidence for the possibility that the two types of cues may be processed independently.

Effects of strobe rearing on vestibular deficits occurring in adulthood

It can be seen from Fig. 4, that with most supports (ladders, double rail and beam), the performances of doubly deprived (POST-OP RAN) cats perfectly matched those of vestibular-deprived cats (POST-OP NOR) under all the visual conditions used. The deficit due to kinetic visual deprivation alone therefore did not increase the effect of the vestibular lesion alone as regards control of balance and paw guidance. The deficit due to strobe-rearing alone apparently affected the processing of vestibular signals, since it disappeared after the vestibular lesion.

On the other hand, on wide supports, the deficit due to strobe-rearing seems to increase the vestibular deficit (dashed areas). This suggests that deficits of visual and vestibular origin were independent and possibly involved in separate functions, such as visual definition of the goal and vestibular stabilization along a straight course, respectively. The possibility that the processing of kinesthetic cues may also have been disturbed, affecting the orientation of strobe-reared cats, may also help to explain these deficits.

Visual recovery

As we have just stated, the performances of strobe cats labyrinthectomized as adults showed the same pattern as a function of visual conditions as that of the control cats with lesions. More specifically, on every type of support, the curves showing the effects of visual conditions in the two groups were either superimposed or parallel. This shows that the role of vision in compensating for the vestibular deficit, which in adults mainly affected the ability to maintain a straight course, was practically independent of visual rearing conditions. It should be noted that this type of recovery was mediated by positional cues, whereas the strobe-reared cats' use of kinetic cues was still deficient (flat curves above 8 Hz).

Discussion

In the present study, the postural and locomotor deficits induced by early labyrinthectomy were found to be no greater than those observed in adult cats with recent lesions. The emergence of standing in kittens is not markedly delayed, moreover [30], and the static aspects of postural control are preserved when these kittens reach adulthood [29]. These and other data [5, 17] do not support the idea that the vestibular system might provide a fundamental reference for the development of spatially oriented behaviour. This seems to be especially true of behaviours requiring static information, such as that which might be provided by the otolith organs, whereas the specific vestibular contribution to dynamic behaviours probably feeds upon information from the vertical semicircular canals [19, 33].

As regards early visual experience, it is remarkable that strobe rearing should induce sensorimotor deficits which are both more prominent and more persistent than those associated with stroboscopic illumination in normal adults [2, 38]. Besides interfering with purely visual mechanisms [7] strobe rearing seems to also impair some processes involving vestibular cues, since normal and strobe-reared cats give similar performances, for instance in dynamic balance and paw visual guidance, when deprived of vestibular information as adults. Kinetic visual cues thus seem to play a prominent role in the development of spatially oriented behaviours (including some vestibular controls), with the exception of dynamic balance, which is not impaired by strobe rearing. Assuming that the vestibular system plays a facilitatory role in locomotor rhythm (labyrinthectomized cats are slower on average than controls), the low speed of strobe cats with intact vestibular receptors might be attributable to kinetic visual cues involved in calibrating the vestibular controls. The finding that vestibular significance benefits from visual information has already been reported in several studies [10, 21, 24].

Compensatory processes can also reveal differences between the vestibular and visual channels: although the strobe-induced deficit is in no way compensated by vestibular cues, visual cues, especially positional ones, do contribute considerably to compensating for some components of locomotor control in animals with vestibular lesions received either early or later in life.

The main component of locomotion involving a specific vestibular contribution is dynamic equilibrium [15, 20, 30]. This body-centred (proprioceptive) role of the vestibular system was reflected here in the particularly poor performance of labyrinthectomized cats on narrow supports. Very little recovery occurred in the animals, whatever the date of their lesions. This type of vestibulomotor mechanism therefore seems to be both specific and independent of visual inputs, both in adults and during maturation, even in strobe-reared cats. Although kinetic visual information has been shown to be especially involved in the control of static balance, at least in man [3, 39], this type of visual contribution to dynamic balance in cats seems to play only a minor role, even in the absence of the corresponding vestibular mechanism.

Another aspect of the vestibular contribution to walking intervenes in the ability to keep a straight course. Walking tests on various species [16, 18], provide very sensitive indicators of vestibular imbalance. The difficulties encountered by a subject deprived bilaterally of vestibular inputs should not be attributed to a lack of postural tonus [27], but may bear some relationship to the coordination between tonic neck and vestibular reflexes [26, 28]. If this is so, these locomotor disorders will be related to head movements. Additionally, on an open surface, they might express the balance deficit demonstrated above on narrow supports. The compensation for impairment of this proprioceptive function probably involves a distinct component of locomotion,

namely a repeated visual definition of the goal, which implies that vision plays an ex-proprioceptive role [25]. Unlike the vestibular deficit itself, the visual compensation depends upon early sensory experience: it is enhanced in early labyrinthectomized cats, and less efficient in strobe-reared cats.

The last component which seems to involve vestibular cues is the control of paw placing while walking over an irregular support. This function apparently requires the combined and simultaneous intervention of vestibular and visual mechanisms, since the absence of vestibular cues impairs visual control (Fig. 3B). At this stage in our investigations, it is not yet clear however whether this complementarity involves oculomotor [4] or postural mechanisms. Hein and his colleagues [17] however found no visual placing deficit in hand-supported early labyrinthectomized kittens.

Taken as a whole, the results presented here support the idea that dynamic balance is the component of locomotion to which the vestibular system contributes most specifically. Balance was the most impaired part of the performance of cats with vestibular lesions, even when these cats were left to recover and tested under normal visual conditions. The balance component was also the least dependent upon visual conditions for its maturation in the kitten. Deficits in other components, such as keeping a straight course or paw guidance, may have partly stemmed from the balance deficit. Visual recovery mainly consisted of an improvement in the control of the general direction of locomotion, provided no balance constraints were imposed. However, in the absence of vision, no particular component of locomotion was found to be differentially recovered in early versus late vestibular-deprived cats.

Acknowledgement

We are grateful to Dr. Jessica Blanc for English version.

References

[1] André-Thomas (1940), *Équilibre et Équilibration*, Masson, Paris, 567 pp.

[2] Amblard, B. and Crémieux, J. (1979) Visually guided reaching in the cat reared in fixed or random frequency stroboscopic light. *Neurosci. Lett.*, 15: 9–14.

[3] Amblard, B., Crémieux, J., Marchand, A.R. and Carblanc, A. (1985) Lateral orientation and stabilization of human stance: static versus dynamic visual cues. *Exp. Brain Res.*, 61: 21–37.

[4] Baker J., Goldberg, J., Peterson, B. and Schor, R. (1982) Oculomotor reflexes after semicircular canal plugging in cats. *Brain Res.*, 252: 151–155.

[5] Blakemore, C. and Papaioannou, J. (1974) Does the vestibular apparatus play a role in the development of the visual system? *J. Physiol. London*, 236: 373–385.

[6] Clément, G., Magnin, M. (1983) Visual influence on postural control in the cat. *Exp. Brain Res.*, 52: 429–438.

[7] Crémieux, J., Orban, G.A., Duysens, J. and Amblard (1987) Response properties of area 17 neurons in cats reared in stroboscopic illumination. *J. Neurophysiol.*, 57: 1511–1535.

[8] Crémieux, J., Veraart, C. and Wanet-Defalque, M.C. (1986) Effects of deprivation of vision and vibrissae on goal-directed locomotion in cats. *Exp. Brain Res.*, 65: 229–234.

[9] Cynader, M. and Chernenko, G. (1976) Abolition of direction selectivity in the visual cortex of the cat. *Science*, 193: 504–505.

[10] Dichgans, J., Schmidt, C.L. and Graf, W. (1973) Visual input improves the speedometer function of the vestibular nuclei in the goldfish. *Exp. Brain Res.*, 18: 319–322.

[11] Diener, H.C., Dichgans, J., Guschlbauer, B. and Bacher, M. (1986) Role of visual and static vestibular influences on dynamic posture control. *Human Neurobiol.*, 5: 105–113.

[12] Dow, R.S. (1938) The effects of unilateral and bilateral labyrinthectomy in monkey, baboon and chimpanzee. *Am. J. Physiol.*, 121: 392–399.

[13] Dufour-Mallet, A., Caston, J. and Parrad, J. (1979) Ontogeny of equilibrium behavior in the rat, with special reference to the influence of vision and training. *Physiol. Behav.*, 22/5: 883–894.

[14] Flandrin, J.M., Kennedy, H. and Amblard, B. (1976) Effects of stroboscopic rearing on the binocularity and directionality of cat superior colliculus neurons. *Brain Res.*, 101: 576–581.

[15] Fregly, A.R. (1974) Vestibular ataxia and its measurement in man. In H.H. Kornhüber (Ed.), *Handbook of Sensory Physiology*, Vol. 6(2), *Vestibular System*, Springer-Verlag, Berlin/Heidelberg/New York, pp. 321–360.

[16] Fukuda, T. (1959) The stepping test: two phases of the labyrinthine reflex. *Acta Otolaryngol. Stockholm*, 50: 26.

[17] Hein, A., Vital-Durand, F., Salinger, W. and Diamond, R. (1979) Eye movements initiate visual-motor development in the cat. *Science*, 204: 1321–1322.

[18] Igarashi, M. (1974) Squirrel monkey platform runway test. *Acta Otolaryngol. Stockholm*, 77: 284–288.

[19] Igarashi, M., Alford, B.R., Watanabe, T. and Maxian, P.M. (1970) Direction of ataxic gait after unilateral partial destruction of the vestibular system in squirrel monkeys. *Laryngoscope*, 80: 896–914.

[20] Igarashi, M., Watanabe, T. and Maxian, P.M. (1970) Dynamic equilibrium in squirrel monkeys after unilateral and bilateral labyrinthectomy. *Acta Otolaryngol. Stockholm*, 69: 247–253.

[21] Kennedy, H., Courjon, J.H. and Flandrin, J.M. (1982) Vestibulo-ocular reflex and optokinetic nystagmus in adult cats reared in stroboscopic illumination. *Exp. Brain Res.*, 48: 279–287.

[22] Kennedy, H., Flandrin, J.M. and Amblard, B. (1980) Afferent visual pathways and receptive field properties of superior colliculus neurons in stroboscopically reared cats. *Neurosci. Lett.*, 19: 283–288.

[23] Kennedy, H. and Orban, G.A. (1983) Visual cortical neurons in cats reared in stroboscopic illumination. *J. Neurophysiol.*, 49: 686–704.

[24] Lacour, M., Vidal, P.P. and Xerri, C. (1981) Visual influences on vestibulospinal reflexes during vertical motion in normal and hemilabyrinthectomized monkeys. *Exp. Brain Res.*, 43: 383–394.

[25] Lee, D.N. (1977) The functions of vision. In H.L. Pick, E. Saltzman (Eds.), *Modes of Perceiving and Processing Information*, Erlbaum Press, Hillsdale N.J., pp. 159–170.

[26] Lindsay, K.W., Roberts, T.D.M. and Rosenberg, J.R. (1976) Asymmetric tonic labyrinth reflexes and their interaction with neck reflexes in the decerebrate cat. *J. Physiol. London*, 261: 583–601.

[27] Magnus, R. (1924) *Körperstellung*, Springer-Verlag, Berlin, 740 pp.

[28] Manzoni, D., Pompeiano, O. and Stampacchia, G. (1979) Tonic cervical influences on posture and reflex movements. *Arch. Ital. Biol.*, 117: 81–110.

[29] Marchand, A. and Amblard, B. (1979) Contrôle postural chez les chats délabyrinthés à la naissance. *Agressologie*, 20: 201–202.

[30] Marchand, A.R. and Amblard, B. (1984) Locomotion in adult cats with early vestibular deprivation: visual cue substitution. *Exp. Brain Res.*, 54: 395–405.

[31] Marchand, A.R., Amblard, B. and Crémieux, J. Early sensory determinants of locomotor speed in adult cats: II Effects of stroberearing on vestibulo–motor function. *Physiol. Behav.*, in press.

[32] Mellier, D. and Jouen, F. (1986) Remarques à propos des déplacements chez le bébé aveugle. *Psychol. Franc.*, 31/1: 43–47

[33] Money, K.E. and Scott, J.W. (1962) Functions of separate

sensory receptors of non-auditory labyrinth of the cat. *Am. J. Physiol.*, 202: 1211–1220.

[34] Nakao, C. and Brookhart, J.M. (1967) Effects of labyrinthine and visual deprivation on postural stability. *Physiologist*, 10: 259.

[35] Nashner, L.M., Black, F.O. and Wall, C. (1982) Adaptation to altered support and visual conditions during stance: patients with vestibular deficits. *J. Neurosci.*, 2: 536–544.

[36] Orban, G.A., Kennedy, H., Maes, H. and Amblard, B. (1978) Cats reared in stroboscopic illumination: velocity characteristics of area 18 neurons. *Arch. Ital. Biol.*, 116: 413–419.

[37] Paillard, J. and Amblard, B. (1985) Static versus kinetic visual cues for the processing of spatial relationships. In D.J. Ingle, M. Jeannerod and D.N. Lee (Eds.), *Brain Mechanisms and Spatial Vision*, Martinus Nijhoff, Dordrecht/Boston/Lancaster, pp. 299–330.

[38] Pasternak, T., Schumer, R.A., Gizzi, M.S. and Movshon, J.A. (1985) Abolition of visual cortical direction sensitivity affects visual behavior in cats. *Exp. Brain Res.*, 61: 214–217.

[39] Paulus, W.M., Straube, A. and Brandt, Th. (1984) Visual stabilization of posture. Physiological stimulus characteristics and clinical aspects. *Brain*, 107: 1143–1163.

[40] Putkonen, P.T.S., Courjon, J.H. and Jeannerod, M. (1977) Compensation of postural effects of hemilabyrinthectomy in the cat: a sensory substitution process? *Exp. Brain Res.*, 28: 249–257.

[41] Rademaker, G.G.J. (1935) *Réactions Labyrinthiques et Équilibre; l'Ataxie Labyrinthique*, Masson, Paris, 262 pp.

[42] Soechting, J.F. and Berthoz, A. (1979) Dynamic role of vision in the control of posture in man. *Exp. Brain Res.*, 36: 551–561.

[43] Villablanca, J.R. and Olmstead, C.E. (1979) Neurological development of kittens. *Dev. Psychobiol.*, 12: 101–127.

[44] Windle, W.F. and Fish, M.W. (1932) The development of the vestibular righting reflex in the cat. *J. Comp. Neurol.*, 54: 89–96.

[45] Xerri, C. and Lacour, M. (1980) Compensation des déficits posturaux et cinétiques après neurectomie vestibulaire unilatérale chez le chat. *Acta Otolaryngol. Stockholm*, 90: 414–424.

SECTION V

Vestibular Control of Posture

O. Pompeiano and J.H.J. Allum (Eds.)
Progress in Brain Research, Vol. 76
© 1988 Elsevier Science Publishers B.V. (Biomedical Division)

Overview

B.W. Peterson

Department of Physiology, Northwestern University Medical School, 303 East Chicago Avenue, Chicago, IL 60611, U.S.A.

Collectively the contributions in this section examined the complex pattern of sensorimotor coordination that serves to maintain standing posture in humans. The topics ranged from electrically activated reflex contractions of leg muscles following the application of galvanic stimuli which would activate labyrinthine afferents (Chapter 25) to the reorganization of postural mechanisms upon exposure to a microgravity environment (Chapter 27). The central focus of the session, however, was the four papers dealing with postural reactions of humans to perturbing stimuli in a normal gravitional environment (Chapters 21-24). The presentation and discussion of these papers led to the resolution or clarification of a number of issues that have arisen in this field in recent years. The following discussion therefore concentrates upon these issues.

The first issue concerns the nature of postural reactions. Publications by Nashner, Black and colleagues in the past have emphasized the discreteness of postural responses to perturbations in the subject's sagittal plane. In particular they identified two 'postural strategies' that appear under different stimulus conditions: (1) Small, relatively slow translations of the support surface elicit an 'ankle strategy' in which muscle activity appears first in ankle muscles and then ascends the body. Nashner and his colleagues claim that the ankle strategy relies primarily on ankle proprioceptive input and does not require vestibular function for its execution. (2) A 'hip strategy' appears in response to translations when the subject stands on a narrow beam, *preventing him from using ankle forces to move the centre of mass of the body* or in response to platform rotations. It is a more complex movement involving approximately simultaneous, coordinated activation of body and neck musculature, which produces translation of the pelvic girdle with head held stable in space. In their papers at this session (Chapters 21 and 23), Drs. Nashner and Black sought to correct the impression that the ankle and hip strategies occur in pure form in an all-or-nothing fashion. They emphasize instead that hybrid mixtures of the two strategies are the rule and that subjects tend to grade continuously from ankle strategy to hip strategy to stepping responses as the velocity and amplitude of translational perturbation increases. The group therefore places itself in agreement with other workers who have emphasized the continuously graded nature of postural responses. In discussions after the session, however, Dr. Nashner maintained that careful attention to the pattern of muscle activity onset times still reveals discrete components within these mixed responses, even when the direction of perturbations is shifted away from the sagittal plane.

In his presentation (Chapter 24) Dr. Allum indicated that he never observed ankle strategy type responses in either normals or in patients with peripheral vestibular deficits. In the discussion Dr. Nashner agreed that the ankle strategy would not be seen in normals under the experimental conditions used by Dr. Allum – rotational perturbations of the platform with the subjects initially leaning backwards to facilitate detection of early reflex responses in the tibialis anterior muscle. Under these conditions a hip or mixed ankle–hip response pattern would be expected. Thus the two groups are in agreement for situations in which both have data from normals. It remains for others to check the observations of the Nashner group that pure ankle strategies are elicited in response to small, slow translational perturbations.

A second issue concerned the role of vestibular signals in triggering and/or modulating the amplitude of postural response. Disagreements in this area were not resolved but the issue was clarified. Dr. Allum reported that he and Emily Keshner observed in patients with bilateral vestibular deficits a highly significant reduction in the stabilizing activity of the tibialis anterior muscle which appears at 120 ms when the support surface is rotated backwards. They concluded that vestibular response to rotational perturbation of the head (which can be recorded 20 ms after the onset of surface rotation) played a major role in initiating postural responses or, at least, in modulating proprioceptively triggered responses. As indicated above, their paradigm evokes a hip strategy response in both normals and vestibular-deficit patients (although the two groups differ in their description of the relation of head and hip motions). Interestingly, Dr. Black reported that bilateral vestibular patients are not able to employ a hip strategy to maintain balance (Chapter 23). This would tend to disagree with Dr. Allum's conclusion. Furthermore, Dr. Nashner and his colleagues remain unconvinced that vestibular reflexes play a causative role in postural reactions. They emphasize instead the subject's requirement to stabilize the head during a hip strategy and the switching of strategies that occurs in vestibular patients.

Dr. Diener, in the experiments described in his contribution (Chapter 22), also tried to address the role of vestibular input by having the subjects execute a postural task with the head tilted backward, thus altering the response of canal and otolith afferents to head rotations. It was pointed out, however, that the receptors continued to respond in this situation and presumably the central nervous system is able to interpret the altered signals correctly. Thus

Dr. Diener's careful documentation that transient postural responses are not altered by head position changes or by ischaemic removal of foot and ankle sensation do not necessarily imply that vestibular reflexes are unimportant in eliciting postural responses.

Conversely, Dr. Tokita's presentation (Chapter 25) provided additional evidence that activation of vestibular afferents can lead to strong electromyographic activity in limb muscles in standing subjects. Also Dr. Diener could confirm Dr. Allum's results that stabilizing ankle muscle activity is reduced in patients with bilateral vestibular deficits. Since these experiments were carried out with subjects standing upright, the initial body position appears not to alter the role of vestibular influences on postural control in standing humans. At the moment the most parsimonious conclusion is that vestibular reflexes do play an important role, at least in the hip strategy. Further experiments will be needed to resolve this key question.

Two important components of future work will be obtaining a complete biomechanical model of standing posture and observing postural reactions in planes other than the sagittal plane. The model will be especially important in interpreting the complex rearrangement of postural responses reported by Drs. Lestienne and Gurfinkel (Chapter 27) in microgravity situations. Their observations provided clear evidence that postural reactions are disrupted by the transition from $1.0 \times g$ to $0 \times g$ and back. As Dr. Lestienne pointed out, however, $0 \times g$ not only alters vestibular otolith signals but also body biomechanics. An obvious and important alteration is the difference in static posture in microgravity. More subtle but equally important are changes in joint loading, which not only alter musculoskeletal kinematics but also proprioceptive responses. Given the need to interpret results from a relatively small number of subjects in space flight studies, it would seem especially crucial to develop models with sufficient sophistication to predict these changes in microgravity, and to develop hypotheses to guide the design and interpretation of experiments.

O. Pompeiano and J.H.J. Allum (Eds.)
Progress in Brain Research, Vol. 76
© 1988 Elsevier Science Publishers B.V. (Biomedical Division)

CHAPTER 21

Head-trunk movement coordination in the standing posture

L.M. Nashner, C.L. Shupert and F.B. Horak

Neurological Sciences Institute, Good Samaritan Hospital and Medical Center, 1120 N.W. 20th Avenue, Portland, OR 97209, U.S.A.

The coordination of head and trunk movement during postural sway in the anterior/posterior plane was examined in three normal adults. Postural sway about the ankles or hips was elicited in two ways: (1) In free-fall sway trials, the subject passively fell forward while the feet remained in place on the support surface (ankle sway). (2) In perturbed sway trials, subjects stood on either a flat surface (ankle sway) or a narrow beam (hip sway) which was displaced backwards at the onset of each trial. In all cases, postural responses were initiated before significant horizontal head motion was recorded. For subjects swaying about the ankles, changes in neck angle followed changes in ankle angle as the effect of the postural movement was propagated up the body. Neck muscle activation for ankle sway thus appeared to be elicited by neck stretch resulting from the postural correction. These results suggest that head and body motions may be controlled independently during active postural movements for ankle sway. For subjects swaying about the hip, however, changes in neck and hip angles were coordinated to approximately stabilize the rotational position of the head, and neck and hip muscles were activated simultaneously. These results, in contrast to those for ankle sway, suggest that control of head and body motion is coordinated on a feedforward basis during hip sway.

Introduction

Standing in equilibrium involves sensing the position of the body's centre of mass and moving the body to adjust the position of the centre of mass over the base of support provided by the feet. Sensing the state of equilibrium is a complex task. Combinations of visual, vestibular, and somatosensory inputs are required, because no single modality directly senses the position of the centre of mass. We use the terms 'sensory organization' to describe the process of combining sensory information from a variety of sources into the complex sense of equilibrium, and 'movement coordination' to describe the coordinated muscular activations which move the body's centre of mass over the base of support.

Previous studies examined the effects on sensory organization of exposing normal subjects[1–3] and patients with peripheral vestibular deficits [4–6] to altered visual and support surface conditions. These studies have demonstrated that the sensory organization of normal subjects is highly adaptable. Normal subjects are able to maintain equilibrium despite unreliable sensory information from either the surface on which they are standing, or their visual world, or both. Vestibular patients, in contrast, demonstrate two types of abnormalities when presented with unreliable sensory information. The first type, which we refer to as *sensory loss*, is characterized by automatic postural responses which are delayed and/or too weak to maintain balance when visual and support surface information is unreliable. Patients with this type of abnormality appear unable to use vestibular information alone to control posture. The second type, *abnormal sensory selection*, is characterized by automatic postural responses to functionally inappropriate sensory information during exposure to inaccurate feedback

---

Abbreviations: AP, anteroposterior; EMG, electromyograph; LED, light-emitting diode.

from the support surface and/or visual surround. Patients with this type of abnormality appear to ignore reliable sensory information from alternative sources and are therefore very unstable in sensory-conflict situations. Based on a comparison of posturographic and clinical findings, we have postulated that distorted vestibular signals may be one cause for the sensory selection problems of the vestibular patients [5–7].

Sensory organization and movement coordination interact during postural control. One cause for interaction is that a given shift in the position of the body's centre of mass can be accomplished using differing combinations of ankle, hip, and head motions [8]. Depending on the combination of body segment motions, the same centre of body mass shift will elicit very different combinations of somatosensory, vestibular, and visual inputs. Nevertheless, these different combinations of sensory input must be correctly interpreted if balance is to be maintained.

A previous report suggested that fixing the rotational orientation of the head in relation to gravity during postural movements simplifies the organization of sensory inputs [9]. Restricting head rotations provides a stable vestibular gravitational reference under all body movement conditions. In the present project, we have observed the body and head motions of subjects performing postural tasks with different movement patterns in order to examine how normal subjects control head position during postural movements.

Methods

Measuring body movements and muscular activations

Body and head motions in the AP plane were measured by three independent means: (1) AP sway about the ankles was measured by a platform-mounted potentiometer attached to the hips with light rods and belt. (2) The velocity of AP head rotation was measured with an angular rate sensor (Watson, Model ARS-C141-1A) attached to a snugly fitting bicycle helmet. The head rotational acceleration and angle were calculated by sampling the angular rate signal (500/s) and performing numerical differentiation and integration, respectively. (3) Body segment positions in the AP plane (3 mm resolution, 100 samples/s) were measured using an opto-electrical movement analyser (Watsmart, Northern Digital). LED targets were placed on the support surface, lateral 5th metatarsal, lateral maleolus, lateral condole, lateral trochanter, acromion, ear lobe, and front and back of the helmet. Neck (atlanto-occipital pivot), hip, knee, and ankle angles were calculated from the LED information.

In addition to AP sway motions, the forces exerted by each foot on the surface were measured by two adjacent 23 cm × 46 cm strain-gauge force-plates incorporated into the support surface. Each forceplate measured AP ankle torque and horizontal AP shear force (see [10]).

Patterns of muscular activation were measured by recording the surface EMG activities of anterior tibialis, gastrocnemius, quadriceps (rectus femoris), hamstrings, lumbar paraspinal, rectus abdominus, upper trapezius (neck extensor), and sternocleido-mastoid (neck flexor) muscles using silver–silver chloride electrode pairs. Raw EMG signals were band-pass filtered (100 and 5000 Hz), full-wave rectified, and then low-pass filtered (0–100 Hz) prior to sampling by digital computer (500/s). EMG latencies were determined from individual records. Patterns of activation were analysed by ensemble averaging groups of trials.

Experimental protocol

Postural sway in the AP plane was induced in two ways (Fig. 1):

(1) In free-fall sway trials, the position of the feet was fixed, while the upper trunk and head accelerated forward under the influence of gravity. Free-fall sway was enhanced by sway-referencing the support surface, i.e. rotating the support surface about an axis colinear with the ankle joints to track the AP sway signal provided by the sway potentiometer [11]. Sway-referencing reduces any passive stability

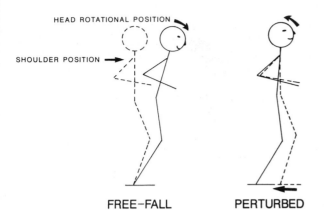

HEAD ROTATIONAL POSITION

SHOULDER POSITION

FREE-FALL   PERTURBED

Fig. 1. Stick figures comparing the patterns of body movement during free-fall and perturbed sway.

provided by the inherent stiffness of the ankle joints [1, 12] and delays active postural responses [4].

(2) In perturbed sway trials, the upper body and head were initially stationary, while the feet were displaced backward by unexpectedly translating the support surface. Two velocities of support surface translation were used; slow perturbations at 15 cm/s for 250 ms and fast perturbations at 30 cm/s for 345 ms.

Subjects were required to alter their patterns of corrective postural responses to perturbations by standing on two different lengths of support surface [8]. The normal support surface was 45 cm, i.e. longer than the feet. The short support surface was 10 cm, approximately one-half the length of a normal adult foot.

Corrective postural movements of the head and body, and associated EMG and forceplate signals, were examined in three subjects ranging in age from 22 to 43 years. All were screened for absence of vestibular and neurological disorders. Each subject was exposed to support-surface perturbations. On the normal-length support surface, both slow and fast translations were used in separate groups of trials. On the short support surface, only the slow perturbations were used. One of the three subjects participated in the free-fall sway trials.

During all types of trials, data was sampled by digital computer (500/s for EMGs, forceplate, and potentiometer signals; 100/s for Watsmart LED signals) and stored for later off-line analysis.

Results

Muscular responses to sway

On the normal-length support surface, EMG responses to free-fall sway (Fig. 2a) were similar to the 'ankle strategy' elicited by slow translations of the support surface in previous studies by Horak and Nashner [8]. In both situations, activity began in the gastrocnemius and radiated proximally to the hamstrings and paraspinal synergists. Translating the normal support surface more rapidly resulted in a complex activation of antagonists (rectus abdominus and quadriceps) resembling a mixed 'ankle' and 'hip' pattern (Fig. 2B). During slow translations of the short surface, in contrast, abdominal and quadriceps muscles were the predominantly active muscles as for the previously reported 'hip strategy' (Fig. 2C).

EMG responses to free-fall and small (not shown) translations of the normal support surface are similar to the 'ankle' response pattern described previously [13]. This muscle response pattern moves the body's centre of mass backward by exerting torque against the support surface and rotating the body backward about the ankle joints while maintaining the knee and hip joint angles approximately fixed [8]. On the short support surface, in contrast, activation of the opposing trunk and thigh muscles moves the centre of body mass backward by rapidly flexing the body forward about the hips and generating horizontal shear force against the support surface. This is the so-called 'hip' response pattern. The complex activation of antagonist muscles during rapid translations of the normal-length support surface moves the centre of mass backward by combining the above described ankle and hip joint motions.

Head and body movements prior to postural responses

Prior to the onset of compensatory responses to

246

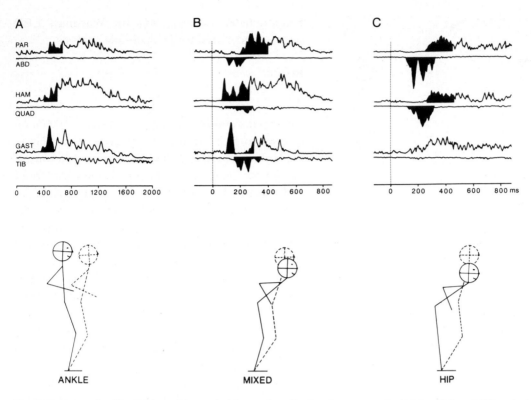

Fig. 2. Patterns of ankle, thigh, and lower trunk muscle activation in response to (A) free-fall and (B) perturbed sway on normal and (C) short-length support surfaces. Gastrocnemius (GAST), hamstrings (HAM), and paraspinal (PAR) records are produced by full-wave rectifying and smoothing surface electrode recordings. Anterior tibialis (TIB), quadriceps (QUAD), and abdominal (ABD) recordings are shown inverted below their respective antagonists. The dotted lines in parts B and C show onsets of support surface translations. Note that the time base in part A is compressed to include twice the time as parts B and C.

free-fall sway, trajectories of forward shoulder displacement and nose-down head rotation were approximately parabolic, although the associated accelerations were too small to measure (Fig. 3A). During both the slow and rapid perturbed sway trials, little if any shoulder or head acceleration was noted during the 90–100 ms latent period prior to the onset of active postural responses (Fig. 3B and 3C).

Head and body movements during postural responses

During responses to free-fall sway on the normal-length support surface, the earliest shoulder and head accelerations followed gastrocnemius activations by 200–300 ms (heavy arrow, Fig. 3A). These

accelerations indicated the time required for the activated leg muscles to generate force against the support surface, and for the propagation of that force to the upper body and head.

When subjects used the ankle response pattern to compensate sway following free fall, trapezius activations were delayed by an average of 292 ± 62 ms relative to the gastrocnemius. These delayed neck muscle activations coincided with the onset of the backward shoulder acceleration, and therefore could have been reactions to local neck stretch inputs.

Despite the fact that movements of the head in space differed during free-fall and perturbed sway trials on the normal-length support surface (Fig. 1), the relative timing of leg, trunk, and head muscle

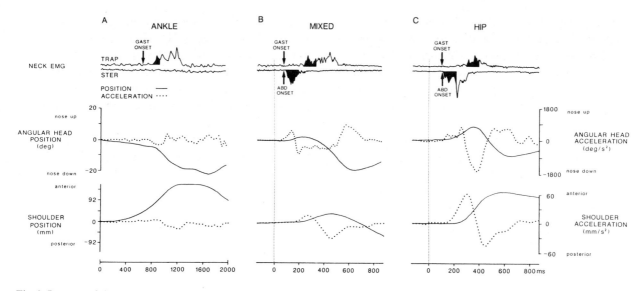

Fig. 3. Patterns of shoulder and head motions and neck muscle activations during active responses to (A) free-falling, (B) large translations of the normal-length support surface, and (C) small translations of the short-length surface. Shoulder linear position (heavy lines) and acceleration (dotted lines) are shown for the AP direction. Head rotational position (heavy lines) and acceleration (dotted lines) are shown for the nose-up direction. Trapezius (TRAP, a neck extensor) and sternocleidomastoid (STER, a neck flexor) activations are shown in the same format as used in Fig. 2.

activations were similar, when subjects used pure ankle response patterns.

The spatial and temporal properties of leg, trunk, and neck muscle activations differed dramatically when subjects on the shortened support surface used the hip response pattern to compensate sway. Now, abdominal (98 ± 11), quadriceps (88 ± 11), and sternocleidomastoid (98 ± 9) activations were approximately simultaneous. Thus, when subjects used the hip response pattern, activations of neck muscles anticipated rather than followed the onset of head accelerations (Fig. 3C).

To determine whether fixation of a visual target influenced neck muscle responses during hip response patterns, we repeated the shortened support surface trials with the subjects' eyes closed. Coordination of leg, trunk, and neck muscles was similar during the eyes open and closed trials.

Rapid translation of the normal support surface activated gastrocnemius (89 ± 8 ms) and abdominal (87 ± 14 ms) muscles approximately simultaneously, producing a mixture of ankle and hip postural movements. In these trials, we observed a

mixture of anticipatory and reactive neck muscle responses, with anticipatory responses related to the hip component of the movement and reactive responses related to the ankle component. During the initial phase of the response, sternocleidomastoid (85 ± ms) activations coincided with abdominals and anticipated the forward shoulder and nose-up head accelerations (Fig. 3B). Trapezius activations, in contrast, were delayed until 288 ± 51 ms, lagging gastrocnemius by approximately the same amount as during the free-fall sway trials.

Control of head orientation

The above results describe two primary and one mixed pattern of leg and trunk muscle activation and associated body segment motions. Our examination of neck muscle EMGs also showed two primary modes of activation, one anticipating and the other reacting to motions of the head. With both response patterns, leg and/or trunk muscles were activated within 100 ms, whereas disruption of the head rotational position lagged these activations by an additional 100 to 200 ms. When the hip pattern was used, thigh, lower trunk, and neck muscle activations were simultaneous, with the neck component anticipating the disruption of head position by 100–150 ms. When the ankle pattern was used, in contrast, neck muscle activations were delayed until onset of the head perturbation.

Our final objective was to determine the relative effectiveness of anticipatory and reactive neck muscle responses in stabilizing the rotational position of the head. We used angle–angle plots of ankle, hip, and neck joint trajectories to assess the rotational stability of the head. During ankle pattern responses to free-fall and small perturbations on the normal-length support surface, movement trajectories in hip angle–neck angle space were approximately circular (Fig. 4A). Additional plots of ankle versus hip angles (not shown) also produced similar trajectories. During both eyes open and eyes closed trials on the shortened support surface, the hip pattern of postural movement produced approximately diagonal straight-line trajectories in neck angle–hip angle space (Fig. 4B).

To fix the orientation of the head during AP swaying, neck rotations must be equal and opposite to the sum of the ankle and hip joint rotations. If plotted in hip–neck angle space, therefore, coordinated motions of the head and body with the head orientation fixed would produce approximately 45° diagonal straight lines, similar to those observed during the hip movement pattern (Fig. 4B). The approximately circular trajectories produced by the ankle movement pattern, in contrast, indicate that head and body motions are approximately 90° out of phase. Phase shifts of 90° would be produced with the head moving passively on the trunk.

Discussion

Two postural movement patterns compensate body sway

Standing in equilibrium requires that the body's centre of mass be positioned within the area of foot support. When the equilibrium position is disturbed by perturbations or destabilizing effects of gravity, two primary postural movement patterns are used by normal subjects. Contractions of leg and lower trunk muscles in a distal-to-proximal sequence move the body's centre of mass by exerting

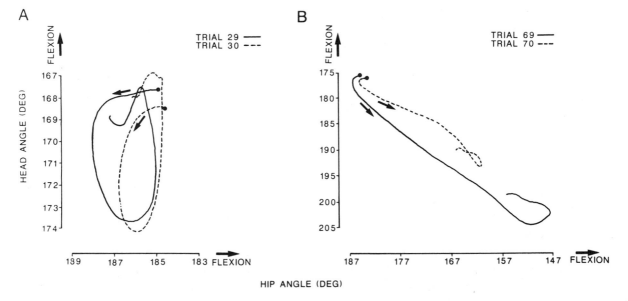

Fig. 4. Plots of head angles (vertical axes) versus hip angles (horizontal axes) for active ankle (A) and hip (B) patterns of postural movement.

torque against the support surface and rotating the body primarily about the ankle joints. Contraction of the antagonistic thigh and lower trunk muscles in a proximal-to-distal sequence shifts the body's centre of mass backwards by rapidly flexing the hips, which generates horizontal shear force against the support surface [8].

Coordinated and independent control of head position

Our present results indicate that, during active postural movements about the hip, trunk and head motions are coordinated approximately to stabilize the rotational position of the head in relation to gravity (Fig. 4B). Stabilization of the head is accomplished on a feedforward basis by the simultaneous activation of hip and neck flexor muscles. Activation of neck flexors anticipates the nose-up head displacements which occur as the mechanical effects of hip flexion propagate to the upper body. These results suggest that, independent of visual influences, control of head and body motions is coordinated during active hip postural movements.

When free-falls and small perturbations on a normal-length support surface allow subjects to compensate sway with the ankle movement pattern, active correction of the rotational position of the head can be delayed until the mechanical effects of rotating the body backward about the ankles propagate to the upper body. During these much slower leg and trunk postural movements, the rotational position of the head is not as well stabilized (Fig. 4A). Thus, our results suggest that head and body motions may be controlled independently during active ankle postural movements.

Other investigators reported simultaneous activations of leg and neck muscles during active responses to backward translations of a normal-length support surface [14]. These authors, however, did not determine whether their subjects used ankle or mixed ankle–hip movement patterns. Their observations are similar to our mixed ankle–hip response patterns, which often result when larger displacements of a normal-length support surface are

used. In other studies, head accelerations occurred within 10–50 ms of rapid support surface tilts, suggesting that local feedback information might be available prior to the onset of automatic postural responses under some perturbation conditions [15, 16]. Differences between horizontal translations and rotations of the platform surface, however, probably account for the much earlier onset of head acceleration. The rapid support surface tilts in the studies by Allum and his coworkers caused large vertical head accelerations with latencies as small as 10 ms. Upward vertical accelerations would cause nose-down head rotations, because the bulk of the head mass is in front of the neck pivot joint. Such head rotations are reported by Allum and his colleagues [15, 16].

The interaction of anticipatory and reactive control of head position was demonstrated when large perturbations forced subjects standing on support surfaces of normal length to use mixtures of ankle and hip movements. In this task, activation of the neck flexor was synchronized with the hip flexor muscles, anticipating the nose-up component of the head perturbation (Fig. 3B). Activation of neck extensors, however, was delayed until the mechanical effects of the active ankle movement propagated to the upper body.

Interactions between sensory and motor mechanisms

Why might the postural system coordinate body and head controls during active hip but not during active ankle postural movements? Several explanations are possible:

(1) *Threshold*. Because shoulder and head accelerations are smaller with active ankle than with active hip movements, head orientation remains within tolerable limits without anticipatory control with the ankle but not with the hip movement pattern.

(2) *Reference sense*. To control the position of the body's centre of mass, a reference sense fixed in relation to gravity is required. When the ankle movement pattern is used to maintain balance, proprioception linked to a stable support surface is used as the fixed reference sense. The head is stabi-

lized with reference to the trunk using stretch-evoked neck activation. When the hip movement pattern is used, in contrast, the rotational orientation of the head is actively fixed with reference to gravity so that the vestibular system can be used as the reference sense.

Several recent observations support a 'reference sense' hypothesis. Patients with bilaterally absent vestibular function appear to rely on surface information to control posture; they are able to stand normally when exposed to a sway-referenced visual surround. These patients perform the posture ankle response pattern normally, but seldom if ever perform the active hip response pattern, even when required by standing on a shortened support surface [7, 17, 18]. Patients with distorted vestibular function, however, appear to rely on visual and vestibular information. Most of these patients become unstable when presented with a sway-referenced visual surround despite normal surface information, and some are able to stand with eyes closed on a sway-referenced surface. These patients appear to rely more heavily on hip motion to control the centre of mass (see [7]). Bilateral ankle ischaemia, which disrupts the proprioceptive information from the feet, causes normal subjects to switch from an ankle to a hip pattern of postural control, even for very small support surface perturbations [17].

In conclusion, our studies show significant interactions between mechanisms for organization of the senses and coordination of movements within the postural control system. Our results suggest that the pattern of postural movement selected by normal individuals depends not only on the configuration of the support surface but also on the available sensory information. These preliminary findings concerning the control of head position during postural movements in normals will provide the background to studies of head control in patients with peripheral vestibular disorders. It is not clear, for example, whether patients with bilaterally absent vestibular function, who appear to use ankle movements to control the position of the centre of mass, and patients with distorted vestibular function, who rely more on hip movements, control

head position in the same way as normal subjects executing the same movements. It is quite likely that patients with abnormalities in coordinating head and body movements will have difficulty in sensing their centre of mass position. Further studies of the control of head and body position in normal subjects and patients may therefore provide important insights into the nature of ataxias associated with vestibular disease.

Acknowledgements

These studies were supported by NIH grants NS 12661 (L.M.N.), NS 12661 and NS 19222 (C.L.S.) and NS 01094 and NS 06457 (F.B.H.).

References

[1] Nashner, L.M. (1976) Adapting reflexes controlling the human posture. *Exp. Brain Res.*, 26: 59–72.

[2] Nashner, L.M. and Berthoz, A. (1978) Visual contribution to rapid motor responses during posture control. *Brain Res.*, 150: 403–407.

[3] Soechting, J. and Berthoz, A. (1979) Dynamic role of vision in the control of posture in man. *Exp. Brain Res.*, 36: 551–561.

[4] Nashner, L.M., Black, F.O. and Wall, C. III (1982) Adaptation to altered support and visual conditions during stance: patients with vestibular deficits. *J. Neurosci.*, 2: 536–544.

[5] Black, F.O. and Nashner, L.M. (1984) Postural disturbances in patients with benign paroxysmal positional nystagmus and vertigo. *Ann. Otol. Rhinol. Laryngol.*, 93: 595–599.

[6] Black, F.O. and Nashner, L.M. (1985) Posture control in four classes of vestibular abnormalities. In M. Igarashi and F.O. Black (Eds.), *Vestibular and Visual Control of Posture and Locomotor Equilibrium*. S. Karger, Basle pp. 271–281.

[7] Black, F.O., Shupert, C.L., Horak, F.B. and Nashner, L.M. (1988) Abnormal postural control associated with peripheral vestibular disorders. In O. Pompeiano and J.H.J. Allum (Eds.), *Vestibulospinal Control of Posture and Locomotion, Progress in Brain Research, Vol. 76*, Elsevier, Amsterdam, pp. 263–275.

[8] Horak, F.B., Nashner, L.M. (1986) Central programming of postural movements: adaptation to altered support-surface configurations. *J. Neurophysiol.*, 55: 1369–1381.

[9] Nashner, L.M. (1985) Strategies for organization of human posture. In M. Igarashi and F.O. Black (Eds.), *Vestibular and Visual Control of Posture and Locomotor Equilibrium*, S. Karger, Basle, pp. 1–8.

[10] Nashner, L.M., Woollacott, M. and Tuma, G. (1979) Organization of rapid responses to postural and locomotor-like

perturbations of standing man. *Exp. Brain Res.*, 36: 463–476.

[11] Nashner, L.M. (1971) A model describing vestibular detection of body sway motion. *Acta Otolaryngol. Stockholm*, 72: 429–436.

[12] Gurfinkel, V.S., Lipshits, M.I. and Popov, K.Y. (1974) Is the stretch reflex the main mechanism in the system of regulation of the vertical posture of man? *Biophysics*, 19: 744–748.

[13] Nashner, L.M. (1977) Fixed patterns of rapid postural responses among leg muscles during stance. *Exp. Brain Res.*, 30: 13–24.

[14] Woollacott, M.H. and Keshner, E. (1984) Upper body responses to postural perturbations in man. *Soc. Neurosci. Abstr.*, 10: 635.

[15] Allum, J.H.J. and Pfaltz, C.R. (1984) Visual and vestibular contributions to pitch sway stabilization in the ankle muscles of normals and patients with bilateral peripheral vestibular deficits. *Exp. Brain Res.*, 58: 82–94.

[16] Allum, J.H.J. and Keshner, E. (1986) Vestibular and proprioceptive control of sway stabilization. In W. Bles and T. Brandt (Eds.), *Disorders of Posture and Gait*, Elsevier, Amsterdam, pp. 19–40.

[17] Nashner, L.M., Diener, H.C. and Horak, F.B. (1985) Selection of human postural synergies differ with peripheral somatosensory versus vestibular loss. *Soc. Neurosci. Abstr.*, 11; 704.

[18] Shumway-Cook, A., Horak, F.B. and Black, F.O. (1986) Contribution of the vestibulospinal system to development of postural coordination. *Soc. Neurosci. Abstr.*, 12: 1301.

O. Pompeiano and J.H.J. Allum (Eds.)
Progress in Brain Research, Vol. 76
© 1988 Elsevier Science Publishers B.V. (Biomedical Division)

CHAPTER 22

On the role of vestibular, visual and somatosensory information for dynamic postural control in humans

H.-C. Diener and J. Dichgans

Neurologische Klinik, Eberhard-Karls Universität, Tübingen, Liebermeisterstrasse 18–20, D-7400 Tübingen, F.R.G.

Postural stabilization in altered visual, vestibular, and somatosensory conditions was investigated in humans subjected to either a fast unidirectional displacement or to a continuous sinusoidal movement of the standing support. Visual inputs were varied in four ways: (1) stroboscopic illumination, (2) stabilizing the visual surround with respect to head movements, (3) inducing apparent body movement in pitch using stripe patterns which moved continuously up or down in front of the subject, (4) eye closure. Static vestibular (and neck) input was modified by bending the head forwards or backwards, or to the right or left shoulder with the eyes closed. Somatosensory input from both feet was reduced by an ischaemic block at a level just above the ankle joints. With fast, transient, toe-up platform displacements (high-frequency test) neither the biomechanical parameters as measured by the displacement of the centre of foot pressure nor the early EMG responses of the anterior tibial and triceps surae muscles were modified by a manipulation of visual, vestibular or somatosensory feedback conditions. Sudden disturbances are obviously compensated by an early set of reflex-like muscle responses that, depending on the starting position, are stereotypically released without feedback control to save time at the expence of accuracy (emergency reaction). Continuous regulation of upright stance during sinusoidal displacement at 1 or 0.3 Hz (low-frequency test), however, clearly depends on visual, vestibular, and somatosensory feedback. Studies in patients should contain both tests, since each examines different functions of the very complex posture stabilizing network. Manipulations of sensory feedback, however, are only recommended in the low-frequency test. The experimental suppression or disturbance by disease of two of the three feedback loops invariably causes a conspicuous postural instability.

Introduction

The stabilization of human stance after external disturbances depends on the integrative evaluation of afferent information from proprioceptive, visual, and vestibular inputs. Nashner [1, 2] indicated that each of the three sensory systems, although with some overlap, is specialized to work within a certain domain of frequencies and amplitudes and that in this respect the three systems are not entirely redundant. Up to now, it is not entirely clear whether the selection of a certain sensory input for postural control is performed in a hierarchical way giving, for example, vestibular priority over visual input or whether all three inputs are used in parallel.

Most experiments performed so far dealt with the influence of the *visual system* on postural control [3]. Results from experiments in which subjects were exposed to large moving visual scenes in order to induce a visual disturbance of posture and self-motion perception [4–6] indicated that visual stabilization of posture operates mainly in the low frequency range at and below 0.1 Hz. The importance of visual information for dynamic posture control was earlier evaluated by applying sinusoidal platform oscillations in pitch with eyes open and

---

Abbreviations: CFP, centre of foot pressure; EMG, electromyogram; RMS, root mean square.

closed. Stabilization of posture by vision in this experiment was best within the frequency range between 0.03 and 0.3 Hz [7]. The unexpected exposure to conflicting information from different sensory channels may extend the frequency range of the visual channel. In the case of a mismatch between visual and vestibular motion inputs, e.g. when the subject is linearly displaced and the visual scene moves together with the head, thus indicating a stable visual surround, postural EMG responses as early as 100 ms after the beginning of the linear displacement are significantly attenuated [8].

The working range of the *vestibular system* for posture control in humans can only be estimated. A model of vestibular motor control by Nashner [9] predicted that the semicircular channels best sense the rate of sway above 0.1 Hz and the otoliths sense sway below this frequency.

The working range of *somatosensory inputs* like pressure receptors, joint receptors, and tendon organs in humans is largely unknown. Proprioception involving muscle spindles includes high frequencies above 1 Hz [10, 11].

The present study was undertaken to investigate the influence of different visual, vestibular, and somatosensory inputs on two experimental tasks testing postural stabilization after sudden or slow displacements of a supporting platform. Sudden disturbances of upright stance are compensated by a set of rapid, mostly automatic motor responses in the stretched muscles and their antagonists of the lower leg [12–14] as well as trunk and neck muscles [15]. Sinusoidal displacements of the support surface also require continuous regulation of postural balance [7]. It was investigated whether both tasks require visual, vestibular, and somatosensory feedback and if so whether this feedback provides information about motion and/or orientation. The question of conflict solution and corroborative action in the case of corresponding or contradictory sensory information was also addressed. The entire study was performed with the goal of not only understanding the postural control system but also exploring the potential clinical usefulness of these tests.

Material and methods

Apparatus

Subjects stood on a movable force-measuring platform (Tönnies Inc.) with their feet 4 cm apart. Strain gauges at the four corners of the platform measured the forces perpendicular to the platform and allowed calculation of the displacement of the CFP in anterior–posterior and lateral directions. EMGs from both legs were recorded with surface electrodes from the anterior tibial and triceps surae muscles. EMG signals were fullwave rectified, band-pass filtered, and amplified.

Changes in visual feedback

The contribution of vision to postural stabilization was measured in the following way:

(1) To assess visual stabilization of the quiet stance, sway parameters were compared while standing with the eyes open and closed respectively.

(2) To investigate whether the important parameter for visual stabilization was the orientation of contours or whether it was motion, the earlier experimental set up by Amblard and Crémieux [26] was applied to our displacement conditions. We used a 4 Hz stroboscopic illumination of the surrounding laboratory.

(3) Conflicting information from the different visual feedback loops were tested using two paradigms:

(a) To study the effect of large field visual motion that contradicts the gravitational input of stationarity, subjects stood in front of a curved projection screen which fully covered the visual field in its vertical extension. The remaining lateral parts of the visual field were covered by flat white projection surfaces. An optokinetic pattern projector above the head of the subject produced a pattern of horizontally oriented black-and-white stripes. These stripes could be moved either up- or downwards with an angular velocity of 65°/s or kept stationary.

(b) To study the reverse conflict, i.e. veridical vestibular feedback about spontaneous sway but visual perception of stationarity, the visual scene was stabilized with respect to head movements. Subjects wore a very light paper dome that surrounded the head entirely and moved with it like a hat. Its inner surface was covered with black and white stripes.

Changes in vestibular conditions

To investigate the vestibular contribution to postural sway, static vestibular input was modified by changing the head position prior to platform displacement. This manoeuvre puts the utricles (and saccules) into in an anomalous position away from the optimal working range. The following conditions were compared: head in its normal position (eyes closed), head tilted forward (30°), head extended as far as posible backwards (45°), or bent to the left or right shoulder (45°) respectively.

Changes in somatosensory input

In order to assess the contribution of somatosensory information from foot and ankle joint receptors, we applied ischaemia. Ischaemia is known to affect the fast-conducting Ia fibres from small foot muscles first. Thus this technique allows for selective (early) measurements of the effects of sensory deprivation [16]. After recording with platform tilts and sinusoidal platform movements under normal physiological conditions, two blood-pressure cuffs were applied above the level of the ankle joints on both sides. The pressure of the two cuffs was increased to 300 mmHg. The effect of ischaemia on motor neurons and somatosensory input was tested every 5 minutes between single trials by manually determining the force of maximal voluntary dorsiflection and plantarflection of the big toe and the foot. The sensitivity for vibration or tactile stimulation and position sense of the big toe and the ankle joint were also tested.

Platform displacements

The equilibrium was perturbed with sudden toe-up ramp rotations of the platform by 4° with a velocity of 80°/s in a sequence with random intervals of eight runs each. The initial body position was monitored by the experimenter (for details see [14, 19]). Sinusoidal toe-up and -down platform displacements around the ankle joint were performed with a frequency of 1 or 0.3 Hz and with an amplitude of ± 4°.

Data analysis

Onset latencies of EMG activity after sudden tilt as well as durations and integrals were calculated after visual identification of the onset and termination of each EMG component in each of eight consecutive single trials. EMG and CFP recordings were then averaged over eight runs and plotted. The anterior–posterior displacements of the CFP during sinusoidal platform movements were fed into a computer for on-line Fourier analysis. The total duration of sampling was 44.1 s. We calculated the RMSs of the power spectrum for the whole frequency range between 0 and 12.5 Hz. Angular displacements of the head and hip in the anterior–posterior direction were recorded by means of goniometers rigidly attached to head and hip belts. These data also were subjected to a Fourier analysis.

Subjects

Ten healthy subjects aged between 18 and 33 years participated in the experiments with altered visual and vestibular conditions and four healthy men aged between 28 and 32 years in the experiment with altered somatosensory input.

Results

Standing on a stable surface

Postural sway increases by about 50% with closed eyes as compared to open eyes. The anterior–posterior sway is invariably greater than sway in the lateral dimension with and without the visual contribution to postural stabilization [17].

Sinusoidal displacements

The sinusoidal movement of the platform provoked a continuous anterior–posterior regulation of upright posture. The Fourier spectra revealed that the greatest power of CFP displacement was at the frequency of the imposed displacement (Fig. 1). Additionally, there were lower- and higher-frequency components of body sway besides the one at the stimulus frequency which contributed to postural control. The total amount of anterior–posterior body sway as measured by the RMSs of Fourier spectra was significantly influenced by the seven dif-

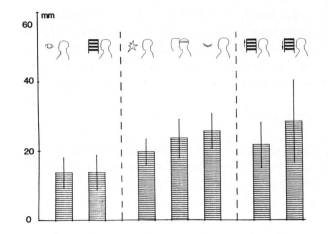

Fig. 2. RMS of body sway from the Fourier power spectra during 1 Hz sinusoidal platform movements (means and standard deviations from 10 subjects). The visual conditions from left to right were: normal visual surround, viewing a stationary stripe pattern, stroboscopic illumination, stabilized vision, eyes closed, stripe movement upwards, and stripe movement downwards.

ferent visual and five different vestibular conditions (for details see [14]). RMSs increased from the eyes-open condition to stroboscopic illumination, stabilized visual surround, and eyes closed. Stripe patterns moving upwards created less postural instability than stripe patterns moving downwards (Fig. 2).

The RMSs of anterior–posterior body sway with the eyes closed were identical for normal head position and head flexed forwards. Body sway was increased with the head bent to the right and left shoulder and was further increased when the head was extended to the neck (Fig. 3).

Body sway as measured by the RMSs of the power spectrum as well as head and hip sway increased with increasing time of ischaemia at the level of the ankle. The biggest effect could be observed after 45 minutes of ischaemia [19]. The mean RMSs increased from 121 to 196 after 45 minutes of ischaemia, the peak amplitude in the Fourier spectrum increased from 39 to 138 mV.

The results indicate that visual, vestibular, and somatosensory feedback are essential for the compensation of continuously applied low-frequency disturbances to the upright standing human. Dis-

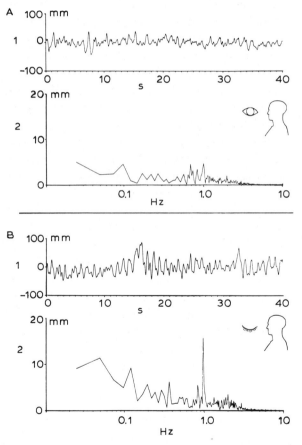

Fig. 1. (1) Original recording of the anterior–posterior body sway during sinusoidal platform movements at 1 Hz over a time period of 40 s. (2) Fourier power spectra of sway with a linear scale for the ordinate with eyes open (A) or eyes closed (B). Note the increased power of body sway around the stimulus frequency (1 Hz) and between 2 and 3 Hz when the eyes are closed.

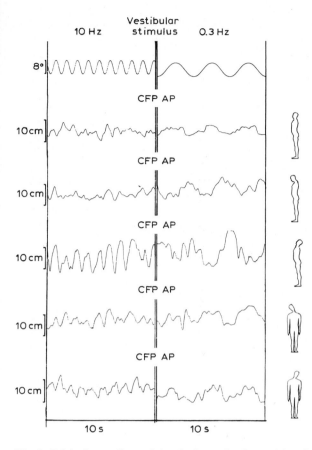

Fig. 3. Original recordings of the platform stimulus at 1.0 and 0.3 Hz and displacements of the anterior–posterior component of the CFP under different static vestibular conditions with the eyes closed. Note the increase of body sway when the head is extended backwards or bent to the right or left shoulder.

turbed somatosensory and vestibular information obviously can be compensated by visual input.

Transient ramp displacements

With the eyes open or closed, sudden tilt of the platform toe-up with a velocity of 80°/s and an amplitude of 4° evokes a short-latency response with the mean latency between 37 and 50 ms and a medium latency response after between 75 and 110 ms in the triceps surae muscle. The long-latency response, with a latency of between 110 and 124 ms, appears in the antagonist, the anterior tibial muscle.

Changing the visual, vestibular, or somatosensory experimental conditions had no significant influence on latency, duration, and integral of each of the three EMG responses or the displacement of the CFP during the first 500 ms (Figs. 4 and 5). Thus phasic EMG responses to rapid ankle rotation and related torque changes reflected through the CFP remained unchanged despite very different visual, vestibular, and somatosensory inputs. In addition,

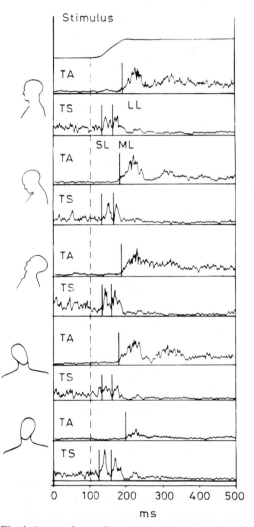

Fig. 4. Averaged recordings (eight trials) of rectified EMGs from the anterior tibial (TA) and triceps surae (TS) after a rapid tilt of the platform toe-up (80°/s, 4°; see upper trace) under different conditions of static vestibular input. SL = short latency; ML = medium latency; LL = long latency response. Note the unchanged EMG recordings under different vestibular conditions.

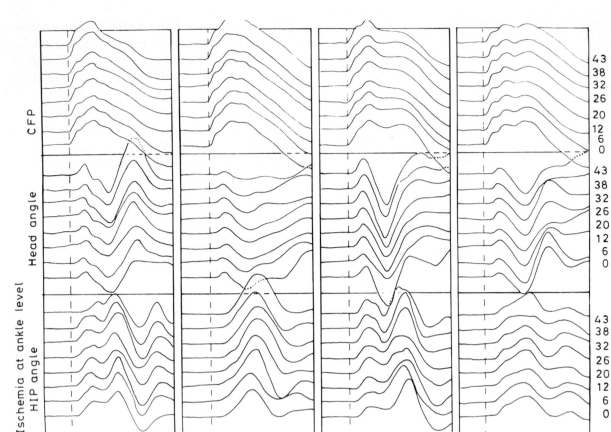

Fig. 5. Averaged recordings (eight runs) of the displacements of the CFP, head angle and hip angle after sudden tilts of the platform toe-up (vertical dotted line) with increasing time after the beginning of ischaemia above the ankle. Upward deflections or the recordings imply an anterior shift of the body or a forward inclination of head and hip. Despite considerable interindividual differences between the four subjects (rows 1–4), there is a close similarity of the induced sway within one subject throughout the entire experiment between minutes 0 and 43.

we observed no side differences between the EMG responses from the right and left legs when the head was tilted to the right or left side respectively.

Experiments in patients

In order to get more insight into the role of the vestibular input for posture control, we performed platform tilts in three patients with a total bilateral loss of vestibular function. In two cases this was due to bilateral surgery of a neurinoma of the VIIIth nerve. In one case, it was due to inherited degeneration of the VIIIth nerve. The missing vestibular function was in all cases proved by absent ca-lorics, and absent vestibulo-ocular reflexes in horizontal and vertical direction with low- and high-frequency stimulation. In the two operated cases, acoustically evoked responses were absent. Lesions outside the vestibular system were excluded by neurological examination, electrophysiological testing, somatosensory evoked potentials, visual evoked potentials, by computed tomography, and nuclear magnetic resonance imaging.

The latencies of short- and medium-latency EMG responses in triceps surae and the long-latency response in anterior tibial muscle were not different in patients with bilateral vestibular deficit than in normals (Fig. 6). The size of the long-latency

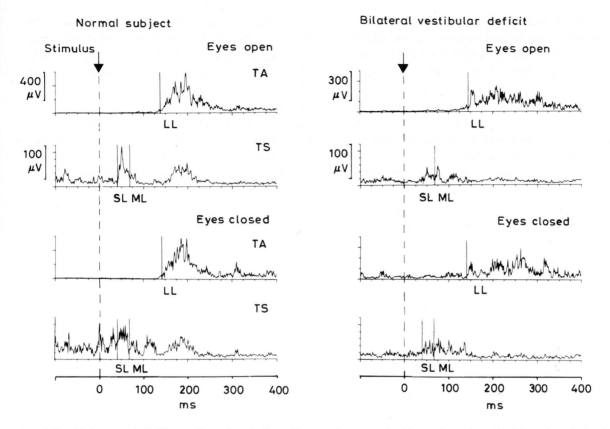

Fig. 6. Rectified averaged EMG recordings after platform tilt toe-up in a normal subject and a patient with bilateral vestibular deficit with eyes open and eyes closed. Short-, medium-, and long-latency reflexes can be observed with normal latency in the patient with bilateral vestibular deficit. The size of the long-latency response, however, is decreased. For abbreviations see Fig. 4.

EMG response, which stabilizes posture, however, was decreased. The number of subjects was too small to perform a statistical analysis. In some of the trials, the patients were not able to keep upright after platform tilt when the eyes were closed. These results confirm that the size of the long-latency EMG response is modulated by vestibulospinal influences [20].

Discussion

The present study confirms that visual, vestibular, and somatosensory feedback contribute to the compensation of a low-frequency disturbance continuously applied to the upright standing human, whereas, provided that proprioceptive feedback through spindle afferents from leg muscles is intact, these additional feedback loops seem to be insignificant for the compensation of transient high-frequency postural disturbances. Visual input can compensate for the deficiency of somatosensory and vestibular input [19].

Our results with stabilized visual conditions are in contrast with those of Nashner and Berthoz [8] and Vidal et al. [21]. In their experiments with linear displacements, EMG responses as early as 100 ms were significantly attenuated when the visual surround moved together with the head, whereas no such attenuation was seen in our experiments. This is most probably due to different stimulus conditions. The angular velocity of displacement around the ankle joint was around 6°/s in their study compared to 80°/s in our experiments. Another explanation could be that visual input is much more important in cases of linear translation (as in Nashner and Vidal's experiment) than with tilt around the ankle joint, as in our experiments. A third alternative could be that our subjects were continuously provided with stabilized visual surrounding even between platform tilts whereas visual stabilization started in Nashner and Berthoz' [8] conditions at the moment of linear surface displacements.

Our results by no means indicate that afferent information is not used for rapid postural control, but that after exclusion or malfunction of one of the three systems the other two are able to compensate completely. At least two of the three senses must be out of order to provoke falling after a sudden disturbance. This was also shown in the experiments with bilaterally labyrinthectomized patients who have normal EMG responses and perfect postural stabilization with rapid tilt as long as the eyes are open but may fall with the eyes closed. The same is true in patients with severe demyelinating polyneuropathy and missing position sense as well as in patients with Friedreich's ataxia who are quite stable with their eyes open but fall backwards with the eyes closed [22, 23].

Considering the possible modulation of stretch reflex amplitudes with head tilt, our results are in disagreement with those obtained in humans who were tilted on a tilting table in pitch with their neck fixed [24, 25]. We were unable to find a significant modulation of stretch reflex amplitudes by alteration of static vestibular input. This can possibly be ascribed to the compensatory effect of neck afferents on tonic labyrinthine reflexes.

Visual, vestibular, and somatosensory afferent information clearly influences the compensation of sinusoidally applied disturbances. Stroboscopic illumination resulted in increased body sway. The importance of visual movement perception as opposed to perception of contour orientation was already evaluated by Amblard and Crémieux [26], who were able to induce postural destabilization in quietly standing humans by stroboscopic illumina-

tion. The fact that postural instability was greater with eyes closed than with stroboscopic illumination may indicate that the intermittent presentation of stationary contours also contributes to postural stability [27]. The most dramatic destabilizing effect was seen when moving patterns induced the perception of being tilted in pitch. The movement pattern induced perceived motion of the body in pitch in the direction opposite to that of the moving stripes. This leads to the perception of falling backwards in the case of stripes moving down. The asymmetry between the two conditions is explained by the fact that normal subjects feel much more uncomfortable and unsafe when tilted backwards than when tilted forwards.

The result with changed afferent input from somatosensory receptors fits well with the assumption that spindle afferents have their working range above 1 Hz, whereas pressure, joint, and skin receptors are more important in the low frequency range. Vision has its working range below 1 Hz [3, 7] and therefore is able to compensate for the deficiency of somatosensory information under ischaemia with low-frequency sinusoidal stimulation.

In summary, the comparison of the results obtained in this study with fast transient ramp and slow continuous sinusoidal platform displacement indicates that there are at least two different modes of postural stabilization.

(1) One mode acts through reflex-like responses that are not immediately modified and possibly not even accessible to modifying inputs from the visual, vestibular, or somatosensory system but are organized in advance according to prior experience about functional objectives. Afferent information from spindle receptors is only used to trigger spinal and transcortical reflexes. Within the system, there is a certain amount of flexibility in both the time and amplitude domains [13, 22] but this, although functionally adaptive, acts through preset modifications of the response pattern and not via feedback. Postural stabilization is performed normally as long as at least two of the three afferent systems contain congruent information. This mode subserves only fast corrections to fast (transient) disturbances.

(2) A continuous mode, highly dependent on visual, vestibular, and proprioceptive feedback that subserves the compensation of low-frequency disturbances on the one side and of continuous displacements on the other. This mode is more subjected to adaptive changes [28].

The results indicate that postural studies in patients with deficits in vestibular, visual, or somatosensory and proprioceptive input should either be performed with low-frequency testing or during conflicting afferent input conditions or excluding at least two of the three afferent systems.

Acknowledgements

This paper has been supported by the Deutsche Forschungsgemeinschaft, SFB 307 A3.

References

[1] Nashner, L.M. (1970) Sensory feedback in human posture control. *Massachusetts Institute of Technology Report*, MVT 70–3.

[2] Nashner, L.M. (1981) Analysis of stance posture in humans. In A.L. Towe and E.S. Luschei (Eds.), *Handbook of Behavioural Neurobiology, Vol. 5*, Plenum, New York, pp. 527–561.

[3] Dichgans, J. and Brandt, Th. (1978) Visual–vestibular interaction. In H.W. Leibowitz and H.L. Teubner (Eds.), *Handbook of Sensory Physiology*, Springer, Berlin, pp. 755–804.

[4] Dichgans, J., Mauritz, K.H., Allum, J.H.J. and Brandt, Th. (1976) Postural sway in normals and ataxic patients: analysis of the stabilizing and destabilizing effects of vision. *Aggressologie*, 17C: 15–24.

[5] Lestienne, F., Soechting, J. and Berthoz, A. (1977) Postural readjustments induced by linear motion of visual scenes. *Exp. Brain Res.*, 28: 363–384.

[6] Mauritz, K.H., Dichgans, J. and Hufschmidt, A. (1977) The angle of visual roll motion determines the displacement of subjective visual vertical. *Percept. Psychophys.*, 22: 557–562.

[7] Diener, H.C., Dichgans, J., Bruzek, W. and Selinka, H. (1982) Stabilization of human posture during induced oscillations of the body. *Exp. Brain Res.*, 45: 126–132.

[8] Nashner, L.M. and Berthoz, A. (1978) Visual contribution to rapid motor responses during postural control. *Brain Res.*, 150: 403–407.

[9] Nashner, L.M. (1972) Vestibular posture control model. *Kybernetik*, 10: 106–110.

[10] Goodwin, G.M., Hulliger, M. and Matthews, W.B. (1976) Studies on muscle spindle primary endings with sinusoidal stretching. In S. Homma (Ed.), *Understanding the Stretch Reflex, Progress in Brain Research, Vol. 44*, Elsevier, Amsterdam, pp. 89–98.

[11] Poppele, R.E. and Kennedy, W.R. (1974) Comparison between behaviour of human and cat muscle spindles recorded in vitro. *Brain Res.*, 75: 316–319.

[12] Diener, H.C., Dichgans, J. and Bruzek, W. (1983) Variability of postural 'reflexes' in humans. *Exp. Brain Res.*, 52: 423–428.

[13] Diener, H.C., Dichgans, J., Bootz, F. and Bacher, M. (1984) Early stabilization of human posture after a sudden disturbance: Influence of rate and amplitude of displacement. *Exp. Brain Res.*, 56: 126–134.

[14] Diener, H.C., Dichgans, J., Guschlbauer, B. and Bacher, M. (1986) Role of vestibular and static vestibular influences on dynamic posture control. *Human Neurobiol.*, 5: 105–113.

[15] Keshner, E.A. and Woollacott, M.H. (1987) Neck and trunk muscle response during postural perturbations in humans. In press.

[16] Mauritz, K.H. and Dietz, V. (1980) Characteristics of postural instability induced by ischemic blocking of leg afferents. *Exp. Brain Res.*, 38: 117–119.

[17] Diener, H.C., Dichgans, J., Bacher, M. and Gompf, B. (1984) Quantification of postural sway in normals and patients with cerebellar diseases. *EEG Clin. Neurophysiol.*, 57: 134–142.

[18] Berthoz, A., Lacour, M., Soechting, J.F. and Vidal, P.P. (1979) The role of vision in the control of posture during linear motion. In R. Granit and O. Pompeiano (Eds.), *Reflex Control of Posture and Movement, Progress in Brain Research, Vol. 50*, Elsevier, Amsterdam, pp. 197–209.

[19] Diener, H.C., Dichgans, J., Guschlbauer, B. and Mau, H. (1984) The significance of proprioception on postural stabilization as assessed by ischemia. *Exp. Brain Res.*, 296: 103–109.

[20] Allum, J.H.J. and Pfaltz, C.R. (1985) Visual and vestibular contributions to pitch sway stabilization in the ankle muscles of normals and patients with bilateral peripheral vestibular deficits. *Exp. Brain Res.*, 58: 82–94.

[21] Vidal, P.P., Gouny, M. and Berthoz, A. (1979) Rôle de la vision dans le déclenchement de réactions posturales rapides. *Arch. Ital. Biol.*, 116: 281–291.

[22] Diener, H.C. and Dichgans, J. (1986) Long loop reflexes and posture. In W. Bles and Th. Brandt (Eds.), *Disorders of Posture and Gait*, Elsevier, Amsterdam, pp. 41–51.

[23] Friedemann, H.H., Noth, J., Diener, H.C. and Bacher, M. (1987) Long latency EMG responses in hand and leg muscles: cerebellar disorders. *J. Neurol. Neurosurg. Psychiatr.*, 50: 71–77.

[24] Chan, C.W.Y. and Kearney, R.E. (1982) Influence of static tilt on soleus motoneuron excitability in man. *Neurosci. Lett.*, 33: 333–338.

[25] Aiello, I., Rosati, G., Serra, G., Jugnoli, V. and Manca, M. (1983) Static vestibular spinal influences in relation to different body tilts in man. *Exp. Brain Res.*, 79: 18–26.

[26] Amblard, B. and Cremieux, J. (1976) Role of visual information in the maintenance of postural equilibrium in man. *Aggressologie*, 17C: 25–36.

[27] Paulus, W.M., Straube, A. and Brandt, Th. (1984) Visual stabilization of posture. *Brain*, 107: 1143–1163.

[28] Black, F.O. and Nashner, L.M. (1984) Vestibulo-spinal control differs in patients with reduced versus distorted vestibular function. *Acta Otolaryngol. Stockholm, Suppl.*, 406: 110–114.

O. Pompeiano and J.H.J. Allum (Eds.)
Progress in Brain Research, Vol. 76
© 1988 Elsevier Science Publishers B.V. (Biomedical Division)

CHAPTER 23

Abnormal postural control associated with peripheral vestibular disorders

F.O. Black[1], C.L. Shupert[1], F.B. Horak[1] and L.M. Nashner[2]

[1]Department of Neuro-otology, Neurological Sciences Institute, Good Samaritan Hospital and Medical Center, 1015 N.W. 22nd Avenue, Portland, OR 97210, and [2]Neurological Sciences Institute, Good Samaritan Hospital and Medical Center, 1120 N.W. 20th Avenue, Portland, OR 97209, U.S.A.

The development of a systematic approach to the diagnosis and management of ataxias of vestibular origin depends critically on the elucidation of the complex sensory and motor interactions involved in human postural control. In this paper, the results of studies of both sensory and motor control of posture in adults and children with peripheral vestibular deficits are summarized and reviewed. In studies of the sensory organization of postural control, normal subjects and patients with peripheral vestibular deficits were exposed to unreliable information from their support surface and/or visual surround during quiet stance. While normal adults and children were able to maintain balance under these conditions, the majority of children and adults with peripheral vestibular deficits showed one or both of the following abnormalities: (1) Vestibular loss patients were unable to maintain equilibrium when forced to rely on vestibular information for postural control. (2) Vestibular distortion patients were unable to select an accurate source of sensory information when exposed to sensory conflicts during quiet stance. Preliminary results of studies of motor coordination in these patients also suggest that vestibular loss patients rely almost exclusively on ankle sway to control posture, even during balance tasks which require hip movements to maintain equilibrium. In contrast, some vestibular distortion patients appear to rely on hip motions, even when not required to do so to maintain balance. The results of these studies are discussed in terms of the implications for both sensory and motor aspects of postural control in patients with ataxias of vestibular origin.

Introduction

Human upright postural stability requires that the body centre of mass be positioned over the support base provided by the feet. Two main components are required for this task: (1) accurate sensory and perceptual information about body movements with respect to orientation references external to the body, and (2) accurate motor system commands to maintain or correct body centre of mass position with respect to earth vertical.

Both the sensory and motor components of the human vestibulo-ocular and vestibulo spinal control systems are extremely complex. While the anatomy and neurophysiology of the vertical and horizontal vestibulo-ocular systems are relatively well understood, the effect of interactions between the canal (angular) and macular (linear) motion sensors on the control of eye movements is less clear. Comparatively little is known about the role of vestibulospinal mechanisms in the control of posture, and even less is known about the anatomical and phy-

---

Abbreviations: AP, anterior–posterior; BPPN, benign paroxysmal positional nystagmus; PI, performance index; VOR, vestibulo-ocular reflex.

siological interrelations among the systems which control eye and body movements. Nevertheless, physiologists and clinicians can obtain important insights into vestibulospinal mechanisms for postural control by studying the contributions of the vestibular, visual and somatosensory systems to postural stability, and how body movements interact with the sensory control of posture and movement in normal subjects and in patients with peripheral vestibular abnormalities.

Complete unilateral loss of vestibular function (opposite ear normal) and complete bilateral loss of vestibular function provide opportunities to examine special cases of altered vestibular sensory input to the brain and how those inputs affect the motor control of posture. Good clinical examples of these types of vestibular deficits are patients who have undergone unilateral labyrinthectomy or complete unilateral vestibular nerve section and ototoxically induced vestibular loss. These types of vestibular losses are essentially sensorineural in nature.

Many naturally occurring vestibular deficits, however, affect only a part of the vestibular system, often leaving function in one or more of the five peripheral receptors intact. Particularly if the disorders results from relatively mild trauma or is progressive, partial vestibular lesions are often associated with pathological changes which result in abnormal vertical canal–otolith functional interactions [1]. The most common type of such an interaction results in BPPN.

It is generally agreed that the underlying abnormal physiology of BPPN arises from any condition which results in loss of zero buoyancy between the endolymph and cupula of a semicircular canal, usually the posterior canal. Schuknecht [1] has presented evidence that such a loss of zero buoyancy can occur when otoconia, dislodged from the macula, accumulate on the ampulla of the posterior canal. In such cases, changes in head position, including head tilts, which normally do not produce cupular deflections, are detected by the posterior canal. This type of vestibular abnormality results in an altered mechanical transfer (or coupling) of head motions to the vestibular hair cells, as opposed to loss of hair cell function. Other pathologies which may result in distorted vestibular input to the central nervous sytem include perilymph fistulas, fluctuating endolymphatic hydrops, including Meniere's disease, and ossicular chain and middle ear abnormalities which can result in sudden alterations in inner ear fluid pressure.

Dividing vestibular pathologies into sensorineural losses and distortions is an oversimplification. Approximately 60% of our patients exhibit some characteristics of each type of disorder, and we therefore classify them as 'mixed'. Vestibular pathologies which result in fluctuating and/or progressive abnormal sensory signals which are poorly correlated with head angular or linear motion may result in very different sensory interaction and postural movement patterns than those associated with vestibular function loss or reduction.

Recent studies from our laboratory have begun to explore the effects of peripheral vestibular deficits upon sensory interactions and body movements in human postural control [2–10]. The results of sensory interaction tests have shown that patients with vestibular disorders use sensory information to control postural sway differently when compared to normal subjects. During these tests, different sensory conditions for standing are created by rotating the subject's visual surround and/or support surface in proportion to the subject's AP body sway, thus producing perceptually absent or misleading ('conflicting') sensory feedback from the visual or the somatosensory systems during postural movements. While normal subjects are capable of standing, albeit with increased body sway, during sensory conflict conditions, patients with losses or acute reductions of peripheral vestibular function usually fall when forced to rely on vestibular information to control posture [2, 3, 5, 8]. Furthermore, some patients with BPPN and other conductive vestibular disorders resulting in distorted vestibular information appear to rely heavily on vision to control posture, at least during the acute period of their disease before compensation has taken place. These patients tend to fall when provided with misleading visual feedback during postural sway [6].

Postural movement patterns of patients with peripheral vestibular pathologies differ significantly from those of normals. Based on theoretical considerations, Nashner and McCollum [11] suggested, and Horak and Nashner [12] demonstrated experimentally, that normal subjects employ two optimal types of postural movements, either discretely or in combinations, in order to achieve or maintain postural stability during AP sway. When standing on a rigid surface longer and wider than the feet, most normal subjects reposition the centre of body mass by exerting torques and rotations primarily around the ankles, resulting in head, hip, and ankle movements in phase with one another. In order to balance while standing crosswise on a narrow beam shorter than the feet, which prevents the effective use of foot torque forces for control of body position, normal subjects reposition the centre of body mass by exerting horizontal shear forces on the support surface. The resultant body rotation occurs primarily around the hips instead of the ankles. During rotation about the hips, however, head and ankle movements are 180° out of phase with hip movements. Normal subjects have been observed to use combinations of hip and ankle movement patterns when subjected to very large translations on a flat surface (see [13]) or when learning to stand on a narrow beam [12].

We have observed that patients with loss of vestibular function employ postural movements very similar to those observed in normal subjects who sway primarily about the ankles [10]. However, patients with severe, bilateral loss of vestibular function appear to be restricted to the use of ankle movements for postural control, even when task constraints render that type of postural movement inefficient or ineffective [9, 10, 14]. Preliminary observations indicate that many patients with distorted or mixed types of vestibular disorders appear to rely paradoxically on postural movements involving excessive hip motion, possibly in an attempt to minimize distorted sensory input from the vestibular system.

In this context is is important to note that sensory disorders affect not only the detection of postural perturbations, but also the interpretation of self-initiated sensory signals generated by postural corrections. The type of postural movements that patients and normals select also necessarily affects the type of sensory input available during postural control. The sensory and motor interactions involved in human postural control are thus quite complex. The development of a systematic approach to the diagnosis and management of ataxias of vestibular origin depends critically on the elucidation of these complex interactions. The purpose of this paper is to review and summarize the results of our previous studies and to present some preliminary research concerning postural control in adults and children with peripheral vestibular disorders.

Methods

Subjects

In these experiments we studied the postural actions of 20 normal adults and 80 adult patients with clinically documented peripheral vestibular deficits. The postural movements of 48 normal and 30 hearing-impaired children ranging in age from 7–12 years were also studied in a separate experiment. Adult patients participating in the study were selected using the following criteria: (1) ability to stand and walk freely, (2) history and clinical signs consistent with peripheral vestibular disorder, and (3) an absence of other central nervous system disorders. The hearing-impaired children were recruited from the public school system and had no known physical handicaps except their hearing loss. All had hearing threshold reductions greater than 30 dB in both ears and acquired their hearing loss within the first two years of life. Four children had congenital losses and 10 lost their hearing as a result of meningitis; the etiology of the hearing loss was unknown in the remaining 16 cases.

Procedure

A brief clinical history of each normal subject was taken to minimize the possibility of peripheral vestibular or central nervous sytem disorders. Each patient was given complete neurologic and neuro-otologic assessments identifying, as far as possible, the presence of vestibular or central nervous sytem postural disorders. Clinical assessment included a VOR test (consisting of sinusoidal body rotations in the horizontal plane at 0.05, 0.2, and 0.8 Hz and a 440-second pseudorandom rotation sequence consisting of a sum of sinusoidal motions at frequencies ranging from 0.01 to 1.5 Hz), a caloric test (peak velocity comparison procedure of Stahle [15]), a Hallpike positional nystagmus test (procedure and diagnostic criteria adopted from Baloh et al. [16]), and a complete hearing assessment. The children also received the standardized Bruninks-Osteresky Test of Balance and Motor Proficiency. (A detailed description of the clinical tests has been published in Black and Nashner [5, 6] and in Horak et al. [8]).

Results of clinical assessments were analysed separately and compared with moving platform results only after both components of the study were completed. In the study of adults, the patients were divided into 3 categories based on their postural response to the sensory conflict tests (see next section). The results of the clinical tests were then independently summarized. In the study of children, the subjects' VOR test results and the results of the clinical tests of balance and motor proficiency were used to divide the children into groups with similar diagnoses. The childrens' postural response to the sensory conflict tests were then independently summarized for each diagnosis category.

Moving platform posturography

Our methods for altering the sensory conditions of standing and quantifying the resulting kinematic and muscular activation characteristics have been described elsewhere [2, 3, 12]. AP sway of the body centre of mass was measured by attaching a potentiometer to the hips with a belt and a system of rigid light rods. This method measured motions of the centre of body mass only approximately, since it did not account for the effects of hip joint motions.

In some patients, a second potentiometer was attached to the back at shoulder height to measure the contributions of hip as well as ankle joint motions to AP sway. Assuming a normally distributed mass in a normally proportioned body [17], and further assuming little motion at the knee during postural sway, it is possible to calculate the sway angle of the patient's centre of gravity from the ankle and hip sway angles. Ankle, hip, and centre of gravity sway angle amplitudes were used both as a measure of postural stability and as descriptors of the body movements during postural control.

For both the children and the adults, the subject's task during posture testing was to maintain an upright stance for 21 seconds with as little postural sway as possible while presented with six different sensory conditions (see Table 1). The subject stood on the footplates facing into a 1 m square enclosure open at the back and bottom sides. Both the footplates and the visual surround could be rotated independently about an axis approximately colinear with the subject's ankle joints. During the first two trials, the patients were instructed to stand on a fixed surface, first with eyes open then with eyes closed (standard Romberg trials). The remaining four trials exposed the patient to sensory-conflict conditions. The conflict conditions were created by rotating either the visual surround and/or the platform support surface in proportion to the subject's ankle sway angle. Under these conditions, the subject could detect no systematic change in visual surround motion and/or ankle position with respect to change in centre of mass position. These test conditions are defined as sway-referenced vision or sway-referenced surface support as opposed to the gravity-referenced vision or surface support which are normally experienced in the standard Romberg condition. The complete test sequence included all combinations of sensory orientation conditions possible in a terrestrial environment (Table 1).

The ability of 7 children and 5 adults with bilaterally absent vestibular function to execute coordinated postural movements in response to brief, constant-velocity platform translations while standing on a normal support surface and across a narrow

TABLE 1
Test condition sequence for moving-platform posturography

Trial	Sensory conflict	Test conditions		Sensory conditions	
		Visual reference	Support reference	Accurate	Inaccurate
1. SnVn	No	Gravity	Gravity	Vision, Vestibular, Support surface	
2. SnVc	No	Eyes closed	Gravity	Vestibular, Support surface	
3. SnVs	Yes	Postural sway	Gravity	Vestibular, Support surface	Vision
4. SnVn	Yes	Gravity	Postural sway	Vestibular, Visual	Support surface
5. SsVc	Yes	Eyes closed	Postural sway	Vestibular	Support surface
6. SsVs	Yes	Postural sway	Postural sway	Vestibular	Vision, Support surface

Sn, normal, earth fixed support surface; Ss, sway referenced support surface; Vn, normal gravity referenced visual reference; Vs, sway referenced visual reference.

beam was assessed. The results of the patients were compared to those of 20 normal adults and 15 normal children. Postural movements were elicited by imposing forward and backward displacements of the footplates in the earth horizontal plane. Displacing the footplates in one direction caused the subject to sway in the other, requiring a rapid compensatory movement to restore equilibrium. All subjects included in the group of vestibular absent patients had horizontal VOR scores outside the 99% confidence limits derived from a study of over 200 normal adults and 52 normal children [8, 18]. The adult patients also had absent caloric responses. Single-frame analysis of videotaped records was used to measure the ankle, knee, and hip joint contributions to sway [12].

Data analysis

A 'performance index' (PI) was calculated for each subject in order to determine the extent to which AP sway approached the limits of stability during each of the 21 second trials. The PI was calculated by numerically integrating the rectified AP sway signal (with steady-state offset removed), and then scaling the result as a percentage of the maximum AP sway possible during in-place standing (approximately 8° forward and 4° backward for adults). PIs near zero indicated a highly stable stance while stance was precariously unstable with PIs approaching 100. A PI of 100 was arbitrarily assigned when a patient lost balance [2].

Results

Sensory test

The mean and standard deviations of postural sway as a percentage of the theoretical maximum are displayed for normal adults (open bars) and adult patients with vestibular disorders (closed bars) in Fig. 1. Regardless of the type of vestibular disorder, the majority of patients with peripheral vestibular dysfunction and normal neurological signs had normal postural sway while standing on a normal surface with eyes open (Condition 1) and eyes closed (Condition 2). However, 77 of the 80 adult patients with vestibular disorders performed significantly differently from normals in at least 2 of the 4 other sensory conditions (Mann–Whitney U tests). We then

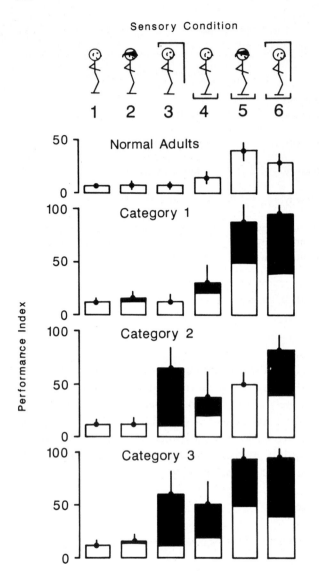

Fig. 1. Performance of normals and patients with peripheral vestibular deficits during 6 sensory conditions categorized into separate groups. The cartoon figures above the graphs indicate the sensory conditions for each trial. Bar graphs show group mean performance indices, and error bars indicate one standard deviation above the mean. The black bars in the patient bar graphs show portions which are greater than one standard deviation above the normal response.

separated 73 of the 77 patients into three categories based on the combination of normal and significantly abnormal scores received under the 6 sensory conditions. In the remaining 4 patients, sway was significantly more than normals in all 6 sensory conditions and therefore could not be categorized.

Patients classified as Category 1 ($n = 28$) swayed well within normal limits in Conditions 1 through 4, but were consistently abnormal or fell in Conditions 5 and 6, which removed all accurate sensory orientation cues except vestibular. This category included a majority of patients with abnormally low VOR gains (81%) and asymmetries (64%). Typical histories included exposure to pharmacological agents known to impair vestibular end organs, loss of sensitivity and dynamic range associated with aging, and diagnoses of Meniere's disease and other degenerative inner ear diseases.

Patients classified as Category 2 ($n = 11$) demonstrated excessive postural sway in Conditions 3 and 6 (sway-referenced vision). Paradoxically, these same patients could maintain normal sway in Condition 5 which requires vestibular sensory input for control of posture [5, 6]. This category included a large number of younger patients (91% under 50 years of age compared to 47% in Category 1), a lower incidence of reduced (64%) and asymmetrical (17%) VOR, and a larger number reporting head trauma as a precipitating factor (63% compared to 14% in Category 1). Head trauma is commonly reported as an etiological factor in BPPN [1].

Category 3 represents the most common abnormal vestibular postural sway pattern observed in this experiment. Patients in this category ($n = 34$) show a combination of the above two patterns, i.e. normal in Conditions 1 and 2, abnormal in Conditions 3, 4, 5 and 6. The clinical findings for Category 3 patients also suggest a combination of pathological mechanisms. The age distribution was bimodal, with approximately half the patients below 45 years, and the other half above 50 years of age. Within the younger group, history of head trauma was frequent (51%), but within the older group head trauma was seldom reported (6%).

The normal 7–12-year-old children and the hearing-impaired children with normal vestibular function performed similarly to the normal adults in the 6 sensory conditions (see Fig. 2). The sensory organization deficits in hearing-impaired children with

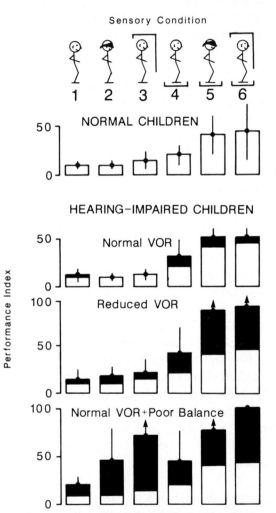

abnormal horizontal VORs were also similar to the Category 1 adults (unilaterally or bilaterally reduced or absent vestibular function), i.e. near normal postural sway in all sensory conditions except Conditions 5 and 6, in which vestibular input is required for orientation (see results for reduced VOR children in Fig. 2). Three hearing-impaired children with normal horizontal VOR, however, who scored at less than the 1st percentile on the Bruninks-Osteresky Test of Motor Proficiency had a different sort of sensory organization deficit. Like the Category 3 adults, these children had excessive sway in all sensory conflict conditions (Conditions 3, 4, 5 and 6). Unlike the adults, however, these children also had excessive sway in the first two standard Romberg conditions.

Postural movements

Generally, in response to support surface translations, the leg and trunk postural movements in adults and children with bilaterally absent vestibular function were normally coordinated ankle sway patterns. However, when standing across a narrow surface for which an ankle movement pattern was no longer effective, all bilaterally absent vestibular patients could not or would not change postural movements to a hip sway pattern. Fig. 3 shows stick-figure representation derived from video images of the successful hip movement patterns for a normal adult and a normal child and for an adult and a child with bilaterally absent vestibular function [9, 10]. It should be noted that the adult and the child with absent vestibular function whose data are displayed here were not able to maintain balance on the narrow surface and fell into the support harness.

Although all the patients with absent vestibular function that we have studied so far appear to control the centre of mass position using ankle sway almost exclusively, some patients with peripheral vestibular disorders which result in distorted, rather than absent, vestibular function appear to rely more heavily on hip movements to control the centre of mass position. Fig. 4 shows the postural movement patterns of two patients with peripheral vestibular disorders during attempts to stand quietly in Condition 3 (sway referenced vision). The subject in Fig. 4a was 55 years old and had bilaterally absent vestibular function due to bilateral temporal bone fractures (Category 1). This subject controlled the position of the centre of mass using primarily

Fig. 2. Performance of normal and hearing-impaired children during 6 sensory conditions categorized into separate groups. The cartoon figures above the graphs indicate the sensory conditions for each trial. Bar graphs show group mean performance indices, and error bars indicate one standard deviation above the mean. Error bars with arrow heads indicate standard deviations which were too large to represent on the graph. The black bars in the hearing impaired childrens' bar graphs show portions which are greater than the normal mean.

ankle motion in all sensory conditions. When the subject sways at the ankles, the ankle angle, calculated centre of gravity position, and hip angle all move in phase (i.e. the subject sways rigidly like an

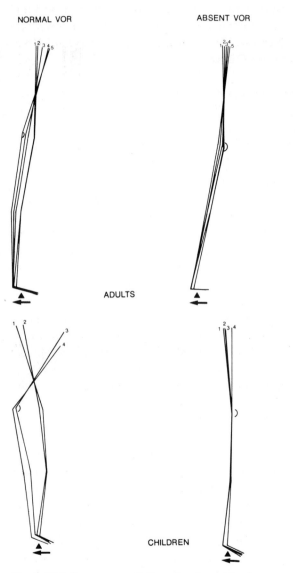

Fig. 3. Stick figure representations showing postural movement patterns for one normal adult and one normal child compared to those for one adult and one child with bilaterally absent vestibular function. The small numerals above the stick figures indicate the time sequence (approximately 250 ms between sticks). Subjects were facing to the right and were standing crosswise on a 4-inch beam, which was moved backward with respect to the subject at 15 cm/s for 250 ms at the onset of the trial.

inverted pendulum). This pattern was typical of the 5 adults with bilaterally absent vestibular function. The subject whose data are depicted in Fig. 4b was a 39 year old patient with unilateral BPPN following head injury in a skiing accident (Category 2 and 3). This subject swayed primarily about the hips, resulting in changes in ankle and hip angle which were 180° out of phase. Comparison of the plots of hip angle versus ankle angle for each patient illustrates both the opposite phase relationships and the much larger hip angle changes for the subject in Fig. 4b.

In our study of 73 patients with peripheral vestibular disorders we also noted differences in sway patterns among the different patient categories. When Category 1 patients, the majority of whom had bilaterally or unilaterally reduced vestibular function, became unstable, they tended to sway about the ankle joints with the hips held rigidly. In contrast, Category 2 and 3 patients, the majority of whom had distortions rather than losses of vestibular function, tend to demonstrate larger amounts of hip sway. In order to quantify this difference, the body motion patterns of 15 patients in each group were selected randomly and analysed in detail. For the 15 Category 1 patients, peak ankle excursions averaged $10.2 \pm 2.8°$ (standard deviation), and the ratio of peak hip to peak ankle motion averaged 0.6 ± 0.3. For the 15 Category 2 and 3 patients, average peak ankle joint excursions were similar at $9.8 \pm 2.7°$, but the average hip/ankle ratio of $1.7 \pm 0.8°$, however, was significantly larger (Mann-Whitney $U, p < 0.001$).

Discussion

Peripheral vestibular deficits can result in various types of abnormalities in the use of sensory information for orientation as well as in the movement patterns used for adjustment of body centre of mass. Both sensory and motor aspects of postural dyscontrol in vestibular deficit patients provide important insights into vestibulospinal system mechanisms.

Postural sway responses under different sensory

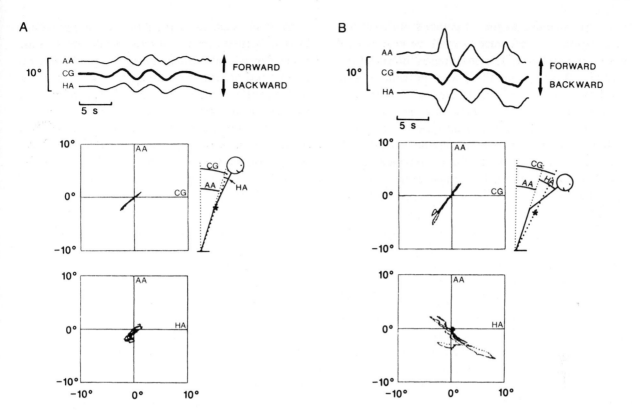

Fig. 4. Example sway records for two patients tested with a normal support surface and inaccurate visual feedback. In the top panel of the figure, hip angle (HA), ankle angle (AA), and centre of gravity position (CG) are plotted as a function of time. Positive angles indicate anterior motion. In the middle panel of the figure, AA changes are plotted as a function of CG motion for the same trial. In the bottom panel of the figure, the HA changes are plotted as a function of AA changes for the same trial. (A) The results of a patient with bilaterally absent vestibular function. Note the small amount of hip motion which is in phase with ankle and centre of gravity motion. (B) The results of a patient with BPPN. Note the large amount of hip motion which is out of phase with ankle and centre of gravity motion.

conditions in adults and children older than seven years with unilateral and bilateral loss of vestibular function support the hypothesis that vestibular, visual and somatosensory inputs provide partially redundant orientation references for the control of posture. When either visual or somatosensory inputs were available and accurate (Conditions 1–4), the vestibular-deficient patients could maintain postural sway within normal limits. Thus, they did not have difficulty selecting the gravity-referenced sense when exposed to other sensory inputs which were sway-referenced. When presented with sensory conditions which removed accurate visual and somatosensory orientation references (Conditions 5

and 6) however, unilateral and bilateral vestibular-deficient patients could not maintain normal sway and consistently free-fell into the support harness. There was a good correlation between the diagnosis of reduced vestibular function based on the VOR and the Category 1 pattern of sensory performance for both the adults and the children, suggesting that a sensorineural loss of vestibular input does not affect the ability to select an alternative gravity-referenced sensory input when available.

Category 2 patients demonstrated excessive postural sway when exposed to a sway-referenced visual surround, which suggests an obligatory dependence upon visual orientation references when standing with eyes open. Category 2 patients preferentially used vision as a reference to earth vertical, even if inaccurate and even if orientation to the visual reference resulted in a fall. These individuals were stable with eyes closed and the support surface sway-referenced (Condition 5), indicating that their vestibular input *in isolation* was adequate to maintain stability. Often, these patients had horizontal VOR gains within normal limits, but complained of motion sickness exacerbated by exposure to sway-referenced vision, and had positional vertigo suggestive of BPPN.

Most posturally unstable patients encountered clinically exhibit a combination of the above two types of sensory deficits in postural control (Category 3). These patients could not rely on vestibular inputs alone for orientation and were visually dependent with eyes open. The majority were unstable in any sensory conflict situation (Conditions 3, 4, 5 and 6). The hearing-impaired children with this pattern also had normal horizontal VOR scores, but scored poorly on clinical tests of balance and coordination.

The sensory selection deficits represented by Category 2 and 3 patients may be due to distorted head-motion signals arising from the peripheral vestibular system. The hypothesis has been proposed by McCollum and Nashner [4] that loading of the posterior canal cupula (for example by otolith displacement following head trauma as proposed by Schuknecht [1]), would phase-shift canal–otolith response interactions toward the otolith response. Keeping in mind the fact that the cupula does not normally respond to linear accelerations, loading of the cupula by otoconia (cupulolithiasis) would cause an increase in the sensitivity of the canal to head rotations in its plane and, in addition, would cause the canal to become sensitive to linear accelerations, thus changing its mode of response. From a sensory input point of view, this would cause the normally independent angular and linear receptive fields to overlap, creating an abnormal peripheral sensory interaction input to the brain. It is hypothesized that such an 'overlap' in peripheral vestibular input could affect visual–vestibular inter-

actions in such a way that an inappropriate 'match' between vestibular and visual inputs would result. Since head trauma and BPPN were frequently reported among the Category 2 and 3 patients, such hypotheses may help to explain their sensory interaction abnormalities during postural control. It is important to note, however, that such sensory interaction abnormalities can also result from central nervous system disorders, such as brainstem, cerebellar, and central vestibular system pathologies [9, 19–21].

From a motor perspective, two main types of postural sway movements could be described in patients with peripheral vestibular disorders. Patients with well-compensated unilateral or bilateral loss of vestibular function exhibited sway primarily around their ankle joints. Many patients with distorted vestibular function, on the other hand, exhibited sway around their hips. Furthermore, although the trunk and leg movement patterns themselves appeared to be normally coordinated, many patients with vestibular deficits seemed to be restricted to the use of one type of movement pattern, even when it was ineffective or inefficient.

It has been demonstrated that most normal subjects use an ankle sway pattern when the foot support surface is broad and firm [12]. Normal subjects will develop a hip sway pattern only under conditions which do not allow development of sufficient torques around the ankle joints to correct sway, for example when cross-wise on a narrow rail or if somatosensory input at the foot is reduced by inducing ankle ischaemia with pressure cuffs [10]. We have observed that children and adults with bilaterally absent vestibular function do not control centre of mass movements with sway about the hips even when hip motions are required by the task, such as when standing or walking on a narrow beam, standing or walking in a tandem Romberg position, or standing on one foot. As a result, the patients with bilaterally absent vestibular function typically fall when attempting to balance under conditions requiring hip motion. In contrast, patients with distorted vestibular function used hip movements to control posture, even while standing on a normally sized firm surface. These patients often appeared unstable or 'ataxic' because of excessive hip motion. It is, however, not clear whether all patients with vestibular distortions use hip motions to control the centre of mass position, and whether these hip motions are normally coordinated; we are currently investigating these questions.

Our experimental results also indicate that the sensory and motor aspects of postural control cannot be studied in isolation from each other, because the type of movement pattern selected affects the type of sensory feedback available during postural movements. Antiphase movements of both the hip and ankle joints, as opposed to movements only about the ankle joints, reverse the relative direction and timing of visual, vestibular and ankle-joint sensory information available for orientation references. The two different types of postural sway therefore provide different sensory feedback conditions. Assume a centre of mass position anterior to the centre of foot support (forward sway). An ankle sway movement pattern would result in backward rotation of both the centre of mass and the head to a position toward postural equilibrium near the centre of the foot support. A hip-sway movement pattern would accomplish the same goal for the centre of mass, but would result in forward, not backward movement of the head, reversing the directions of the visual field and the linear and angular vestibular inputs generated by an ankle sway pattern. The somatosensory information provided by the feet and ankles during hip sway would also be altered, since the centre of body mass position would no longer be correlated with centre of pressure inputs from the feet.

Given that movement about the hips requires correct interpretation (or reinterpretation) of sensory inputs, which would appear to place heavy demands on an accurate vestibular signal, why might patients with distorted vestibular function adopt hip sway patterns to control centre of mass position? One possible answer is suggested by considering the sensory consequences of hip movements in patients with one particular type of vestibular distortion. BPPN is thought to result from loss of zero buoyancy between the cupula and endolymph of the posterior canal, causing the canal to respond to linear as well as angular stimuli. Any change of head position with respect to gravity, in these patients, results in an abnormal canal response. Since the relationship between linear and angular head motion and the direction of centre of mass movement are different for ankle and hip sway, it may be possible that patients with BPPN adopt hip sway patterns in an attempt to reestablish a more normal relationship between their head motion signals and their centre of mass movements. Thus, they may adopt a hip motion pattern in order to compensate for their vestibular deficit. This change in postural movement pattern is, however, not without cost. Hip movement patterns require a reinterpretation of the visual, vestibular, and somatosensory feedback if they are to be used successfully for postural control. From a clinical perspective, the altered movement pattern observed in BPPN patients, i.e. a shift from ankle to hip movements, almost invariably results in sensory conflict and symptoms of spatial disorientation and/or motion sickness.

Another possible answer is suggested by the observation that normal subjects use hip movements for correction of postural sway when surface somatosensory inputs are reduced or distorted by standing on a narrow surface or with ankle ischaemia [10, 12]. Category 2 and 3 patients, who are likely to produce hip postural movements even when standing on a normal surface, also appear not to use somatosensory inputs from the surface for orientation, even when they are available. That is, they fall in Condition 3 (sway-referenced vision only) despite the fact that they have normal gravity-referenced orientation information available from the surface. It remains unclear, however, why patients with distorted vestibular function might ignore these veridical surface inputs. The Category 1 patients with absent vestibular function, on the other hand, appear to rely more heavily on surface inputs and preferentially use an ankle sway pattern. The results of these studies of patients with peripheral vestibular disorders appear to imply that vestibular input, even if abnormal, is critical for the use of hip movements to control postural sway.

A great many questions concerning vestibulospinal control of posture remain to be answered. Little is known, for example, about vertical canal–ocular and otolith–ocular function in patients with postural dyscontrol of vestibular origin. It is possible that measurement of vertical canal and otolith function as reflected by these eye movements may provide further insight into why some patients become unstable only when forced to rely upon vestibular input for postural control (Category 1), and others become unstable whenever sensory conflicts are present (Category 3). It is also possible that measurement of eye-head coordination during postural movements may help us understand both the sensory and movement disorders of patients with postural dyscontrol. We are also currently studying whether normal subjects and patients who are employing hip or ankle movements stabilize their heads with respect to gravity or with respect to their bodies [13, 22]. Careful analysis of leg, trunk, head, and eye position control in patients with all types of vestibular deficiencies under carefully controlled visual and somatosensory feedback conditions need to be carried out. Postural sensorimotor function cannot be fully understood until studies consider both sensory inputs and postural movements as well as their interactions.

Acknowledgements

These studies were supported by a fellowship from the National Institute of Handicapped Research and by grants from the Deafness Research Foundation, the Medical Research Foundation of Oregon to F.B.H., and the National Institutes of Health (NS19222 to F.O.B., NS12661 to L.M.N., and AG06457 and NS01094 to F.B.H.). The studies of hearing impaired children were carried out in collaboration with Anne Shumway-Cook and Terry Crowe. The technical assistance of Robert J. Peterka, without which this work would not have been possible, is also gratefully acknowledged.

References

[1] Schuknecht, H.F. (1974) *Pathology of the Ear*, Harvard University Press, Cambridge MA pp. 475–478.

[2] Nashner, L.M., Black, F.O. and Wall, C. III (1982) Adaptation to altered support surface and visual conditions during stance: Patients with vestibular deficits. *J. Neurosci.*, 2: 536–544.

[3] Black, F.O., Wall, C. III and Nashner, L.M. (1983) Effects of visual and support surface orientation references upon postural control in vestibular deficient subjects. *Acta Otolaryngol. Stockholm*, 95: 199–210.

[4] McCollum, G. and Nashner, L.M. (1983) Geometrical analysis of postural instability in BPPN patients. *Soc. Neurosci. Abstr.*, 9: 317.

[5] Black, F.O. and Nashner, L.M. (1984) Vestibulo-spinal control differs in patients with reduced versus distorted vestibular function. *Acta Otolaryngol. Stockholm Suppl.* 406: 110–114.

[6] Black, F.O. and Nashner, L.M. (1984) Postural disturbances in patients with benign paroxysmal positional nystagmus. *Ann. Otol. Rhinol. Laryngol.*, 93: 595–599.

[7] Black, F.O. (1985) Vestibulospinal function assessment by moving platform posturography. *Am. J. Otol. Suppl.*, 39–46.

[8] Horak, F.B., Shumway-Cook, A., Crowe, T. and Black, F.O. (1988) Vestibular function and motor proficiency in children with hearing impairments and in learning disabled children with motor impairments. *Dev. Med. Child Neurol.*, 30: 64–79.

[9] Shumway-Cook, A., Horak, F.B. and Black, F.O. (1986) Contribution of the vestibulo-spinal systems to postural coordination. *Soc. Neurosci. Abstr.*, 12: 1301.

[10] Nashner, L.M., Diener, H.-C. and Horak, F.B. (1985) Selection of human postural synergies differ with peripheral somatosensory vs. vestibular loss. *Soc. Neurosci. Abstr.*, 11: 704.

[11] Nashner, L.M. and McCollum, G. (1984) The organization of human postural movements: a formal basis and experimental synthesis. *Behav. Brain Sci.*, 8: 135–172.

[12] Horak, F.B. and Nashner, L.M. (1986) Central programming of postural movements: adaptation to altered support-surface conditions. *J. Neurophysiol.*, 55: 1369–1381.

[13] Nashner, L.M., Shupert, C.L. and Horak, F.B. (1988) Head-trunk coordination in the standing posture. In O. Pompeiano and J.H.J. Alum (Eds.), *Vestibulospinal Control of Posture and Locomotion, Progress in Brain Research, Vol. 76*, Elsevier, Amsterdam, pp. 243–251.

[14] Diener, H.C. and Dichgans, J. (1988) Vestibulo-spinal mechanisms for the maintenance of human upright posture. In M.A. Gresty (Ed.), *Movement Disorders of the Extrapyramidal Systems*, McMillan Press, London, in press.

[15] Stahle J. (1956) Electronystagmography in the caloric test. *Acta Societatis Medicorum Uppsaliensis*, 61: 307–332.

[16] Baloh, R.W., Sakala, S.M. and Honrubia, V. (1979) Benign paroxysmal positional nystagmus. *Am. J. Otolaryngol.*, 1: 1–5.

[17] Diffrient, N., Tilley, A.R. and Bardagjy, J.C. (1974) *Humanscale 1/2/3*, MIT Press, Cambridge MA, 43 pp.

[18] Peterka, R.J. and Black, F.O. (1986) *Normal and Abnormal Human Vestibular Ocular Function*, Final technical report: NASA cooperative agreement NCC9–8, 65 pp.

[19] Shumway-Cook, A., Horak, F.B. and Black, F.O. (1988) A critical examination of vestibular function in motor-impaired learning disabled children. *Int. J. Pediatr.Otorhinolaryngol.*, in press.

[20] Horak, F.B., Diener, H.C. and Nashner, L.M. (1986) Abnormal scaling of postural responses in cerebellar patients. *Soc. Neurosci. Abstr.*, 12: 1419.

[21] Nashner, L.M., Shumway-Cook, A. and Marin, O. (1983) Stance posture control in select groups of children with cerebral palsy: deficits in sensory organization and muscular coordination. *Exp. Brain. Res.*, 49: 393–409.

[22] Nashner, L.M. (1985) Strategies for organization of human posture. In M. Igarashi and F.O. Black (Eds.), *Vestibular and Visual Control of Posture and Locomotor Equilibrium.* S. Karger, Basel, pp. 1–8.

O. Pompeiano and J.H.J. Allum (Eds.)
Progress in Brain Research, Vol. 76
© 1988 Elsevier Science Publishers B.V. (Biomedical Division)

CHAPTER 24

Organization of leg–trunk–head equilibrium movements in normals and patients with peripheral vestibular deficits

J.H.J. Allum, E.A. Keshner*, F. Honegger and C.R. Pfaltz

Division of Experimental Audiology and Neurootology, Department of Otorhinolaryngology, University Hospital, CH-4031 Basel, Switzerland

Equilibrium movements of the leg, trunk and head and the underlying organization of EMG activity in ankle and neck muscles was examined during the restabilization of posture required after the support surface of a standing subject is rapidly rotated about the ankle joints. Differences in restabilizing responses were investigated between three populations: normals, patients with acute unilateral peripheral vestibular deficit, and patients with compensated bilateral deficit, in order to quantify the influence of vestibulospinal reflexes on EMG activity and ensuing postural movements. This influence was profound on EMG activity and torque at the ankle joint, particularly when patients were tested under eyes-closed conditions. Patients' response amplitudes at the ankle joint were significantly less than those of normals and were correlated with the extent of the clinically defined vestibular deficit. Thus body equilibriating movements at the ankle joint are overwhelmingly under vestibulospinal control. However, several findings indicated only a minor influence of vestibular deficit on trunk and head movements. Instead, the results suggest that the pattern of restabilizing trunk and head movements results from righting reactions predominately controlled by muscle stretch reflexes.

Introduction

To what extent are vestibulospinal reflexes involved in the control of human stance? In order to answer this question, the organization of body movements after a stance disturbance must be understood. Conventional approaches to understanding the postural control of the upright stance assume either that the body acts as a simple inverted pendulum rotating about the ankle joints [1, 2] or, if movements about the hip and neck joints occur, that the CNS coordinates muscle activity at these joints to ensure a functionally related co-activation with ankle joint muscles [3, 4]. In the event of intersegmental movements when upright stance is perturbed, Bernstein [5] and other authors have argued that it would be difficult for the CNS to independently control rotations about each joint. Rather, it would be more efficient if a fixed pattern of muscle co-activation were employed to restabilize posture. In other words, the number of degrees of freedom of movement is reduced by linking patterns of muscle activity at each joint together. Then central neuronal circuits controlling body stance could estimate in advance the expected visual and vestibular feedback when, for example, the head rotates in accordance with ankle rotation to maintain a stable gaze.

The inverted pendulum theory of postural control in which most stabilizing action is assumed to occur

---

*Present address: Department of Physiology, Northwestern University Medical School, 303 East Chicago Avenue, Chicago, IL 60611, U.S.A.

Abbreviations: CNS, central nervous system; EMG, electromyogram; LL, long latency; ML, medium latency; SL, short latency; SOL, soleus; TA, tibialis anterior; TRAP, trapezius.

at the ankle joints is conceptually supported by evidence indicating a powerful influence of vestibulospinal reflexes on sway-stabilizing ankle torque [6, 7]. These studies have demonstrated a significant difference between the amplitudes of stabilizing reflex EMG activity occurring in the ankle muscles of normals and patients with bilateral peripheral vestibular deficits after their support surface is tipped backwards. Application of the inverted pendulum model to the ensuing sway stabilization, however, is limited since trunk and head movements are antiphasic and more appropriately modelled as part of a multi-link control of posture [7, 8]. In this case the question arises whether the control of posture is centrally programmed, as Bernstein suggested, with dependent activation occurring at joints. For example, whether muscle activity at the neck is correlated with that at the ankle joint. An alternative model would be that vestibulospinal reflexes produce sufficient torque about the ankle joint to stabilize the vertical projection of the body's centre of mass over the support base in an inverted-pendulum mode of action, while rotations of the upper body and head are linked together by proprioceptive reflex systems.

In the current study we have attempted to distinguish between these three proposed models of postural control using measurements of the angular velocities of the lower leg, trunk and head recorded from normals and patients with vestibular deficits. To extend the validity of the results to the complete spectrum of peripheral vestibular deficits, observations from patients with acute and compensated unilateral deficit have been included with those at the two extremes of the vestibular system continuum: normals and patients with bilateral deficit.

Methods

The methods and measurement techniques employed in this study duplicate those described in detail elsewhere [7]. The postural reflexes were elicited by 10 consecutive $40°/s$ ankle dorsiflexion rotations of the support surface on which the subject stood. Two types of recordings were employed. Surface EMG signals were registered from the ankle muscles, tibialis anterior (TA) and soleus (SOL), and from the upper fibres of trapezius (TRAP) covering neck extensor muscles. Supplementary recordings of EMG activity were obtained in the paraspinalis and rectus femoris (quadriceps) muscles of four normal subjects. Biomechanical recordings included platform and lower leg rotations measured with potentiometers, and torque about the ankle joint as registered by a strain gauge system imbedded in the support platform. Absolute head and trunk angular accelerations were measured, with respect to earth-fixed coordinates, using angular acceleration transducers mounted respectively on a helmet and a breast plate harnessed to the chest.

The areas under the EMG records were calculated off-line over two short latency intervals (SLa and SLb), each 40 ms long, commencing 40 and 80 ms after the onset of platform rotation, and over a medium latency (ML) and long latency (LL) interval, each 80 ms long, occurring consecutively after the SL intervals (see Fig. 2). Changes in incremental ankle torque were measured over the same intervals with a 25 ms delay in order to account for the time between appearance of EMG activity in a muscle and its development into a force response. The amplitudes and times of peak forward- and backward-pitching angular velocities were obtained by integration of angular acceleration responses. Lower leg angular velocity was calculated from the angle recording using numerical differentiation (see Fig. 1). EMG areas and torque measurements were taken from individual trials and then averaged, whereas angular velocity peaks were determined after averaging. To account for adaptation effects [2, 7, 9] the averages of the 10 consecutive trials were split into two; one average for the first 3 trials, another for the second 7 trials.

A stepwise linear regression analysis was applied to individual mean values of the average ML and LL EMG areas. With ankle torque as the dependent variable and TA and SOL response areas as predictor variables, the respective bivariate linear regression of torque on each and both muscles was calculated. In order to represent the bivariate regression in two dimensions (see Figs. 5 and 6), the predictor constant that emerged from the bivariate regression of the muscle with the lesser correlation was held constant during a univariate regression of torque on the muscle with the stronger correlation

(see [7] for more specific details of this technique). Possible correlations between the activity of TA and neck extensors and SOL and neck extensors were tested by means of a linear regression analysis on the ML EMG response areas of the respective

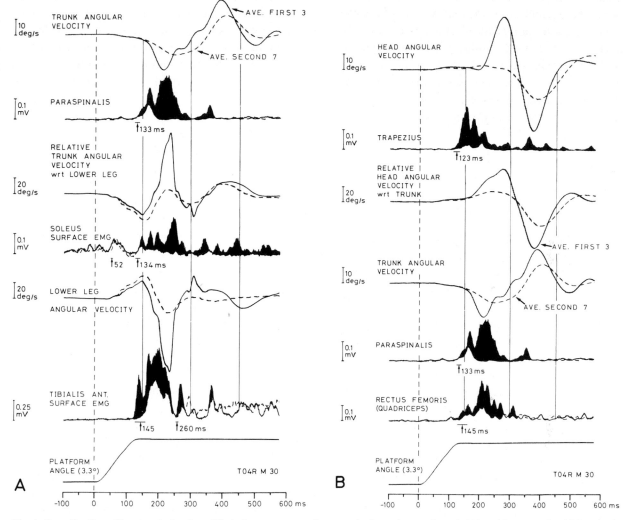

Fig. 1. Coordination of leg–trunk–head equilibriating movements between the lower legs and trunk (A) and between the thighs, trunk and head (B) of a normal 30-year-old to toe-up rotations. The two parts of the figure illustrate average responses of electromyographic and biomechanical measurements recorded from a 30-year-old normal subject compensating for backwards tilt of the support surface while standing upright with eyes open. The averages of the first 3 trials (solid line) and next 7 trials (broken line) are plotted. The decrease in EMG activity, or response adaptation, between the two sets of trials is shown by filled areas on the EMG traces. Average values of the onset latencies for bursts of EMG activity are marked by a vertical arrow, with one standard deviation indicated by a horizontal bar on the arrow. The zero latency reference is the vertical dashed line and corresponds to the first inflexion of platform velocity. Note that for TA these latencies are longer and their deviation larger compared to latencies obtained when the subject is leaning back, preactivating TA prior to the support surface rotation (see Fig. 2). An upward deflection in all angle and angular velocity traces indicates backwards pitching. All angular velocity measurements are with respect to earth-fixed coordinates. The equilibriating reactions have been divided into three phases, each 150 ms in duration as indicated by the thin vertical lines.

muscle pairs. In addition to the normal and bilateral deficit population studied previously [7], 15 patients with unilateral vestibular deficit were examined twice. The first examination occurred in the acute stage of the deficit as soon as the patients' state of vertigo permitted quiet stance for 10 mins. A second examination was performed after central compensation had reduced the horizontal VOR asymmetry to a normal value, usually after a period of 2 months [10]. At this stage of compensation the vertical VOR gain in the pitch plane had changed from, on average, a 66% symmetrical reduction of the normal response to 85% of normal.

Results

Multi-link movements of the legs, trunk and head

Fig. 1 shows a typical set of recordings of lower leg sway angle, and trunk and head angular velocity from a normal subject, regaining upright stance after a dorsiflexion rotation of the support surface. The equilibriating reactions after the onset of platform rotation have been divided into three intervals, each 150 ms in duration on the basis of inflexion points in the flower leg and trunk angular velocity traces. Thus each interval presents a different pattern of mulit-linked movements of body segments. The relative velocity traces in Fig. 1 provide no evidence that the body moves as an inverted pendulum during these intervals. This despite a general stiffening of the body linkage over trials for all three intervals as indicated by the dashed trajectories in Fig. 1.

The first interval of movement is dominated by passive biomechanical properties of the body. Lower legs and trunk are forced in opposite directions by the stimulus. Initially, as Fig. 1 documents, the stimulus-imposed rotation of the support surface moves the toes up and stretches the triceps surae muscles without affecting the position of the body links. The acceleration of the support surface, however, is transmitted mechanically through the body to the head to produce a suprathreshold an-

gular acceleration stimulus to the vestibular system 20 ms after rotation onset [6]. Essentially the ankle muscles act in the first 100 ms like stretched springs and impose a torque on the platform roughly proportional to their displacement. As the platform movement terminates, rotation of the body segments in different directions is observed (see relative velocity traces in Fig. 1). The hips can be assumed to move backwards since the legs rotate backwards about the ankle joint as the trunk rotates forwards. Presumably this action on the hips results from the stretch response of the triceps surae muscles: a combination of the elastic forces noted above and active contraction generated by the short latency (SL) response of triceps surae [11]. In Figs. 2 and 3, the SL response occurred in SOL at 77 and 46 ms respectively, though, on average, the SL response commenced at 56 ms standard deviation 14 ms; [7]). As the trunk rotates forwards the head is held relatively stable since head angular velocity changes little with respect to gravity (Fig. 1), due to the biphasic profile of head angular acceleration (Fig. 2).

The second phase of stimulus-induced movement (150 to 300 ms) is characterized by the lower legs and trunk moving forward. Trunk movements are less rapid than those of the legs. As illustrated in Fig. 1, the relative velocity of the trunk with respect to the lower legs is less than the leg velocity. The rearward velocity of the legs and hips occurring during the first 150 ms is arrested and reversed in direction primarily by a large burst of TA and quadriceps activity commencing after 120 ms (see Fig. 1). At about the same time a ML burst of SOL activity occurs (see Fig. 2). The change in ankle torque beginning 25 ms after this ML burst of TA activity (see Fig. 2) precipitates a marked equilibriating effect on body posture. It aligns the lower leg angle with the vertical and would rapidly increase the prior forward angular velocity of the trunk if the paraspinal activity commencing at 130 ms did not resist further forward trunk motion (see Fig. 1). As the ankle torque levels off, bursts of LL activity occur almost simultaneously in SOL and TA at circa 220 ms (see Fig. 2). At the same time

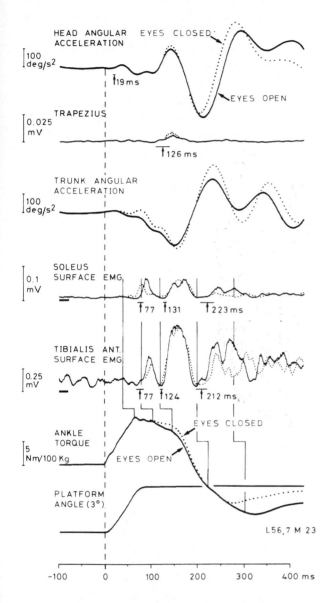

HEAD ANGULAR   EYES CLOSED
ACCELERATION

100 deg/s²

19 ms

EYES OPEN

TRAPEZIUS

0.025 mV

126 ms

TRUNK ANGULAR
ACCELERATION

100 deg/s²

SOLEUS
SURFACE EMG

0.1 mV

77   131   223 ms

TIBIALIS ANT.
SURFACE EMG

0.25 mV

77   124   212 ms

ANKLE
TORQUE   EYES CLOSED

5 Nm/100 Kg   EYES OPEN

PLATFORM
ANGLE (3°)

L 56,7 M 23

-100   0   100   200   300   400 ms

Fig. 2. Average responses of a 23-year-old normal subject to toe-up rotations of the support surface when standing slightly leaning back under eyes-open (solid lines) and eyes-closed (dotted lines) conditions. The averages are for trials 4–10 of a series of 10. Backwards pitch of head and trunk angular acceleration is indicated by an upward deflection of the traces as is increasing plantar flexion force on the platform. The 40 and 80 ms intervals over which EMG areas were calculated are marked by thin full vertical lines on SOL and TA traces. For measurements of ankle torque changes these intervals were delayed 25 ms as shown. (From [14].)

the lower leg but not the trunk angular velocity is slowed to zero.

Evidence from normals and patients with vestibular deficits will be presented below suggesting that the two sets of ML and LL bursts in TA and SOL are co-activated and functionally have first a restabilizing and then a braking action on the body. The recordings of angular velocity taken at different places on the body from the normal case study in Fig. 1 support this hypothesis. Although the combined action of TA and quadriceps results in a forward motion of legs and trunk, the complete body does not move as a rigid inverted pendulum. Fig. 1 shows that the head moves backward on the trunk during the second interval of movement (as defined in Fig. 1). Presumably this action results from the neck extensor activity labelled as TRAP in Figs. 2 and 3.

Once the legs are vertical, two righting actions are required to complete the restabilization task. It remains for the trunk to rotate backwards about the hips and the head to rotate forward about the trunk in order to re-acquire a completely vertical posture. Fig. 1 shows that the last 150 ms of movement is accomplished without major alterations in the lower leg sway angle. Angular movements of the trunk with respect to the lower leg are composed almost entirely of trunk movements. Movements of the head with respect to the trunk are large because these two segments move in opposite directions. After some 450 ms from onset of the support surface rotation, stimulus-related angular velocities of the body segments are practically small. In summary, the recordings of Fig. 1 provide no evidence supporting the hypothesis that the body links (lower leg, trunk and head) ever move together as a simple inverted pendulum following rotation of the support surface although, during the major equilibrating phase, the lower legs and trunk rotate forward as a unit about the ankle joints.

Vestibular influences on righting reactions

The temporal organization of the postural response correcting for the support-surface rotation is characterized by a forward rotation of the legs and trunk about the ankle joint which is braked in an upright lower leg position. The extent to which

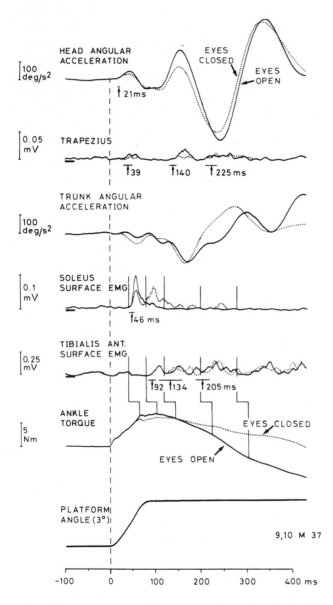

Fig. 3. Average responses of eyes-open and eyes-closed trials of a 37-year-old patient with a bilateral peripheral vestibular deficit of unknown etiology which commenced 1.5 years prior to the examination. The layout of the figure is identical to that of Fig. 2. Note the diminished EMG activity and more shallow torque trace compared to Fig. 2, particularly for eyes-closed trials. (From [14].)

lower leg muscle activity responsible for this postural response is altered by a vestibular deficit can be judged from Figs. 2 and 3. Fig. 2 depicts normal responses under eyes-open (full lines) and eyes-closed (dotted lines) conditions, and Fig. 3 shows responses from a subject with absent vestibular function (as defined by clinical tests).

The major differences between Figs. 2 and 3 are quite apparent in the amplitudes of all SOL and TA bursts of activity following the SL stretch reflex response in SOL. These differences are particularly striking for the ML responses commencing at ca. 120 ms. Over the ML response period, as defined by the thin vertical lines between 120 (145 for torque) and 200 (225) ms on the figures, the patient's ankle torque responses are characterized by a flatter profile, i.e. a smaller torque than normal to correct the induced hip and lower leg backwards sway. As a result, the pulse of fowards trunk acceleration in Fig. 3 peaks later and has a smaller amplitude than that of the normal (Fig. 2).

Figs. 2 and 3 present cases at diametric ends of vestibular system efficacy. The complete spectrum of vestibular influences on ML responses is presented as population statistics in Fig. 4. Here the average responses of three gradations of vestibular system deficiency are presented. These are, in increasing order of deficit severity; compensated unilateral deficit, acute unilateral deficit, and compensated bilateral deficit. The response size (ML EMG area or ML torque change) decrease stepwise with deficit severity. This correlation is very evident for the average of the 2nd 7 trials under eyes-closed conditions (lower right, Fig. 4). The averages are split into two sets in Fig. 4, apart from being considered for either eyes-open (left half of figure) and eyes-closed (right) conditions. Those for the 1st 3 trials are displayed separately from those for the 2nd 7 trials because the first set are significantly larger in amplitude for both normals and patients [7]. An example of the change in EMG amplitudes between the two sets of trials is shown in Fig. 1 for a normal subject. Contrary to previous reports [9, 12] the ratio of these two averages is not different between normals and patients [7, 13, 14].

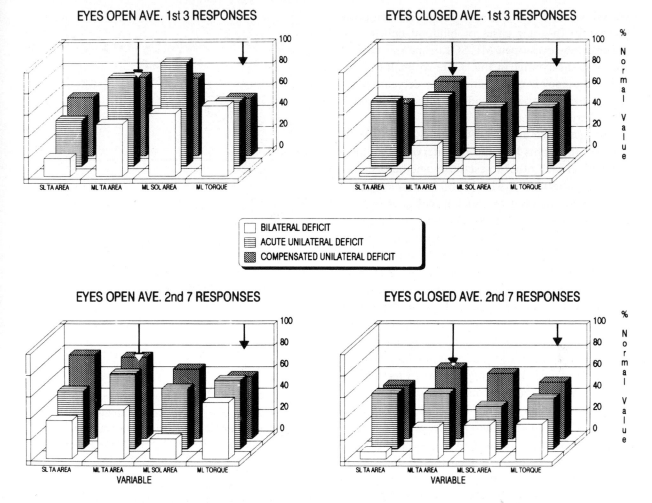

Fig. 4. Vestibulospinal reflexes. Percentage reduction of population mean values of EMG and torque responses in comparison to normal values. Three populations are illustrated; bilateral-deficit patients and patients having either acute or compensated unilateral deficit. Response variables compared, in order from left to right in each bar diagram, are SL TA EMG area (between 80 and 120 ms after onset of platform rotation), ML SOL and TA area (120–200 ms) and ML torque (145–225 ms). Eyes-open trials are on the left, eyes-closed on the right, average of 1st 3 trials in the upper portion of the figure, average of 2nd 7 trials in the lower portion. The vertical arrows above ML TA area and ML torque area indicate one standard deviation of the normal responses. Note the stepwise graduation of responses with deficit severity for eyes-closed trials. (From [14].)

Muscle co-activation at the ankle joint

Having established that the strength of the righting ankle torque generated by TA activity is correlated with the clinically defined severity of a vestibular deficit, the question arises if the co-activation pattern of ML and LL responses in the ankle muscles is also altered by a vestibular deficit.

In order to justify calling the overlapping activity patterns of the antagonist TA and SOL muscles depicted in Figs. 2 and 3 a 'co-activation', two criteria must be satisfied. Firstly the time between the onset of TA and SOL ML responses must be nonsignificant (within 1 S.D. of each other) and secondly the size of the responses must increase or decrease together. The ML response onset latencies always occurred within one standard deviation of each other [7], except in some cases of bilateral deficit. For example, the eyes-open ML SOL responses used to compose the average in Fig. 3, are so small that defining a latency is not practical. The decrease in response size over trials provided a suitable test of the second criterion.

The mean area under the TA and SOL EMG curves over the 80 ms ML and LL intervals were plotted against each other to establish whether a co-activation pattern occurs in the ankle muscles. These intervals are marked by thin vertical lines in Figs. 2 and 3. As shown in these two figures, data were considered separately for eyes-open and -closed conditions. Under each of these conditions every subject had two data points: that for the average of the 1st 3 and that for the 2nd 7 trials. Linear correlation coefficients were derived as in a previous publication [7] with normals and bilateral deficit patients data regressed together. The unilateral deficit data (acute and compensated amalgamated together) provided further regressions to test for co-activation in this population.

The areas under the ML bursts of TA and SOL are plotted in the lower half of Fig. 5. These antagonistic muscles exhibited a strongly correlated action in magnitude for combined normal and bilateral-deficit data both with eyes open ($r = 0.86$) and eyes closed ($r = 0.73$). Eyes-open unilateral data had an equally strong correlation; however, eyes-closed data was clearly less well correlated ($r = 0.36$, $p = 0.005$). Highly correlated LL responses acting to brake the body in an upright position were also observed (see lower half of Fig. 6). Again it was the unilateral-deficit, eyes-closed data that showed a lower correlation ($r = 0.5$). For the other data exhibited in the lower part of Fig. 6, the correlation was greater than 0.7. Thus for both ML and LL activity, the patient data contributed to a highly correlated pattern of co-activation with vision having little effect on the correlations except for the unilateral data. If the location of individual data points are examined in the lower half of Figs. 5 and 6, two aspects of the data are noteworthy. Firstly, as documented in Fig. 4, ML patient data size is

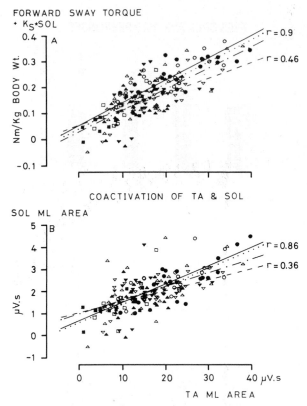

Fig. 5. Medium latency restabilizing action. Coupled activity of SOL and TA and their joint influence on ankle torque at medium latencies. (A) Linear regression of the average area under the EMG burst of TA (x axis) on the average area of ankle torque after controlling for SOL ML area (the term $K_{SOL} \times SOL$) (y axis) for each subject's 1st 3 and 2nd 7 trials at ML. Individual ankle torque values have been divided by the subject's body weight; then the average ML activity of SOL multiplied by its bivariate regression coefficient, is added to the score (forward sway torque + $K_{SOL} \times SOL$). Data for normals and patients is again combined as described above and the correlation coefficients are printed next to the regression lines. (B) The average areas under the ML burst of TA activity (x axis) of each subject's 1st 3 and 2nd 7 trials of dorsiflexion rotations are plotted against the average areas under the ML EMG burst of SOL. Open and filled symbols represent the data for eyes-open and eyes-closed conditions, respectively: $\bigcirc/\bullet$, normals; $\square/\blacksquare$, bilateral-deficit patients; $\triangle/\blacktriangle$, unilateral-deficit patients at onset; $\bigtriangledown/\blacktriangledown$, unilateral-deficit patients after 2 months. The linear regression lines have been drawn for the combined eyes-open (EO) normal and bilateral-deficit patient data (solid line) and the combined eyes-closed (EC) data (dotted line). The dash-dot and dashed lines indicate the linear regression lines fitted to the combined EO and EC unilateral data respectively. The respective correlation coefficient of the combined normal and bilateral group data for EO and unilateral EC data is printed next to the respective regression of each line.

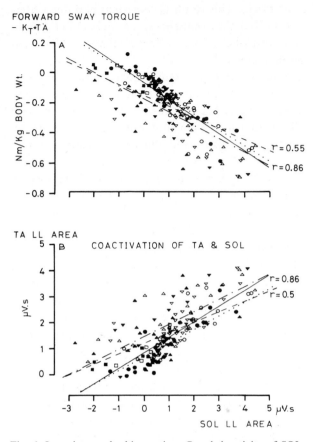

FORWARD SWAY TORQUE
$- K_T \cdot \dot{T} A$

COACTIVATION OF TA & SOL

Fig. 6. Long-latency braking action. Coupled activity of SOL and TA and their joint influence on ankle torque at long latencies. The layout is identical to Fig. 5, as are the symbols. (A) Linear regression of SOL (x axis) on ankle torque after controlling for TA area (the term, $- K_{TA} \times TA$) (y axis). As in Fig. 5, individual ankle torque values were divided by the subject's body weight. The average activity of TA is multiplied by its regression coefficient and subtracted from the values of torque (forward sway torque $- K_{TA} \times TA$). (B) Average SOL LL area (x axis) plotted against average TA LL area (y axis). Normal and patient data have again been combined to produce the linear regression.

conspicuously smaller than normal, and secondly the range of patients' LL responses overlap that of normals. The question arises as to what extent these aspects are replicated in ankle torque.

If both ankle muscles, SOL and TA are co-activated, then both will influence ankle torque, but in opposite directions. Neither alone can be uniquely

correlated with torque. When torque output at the ankle, after division by the subject's weight to remove intersubject variability, was plotted against EMG ML of LL area of either muscle, weak correlations resulted. When, however, the concerted action of both muscles was taken into account using a multiple linear regression; viz,

$$Torque = K_{TA} \times TA - K_{SOL} \times SOL + a \; constant;$$

extremely significant correlations between ankle torque and EMG area were obtained (see upper part of Figs. 5 and 6).

For the ML data (Fig. 5), the magnitude of the slope (K_{TA}) and its associated correlation coefficient indicated that TA exerted the strongest influence on torque when SOL action was accounted for. As mentioned earlier, the action of TA was clearly to increase forward sway torque about the ankle joint and bring the body forwards after the hips were thrust back by the platform rotation. The patients' torque data points are noticeably smaller in amplitude than those of normals (as documented in Fig. 4). The weaker correlation seen in unilateral-deficit patients' co-activation under eyes-closed conditions was replicated as a weaker correlation of TA ML EMG area with ankle torque.

Longer-latency torque was best predicted by SOL LL EMG area when controlling for TA activity (see upper part of Fig. 6). The more influential SOL action produced a negative sloping regression line, suggesting a braking action on the forward sway produced by ML TA activity. A clear separation of patient and normal data in the breaking torque action is not observed in Fig. 6. In contrast to the vestibular influence on equilibrating torque, the braking action follows automatically, whether a vestibular deficit is present or not. The expected consequence for trunk angular velocity would be a smaller and later peak of forward angular velocity but normal peak backward angular velocity for the patients. In total, a more unstable response for the patients would be predicted because the net backward velocity would be greater for the patients. This prediction is explored below.

Patterns of trunk and head movements in normals and vestibular-deficit patients

In contrast to the significant influences of a vestibular deficit on ankle torque, data on the pattern of trunk and head angular velocities showed, with minor exceptions, no conclusive differences between normal and vestibular-deficit subjects. The data in Fig. 7, which depicts the time and amplitude of each subject's minimum (maximum forward pitching) and maximum backward pitching trunk angular velocity, provides no distinguishing features separating normals from patients. Rather, the boundaries enclosing 95% of the normal data includes many data points from patients. The peak of forward pitching trunk velocity occurring between 180 and 250 ms after support surface rotation onset is replicated by all subjects tested except by a few unilateral-deficit patients. For the backwards pitching pulse of trunk angular velocity which effectively straightens the body during the third phase of movement (see Fig. 1), somewhat more of the patients data points lie outside the normal bounds (Fig. 7). Particularly the bilateral-deficit patients have data points indicating peak backward pitching times outside the normal range of 350 to 500 ms or larger than normal amplitudes within the normal

time range. This result is consistent with the observation that these patients under eyes-closed conditions must be stabilized by the examiner to prevent a fall backwards.

The data in Fig. 7, which quantify the maximum and minimum points of the biphasic wave of trunk angular velocity, document, in conjunction with Fig. 1, that intersegmental movements of the trunk on the hips also occur during the third phase of movement. Thus a 'hip strategy' and not a 'ankle strategy' is a common component of the latter part of both normal and vestibular-deficit equilibrating reactions. The observed forwards and then backwards movement of the trunk in response to support surface movement presents the CNS with a choice of head movement strategies. If the head is held constant in space, stable gaze is maintained, but if it is aligned with the body, movements of the centre of mass can be better predicted. As the trajectories in Fig. 1 show, head movements compensate for those of the trunk rather than following them. The data in Fig. 8 support this finding for both normal and vestibular-deficit populations. Fig. 8 illustrates the relation between maximum head angular velocity which shortly follows minimum trunk angular velocity (lower half of Fig. 8) and the relation between the minimum head velocity and maximum trunk velocity (upper part of Fig. 8) during the latter part of the equilibrating reaction. The peak amplitudes of these movements have approximately equal magnitudes of 5°/s indicating that head movements are equal and opposite in direction to trunk movements.

The scatter plots of Fig. 8 also indicate a weak influence of a vestibular deficit or of the absence of vision on head movements. A separation of the data points into clusters for normals and deficit patients is not apparent, though data points well away from the main cluster are observed for patients but not for normals. This finding on the relation of head movements to trunk movements is consistent with the weakly significant influence of a vestibular deficit on neck extensor activity commencing at 120 ms [7, 13].

To examine whether the head movements were

Fig. 7. Times and amplitudes of minimum (maximum forward pitching) and maximum backwards pitching trunk angular velocity in response to platform backwards tilt. Data from normal and vestibular-deficit populations are represented with the same symbols as in Figs. 5 and 6. The dashed lines represent approximate 95% confidence areas for the normals.

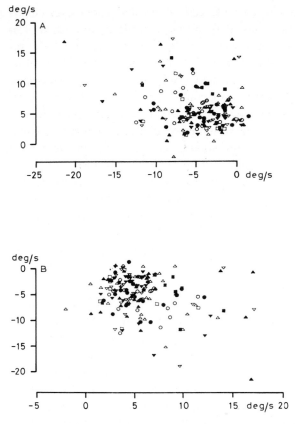

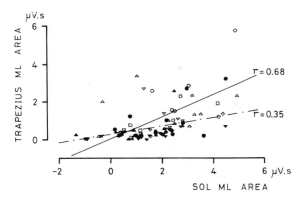

Fig. 8. (A) The relationship between minimum head and maximum trunk angular velocity whose relative times vary from subject to subject and between the averages of the 1st 3 and 2nd 7 trials (see Fig. 1). (B) Amplitude relationship of the maximum amplitude of backwards pitching head angular velocity to the preceding minimum trunk angular velocity. Symbols representing normal and patient data are identical to those used in other figures.

complicated by the more rapid adaptation of neck muscle EMG responses than in the ankle muscles [7]. For this reason, linear correlations were considered only for data representing the average of the 1st 3 trials, rather than including the averages of the 2nd 7 trials as in Figs. 5 and 6. The strongest correlation found was, as shown in Fig. 9, between SOL and TRAP. However, here the best correlation did not yield higher regression coefficients than 0.68. It is difficult, on the basis of these results, to conclude that a single afferently generated program controls both ankle muscle activity and neck muscle activation.

Discussion

When the body position is either disturbed experimentally, as in this study by rotating the support surface, or in more natural circumstances, a number of motor tasks are encountered. Firstly the centre of body mass must be stably positioned within the area of foot support, secondly movements of the body links imposed by the disturbance should be corrected into an upright stance, and finally,

Fig. 9. Questionable co-activation between neck extensor muscles and SOL tested using ML EMG response areas. Data for the average of the first 3 eyes-open (open symbols) and eyes-closed (filled symbols) trials have been plotted for normals (○/●) and patients (bilateral deficit, □/■ squares; unilateral, △/▲, as in Fig. 6). The linear regression lines were fitted to the combined normal and patient data (the unilateral data was not considered separately as in Figs. 5 and 6). The solid line is the regression line for eyes-open and the dash-dot line for eyes-closed conditions.

related to the same vestibulospinal inputs as ankle muscle EMG activity, co-activation between neck and ankle muscles was investigated in a manner similar to that used to investigate co-activation between ankle muscles. As before, two criteria were employed: overlapping of onset latencies and correlation of areas under ML EMG responses. Figs. 2 and 3 illustrate that the onset latencies of ML TRAP activity are within one standard deviation of the corresponding latencies in ankle muscles (see also Table 1 in [7]). The correlation between ankle and neck muscle ML areas was, however, weak and

throughout these movements the head must be steadied so that gaze is stable. The purposes of this study have been twofold. To determine the type of movements underlying these motor tasks and to establish how dependent they are on vestibular inputs.

Our evidence suggests that the functionally more important task of replacing the centre of mass over the base of support is accomplished between 150 and 300 ms after the onset of the disturbance and then the upper body is straightened out with respect to the legs in the following 150 ms in order to complete the restabilization within 500 ms. Throughout these two phases of movements, head rotations compensate for trunk rotations in order to maintain gaze fixation. Patients with vestibular deficits respond at the neck, ankle, and presumably at the hips as a result of induced destabilization (EMG responses of thigh and lower trunk muscles were not recorded from patients in this study). It is, however, the ankle muscle responses that are significantly weaker as a result of vestibular deficit and therefore are not as effective in producing the necessary forward torque that would place the body mass over the foot support. Rotation of the trunk about the hip and the head on the neck are not so significantly altered by a deficit of the vestibular system.

Contractions of lower leg muscles move the body centre of mass (trunk and legs) over the foot support by creating torque against the support surface, thereby rotating the body about the ankle joints. This study indicates that a pathological decrease in the strength of peripheral vestibular signals (as tested in standard clinical tests) will produce a correlated reduction in the stabilizing response in the ankle muscles at 120 ms (ML responses) followed by a correspondingly reduced ankle torque. The early excitation of semicircular canal afferents to pitch angular accelerations, ca. 20 ms following the onset of platform rotations, would supply the necessary vestibulospinal signals for the sway-stabilizing responses in the ankle muscles [6]. Although the ankle muscle and ankle torque ML responses of the bilateral-deficit patients are fundamentally reduced

to, on average, 30% of normal under eyes-closed conditions, they are not completely abolished. The onset latencies of these pathological EMG responses are also only marginally delayed by some 6 ms [7]. This evidence establishes a vestibulogenic origin for a substantial portion of the ML ankle responses. Because these ML responses have not yet been observed to be completely absent for a patient lacking a functioning vestibular system, we cannot exclude the possibility that the ML response is preprogrammed. In this case, the ML response would be initiated by proprioceptive reflexes when destabilization causes muscle stretch (in the lower leg, hip or neck muscles), and then would require vestibulospinal signals to modulate its amplitude. A likely pathway for such a modulation could be the powerful inhibition of lumbar Renshaw cells induced by ipsilateral posterior vertical semicircular canal afferents [15]. An additional modulating influence on the Renshaw cells could include the inhibitory recticulospinal cells in the medulla which receive contralateral vestibular inputs [16]. With Renshaw cells temporarily inhibited as a result of vestibular input, signals from other reflex arcs, such as muscle stretch reflexes, as well as direct vestibulospinal inputs to motoneurons, would have a substantially greater excitatory influence on lumbar motoneurons.

The straightening of the body by rotating the trunk backwards about the hip joint compensates for the forward trunk movement imposed by the stimulus and that caused by rotating the body forward as the centre of mass is placed over the base of support. Our present results indicate that this active trunk rotation is not significantly influenced by a vestibular deficit. Thus the question arises as to which neuronal mechanisms are responsible for this action given that the trunk movements are not correlated with the amplitude (EMG area) of stabilizing ankle muscle activity. This latter finding effectively rules out the possibility that the last phase of the movement dominated by trunk rotations is somehow linked by the CNS to the torque generated at the ankle in order to reduce the number of degrees of joint freedom that must be controlled.

Rather, our results indicate an independent control of trunk movements on the hip from control of rotations of the body about the ankle joint. The most parsimonious explanation for the rearwards trunk movements straightening the body, is that they occur as a result of stretch reflexes elicited in hip extensor muscles following stimulus imposed hip flexion. According to this explanation such hip stretch reflexes would functionally assist stabilization of the body, in contrast to particularly the SL stretch reflexes of the triceps surae muscles, the action of which would be to further destabilize sway after platform rotations if not opposed by TA SL and ML activity. Presumably these hip responses require no vestibulospinal modulation in order to effectively perform their righting reaction.

The rotational velocity of the head is not stable in relation to gravity. Head movements appear to be coordinated with those of the trunk so that this goal is partially achieved and gaze thereby held approximately stable in space. As shown in Figs. 1, 2, and 3, the head rotations with respect to gravity are equal to but more than $180°$ out-of-phase with trunk rotations. Although the major ML stabilizing responses occur at approximately the same latency in the neck and ankle muscles, suggestive of some central coordination of muscle activation at both body segments, these muscle groups appear from three considerations not to be co-activated. First the decrease in ML areas over trials is different at the neck and ankle, secondly the sizes of the response areas are not correlated, and lastly neck activity is not so significantly altered as ankle muscles by the absence or reduction of vestibular afferent signals [7]. Thus, as with the trunk, separate systems from those of the ankle muscles must be considered for the control of head movements. It has already been noted that the afferent origin of the neck muscle responses during postural restabilization has not been clearly identified, though, as apparent in Fig. 3, early, presumably stretch-evoked, responses are ummasked following a bilateral vestibular deficit [6]. Cervical stretch reflex mechanisms appear to be the most parsimonious explanation for the neuronal mechanisms underlying head stabilization on the trunk, with vestibular afferent and visual signals providing a secondary contribution.

It is somewhat intriguing that the CNS appears to rely on different sensory inputs to control the two active phases of the equilibriating reaction to support surface tilt. Vestibulospinal reflexes are used to replace the body's centre of mass over the support surface by activating the ankle muscles, whereas hip and head rotations appear to be primarily under the control of other sensory systems, of which muscle proprioceptive reflexes are the most likely candidate. It is equally intriguing that in the event of a vestibular deficit a different movement strategy, for example more hip movement, is not used to align the centre of mass over the base of support rather than rotation about the ankle joint. Instead the double mode of restabilization, first ankle rotation and then hip rotation is used by both normals and patients with peripheral vestibular deficits, suggesting a generalized central program controlling the structure of the equilibriating response. The separation of one sensory input for one mode of movement is maintained despite a vestibular deficit. For tilts of the support surface, at least, visual rather than proprioceptive signals are used to compensate for the absence of vestibulospinal activation of ankle muscles [6, 7]. Given the availability of visual signals in vestibular nuclei neurons [17] and the destabilizing influence of early SL stretch reflexes in the ankle muscles if these stretch reflexes were enhanced, the use of visual signals is clearly appropriate. Whether our hypothesis of the two active phases of the equilibriating reactions to support surface tilts being controlled separately by different sensory channels is also applicable to support surface translations remains to be investigated. If so it might imply that the development of man's unique upright stance occurred in two stages, each dependent on a different sensory input.

Acknowledgements

This research was supported by the Swiss National Science Foundation grant number 3.148-0.85. We are indebted to P. Abt for electronic engineering assistance and to W. Brunetti for typing the manuscript.

References

[1] Gurfinkel, E.V. (1973) Physical foundations of the stabilography. *Agressologie*, 14c: 9–14.

[2] Nashner, L.N. (1976) Adapting reflexes controlling the human posture. *Exp. Brain Res.*, 26: 59–72.

[3] Nashner, L.M., Woollacott, M. and Tuma, G. (1979) Organization of rapid responses to postural and locomotor-like perturbations of standing man. *Exp. Brain Res.*, 36: 463–476.

[4] Horak, F.B. and Nashner, L.M. (1986) Central programming of postural movements: adaptation to altered support-surface configurations. *J. Neurophysiol.*, 55: 1369–1381.

[5] Bernstein, N. (1967) *The Coordination and Regulation of Movement*, Pergamon, New York.

[6] Allum, J.H.J. and Pfaltz, C.R. (1985) Visual and vestibular contributions to pitch sway stabilization in the ankle muscles of normals and patients with bilateral peripheral deficits. *Exp. Brain Res.*, 58: 82–94.

[7] Keshner, E.A., Allum, J.H.J. and Pfaltz, C.R. (1987) Postural coactivation and adaptation in the sway stabilizing responses of normals and patients with bilateral vestibular deficit. *Exp. Brain Res.*, 69: 77–92.

[8] Diener, H.C., Bootz, F., Dichgans, J. and Bruzek W. (1983) Variability of postural 'reflexes' in humans. *Exp. Brain Res.*, 52: 423–428.

[9] Nashner, L.M., Black, F.O. and Wall, C. III (1982) Adaptation to altered support and visual conditions during stance: patients with vestibular deficits. *J. Neurosci.*, 2: 536–544.

[10] Allum, J.H.J., Yamane, M. and Pfaltz, C.R. (1988) Long-term modifications of vertical and horizontal vestibulo-ocular reflex dynamics in man. I. After acute unilateral peripheral vestibular paralysis. *Acta Otolaryngol. Stockholm*, 105: 328–337.

[11] Allum, J.H.J. and Mauritz, K.-H. (1984) Compensation for intrinsic muscle stiffness by short latency reflexes in human triceps surae muscles. *J. Neurophysiol.*, 52: 797–818.

[12] Black, F.O., Wall, C. III and Nashner, L.M. (1983) Effects of visual and support surface orientation references upon postural control in vestibular deficient subjects. *Acta Otolaryngol. Stockholm*, 95: 199–210.

[13] Keshner, E.A. and Allum, J.H.J. (1986) Plasticity in pitch sway stabilization: normal habituation and compensation for peripheral vestibular deficits. In W. Bles and T. Brandt (Eds.), *Disorders of Posture and Gait*, Elsevier, Amsterdam, pp. 289–314.

[14] Allum, J.H.J., Keshner, E.A., Honegger, F. and Pfaltz, C.R. (1988) Indicators of the influence of a peripheral vestibular deficit has on vestibulo-spinal reflex responses controlling postural stability. *Acta Otolaryngol. Stockholm*, in press.

[15] Ross, H.-G. and Thewissen, M. (1987) Inhibitory connections of ipsilateral semicircular canal afferents onto Renshaw cells in the lumbar spinal cord of the cat. *J. Physiol. London*, 388: 83–99.

[16] Pompeiano, O., Wand, P. and Srivastava, U.C. (1985) Influence of Renshaw cells on the response gain of hindlimb extensor muscles to sinusoidal labyrinth stimulation. *Pflügers Arch.*, 404: 107–118.

[17] Waespe, W. and Henn, V. (1977) Neuronal activity in the vestibular nuclei of the alert monkey during vestibular and optokinetic stimulation. *Exp. Brain Res.*, 27: 523–538.

O. Pompeiano and J.H.J. Allum (Eds.)
Progress in Brain Research, Vol. 76
© 1988 Elsevier Science Publishers B.V. (Biomedical Division)

CHAPTER 25

Labyrinthine control of upright standing posture in humans

T. Tokita, Y. Ito, H. Miyata and H. Koizumi

Department of Otorhinolaryngology, Gifu University School of Medicine, Tsukasamachi 40, Gifu 500, Japan

To clarify the role of the labyrinth in the regulation of upright standing posture, vestibular control of the soleus muscle was studied by reference to the evoked EMG induced by galvanic stimulation of the labyrinth in humans. Galvanic labyrinthine stimulation induced ipsilateral excitation and contralateral inhibition of soleus muscle activity with a latency of about 100 ms. The inhibition was stronger than the excitation and showed predominance of the long-latency component in the evoked responses. These results indicated that the labyrinthine system exerts a prominent inhibitory influence on spinal extensor mechanisms. The predominance of this inhibitory control explained the peculiar forward–backward sway observed in the upright standing posture of patients with bilateral loss of labyrinthine function. In general, the role of the labyrinth in postural regulation has been explained on the basis of the facilitatory effect exerted by the lateral vestibulospinal tract on the extensor muscles. However, for the total labyrinthine system, the inhibitory influence upon the extensor is more important for postural regulation.

Introduction

The role of the labyrinth in postural regulation has been explained on the basis of the facilitatory effect upon the extensor by the lateral vestibulospinal tract. Brodal et al. [1] described that the vestibular apparatus, particularly the vestibular nuclei, exerts a facilitatory effect on the extensor tonus and extensor reflexes, accompanied by reciprocal influences on the antagonistic muscles. However, patients with bilateral loss of labyrinthine excitability show a characteristic forward–backward sway in stabilograms. A similar forward–backward sway has been observed in patients with increased spinal reflexes. These findings suggest the importance of the inhibitory influence of the labyrinth upon the extensor muscles [2].

The purpose of the present study was to clarify the nature of vestibular control upon the antigravity muscles using an evoked EMG induced by galvanic stimulation of the labyrinth in an upright standing posture in humans.

Methods

Fig. 1. shows the experimental procedure used. A subject was asked to stand with eyes closed on a stabilometer, and was stimulated with galvanic current. The stimulation was performed using both monopolar–monoaural and monopolar–biaural methods. The intensity was 1 mA for the former and 2 mA for the latter. The duration was 4 or 6 s.

The vestibulospinal responses induced by the stimulation were observed in terms of the CG sway and the activities of both soleus muscles. The muscle activities were recorded as integrated EMG with surface electrodes. The reactions induced by repetitive stimulation between 5 and 10 times were averaged using a microcomputer and displayed on a cathode ray tube.

Abbreviations: CG, centre of gravity of the body; DR, deviation response; EMG, electromyogram; EPSP, excitatory postsynaptic potential; IR, initial response.

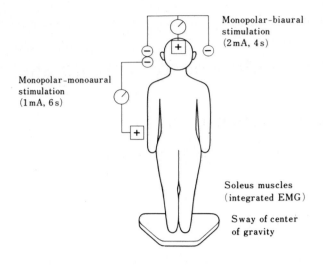

Fig. 1. Examination of galvanic vestibulospinal reflexes.

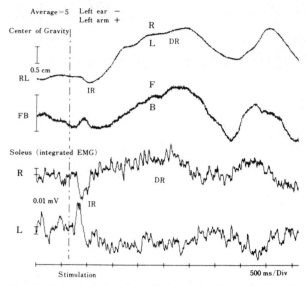

Fig. 2. Galvanic induced vestibulospinal reflexes. L, left; R, right; F, forwards; B, backwards.

The examination was performed on 6 healthy males.

Results

Responses induced by monopolar–monoaural stimulation

Fig. 2 indicates the CG sway and the evoked EMGs of the right and left soleus muscles when galvanic stimulation was carried out with the cathode on the left ear. The first and second lines are records of the right–left (R–L) and forward–backward (F–B) sway of the CG, respectively. The third and fourth lines indicate the activities of the right and left soleus muscles. The abscissa shows the time course. One division is 500 ms. The vertical dashed line indicates the time of stimulation. The ordinate is the amplitude of the reaction. The R–L sway of the CG indicated an initial response (IR) toward the left, i.e. the stimulated side, with a latency of about 200 ms. The IR was followed by a deviation response (DR) toward the right side, which continued during the stimulation. In the soleus muscles, the activity increased with a latency of about 100 ms on the left, i.e. the stimulated side, and decreased on the right, i.e. the contralateral side. These were the IRs of the

soleus muscles. Following the IRs, the activities of the soleus muscles increased on the right side and decreased on the left side. These were the DRs of the soleus muscles.

The IRs are considered to be indicating direct evoked responses of the vestibulospinal pathways. On the other hand, the DRs of the muscles are secondary responses produced by body deviation toward the contralateral side of the stimulation. Thereafter, the IRs of the soleus muscles were subjected to study.

Latency and duration of labyrinthine-evoked EMG

Fig. 3 indicates the latency and duration of the IR for both soleus muscles. The left ear was stimulated by cathodal current at 1 mA. The time scale is 200 ms per division. The latency of the IR was 108 ms on the right side and 106 ms on the left side, and the duration was longer on the right inhibitory side than the left excitatory side. The contralateral inhibition was stronger than the ipsilateral excitation for the soleus activities induced by galvanic labyrinthine stimulation. The excitation of the stimulated side seemed to be effected through the lateral vesti-

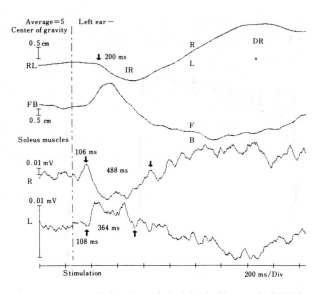

Fig. 3. Latency and duration of the labyrinthine-evoked EMG of the soleus muscles.

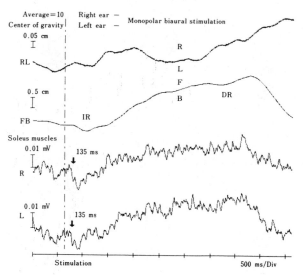

Fig. 4. Evoked EMG induced by monopolar–biaural stimulation.

bulospinal pathway. For the inhibitory effect, other pathways such as the reticulospinal pathway should be considered. For the IR of the soleus, solely an inhibitory effect was observed in 3 of 12 ears tested (6 subjects). None of the subjects indicated only an excitatory effect. These results indicate that the labyrinth produces strong contralateral inhibition of the soleus muscles compared with ipsilateral excitation. In order to confirm these results, the following monopolar–biaural stimulation experiment was carried out.

Labyrinthine-evoked EMG induced by monopolar–biaural stimulation

Fig. 4 shows the result of monopolar–biaural stimulation by application of the cathode to both ears, resulting in stimulation of the bilateral labyrinths. The intensity of the galvanic current was 2 mA. Following the stimulation, the activity of both soleus muscles decreased with a latency of 135 ms, which was longer than that for monopolar–monoaural stimulation. This result indicated that the inhibitory influence was stronger than the excitatory influence upon the soleus muscles. A difference in

intensity between inhibition and excitation appeared as a longer response latency compared with that seen in monopolar–monoaural stimulation. This observation indicated that the predominance of the inhibition is dependent on the long-latency components in the labyrinthine-evoked responses.

Discussion

The results obtained from the present studies on the labyrinthine-evoked EMG were as follows.

(1) Galvanic labyrinthine stimulation induced ipsilateral excitation and contralateral inhibition of soleus muscle activity with a latency of about 100 ms.

(2) The evoked EMG induced by monopolar–monoaural stimulation provided evidence of predominance of inhibitory control. This predominance was based on the long-latency component in the evoked EMG.

(3) The labyrinthine spinal system as a whole appeared to have an inhibitory effect on the antigravity muscles.

These results modify the concept that impulses of vestibular origin exert only a tonic excitatory influ-

294

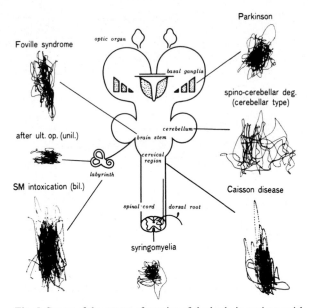

Fig. 5. Sways of the centre of gravity of the body in patients with equilibrium disturbances (stabilograms with eyes closed). deg., degeneration; unil., unilateral; bil., bilateral; ult. op, ultrasonic operation.

ence on postural tonus and spinal extensor mechanisms. In particular, it appears that the labyrinthine input exerts a prominent inhibitory influence on the spinal cord. Patients with bilateral loss of labyrinthine excitability indicates a characteristic forward–backward sway in upright standing posture. Fig. 5 shows stabilograms, i.e. CG sways in an upright standing posture, in patients with equilibrium disturbances due to dysfunction of the labyrinth, brainstem, cerebellum and spinal cord. A patient with bilateral loss of labyrinthine excitability due to streptomycin intoxication shows a forward–backward sway. Similar forward–backward sways were also observed in patients with Foville's syndrome and Caisson disease accompanied by increased spinal reflexes This forward–backward sway in patients with loss of labyrinthine function is interpreted as being caused by increased spinal reflexes due to loss of inhibitory control of the extensor muscles.

These results indicate that the crossed inhibitory pathway is important in vestibulospinal control. On the crossed pathways from the vestibular nuclei to the spinal cord, the following pathways have been described. Grillner and Hongo [3] reported that the vestibulospinal tract gives disynaptic excitation and trisynaptic inhibition to contralateral α motoneurons through interneurons which are located in the ventromedial part of the gray matter and send their axons to the contralateral side of the spinal cord. The reticulospinal pathway can also greatly contribute to the contralateral inhibition observed during labyrinthine stimulation. The vestibular nuclei project, in fact, to reticulospinal and propriospinal neurons, which may thus collaborate with the vestibulospinal projections to the labyrinthine control of different spinal mechanisms [4]. The pontine reticulospinal pathway descends ipsilaterally, while the medullary pathway is both crossed and uncrossed [5]. Stimulation of the medial brainstem region evokes reciprocal effects; excitation of the flexor and inhibition of the extensor motoneurons, and the pathway evoking monosynaptic EPSPs in lumbar flexor motoneurons originates from the ipsilateral nucleus reticularis pontis caudalis [6]. However, the reticulospinal projection cannot by itself explain the predominance of the contralateral inhibition observed during vestibular stimulation. Pompeiano [7] reported that the vestibulospinal tract acting on neurons of the crossed spinoreticulocerebellar pathway and the olivocerebellar projection may send labyrinthine influences to the contralateral cerebellar vermis. The possibility therefore exists that these crossed pathways passing through the cerebellum are in part at least responsible for the inhibitory component of the labyrinthine responses acting on contralateral extensor muscles. However, the neural mechanism responsible for predominance of contralateral inhibition remains to be determined.

References

[1] Brodal, A., Pompeiano, O. and Walberg, F. (1962) *The Vestibular Nuclei and their Connections, Anatomy and Functional Correlations*, Oliver and Boyd, Edinburgh/London, pp. 109–126.
[2] Tokita, T., Maeda, M. and Miyata, H. (1981) The role of the labyrinth in standing posture regulation. *Acta Otolaryngol. Stockholm*, 91:521–527.

[3] Grillner, S. and Hongo, T. (1972) Vestibulospinal effects on motoneurones and interneurones in the lumbosacral cord. In A. Brodal and O. Pompeiano (Eds.), *Basic Aspects of Control Vestibular Mechanisms, Progress of Brain Research, Vol. 37*, Elsevier, Amsterdam, pp. 243–262.

[4] Pompeiano, O. (1972) Vestibulospinal relations: vestibular influences on gamma motoneurons and primary afferents. In A. Brodal and O. Pompeiano (Eds.), *Basic Aspects of Control Vestibular Mechanisms, Progress in Brain Research, Vol. 37*, Elsevier, Amsterdam, pp. 197–232.

[5] Brodal, A. (1957) *The Reticular Formation of the Brain Stem. Anatomical Aspects and Functional Correlations*, Oliver and Boyd, Edinburgh/London, pp. 12–31.

[6] Grillner, S. and Lund, S. (1968) The origin of a descending pathway with monosynaptic action on flexor motoneurones. *Acta Physiol. Scand.*, 74:274–284.

[7] Pompeiano, O. (1985) Experimental central nervous system lesions and posture. In M. Igarashi and O. Black (Eds.), *Vestibular and Visual Control on Posture and Locomotor Equilibrium*, Karger, Basel, pp. 218–231.

O. Pompeiano and J.H.J. Allum (Eds.)
Progress in Brain Research, Vol. 76
© 1988 Elsevier Science Publishers B.V. (Biomedical Division)

CHAPTER 26

A system identification approach to balance testing

B.E. Maki and G.R. Fernie

Centre for Studies in Aging, Sunnybrook Medical Centre and Department of Surgery, University of Toronto,
2075 Bayview Avenue, Toronto, Ontario, M4N 3M5 Canada

By modelling the posture control system as a linear transfer function cascaded with a saturation-like nonlinearity, the problem of quantifying relative stability was reduced to a linear system identification problem. The relative stability of different individuals was quantified in terms of the nominal 'saturation amplitude' (SA), the transient perturbation amplitude at which the resulting COP displacement would saturate (or equal the length of) the BOS. To ensure subject safety and to minimize anticipatory adaptations, the transient response was determined indirectly. A small-amplitude pseudorandom perturbation was applied and the results used to identify the linear component of the cascade model. The linear transfer function was then used to predict the large-amplitude transient response, thereby allowing the saturation amplitude to be estimated. Three system identification methods were used: cross spectral, least squares and maximum likelihood. In order to approximate the kinematics and sensory input of typical falling situations, the test perturbation was selected to be an anterior–posterior acceleration of the platform on which the subject stood, with a visual field that moved with the platform. The perturbation waveform, power spectrum, bandwidth, duration and amplitude were selected to meet requirements for persistent excitation, accurate identification, stationarity and subject safety and tolerance. Pilot experiments were performed to aid in the selection of the perturbation parameters. Testing of 64 young and elderly normal adults has shown the balance test to be a sensitive measure of the deterioration in postural control known to occur in normal ageing. Depending on the system identification method used, the balance test has been able to identify up to three of five patients with peripheral vestibular lesions and five of five elderly subjects with a history of falling, at a false positive rate of 25%. Comparison of the model predictions with direct measurements of transient response has indicated that the model may overestimate the response to large transient perturbations; however, the transient test results may have been confounded by adaptive effects. The balance test results have shown no significant correlation with measures of spontaneous postural sway, except in normal young adults.

Introduction

One of the simplest and most widely used quantitative balance tests involves measurement of spontaneous postural sway during quiet standing. An alternate approach is to measure the response to an applied postural perturbation.

In perturbation experiments, the responses may be evaluated in a comparative manner, viewing the perturbation primarily as a stimulus, i.e. a means to elicit balancing responses. This is the approach used in many neurophysiological experiments. In contrast, in the system identification approach, measurements of the applied perturbation and the resulting balancing response are used to identify an input/output model of the posture control system.

An input/output model is desirable because it characterizes the system itself and can be used to predict the response of the system to other inputs, i.e. inputs that may differ from those used in the ex-

---

Abbreviations: ANOVA, analysis of variance; BOS, base of support; COP, centre of pressure; SA, saturation amplitude.

periments. The other approaches may yield results that are less generalizable. Spontaneous sway measurements characterize the response to an unknown input, measured over an arbitrary time interval. In the 'comparative response' approach, the results are specific to the particular perturbation used in the tests.

In theory, spontaneous sway measurements can be used to identify input/output models of components of the posture control loop. Ishida and Miyazaki [1] used this approach, treating ankle angle and moment as the input and output. However, the lack of an independent input can create serious bias errors in the model estimates [2].

Spontaneous sway tests have another potential disadvantage. It can be argued that a functional balance test should characterize the relative stability of the individual in actual falling situations. However, the small-amplitude spontaneous sway measures may bear little relation to the postural performance in typical falling situations, which involve much larger amplitudes of sway. Small- and large-amplitude responses may differ because of nonlinearities in the posture control system, e.g. sensory thresholds, nonlinear muscle stiffness.

The purpose of this paper is to outline a system identification approach to balance testing. The details of a new testing methodology are presented, as well as the underlying rationale, and early experimental results are summarized.

The stability criterion

Typically, in system identification studies, linear transfer function models have been used to characterize postural performance (e.g. [3–5]). A linear model may be a reasonable approximation for a limited range of perturbation amplitudes; however, this approach may fail to yield accurate predictions of stability. A fall occurs when a relatively large perturbation causes the posture control system to become unstable. In this situation, the linear approximation may no longer be valid, as saturation-like nonlinearities come into play, i.e. limitations on muscle strength, joint range of motion, support sur-face friction, COP displacement, etc.

The limitation on COP displacement imposed by the finite length of the BOS (i.e. the feet) is hypothesized to be the dominant saturation-like nonlinearity that affects postural stability. Once the COP reaches the perimeter of the BOS, further increases in stabilizing ankle moment or shear force will cause the foot to rotate. In general, at this point (or soon after), a more complex balance-recovery manoeuvre must be executed in order to avoid falling (e.g. grab a handrail, initiate a step, or modify a step already in progress).

Treating the postural perturbation as the input and the resulting COP displacement as the output, the posture control system can be modelled as a 'linear–nonlinear cascade': a linear, time-invariant transfer function cascaded with a saturation-like nonlinearity, where the saturation limits are defined by the length of the BOS. When BOS saturation occurs, the system must switch to a new control mode in order to maintain stability, i.e. a more complex balance-recovery manoeuvre must be initiated. Within the framework of the posture control model postulated by Droulez et al. [6], the system operates in a 'conservative' mode at subsaturation amplitudes, i.e. continuous closed-loop servocontrol. When BOS saturation occurs, the system switches to a 'projective' mode, selecting an appropriate motor program from a pre-established repertoire.

Because of the time delays expected to occur in selecting and initiating the more complex projective manoeuvres, it can be argued that optimal postural stability will be achieved by minimizing reliance on these manoeuvres, instead utilizing the conservative mode of operation to the greatest extent possible. If this is true, then relative postural stability can be defined in terms of the size of the conservative operating range, i.e. the range of perturbations that each individual can withstand without saturating the BOS.

System identification

By separating the posture control model into linear and nonlinear components in the manner described above, the problem of quantifying relative stability is reduced to a linear system identification problem. Although a linear time-invariant model is a gross approximation of the posture control system, the approximation may well be sufficiently accurate for the purposes of a functional balance test. The capabilities of the linear approach were fully exploited by giving careful consideration to the selection and design of the perturbation input signal and by utilizing sophisticated system identification methods.

Selection and design of the perturbation input

Transient versus continuous waveforms

Extrapolation of the balance test results to everyday balancing performance depends on the degree to which the test perturbation simulates common causes of falling, such as slips, trips, missteps and self-induced displacements. A transient waveform would provide the best stimulation of these types of perturbations; however, a transient balance test presents several difficulties.

The safety of such a test is a major concern, particularily in dealing with 'frail' elderly subjects. Even if the risk of injury is reduced through the use of a safety harness, handrails or padded surfaces, anticipatory adaptations may lead to responses that are unlikely to occur in actual falling situations, where balance is perturbed suddenly and unexpectedly. This problem is compounded because repetitive testing is needed in order to achieve accurate system identification when using transient inputs [7]. Repeated testing with transient waveforms can lead to adaptive changes in postural synergies and/ or initial posture [8–10]. These adaptations degrade the identification of a time-invariant model. Moreover, they represent anticipatory effects that are unlikely to occur in actual falls.

One solution to the problems associated with transient perturbations is to use a safe small-amplitude continuous-waveform perturbation in the balance test and to predict large-amplitude transient response using the continuous-waveform test results. Through appropriate choice of amplitude, power spectrum and bandwidth, a continuous perturbation can be designed to minimize apprehension and risk of falling. Large-amplitude response can be predicted from small-amplitude tests provided that the posture control system is approximately linear over the range of perturbation amplitudes used in the measurements and predictions. If the waveform is unpredictable to the subject, then the test should elicit posture control system behaviour similar to that occurring in actual falling situations.

Simulation of falling situations

To allow extrapolation of the balance test results to everyday postural performance, the test perturbation should simulate the kinematics and sensory input of a typical falling circumstance.

A translational acceleration of a platform on which the subject stands approximates the kinematics of typical falling situations in that it creates a relative acceleration between the feet and the upper body. Provided that the visual field moves with the platform, the predominant visual, somatosensory and vestibular sensory feedback is derived from the swaying motion of the body relative to the platform, consistent with a fall relative to the platform frame of reference.

One exception lies in the vestibular otoliths, which record the linear acceleration of the head in an absolute reference frame. It is not clear, at present, to what extent the discongruence in the otolith inputs will affect relatively rapid balancing responses. Nashner [11] has argued that the otoliths do not contribute to rapid responses, because of their slow dynamic response and their inability to distinguish between inertial and gravitational stimuli; however, experimental evidence has suggested that the opposite may be true, at least for vertical accelerations [12].

In any balancing task, the postural responses will depend on the 'sensory context', i.e. the manner in which the data from the different sensory modalities is interpreted and utilized. The moving-field moving-platform test stimulates the sensory context of falls that occur during quasistatic activities, in that the predominant (nonotolith) sensory input is derived from the relative swaying motion of the body. In contrast, the visual input during stationary-field moving-platform tests provides absolute-motion information. Although this type of test might simulate the sensory context of a fall during gait, faithful stimulation of the gait-related sensory inputs is not achieved. Furthermore, in using a continuous waveform, the stationary-field test may suffer from a loss of unpredictability, as subjects are able to estimate the limits of the platform motion and thereby anticipate when changes in direction are imminent.

Selection of the perturbation parameters

To simulate the unpredictable nature of fall-provoking perturbations, a pseudorandom waveform was selected. Pseudorandom waveforms are preferred to random waveforms, because random tests require longer measurement times in order to 'average out' the inherent statistical variability. By designing the pseudorandom signal to include a relatively small number of frequency components, none of which are small-integer multiples, it is possible to minimize harmonic and intermodulation distortion (due to nonlinearity) in the linear transfer function estimates [13,14]. In selecting the power spectrum, bandwidth, amplitude and duration of the test perturbation, consideration was given to the need for persistent excitation, accurate system identification, stationarity, and subject safety and tolerance [15]. Pilot experiments were performed to aid in selecting the perturbation parameters.

Although the same spectrum (flat acceleration), bandwidth (0.1–5.0 Hz) and duration (3 minutes) were selected for all subjects, the most appropriate perturbation amplitude was expected to be subject-dependent. In general, the perturbation amplitude should be as large as possible, within the constraints of subject safety and tolerance, in order to maximize the signal-to-noise ratio in the measurements and to minimize the influence of sensory threshold nonlinearities. In addition, if the assumed linear subsaturation operating range of the posture control system is in fact substantially nonlinear, then it may be desirable to maximize the perturbation amplitude in order to minimize errors in the prediction of large-amplitude transient response. The testing protocol was designed to iterate toward the most appropriate amplitude for each subject, starting with a conservatively small value estimated from the pilot tests (RMS acceleration of 0.1 m/s^2).

System identification methods

Initial exploration of the data was performed by generating nonparametric frequency-response plots, using the cross spectral method [16]. To allow predictions of transient response, the frequency-response estimates were fitted with a parametric transfer function model, using the coherence function as a weighting factor. For the 'nonharmonic' pseudorandom inputs used here, the coherence indicates approximately the amount of 'noise' in the output (due to measurement error and/or unmeasured inputs) [13,14] and therefore reflects the degree of confidence in the frequency-response estimate at each frequency. The general form of the model is:

$$H(s) = Ke^{-\tau s}\, N(s)/D(s),$$

where $N(s)$ and $D(s)$ are polynomials in s, the Laplace operator.

The cross spectral method is an example of the 'classical' frequency-response approach to system identification. In recent years, a plethora of sophisticated time-domain methods has appeared [17]. The data were re-analysed using two of these methods, least squares [18] and maximum likelihood [19], to determine whether the cross spectral results could be improved.

Much of the work in this field has been highly theoretical, and relatively few discussions of practical engineering applications are available. Åström and Wittenmark [20] have concluded that there is no method that is universally the best and that the choice of method is not crucial. Their recommendations included the maximum likelihood method. The least squares method is useful for generating the initial parameter estimates required for the maximum likelihood method, and can be used as a system identification method in its own right, although certain estimation errors can arise [21]. The general form of these models is:

$$A(d)\, y(n) = d^k\, B(d)\, x(n) + \lambda\, C(d)\, e(n),$$

where $y(n)$ and $x(n)$ are the sampled COP and acceleration data, $e(n)$ are the residuals, and A, B and C are polynomials in d, the backward time shift operator. In the least squares model, $\lambda \equiv 1$ and $C(d) \equiv 1$.

Based on the considerations discussed earlier, the subsaturation model was constrained to be a linear, time-invariant, single-input/single-output transfer function. For each test, however, it was necessary to determine the most appropriate model order and dead time (i.e. time delay or latency). Of the several methods that exist for determining model structure [22], the Akaike method was chosen because of its simplicity. The Akaike criterion avoids the problem of 'overfitting' by penalizing model complexity. Upper bounds for the equation order and dead time were estimated through inspection of the nonparametric frequency-response plots. For the least squares and maximum likelihood methods, the maximum equation order was set at a higher value (i.e. the limit imposed by the system identification software) in order to 'whiten' the residuals, if necessary, in order to prevent bias errors in the estimates [21].

The balance testing methodology

The balance test is based on the linear–nonlinear cascade posture control model. The relative stability of different individuals is quantified in terms of the nominal SA, the transient perturbation amplitude at which the resulting COP displacement would saturate (or equal the length of) the BOS.

To ensure subject safety and to minimize anticipatory adaptations, the transient response is determined indirectly. A small-amplitude pseudorandom perturbation is applied by accelerating the platform on which the subject stands, and the resulting acceleration and COP measurements are used to identify the linear component of the model.

The linear transfer function is then used to predict the transient response to a 'unit-area' pulse in platform acceleration. The nominal saturation amplitude is estimated as follows: SA = BOS/ΔCOP, where ΔCOP is the peak COP displacement in the predicted unit pulse response (see Fig. 3) and BOS is the average anterior–posterior foot length.

In an actual fall, BOS saturation will depend on the initial COP location, as well as the dynamic COP displacement associated with the balancing response. Lacking information about the most probable initial COP location, the nominal SA estimates do not account for this factor. The ability to generate stabilizing ankle moment or shear force during the balance test will not be fully compromised until both feet saturate; therefore, the SA is defined using the overall COP, rather than analysing each foot separately. Since the return overshoot is much smaller than the initial COP displacement and therefore less likely to cause BOS saturation, the SA estimates are based on the initial COP displacement alone (see Fig. 3). The length of the BOS is defined as the foot length, since analysis of transient tests failed to provide a more accurate functional definition [23].

Experimental methods

The experimental methods are outlined below. More detailed descriptions are provided elsewhere [15,23–25].

The perturbation platform

The perturbation platform generates one degree-of-freedom of anterior–posterior translational motion. It is capable of generating accelerations of up to 20 m/s^2, with a peak velocity of 2 m/s and a range of 0.6 m. For the perturbation amplitudes used in the balance test, the frequency response of the platform is flat to within 3 dB for frequencies up to 5 Hz. A visual surround, safety handrails and foam-padded enclosure move with the platform. Mounted on the platform are two force plates, which record the location of the COP on each foot to within approximately 1 mm, and an accelerometer, which records

302

the platform acceleration to within approximately 0.05 m/s² (error standard deviation).

The testing procedure

For each test, the subjects are instructed to stand relaxed, with feet comfortably spaced (unshod), and arms at sides. To ensure consistent visual and vestibular input, the subjects are instructed to look straight ahead, using a poster as a visual target (eye–object distance of 0.7 m). 'Muzak'® (i.e. bland monotonous music) is played (through headphones) to mask auditory cues from the platform motor, as well as distracting sounds from the laboratory environment.

The platform motion is controlled to start and end gradually, with no sudden changes in acceleration. During the tests, the subjects are observed to determine whether they grabbed the safety handrail, moved their feet or waved their arms. Foot tracings are used to detect changes from the initial foot position and to allow the feet to be repositioned identically in subsequent tests. Fatigue-related changes in response are minimized by allowing seated rests (2–3 minutes) between tests.

Protocol

To date, the balance test methodology has been used to test 32 young (20–40) and 32 elderly (61–79) healthy normal subjects, as well as 5 patients with unilateral peripheral vestibular lesions and 5 elderly subjects with a documented history of falling.

The protocol included a learning trial, tests at two different amplitudes, and a blindfolded test. Initially, a conservatively small amplitude was used (RMS acceleration of 0.1 m/s²). The amplitude was either increased (to 0.15 m/s²) or decreased (to 0.075 m/s²) in the next test, depending on the tolerance of the subject. Spontaneous sway was also measured, to allow the balance test responses to be compared to more traditional measures of postural stability.

In addition to the tests described above, the young normal subjects were tested using transient (acceleration pulse) waveforms. The amplitudes ranged from 0.5 to 3 m/s²; three trials were performed at each amplitude. The primary objective of these tests was to provide data that would allow the ability of the continuous-waveform tests to predict transient response to be evaluated. For safety reasons, the elderly subjects were not tested. Furthermore, only backward platform translations were used, and the perturbation amplitudes were tested in ascending order, stopping when the subject could no longer maintain balance.

Results and discussion

Example experimental results are shown in Figs. 1–4. Fig. 1 shows a 20 s segment of the measured input (acceleration) and output (COP) data. The resulting frequency response estimate (cross spectral method) and unit pulse response prediction are shown in Figs. 2 and 3, respectively. Example transient response predictions and measurements are compared in Fig. 4.

In general, the three system identification methods produced ΔCOP estimates that were in fairly

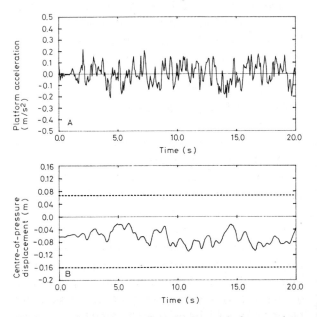

Fig. 1. Example input/output data. (A) Input (platform acceleration); (B) output (centre-of-pressure displacement); broken lines indicate anterior and posterior boundaries of the BOS.

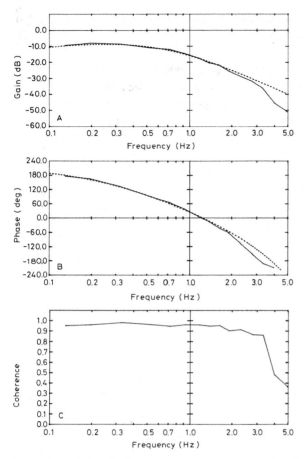

Fig. 2. Example transfer function estimates (cross spectral method): (A) gain; (B) phase; (C) coherence; solid line, nonparametric frequency response; broken line, parametric transfer function.

close agreement (mean difference $\simeq 2\%$, standard deviation $\simeq 5\%$). Occasionally, however, selection of an inappropriate model structure caused the cross spectral method to produce results that differed by 20–30%. For this reason, the cross spectral method is not recommended, except for initial data exploration and in cases where computational expense must be minimized.

The experimental results are summarized below. More detailed discussions are presented elsewhere [23–25].

Age and sex differences in normal subjects

ANOVA demonstrated highly significant ($p <$

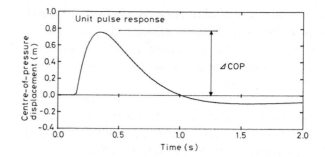

Fig. 3. Example transient response prediction: centre-of-pressure displacement resulting from 'unit-area' acceleration pulse at time $= 0.0$ seconds (saturation amplitude, SA $=$ BOS$/\Delta$COP, where BOS $=$ average foot length).

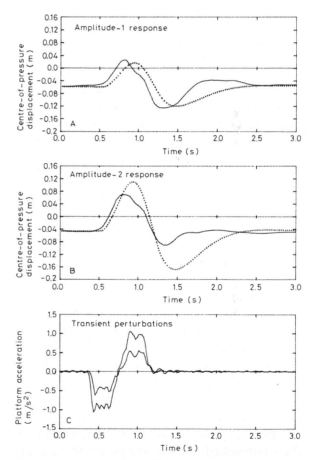

Fig. 4. Comparison of predictions and measurements of transient response, example results: (A) COP response to amplitude-1 perturbation (0.5 m/s^2), (B) COP response to amplitude-2 perturbation (1.0 m/s^2) (solid line, measured response; broken line, predicted response); (C) amplitude-1 and amplitude-2 platform accelerations.

< 0.001) differences between young and elderly normals, with reduced stability (i.e. smaller SA) predicted for the elderly under both eyes-open and blindfolded conditions. No significant sex-related differences were found ($p > 0.1$). ANOVA of the dead time parameter in the model showed significantly higher values in the elderly subjects (e.g. mean of 0.117 s versus 0.091 s; $p < 0.001$); therefore, at least some of the age-related differences in SA can be attributed to slowing of the postural responses.

Influence of vision

The experiments demonstrated a significant increase in predicted stability in the blindfolded test ($p < 0.01$). Approximately 85–90% of the normal subjects showed an increase in SA when blindfolded. Possibly, subjects overcompensate for the loss of visual input by increasing the 'stiffness' of the posture control system, through increases in the gain of the vestibular and somatosensory feedback or through various other mechanisms (e.g. cocontraction). Increases in reflex gain with eyes closed have in fact been demonstrated [1,3].

Identification of balance-impaired individuals

With the exception of one vestibular patient, the eyes-open balancing performance of the balance-impaired subjects was similar to that of the normal subjects. The major differences appeared in the blindfolded tests and in the eyes-open/blindfolded ratio. Using the eyes-open/blindfolded ratio, the balance test was able to identify correctly up to 3 of the 5 vestibular patients, and 5 of the 5 elderly fallers, at a false positive rate of 25% in the normal subjects.

It should be emphasized that the testing of the balance-impaired subjects performed to date has been intended to provide only a preliminary evaluation of the balance test. The small numbers of balance-impaired subjects tested severely limit the accuracy with which the true misclassification rates can be estimated [26].

Comparison of spontaneous sway with balance test responses

For amplitude measures of spontaneous sway, larger values are expected to be indicative of greater instability. Because the SA is instead a measure of stability, one would expect a negative correlation between these measures of spontaneous sway and the SA. Only in the young normal subjects was this found to be the case. The elderly normals, vestibular patients and elderly fallers either failed to show this trend or showed the opposite trend.

Conceivably, the elderly normal, vestibular patient and elderly faller subjects may show a greater tendency to modulate their balancing strategy. Thus, for example, the more unstable individuals may increase their 'stiffness' during the balance tests in order to prevent themselves from falling, but may show relatively normal levels of 'stiffness' during the spontaneous sway test, in the absence of a serious postural threat. Conversely, for the young normals, the two testing situations may represent equally low levels of postural threat: therefore, these subjects may tend to show similar balancing strategies in both types of tests.

Ideally, in order to accurately predict falling liability, the balance test should evoke the balancing strategy that would occur in an actual falling situation. In balance tests that lack an adequate postural threat, relatively stable subjects may tend to adopt a 'sloppy' control strategy. In order to evoke realistic responses in the balance test, it may be necessary to more closely match the level of perturbation to the balancing capabilities of each subject.

Comparison with transient test responses

The results of the transient tests showed a strong amplitude dependence in the subsaturation balancing performance. In particular, the gain of the response (i.e. the peak COP displacement divided by the peak acceleration) was found to decrease as the perturbation amplitude was increased. For the smallest transient amplitude, the input–output model derived from the balance test predicted the peak transient response to a reasonable degree of accuracy (mean error $\simeq 15\%$, standard deviation $\simeq 20\%$). For larger transient perturbations, however, the predictions derived from the balance test sustantially overestimated the measured transient responses (e.g. see Fig. 4).

However, because the transient amplitudes were tested in ascending order, amplitude-dependent effects may have been confounded by adaptive 'order effects'. For the first few trials, there was a progressive decrease in the response gain with each new trial ($p < 0.01$). In many subjects, the initial COP location tended to shift backward as the tests progressed, i.e. subjects increasingly leaned in a direction opposite to the anticipated centre-of-gravity displacement.

Order effects notwithstanding, at least some of the observed amplitude dependence may be due to real amplitude-dependent effects, resulting either from nonlinearity intrinsic to the control loop or from amplitude-dependent modulation of balancing strategy. Although amplitude dependence will degrade the absolute accuracy with which the small-amplitude balance test can be used to predict large-amplitude transient response, the balance test may nonetheless allow for useful comparative evaluations of relative postural performance.

Acknowledgements

This work was supported by the Medical Research Council of Canada (grant MA-8025). Advice and assistance were provided by P.J. Holliday of West Park Research (Toronto) and by J.P. Paul and A.C. Nicol of the University of Strathclyde (Glasgow).

References

[1] Ishida, A. and Miyazaki, S. (1985) Identification of the posture control system using records during quiet stance. In M. Igarishi and F.O. Black (Eds.), *Vestibular and Visual Control on Posture and Locomotor Equilibrium*, Karger, Basel, pp. 70–73.

[2] Van Lunteren, A. (1979) *Identification of Human Operator Describing Function Models with One or Two Inputs in Closed Loop Systems*, PhD thesis, Delft University of Technology, The Netherlands, pp. 32–66.

[3] Ishida, A. and Imai, S. (1980) Responses of the posture-control system to pseudo-random acceleration disturbances. *Med. Biol. Eng. Comp.*, 18:433–438.

[4] Andres, R.O. (1982) Diagnostic implications of induced body sway. In V. Honrubia and M.A.B. Brazier (Eds.), *Nystagmus and Vertigo*, Academic Press, New York, pp. 191–204.

[5] Tokita, T., Miyata, H. and Fujiwara, H. (1984) Postural response induced by horizontal motion of a platform. *Acta Otolaryngol. Stockholm Suppl.*, 406: 120–124.

[6] Droulez, J., Berthoz, A. and Vidal, P.P. (1985) Use and limits of visual vestibular interaction in the control of posture, In: M. Igarishi and F.O. Black (Eds.), *Vestibular and Visual Control on Posture and Locomotor Equilibrium*, Karger, Basel, pp. 14–21.

[7] Rake, H. (1980) Step response and frequency response methods. *Automatica*, 16: 519–526.

[8] Nashner, L.M. (1976) Adapting reflexes controlling the human posture. *Exp. Brain Res.*, 26: 59–72.

[9] Horak, F.B., Diener, HC. and Nashner, L.M. (1985) Influence of stimulus parameter and set on human postural strategies. *Soc Neurosci. Abstr.*, 7: 704.

[10] Moore, S.P., Horak, F.B. and Nashner, L.M. (1986) *Influence of Stimulus Anticipation on Human Postural Responses*, Meeting at the North American Society for Psychology of Sport and Physical Activity, Phoenix.

[11] Nashner, L.M (1971) A model describing vestibular detection of body sway motion. *Acta Otolaryngol. Stockholm*, 72: 429–436.

[12] Wilson, V.J. (1985) Otolith-spinal reflexes. In M. Igarashi and F.O. Black (Eds.), *Vestibular and Visual Control on Posture and Locomotor Equilibrium*. Karger, Basel, pp. 177–185.

[13] Maki, B.E. (1986) Interpretation of the coherence function when using pseudorandom inputs to identify non-linear systems. *IEEE Trans. Biomed. Eng.*, BME-33: 775–779.

[14] Maki, B.E. (1988) Addendum to 'Interpretation of the coherence function when using pseudorandom inputs to identify non-linear systems'. *IEEE Trans. Biomed. Eng.*, BME-35: 279–280.

[15] Maki, B.E. (1986) Selection of perturbation parameters for identification of the posture control system. *Med. Biol. Eng. Comp.*, 24: 561–568.

[16] Bendat, J.S. and Piersol, A.G. (1980) *Engineering Applications of Correlation and Spectral Analysis*, Wiley-Interscience, New York, pp. 78–120.

[17] Eykhoff, P. (1982) On the coherence among the multitude of system identification methods. In G.A. Bekey and G.N. Saridis (Eds.), *Identification and System Parameter Estimation*, Pergamon Press, Oxford, pp. 31–42.

[18] Strejc, V. (1980) Least squares parameter estimation. *Automatica*, 16: 535–550.

[19] Åström, K.J. (1980) Maximum likelihood and prediction error methods. *Automatica*, 16: 551–574.

306

[20] Åström, K.J. and Wittenmark, B. (1984) *Computer Controlled Systems: Theory and Design*, Prentice-Hall, Englewood Cliffs, pp. 324–342.

[21] Hsia, T.C. (1978) *System Identification: Least-Squares Methods*, Lexington Books, Lexington, pp. 97–139.

[22] Söderström, T. (1977) On model structure testing in system identification. *Int. J. Control*, 26: 1–18.

[23] Maki, B.E. (1987) *A Posture Control Model and Balance Test for the Prediction of Relative Postural Stability*, PhD Thesis, University of Strathclyde, Glasgow, 209 pp.

[24] Maki, B.E., Holliday, P.J. and Fernie G.R. (1987) A posture control model and balance test for the prediction of relative postural stability. *IEEE Trans. Biomed. Eng.*, BME-34: 797–810.

[25] Maki, B.E, Holliday, P.J. and Fernie, G.R. (1988) Ageing and postural control: a comparison of spontaneous and induced sway measures, in preparation.

[26] Bartlett, S.A., Holliday, P.J., Maki, B.E. and Fernie, G.R. (1986) On the classification of a geriatric subject as a faller or non-faller. *Med. Biol. Eng. Comp.*, 24: 219–222.

O. Pompeiano and J.H.J. Allum (Eds.)
Progress in Brain Research, Vol. 76
© 1988 Elsevier Science Publishers B.V. (Biomedical Division)

CHAPTER 27

Posture as an organizational structure based on a dual process: a formal basis to interpret changes of posture in weightlessness

F.G. Lestienne[1] and V.S. Gurfinkel[2]

[1]Laboratoire de Physiologie Neurosensorielle, C.N.R.S., 15 rue de l'École de Médecine, 75270 Paris CEDEX 06, France and [2]Institute for Problems of Information Transmission, Academy of Sciences of the U.S.S.R., Ermolovoy Street 19, SU-103051 Moscow E24, U.S.S.R.

The purpose of this paper is to advance a formal principle for describing the organizational structure of a multicomponent system governing the control of posture. From this theoretical framework, we shall try to show that this structure, based on two processes – one conservative and one operative – and on a postulated 'body scheme', contributes to solving the problem of adaption and stability in unusual environmental contexts. We present a selection of the findings, collected during postural acitivity during three prolonged spaceflights, which we think may provide a physiological basis for the theoretical model developed here.

Introduction

Since the early days of the cybernetic revolution and the fundamental contribution of Berstein [1], remarkably little progress has been made towards a convincing theoretical framework concerning the practical problem of interaction between living organisms and the external environment, i.e. the ability to solve the problems of adaptation and stability. Questions are not only restricted to the ability to react normally to the usual variability in the environment or to uncertainties, but also to the ability to adapt to the unusual and continuous changes affecting the information content of sensations and changing the mechanical constraints and properties of the motor system.

Starting with the pioneering work of Sherrington, postural activities afford a very fruitful paradigm to generate principles and data on the nature of adaptation. However, considering that real-life skills cannot be investigated by separating the different mechanisms, which are normally simultaneously mobilized in perceptuomotor performance, the majority of models to be found in the literature are severely limited when compared to the complex and rich diversity of postural behaviours [2]. In animals of different species, depending upon the architecture of their body, their locomotor organs, and the influence of the external environment, the repertoire of postural activities is absolutely correlated with the active function of the neuromuscular apparatus: examples range from the simple prolonged maintenance of mollusk's valves in the closed position to the complex and beautiful posture of the human ballet danser.

Structure of the mechanisms governing the control of posture

The posture of the normal human body can be regarded as a complex multicomponent mobile system of inverted pendulums one resting on the other. This system is further complicated by the centre of gravity being located high above the support and the area of the supporting contour being comparatively small. In this chapter we wish to advance a formal principle for describing the organizational structure controlling such a system. We believe that this conceptual scheme, which is based on the consideration that it is reasonable to distinguish two main elements in the structure of the mechanisms governing different physiological systems, namely conservative and operative processes [3], provides a useful framework compatible with the logical processes underlying the organization of human posture (Fig. 1).

The conservative process

This process is responsible for bringing the multicomponent system to *equilibrium* with a minimum of effort. Appropriate muscle activations have to be exerted at each of numerous joints to counteract the static torque. Considering the complexity of the multijoint kinematic chain, it is possible to predict the existence of an infinite number of temporal and spatial combinations of muscle torques which depend upon the position of each body segment relative to the vector of gravity. However, there are internal constraints which limits the possible number of combinations of muscle torques. Indeed, it is a

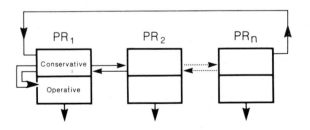

Fig. 1. Schematic description of the multicomponent system underlying the organization of postural control. The structure of each PR (physiological regulator) is divided into two levels: conservative and operative. It is important to note that (1) PR are interconnected and (2) the operative process receives the prescribed value (midposition of the body segment for example) from the conservative process and not from the outside. In other words the multicomponent system creates the prescribed values itself (see explanation in the text).

somewhat trivial observation that each particular subject is perfectly characterized by his 'silhouette'. This individual postural expression is generally innate but can be slightly and slowly changed depending on everyday experience and the environmental context. This silhouette is defined by a specific midposition of each individual segment. The conservative process is responsible for prescribing the value of the midposition of each component of the postural attitude taking into account the knowledge of the physical constraints which drastically limit the boundaries beyond which the state of metastable equilibrium is not possible. This process is a highly predetermined reference, based on and formed by past knowledge such as everyday experiences and, to a certain degree, genetic memory. This conservative process is stable for more-or-less short-term changes in the environment even if they are of high intensity. Conversely, modifications in its level of functioning can be caused by some factors of low intensity but long duration. The formation of stable habits and long-term adaptation can be assumed to depend on this conservative process.

The operative process

Counterbalancing the body weight while standing upright at ease or during voluntary movements such as raising the arm or rising onto the toes requires the existence of an operative process. This process is a mechanism for quickly *stabilizing* the equilibrium of the inverted pendulums by bringing the whole body back in the vicinity of the vertical. The basic function ascribed to the operative process is to provide great changes in the regulated parameters within the dynamic range. These changes are evoked by the action of natural factors and as a rule they have a transistory character. This part of the regulator system can produce fast responses which can even cope with large disturbances provoked by external events. In other words, the operative process works through the regulation of thresholds and enhancement of rapid muscle action on the basis of integrated information from the vestibular, visual, proprioceptive and kinesthetic systems.

The trunk, the main object of regulation for control of upright posture

The important question that arises from the existence of an operative process which tends to keep the multijoint system within the limits of stability is which component of the body is the main object of regulation. The maintenance of stability of the body can be reduced to insuring that the projection of the general centre of gravity onto the supporting surface does not go outside the limits of a defined region of the supporting contour. However, the position of the centre of gravity does not unambiguously define the position of the components of the body or of the body as a whole in space. Considering also the biochemical peculiarities of the upright posture in humans – the small supporting area, the high position of the centre of gravity, the irregular distribution of the masses, and the static moment attaining its highest value in the ankle joints – and according to the view that, in humans, stabilization of the position of the head does not play the leading role for the maintenance of balance in the vertical posture, two solutions seem to be possible. The first would be the stabilization of the angles in the joints of the lower limbs and, in particular, in the ankles. The second would be the stabilization of the position of the upper, heaviest part of the body, i.e. the trunk, which represents, with the upper limbs and the head, about 63% of the total mass of the body.

Intensive studies using periodic disturbance of posture by rhythmic tilting of the supporting platform clearly demonstrate that the stabilizing reactions of the leg muscles were not the result of changes in the length of the muscles but occurred in response to the movement of the trunk [4]. Furthermore, the stabilizing activity of the leg muscles was not connected with the stimulation of vestibular and visual receptors but was due to displacement of the trunk. Taken together with the persistence of muscular reactions to postural imbalance even in the absence of muscle stretch in the standing subject [5], these results reveal that the component of the body which is the main object for maintenance of a stable vertical posture is the trunk. From this point of view the lower limbs can be regarded as levers; a mechanical contrivance for stabilizing the position of the trunk.

Body scheme

From the proposed model of sensorimotor control based on the existence of two different processes some interesting aspects emerge which can be used to clarify the role of a postulated body scheme in the control of postural activity and its implication in the process of adaptation to an unusual environment [6].

In order to introduce the concept of a body scheme which is implicitly connected with the conservative system let us mention some compelling examples of the supporting evidence.

One of the examples illustrating the conservative character of regulation is Walter Cannon's theory of homeostasis, Homeostasis is a result of '... coordinated physiological processes which maintain most of the steady state in the organism'. Cannon characterized homeostasis by the existence of a close connection between two qualities: variability and stability.

Secondly, from clinical and experimental observations, it is well known that the basic features of motor skills persist even after extensive lesions in the central nervous system or in the peripheral skeletomotor apparatus. On the other hand, motor skills are very sensitive to small changes in the conditions of their realization. Paraphrasing Berstein, we can say that the principal characteristics of motor skills are stable, like the features of a face, whereas their realizations are transient, like a facial expression.

The last example, taken from automatic control theory, illustrates more precisely the concept of a body scheme. Modern artificial controllers are based on the use of complex algorithms – mathematical models of the object to be controlled – in order to estimate the vector of state. Measurements of actual output parameters of the object are continuously compared with the predictions of the mo-

310

del. In this example it is possible to see a certain analogy with the body scheme. However, the essential difference between an artificial controller and the physiological regulator lies in the fact that, whereas the first receives the prescribed value from the outside, the second creates it itself (see Figs. 1 and 2).

From the proposed logical organization of the mechanisms governing different physiological systems, it is reasonable to suggest the existence of a central organization of postural regulation based on an internal model of the body. This model is known as the 'body scheme' [7], a somewhat ambiguous term [8].

On the first level, the body scheme is considered to be an inborn basis for the structural organization of the body incorporating the upper and lower end of the body, the left and right side, and the dorsal and ventral surface. The next stage of development

of the body scheme is related to the system of references: one is connected with the vestibular system – an absolute vertical – and the other is formed from visual and proprioceptive information – a proprioceptive vertical. This system of references is characterized by an important property: they are invariant relative to the position of the body itself. The last stage is a higher form of sensory organization which projects the body scheme onto the external space. Active movements and everyday experiences play a major role in the formation of this sensory organization similar to a 'sensory envelope'. This sensory envelope is a complex processing of information not only connected with posture and movement but also related to the body coordinates in correlation with the external space. In this frame of thought we propose that the main functions of the body scheme which is, in the particular case of posture, set into action to maintain the indi-

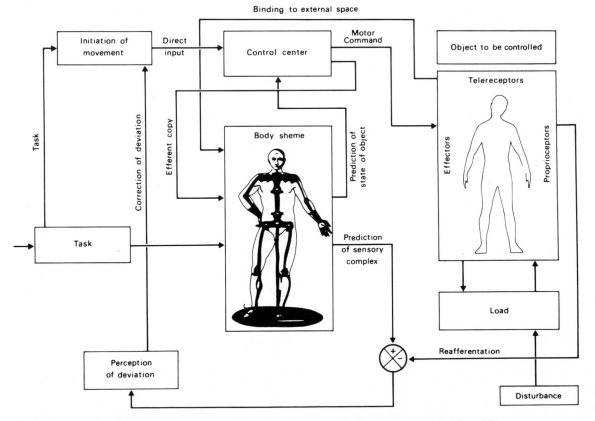

Fig. 2. Conceptual model of sensorimotor control based on a postulated body scheme. (Modified from [6].)

vidual midposition of the multipendulum structure and stabilize the precarious equilibrium, include: (1) perception of the sensory envelope to update the process of multidimensional analysis of the borders between the body and the external space and (2) knowledge of the parameters of the whole body configuration which cannot be directly detected by specific receptors. These parameters are supposed to reflect a simplified but true model taking into account: the lengths of the body segments, the sequence of their linkage, their mass–inertial properties, and the configuration and dimensions of the support surface and the muscle torque.

The diagram of Fig. 2 illustrates the main properties of the body scheme involved in the control of movement, which obviously includes posture. In this diagram, which has been discussed in more detail in a previous paper [6], we will pay special attention to its structure. The organization of this sensorimotor interaction is conceived as a dialogue between the external world, the state of the body segments and the body scheme. As a rule, a standard model is characterized by only one output and it predicts the value of the output parameter of the object and generates an afferent pattern. In contrast, the body scheme is characterized by two outputs predicting: (1) the state of the object in order to organize the motor command by using the controller centre and (2) the afferent pattern of the movement, which is compared with real reafferentation. An important property ascribed to this second output is the correction of the parameters of the model in the case of detection of differences between the predicted afferent pattern and the reafferentation. Furthermore, even after deafferentation, the existence of the double outputs allows the system to predict the state of the object.

What can we learn from postural adaptation in weightlessness?

From data collected during postural activity in prolonged spaceflights [9–11], the most pertinent results support the view of the existence of a dual process – conservative and operative – underlying the

postural adaptation to an unusual environment.

It has been shown that to face this novel mechanical situation – suppression of the longitudinal constraint and the static torque in the multijoint kinematic chain – a redistribution of the tonic EMG activity between extensor and flexor of the ankle is observed throughout the flight [9,11]. Indeed, in contrast to the ground-based situation, erectness of posture, with the feet attached, was maintained primarily by contaction of the ankle flexor muscles. Recently, it has been shown from extensive postural studies performed during parabolic flights, that the redistribution of tonic activity took place instantaneously and not progressively during the maintenance of an upright posture [12]. This quasi-instantaneous redistribution is thought to be attributed to the operative process whereas a slower process – the conservative process responsible for the 'real adaptation' – is involved in correcting the postural attitude. The latter is done by combining existing strategies derived from a repertoire of terrestrial postural strategies based on a postulated body scheme. Fig. 3 illustrates this assumption. This series of three sketches shows the postural attitude observed before and during a 7-day flight when the subject is instructed to maintain an upright posture with the feet attached to the floor. It is clear that on day 2 the exaggerated forward tilt of the whole body was totally incompatible with the existence of a gravity field, However, on day 7 the resulting angular combination between the four joints bring the centre of body mass in the vicinity of the foot support. In other words, the body is in equilibrium with respect to a hypothetical field of terrestrial gravity. These results demonstrate that the elimination of the gravitational torque failed to result in dramatic changes in the usual postural attitude although the tonic postural muscle activity was drastically modified from that observed in the terrestrial gravity condition.

Considering the dynamic nature of posture maintenance, we observed that the two components of the leg muscle activity – anticipatory and compensatory – associated with voluntary rising on the toes and arm movements were very similar to those ob-

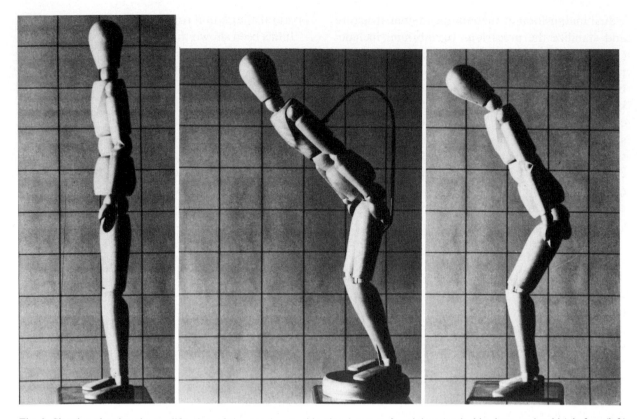

Fig. 3. Sketches showing the modification of the angular combination between four joints (neck, hip, knee and ankle) before (left) and on day 2 (middle) and day 7 (right) of a 7-day spaceflight during the maintenance of an upright posture with the feet attached to the floor.

served at one-G. These two well-structured sequences of EMG activity persist throughout the flight and are enhanced when the feet are free to move [9]. With regard to the perturbation of the whole kinematic chain consecutively to the rapid elevation of the arm, it is important to stress that the hip trajectory was practically the same as in terrestrial conditions, whereas the pathway of the head was significantly longer [10]. This result suggests that in weightlessness the postural control mechanism functions mainly to stabilize the trunk as in the terrestrial condition [5].

Taken together, all these data collected during prolonged weightlessness on five subjects* converge to support the hypothesis of the existence of a dual process underlying the structure of the mechanisms governing the control of posture. According to this idea, our results indicate that the mechanisms of postural adaptation presuppose that the conservative process would offer a certain 'resistance' to an unusual environment. Consequently, depending upon the degree of this resistance this process would produce a more-or-less long-term adaptation. Conversely, the operative process would provide rapid correction of the regulated parameters within the dynamic range. These corrections are evoked by the action of a natural factor and as a rule they are of transitory character.

*Two first experiments were performed on three cosmonauts in June and October 1982 aboard the soviet Salyut spacecraft; the third experiment was carried out on two astronauts during the 51G mission of the US shuttle in June 1985.

Based upon the structure of the conceptual model presented at the beginning of this chapter (Fig. 1), we can speculate the extent to which this scheme can provide a useful framework for a reasonable approach to the problem of adaptation to space flights. Considering that the control of posture is subserved by the multicomponent system illustrated in Fig. 1 and according to the existence of a functional link between the different physiological regulators (PR), it can be proposed that space adaptation is a result of the integrative action of the different PRs receiving information about the distribution of axial load along the skeletomuscular system (PR1), the positions of the internal organs (PR2), the vessel wall distension (PRn). For example, the distension of the vena by a negative pressure applied to the lower part of the body evokes a sensation of a change in the orientation of the whole body.

According to the main hypothesis developed by Barkroft [13] that 'every adaptation is an integration and consequently ... rather large effects may result from the cumulative action of a number of factors, each of which alters in a lesser degree', it seems reasonable to reconsider the idea that the vestibular system can play the leading role in the process of adaptation to weightlessness [14].

Acknowledgements

This work was supported in part by the 'Centre National de la Recherche Spatial' Grant No. 84-1285, 85-1243, 86-1243, 87-1228.

References

[1] Bernstein, N.A. (1967) The Coordination and Regulation of Movements, Pergamon Press, New York, 186 pp.

[2] Gelfand, I.M. and Tsetlin, M.L. (1971) Mathematical modeling of mechanisms of the central nervous system. In I.M. Gelfand, V.S. Gurfinkel, S.V. Fomin and M.L. Tsetlin (Eds.), Models of the Structural-Functional Organization of Certain Biological Systems, MIT Press, Cambridge MA, pp. 1–22.

[3] Lestienne, F. and Gurfinkel, V.S. (1986) Postural adaptation to weightlessness; role of the 'body scheme' in postural control. In Proceedings of EBBS Workshop on Sensory to Motor Transformation, Premotor Mechanism, Zichron Yaacov, 0–23.

[4] Gurfinkel, V.S., Lipshits, M.I., Mori, S. and Popov, K.E. (1976) Postural reactions to the controlled sinusoidal displacement of the supporting plateform. Agressologie, 17B: 71–76.

[5] Gurfinkel, V.S., Lipshits, M.I. and Popov, K.E. (1981) Stabilization of body position as the main task of postural regulation. Fiziologya Cheloveka 7: 400–410 (translated from Russian).

[6] Gurfinkel, V.S. and Levik, Y.S. (1978) Sensory complexes and sensomotor integration. Fiziologya Cheloveka 5/3: 399–414 (translated from Russian).

[7] Head, H. and Holmes, G. (1911) Sensory disturbances from cerebral lesions. Brain, 34: 102–245.

[8] Paillard, J. (1980) Le corps situé et le corps identifié. Une approche psychophysiologique de la notion de schéma corporel. Rev. Med. Suisse Romande, 100: 129–141.

[9] Clement, G., Gurfinkel, V.S., Lestienne, G., Lipshits, M.I. and Popov, K.E. (1984) Adaptation of postural control to weightlessness. Exp. Brain Res., 57: 61–72.

[10] Clement, G., Gurfinkel, V.S., Lestienne, F., Lipshits, M.I. and Popov, K.E. (1985) Changes of posture during transient perturbations in microgravity. Aviat. Space Environ. Med., 56: 666–671.

[11] Clement, G., Vieville, T., Lestienne, F. and Berthoz, A. (1986) Preliminary results of the 'equilibrium and vertigo' experiment performed during STS-51-G shuttle flight. In J.J. Hunt (Ed.), Space and Physiology, ESA Publ. Division, Nordwijk, pp. 129–135.

[12] Clement, G. and André-Deshays, C. (1987) Motor activity and visually induced postural reactions during two-G and zero-G phases of parabolic flight. Neurosci. Lett., 79: 113–116.

[13] Barkroft, J. (1935) Feature in the Architecture of Physiological Functions, Medgiz, Moscow, 224 pp.

[14] Lestienne, F. and Droulez, J. (1983) Les problèmes sensorimoteurs en apesanteur. Rev. Med. Fonctionelle, 16: 195–225.

Mechanisms of Eye–Head–Trunk Coordination

O. Pompeiano and J.H.J. Allum (Eds.)
Progress in Brain Research, Vol. 76
© 1988 Elsevier Science Publishers B.V. (Biomedical Division)

Overview

N. Dieringer*

Institüt für Hirnforschung, Universität Zürich, August-Forel Strasse 1, CH-8029 Zürich, Switzerland

Detailed visual inspection of an object requires a rather stable image of this object on the retina. Such a stable relationship is perturbed by movements of either the object, the subject or both of them. These perturbations are reduced by reflex movements that either pursue the object or counteract any head movement sensed by the vestibular apparatus. Image stabilization is a complex process that involves the interaction of ocular and collicular reflexes elicited by vestibular, visual and proprioceptive signals. Some of the basic features of the central organization of voluntary and compensatory head movements and of the accompanying eye movements in man were described in this section.

As the head tracks an object of interest during pursuit, eye movements in the opposite direction due to vestibular and optokinetic reflexes have to be suppressed. The same reflexes, however, have to be fully compensatory during the next active gaze shift towards a new object of interest. In his contribution (Chapter 28), Dr. Barnes investigated the control of the gain of the vestibulo-ocular reflex in different behavioural contexts. In particular, the role of feedback loops provided by visual inputs and by efference copy is discussed.

In the face of the multiple joints and the many muscles of the neck, head stabilization is a considerably more complex process than that of the eye. It is therefore rather reassuring to see that a number of simplifying features and restrictions exist which reduce the degree of possible complexity. For in-

stance, the results described in the contribution by Drs. Keshner and Peterson (Chapter 29) suggest that not all of the 23 different neck muscles of man are activated for a given task. Rather a given muscle or groups of muscles are most activated in a unique direction. The selection of these directional properties depends on the behavioural context (voluntary or reflex) and on parametric requirements, such as increased levels of force. Selection of more voluntary or more reflex action, on the other hand, appears to be determined by the available sensory feedback.

Dr. Pellionisz' contribution (Chapter 30) suggests a solution to the question raised by Drs. Keshner and Peterson. Namely, how does the CNS transform the three-dimensional sensory information made available by the semicircular canal system into a set of muscle commands when these commands can be distributed in an infinite number of ways to the 30 neck muscles? The rather elegant solution proposed by Dr. Pellionisz is based on the eigen vectors of the matrix representing the pulling directions of each muscle. The advantage of the proposed solution is its physiological feasibility, since it minimizes the sums of squares of muscle activity during any movement. For the neurophysiologist the work of Dr. Pellionisz may present a breakthrough in understanding how the CNS controls complex movements. However, many practical details of this model need to be elaborated upon before it can be tested experimentally.

*Present address: Physiologisches Institut, Universität München, Pettenkoferstrasse 12, D-8000 München 2, F.R.G.

O. Pompeiano and J.H.J. Allum (Eds.)
Progress in Brain Research, Vol. 76
© 1988 Elsevier Science Publishers B.V. (Biomedical Division)

CHAPTER 28

Head–eye co-ordination: visual and nonvisual mechanisms of vestibulo-ocular reflex slow-phase modification

G.R. Barnes

Vestibular Physiology Section, R.A.F. Institute of Aviation Medicine, Farnborough, Hantshire GU14 6SZ, U.K.

During normal head and body manoeuvres there is a continual requirement to modify the gain of the slow-phase component of the vestibulo-ocular response. The acquisition and fixation of earth-fixed targets requires a gain close to unity, whereas head-free tracking of moving targets necessitates a maximal suppression of the VOR in order to maintain visual acuity. Two mechanisms are available for the modification of VOR gain which appear to be quite distinct in their response to pseudorandom motion stimuli. Visual feedback forms the most important mechanism of suppression, but its effectiveness is governed in a nonlinear manner by the frequency composition of the stimulus. This nonlinear characteristic, which has been associated with stimulus predictability, appears to be inherent in the visual feedback and may also be observed in the pursuit reflex response. Modification of VOR gain can also be achieved by nonvisual means, but this is brought about by a separate mechanism to that used for pursuit, which is not affected by the frequency composition or predictability of the stimulus. Suppression of the VOR during voluntary head movements is no better and, indeed, may be worse than during whole-body rotation despite the fact that the motion is predetermined. This underlines the fact that the changes in gain associated with the predictability of stimulus motion probably arise as a function of the nonlinear visual feedback characteristics.

Introduction

When the human subject makes voluntary combined head and eye movements to search the visual field, two types of purposeful eye movements may be identified. First there are rapid saccadic eye movements in the same direction as the head movement which serve to realign the direction of gaze. Such saccadic eye movements are followed by a slower return of the eye toward orbital centre which serves to compensate for the remaining head movement [1], and thus to stabilize eye position in space after the termination of the saccade. This pattern of response is typical of that evoked in response to the sudden appearance of a discrete visual target in the peripheral visual field, or in response to an auditory stimulus which may lie well outside the normal range of the oculomotor system itself. The slower compensatory component of the response is almost certainly generated by the VOR in response to the rotational movement of the head, at least in normal human subjects. To achieve effective stabilization of the visual image at the end of the saccade the gain of the slow-phase component of the VOR should be close to unity.

In contrast, when the subject tracks a moving target with the head free the slow-phase component of the VOR becomes completely inappropriate and must be suppressed in order for effective image stabilization to be achieved [2,3]. When the subject tracks target movements of low frequency (< 1 Hz) and low velocity ($< 40°/s$), suppression is almost complete so that eye movements appear smooth (Fig. 1). In fact, recording of eye movement with a

---

Abbreviations: EOG, electro-oculogram; VOR, vestibulo-ocular reflex.

320

sensitivity better than that offered by the EOG recordings of Fig. 1 indicates the presence of a fine nystagmus in these conditions. At higher target velocity this nystagmus becomes more evident (Fig. 1) although the velocity of the slow-phase component of the eye, which is almost in anti-phase with the head movement, may still be considerably less than that of the head. When the frequency of target motion is increased to 1 Hz it becomes even more difficult to suppress the compensatory slow-phase components. As a consequence, when the head and eye movements are summated to obtain gaze displacement in space it can be seen that the eye no longer follows the target smoothly, but makes a square

wave response (Fig. 1) in which instantaneous retinal velocity error is always very high.

It is evident, therefore, that the ability to modify the activity of the basic VOR is an essential everyday requirement and it is the objective of this paper to discuss the means by which this may be accomplished. The principal mechanism is by the use of a visual feedback mechanisms similar to those used in the pursuit reflex response as indicated by a number of experiments in which visual–vestibular interaction in the control of eye movement has been investigated [4–7]. These experiments have revealed a remarkable similarity in the frequency and velocity limitations of pursuit and VOR suppression.

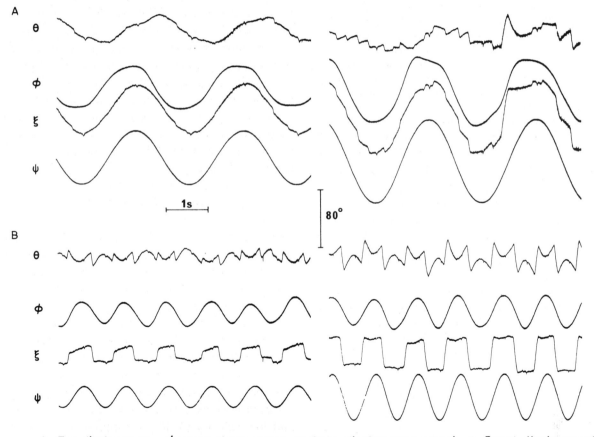

θ – Eye displacement   φ – Head displacement   ξ – Gaze displacement = θ + φ   ψ – Target displacement

Fig. 1. The response of the head and eyes during head-free tracking of a target oscillating sinusoidally in the horizontal plane with differing peak displacement at frequencies of 0.4 Hz (A) and 1.0 Hz (B) and various amplitudes. Eye movements recorded by electrooculography. θ, eye displacement; φ, head displacement; ξ, gaze displacement ($= θ + φ$); ψ, target displacement.

However, experiments by Barr et al. [8] have indicated that the gain of the VOR (i.e. the ratio of slow-phase eye velocity to head velocity) may be suppressed or enhanced when the subject imagines the presence of a head-fixed or earth-fixed target respectively, in complete darkness. The extent to which this nonvisual suppression can be carried out during voluntary head movements is uncertain [9], although it is more certain that gain enhancement can take place when imagining an earth-fixed target.

The results of experiments discussed in this paper show that visual and nonvisual mechanisms may be easily identified because of their differing response to pseudorandom motion stimuli.

The effects of visual suppression on the response to voluntary head movements

The effect of visual stimulation on the suppression of the vestibulo-ocular response to voluntary head movement in yaw was assessed during oscillation of the head at two frequencies, 0.5 and 1.0 Hz with a mean peak velocity of 29°/s and 42°/s. The frequency of oscillation was initially set by synchronization of the head movement with an audio cue which was then silenced during the period of recording. Subjects made head movements, (a) in darkness, whilst carrying out mental arithmetic, (b) whilst viewing a small earth-fixed target light and (c) whilst viewing a similar target attached to the head. In the head-fixed-target condition the target was tachistoscopically illuminated for a period of 100 μs at regular intervals which ranged from 2 ms to 3000 ms. In this, and other experiments described here, eye movements were recorded by an infra-red limbus tracking system rigidly located on the head through a helmet and dental bite.

In darkness, the mean gain of the slow-phase component of eye velocity was 0.75 at 0.5 Hz and 0.84 at 1.0 Hz, but the gains increased to 1.04 and 1.02 respectively during fixation of the earth-fixed target (Fig. 2). When subjects fixated the head-fixed target the degree of suppression of the eye velocity recorded in darkness was greatest when the inter-

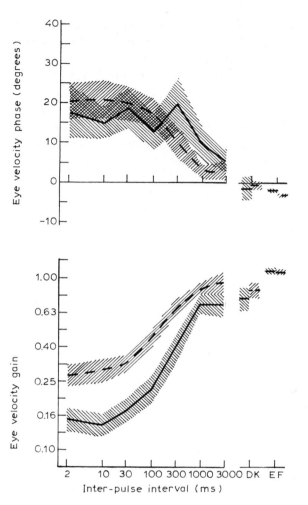

Fig. 2. Eye velocity gain and phase of the VOR during voluntary oscillation of the head in yaw at a frequency of 0.5 Hz (solid line) and 1.0 Hz (broken line). Inter-pulse interval represents the duration between successive presentations of a head-fixed target light. DK, response of VOR in darkness; EF, response during fixation of earth-fixed target.

pulse interval was between 2 and 30 ms (mean gains: 0.15 at 0.5 Hz; 0.29 at 1.0 Hz), in which conditions the target appeared to be almost continuously illuminated. But as the interpulse interval was increased and the retinal velocity error signal was consequently degraded, suppression was progressively impaired (Fig. 2). When the interpulse interval exceeded 1000 ms there was no significant reduction of eye velocity gain compared with that recorded in darkness for either stimulus frequency (Fig. 2). The phase relationship exhibited a considerable advance at the shortest interpulse interval, which was gradually reduced as the interpulse interval was increased and suppression became less effective (Fig. 2).

These findings emphasize the important role of retinal velocity error information in the suppression of the vestibulo-ocular response to voluntary head movement, and accord with the results of a similar experiment in which VOR suppression during passive whole-body rotation was assessed [10]. Note that the responses to the longest interpulse intervals do not show any suppression of the dark response, even though this is a condition which is similar to the instruction to imagine a head-fixed target in darkness. That the suppression achieved by non-visual means is somewhat different to that induced by visual feedback is emphasized in the following experiments.

The effects of pseudorandom motion stimuli on VOR suppression

Experiments on suppression of the VOR induced by passive whole-body rotation were carried out using angular motion stimuli composed of four sinusoids, each of peak velocity $\pm 17.5°/s$. The three low frequencies were held constant at 0.11, 0.24 and 0.37 Hz, whilst the highest frequency (F_4) took values from 0.39 Hz to 2.08 Hz. The vestibulo-ocular response was recorded in three visual stimulus conditions: (a) in darkness, whilst the subject was kept alert by performing a simple auditory-pitch discrimination task; (b) during fixation of a small head-fixed target, and (c) during attempted fixation in the dark of an imagined head-fixed target.

In the dark, the gain of the three lower frequency components was not significantly modified by the frequency of the highest frequency component as it increased from 0.39 Hz to 2.08 Hz (Fig. 3). However, during fixation of the head-fixed target the degree of VOR suppression was significantly modified by the frequency of F_4. When all frequency components were less than 0.39 Hz, the level of eye velocity gain, which had a mean of 0.06 for the three lower frequency components, was not significantly different from that evoked by discrete sinusoids of corresponding frequency (Fig. 3). But, as the highest frequency was increased to 2.08 Hz, mean eye velocity gain for the three low frequencies increased to 0.17, although the gain of the highest frequency component itself remained comparable to that for a discrete sinusoid of identical frequency (Fig. 3).

In contrast, when subjects attempted to suppress the VOR response by imagining the presence of a head-fixed target in darkness, eye velocity gain for the three lower frequencies was not significantly modified by the frequency of the highest frequency component. All subjects achieved some degree of suppression of the dark reponse in this condition, although there was considerable variability and the mean reduction in gain (28%) was not as great as that reported previously [8,11,12]. A more consistent and effective suppression was achieved when the subjects were instructed to fixate the mid-point between two isolated, head-fixed targets placed at $\pm 10°$ in the periphery that were tachistoscopically illuminated at intervals of 1000 ms (THFT condition in Fig. 3). However, even when suppression was aided in this way, eye velocity gain for the low frequencies was not significantly modified as F_4 was increased.

VOR gain enhancement during pseudorandom head movement

In a further experiment the ability to enhance the gain of the VOR was assessed using a less complex turntable motion stimulus composed of only two sinusoids. Previous experiments on the pursuit reflex [13] had established that such a stimulus was adequate to demonstrate the effects of the breakdown in performance associated with the effects of prediction. The stimulus was composed of two sinusoids of equal peak velocity (25°/s). The lower frequency (F_1) was maintained at 0.22 Hz whilst the higher frequency (F_2) was varied from 0.39 Hz to 2.78 Hz in eight increments. In two separate sessions, the vestibulo-ocular response was recorded in four visual stimulus conditions: (*a*) in darkness, whilst the subject was kept alert by performing a simple auditory pitch discrimination task; (*b*) during fixation of a small head-fixed target; (*c*) during attempted fixa-

tion of an imagined head-fixed target in darkness, and (*d*) during attempted fixation of an imagined earth-fixed target in darkness.

In the dark, the gain of the lower-frequency com-

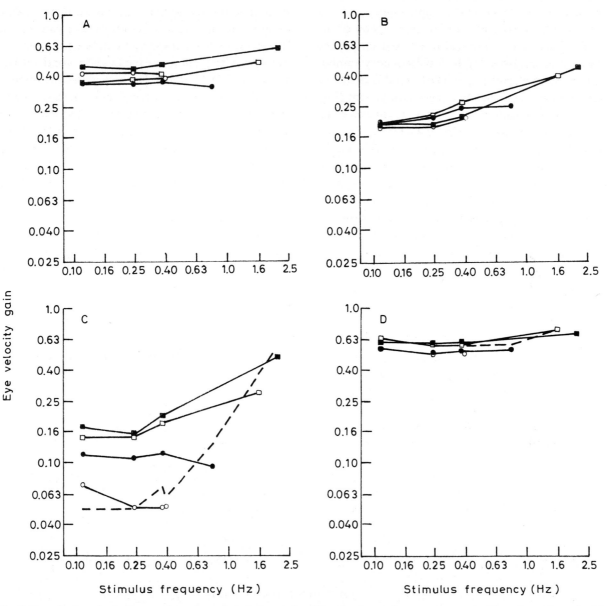

Fig. 3. Eye velocity gain during pseudorandom whole-body rotation. The stimulus motion was composed of four sinusoids, each with peak velocity of $\pm 17.5°/s$. The three lowest frequencies remained constant (0.112 Hz, 0.240 Hz and 0.368 Hz), whilst the highest frequency was varied: $\bigcirc$, 0.39 Hz; $\bullet$, 0.78 Hz; $\square$, 1.56 Hz; $\blacksquare$, 2.08 Hz. Responses were examined in four conditions A, attempted fixation of imaginary target; B, attempted fixation mid-way between tachistoscopically illuminated peripheral targets; C, fixation of a head-fixed target; D, darkness. The broken lines in C and D indicate responses to discrete frequency sinusoidal stimuli (peak velocity $\pm 35°/s$). Mean of 8 subjects.

ponent (Fig. 4A) was not significantly modified by the frequency of the higher-frequency component as it increased from 0.39 to 2.78 Hz. The gain of the higher-frequency component itself (Fig. 4B) exhibited a steady increase as its own frequency increased beyond 0.6 Hz in the manner described previously [14]. In contrast, during suppression of the VOR by fixation of the real head-fixed target, the degree of suppression of the low-frequency component was significantly ($p < 0.001$) modified by the frequency of the higher-frequency component (Fig. 4A). Minimum gain (mean 0.03) was achieved when both frequencies were below 0.4 Hz but gain increased progressively as the frequency (F_2) of the higher-frequency component was increased to reach an asymptotic level of 0.16 when F_2 was above 1.04 Hz. The gain of the higher-frequency component showed a steady increase with its own frequency in the manner described previously [7].

When the subjects attempted to suppress the VOR response in darkness by imagining a head-fixed target, there was little change in the gain of the low-frequency component as the frequency of the higher-frequency component was varied (Fig. 4A). Mean gain for the low-frequency component was reduced to 0.33 compared with the mean gain of 0.6 obtained in darkness. In contrast, the gain of the higher-frequency component exhibited an increase as its own frequency was increased beyond 1.0 Hz, so that at 2.78 Hz there was no significant suppression of the response recorded in darkness. Similar effects were observed during attempted fixation of an imagined earth-fixed target. Mean gain of the low-frequency component was close to unity and was always significantly greater than that recorded in darkness, although it declined slightly as F_2 was increased. The gain of the higher-frequency component was similar to that of the low-frequency component, but there was no significant difference from the dark response at frequencies above 2 Hz.

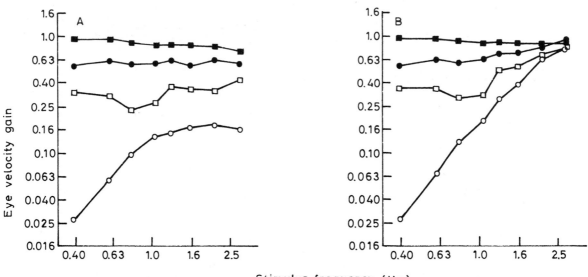

Fig. 4. Eye velocity gain of the VOR in response to angular motion on a turntable in four visual stimulus conditions: ●, rotation darkness; ○, fixation of head-fixed target; □, attempted fixation of imagined head-fixed target; ■, attempted fixation of imagined earth-fixed target. The stimulus was composed of two sinusoids. Responses for the lower frequency component (F1 = 0.22 Hz) are plotted in A, those for the higher frequency component (F2) in B. Both are plotted as a function of the frequency of F2, which varied from 0.39 Hz to 2.78 Hz. Summary of results from two experiments on two separate groups of eight subjects.

Discussion

The mechanism of visual suppression and its relationship to pursuit

It is evident from the experiments described here that the mechanisms responsible for visual suppression of the VOR are very different from those used during nonvisual modification of the vestibular response. During nonvisual changes the modifying element appears to act as a low-pass filter on all frequency components of the stimulus in such a way that modification is progressively reduced at frequencies above 1 Hz. In contrast, visual suppression of the VOR is significantly modified by the frequency composition of the stimulus in a complex,

nonlinear manner. The changes in gain observed during visual suppression of the VOR as the frequency composition of the pseudorandom stimulus is changed are directly comparable to those observed previously for the pursuit reflex [13]. This almost certainly indicates that the same nonlinear visual feedback mechanisms are responsible for reducing retinal velocity error in both pursuit and visual suppression of the VOR, a concept which has been embodied in the model shown in Fig. 5 (pathways 2 and 3).

There appear to be two principal factors which cause a breakdown in oculomotor performance to occur as the frequency composition of the stimulus is changed. First, when the frequency of the highest-frequency component of the stimulus increases

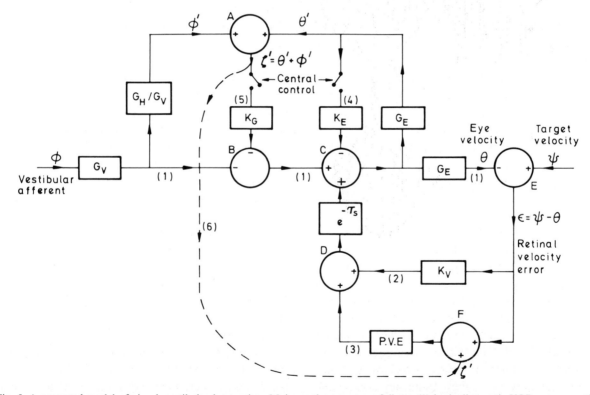

Fig. 5. A proposed model of visual–vestibular interaction. Major pathways are as follows: (1) basic disynaptic VOR arc emanating from semicircular canals; (2) continuous retinal velocity error feedback; (3) predictive velocity estimation; (4) oculomotor efference copy feedback; (5) gaze velocity estimation derived from vestibular afference and oculomotor efference; (6) positive feedback of central gaze velocity estimate to provide estimate of target velocity in space. φ, head velocity; ψ, target velocity with respect to the head; θ, eye velocity; ε, retinal velocity error; ζ, estimate of gaze velocity. $K_V = 1–2$; $G_V = 0.6$; $\tau = 0.08$ s; $G_E = (1 + sT_E)^{-1}$, where $T_E = 0.2$ s.

beyond 0.4 Hz the effectiveness of the visual feedback becomes progressively degraded, resulting in a reduction in eye velocity gain during pursuit or, conversely, an increase in eye velocity gain during VOR suppression. Although the gain of the low-frequency components is impaired in this manner, the gain of the highest-frequency component itself remains enhanced, at a level comparable to that for the response to a predictable discrete sinusoidal stimulus of the same frequency. A secondary factor leading to a breakdown in performance, which has been tested only for pursuit, is that an increase in the velocity ratio between the highest frequency and those which lie below it accentuates the breakdown in gain of the low-frequency components whenever the highest frequency lies in the critical range beyond 0.4 Hz. The absolute velocity of the highest frequency does not appear to influence the gain of the low frequencies [15], except, perhaps, when the velocity is sufficiently high (greater than approximately 40°/s) that the nonlinear velocity feedback characteristics are invoked [16,17].

The mechanism by which these nonlinear changes in gain and phase are brought about by the differing frequency content of the stimulus remains obscure. The conceptual model shown in Fig. 5 indicates one way in which the system may be organized. It is postulated that two feedback mechanisms combine in an attempt to minimize retinal velocity error; (a) a direct low-gain retinal velocity error feedback (pathway 2 in Fig. 5) and (b) a predictive velocity-estimation mechanism (pathway 3). In response to any motion stimulus, in which all frequencies are less than 0.4 Hz, the secondary pathway is able to enhance the gain of all frequency components of the response so as to provide gains comparable to those evoked by discrete frequency sinusoids. In contrast, when the highest frequency rises above 0.4 Hz, the frequency characteristics of the velocity estimation mechanism change in such a way that only the highest frequency component of the stimulus is enhanced. As a consequence, the response at low frequencies becomes more dependent on continuous retinal velocity error feedback (pathway 2) and the gains of the low-frequency

components fall to a common base level (Fig. 5a). These nonlinear features of the response may imply the existence of a set of frequency-tuned channels within the secondary pathway which individually sense the various frequency components of the stimulus and, depending on the relative magnitude of the output from each channel, modify the dynamic characteristics of the secondary pathway so as to limit low-frequency gain and accentuate the gain of the highest-frequency component. Previously [13], it had been suggested that this process of highest frequency gain enhancement might arise from volitional potentiation, but more recent observations [15] indicate that this feature also occurs during passive stimulation of the oculomotor system, implying that it must be an inherent feature of the visual feedback, and not dependent on active participation.

The mechanism of voluntary, nonvisual VOR suppression

Unlike the responses observed with a real head-fixed target, the suppression of the VOR by imagined head-fixed targets was affected very little by the frequency composition of the stimulus, a finding that is in accord with that of McKinley and Peterson [11]. Nevertheless, the gain was frequency dependent, tending towards the gain for the dark condition at any frequency above 1 Hz. In other words, the modifying element during voluntary, nonvisual changes exhibited the characteristics of a low-pass filter, as previously demonstrated by Barr et al. [8].

One way in which nonvisual suppression might be achieved is by the negative feedback of the efference copy of eye velocity to inhibit the vestibular drive, as shown in the model (pathway 4 in Fig. 5). This would serve to minimize the unwanted eye velocity. If an internal representation of the oculomotor dynamics were included in this feedback loop it would exhibit the required characteristics of a low-pass filter. At low frequencies the ratio between the eye velocity during nonvisual suppression and eye velocity in the dark would be equal to $1/(1+K_E)$, where K_E is the gain of efferent feedback, whereas at frequencies beyond 1 Hz the ratio would be close to unity, and there would be little suppression, as is evidenced by the results shown in Fig. 4. McKinley and Peterson [11] discounted the concept of filtering on the basis that the observed changes in gain were not compatible with the lack of change in phase in their results. But our results do show phase changes (data not here presented) which are reasonably compatible with this hypothesis.

The mechanism of VOR gain enhancement

When the subject is instructed to imagine an earth-fixed target during rotation in the dark, the perceptual concept used is similar to that when imagining a head-fixed target, except that the objective is to maintain eye position in a specific direction in space. In the absence of other sensory cues, information concerning orientation must be derived from the semicircular canals. Experiments by Guedry et al. [18] have established that such sensory information is available to the subject, since reasonably accurate estimates of rotational displacement can be made in darkness, at least for small ($<50°$) displacements. This implies that the gain of the vestibular sensory system subserving the perception of whole-body rotation is close to unity even though the vestibulo-ocular gain is rarely greater than 0.6 at low frequencies. In order to provide a good estimate of head velocity (Φ in the model of Fig. 5) the output of the vestibular sensory pathway must be calibrated (i.e. G_H in Fig. 5 must tend towards unity). Such a function is presumably carried out on the basis of continual sensory input derived from the coordination of voluntary head and eye movements in everyday life.

There are a number of ways in which this central percept of head velocity might be used to generate the appropriate eye movements. One possibility, suggested previously by a number of authors [8,19,20], is that the head velocity estimate is combined with an efference copy of eye velocity (as indicated at junction B in Fig. 5) to give a central estimate of gaze velocity. The objective in the imagined earth-fixed target (IEFT) condition would then be to minimize gaze velocity error and this could be achieved by a direct high-gain inhibitory influence at junction B in the model. Assuming $G_H = 1$ and $G_V = 0.6$ the ratio between eye velocity and head velocity (gain) would be equal to $(0.6 + K_G)/(1 + K_G)$.

The ability to achieve near unity gain during attempted fixation of an imagined earth-fixed target would thus be dependent on the efficacy of the inhibitory feedback gain (K_G), a value for K_G of 5–10 being sufficient to account for the levels of eye velocity gain obtained experimentally.

References

[1] Bizzi, E., Kalil, R.E., Morasso, P. and Tagliasco, V. (1972) Central programming and peripheral feedback during eye-head coordination in monkeys. In J. Dichgans and E. Bizzi (Eds.), *Cerebral Control of Eye Movements and Motion Perception, Bibl. Ophthalmol., Vol. 82*, Karger, Basle, pp. 220–232.
[2] Gresty, M.A. and Leech, J. (1977) Co-ordination of the head and eyes in pursuit of predictable and random target motion. *Aviat. Space Environ. Med.*, 48: 741–744.
[3] Barnes, G.R. (1981) Visual-vestibular interaction in the coordination of voluntary eye and head movements. In A. Fuchs and W. Becker (Eds.), *Progress in Oculomotor Research*, Elsevier/North-Holland, Amsterdam, pp. 299–308.
[4] Barnes, G.R., Benson, A.J. and Prior, A.R.J. (1978) Visual-vestibular interaction in the control of eye movement. *Aviat. Space Environ. Med.*, 49: 557–564.
[5] Lau, C.G.Y., Honrubia, V., Jenkins, H.A., Baloh, R.W. and Yee, R.D. (1978) Linear model for visual-vestibular interaction. *Aviat. Space Environ. Med.*, 49: 880–885.
[6] Paige, G.D. (1983) Vestibulo-ocular reflex and its interactions with visual following mechanisms in the squirrel monkey. I. Response characteristics in normal animals. *J. Neurophysiol.*, 49: 134–151.
[7] Barnes, G.R. (1983) The effects of retinal target location on suppression of the vestibulo-ocular reflex. *Exp. Brain Res.*, 49: 257–268.
[8] Barr, C.C., Schultheis, L.W. and Robinson, D.A. (1976) Voluntary, non-visual control of the human vestibulo-ocular reflex. *Acta Otolaryngol. Stockholm*, 81: 365–375.
[9] Takahashi, M., Uemura, T. and Fujishiro, T. (1980) Studies of the vestibulo-ocular reflex and visual-vestibular interactions during active head movements. *Acta Otolaryngol. Stockholm*, 90: 115–124.
[10] Barnes, G.R. and Edge, A. (1983) The effect of strobe rate

328

of head-fixed visual targets on suppression of vestibular nystagmus. *Exp. Brain Res.*, 50: 228–236.

[11] McKinley, P.A. and Peterson, B.W. (1985) Voluntary modulation of the vestibulo-ocular reflex in humans and its relation to smooth pursuit. *Exp. Brain Res.*, 60: 454–464.

[12] Larsby, B., Hyden, D. and Odkvist, L.M. (1984) Gain and phase characteristics of compensatory eye movements in light and darkness. A study with a broad frequency band rotatory test. *Acta Otolaryngol. Stockholm*, 97: 223–232.

[13] Barnes, G.R., Donnelly, S.F. and Eason, R.D. (1987) The role of predictive velocity estimation in the pursuit reflex response to pseudo-random and step displacement stimuli. *J. Physiol. London*, 389: 111–136.

[14] Benson, A.J. (1970) Interactions between semicircular canals and gravireceptors. In D. Busby (Ed.), *Recent Advances in Aerospace Medicine*, Reidel, Dordrecht, pp. 249–261.

[15] Barnes, G.R. and Ruddock, C.J.S. (1987) Characteristic features of the ocular pursuit response to an unpredictable target motion stimulus in man. *Proc. Physiol. Soc.*, Oxford, July 1987.

[16] Dubois, M.F.W. and Collewijn, H. (1979) Optokinetic reactions in man elicited by localised retinal motion stimuli. *Vision Res.*, 19: 1105–1115.

[17] Barnes, G.R. and Crombie, J.W. (1983) The interaction of conflicting retinal motion stimuli in oculomotor control. *Exp. Brain Res.*, 59: 548–558.

[18] Guedry, F.E, Stockwell, L.W., Norman, J.W. and Owens, G.G. (1971) Use of triangular waveforms of angular velocity in the study of vestibular function. *Acta Otolaryngol. Stockholm*, 71: 439–448.

[19] Yasui, S. and Young, L.R. (1975) Perceived visual motion as effective stimulus to pursuit eye movement system. *Science*, 190: 906–908.

[20] Miles, F.A. and Lisberger, S.G. (1981) Plasticity in the vestibulo-ocular reflex: a new hypothesis. *Annu. Rev. Neurosci.*, 4: 273–299.

O. Pompeiano and J.H.J. Allum (Eds.)
Progress in Brain Research, Vol. 76
© 1988 Elsevier Science Publishers B.V. (Biomedical Division)

CHAPTER 29

Motor control strategies underlying head stabilization and voluntary head movements in humans and cats

E.A. Keshner and B.W. Peterson

Department of Physiology, Northwestern University Medical School, 303 East Chicago Avenue, Chicago, IL 60611, U.S.A.

Strategies for movement and stabilization of the head were examined within several paradigms to determine which CNS mechanisms were responsible. Patterns of muscle activation were observed during the performance of reflex (head-fixed) and voluntary (head-free) movements in the cat. Spatial patterns of human neck muscles were also observed during an isometric head stabilization task. Both studies indicated that, although the neck muscles have the potential to respond in multiple directions, they were actually programmed to respond maximally in a single preferential direction that was task dependent. Measures of head position, head velocity, and EMG response during rotations of the body about the vertical axis suggested a predominance of voluntarily organized responses at low frequencies with the possibility of participation of the vestibular reflexes at frequencies in the range of 1 to 5 Hz.

Introduction

In the process of stabilizing the multisegmental body following momentary instability, the human performer encounters several immediate motor tasks. The head must be steadied in order that gaze remain fixed in space. The mass of the head must be aligned with the body, and the centre of mass of the body replaced over the base of support. Each of these tasks might be achieved through more than one central mechanism. Reflexes such as the VCR, CCR, and vestibulo-ocular reflexes at the neck and eyes would oppose undesired motions of the head [1]. Triggered reactions elicited at various body segments [2,3] would act to maintain each body part over the centre of mass. Once the individual received the sensory information indicating that balance had been disturbed, even voluntary actions would be organized so as to effect restabilization. Thus the analysis of such a simple task as maintaining the upright position of the body encounters the complexity of control mechanisms available to the performer in response to a specific pattern of sensory stimuli.

Definitions of the central mechanisms are usually based upon three properties of the response: latency, task dependence, and invariance of motor output. Reflexes are assumed to have the shortest latencies (less than 70 ms) [4], to be independent of the task demands, and to be organized as an invariant output to a specific pattern of sensory inputs [5]. Triggered reactions have longer latencies (80–120 ms), are modified by the demands of the task, but still present a relatively invariant output of motor response [6,7]. Voluntary responses are believed to have the longest latencies (greater than 150 ms), are dependent upon the specific task, and are highly variable in their response organization [4,7]. The difficulty with these definitions arises when complex movements that permit prediction and the elicita-

---

Abbreviations: CCR, cervicocollic reflex; CNS, central nervous system; EMG, electromyogram; (I)GU, (imaginary) gunsight; MA, mental arithmetic; SCM, sternocleidomastoid; SEMI, semispinalis capitis; SPL, splenius capitis; TRAP, trapezius; VCR, vestibulocollic reflex; VT, visual tracking.

tion of preprogrammed responses are measured. Then, the voluntary responses might occur at latencies as early as those of reflexes, and automatic reflexes could serve as the subroutines of voluntary motor programs [8,9].

Evaluating the participation of reflex versus voluntarily organized responses during movement is an important facet of understanding motor control and motor learning strategies. Presumably, the performer's ability to learn or modify movement depends upon his or her capacity for error correction and the inhibition of primitive reflexes that could dominate the movement [10–12]. This problem has come into particularly sharp focus in studies dealing with head stabilization. Studies on decerebrate cats have demonstrated that the short-latency reflexes work together in a linear fashion to stabilize the head over a broad frequency range [13–15]. Studies in alert cats [14], labyrinthectomized monkeys [16], and humans [17,18], however, have presented conflicting representations of the stabilization of head motion as primarily reliant upon either reflex or voluntary motor commands, or the mechanical properties of the head (i.e. inertial and visco-elastic forces).

Head position control is actually an ideal paradigm for studying how CNS mechanisms interact when stabilizing a multidimensional motor system. The VCR and CCR are compensatory short-latency reflexes acting on the head. Longer-latency neck muscle responses, sensitive to changes in task constraints but occurring at latencies shorter than those of voluntarily organized responses, have been reported during a head stabilization task [17], and induced whole-body instability [2,19]. The participation of voluntarily organized head movements can be inferred through studies on anticipatory [20] and centrally preprogrammed [16] movements.

Although the head represents only 7% of the body's total weight [21], 23 different muscles directly link the skull on either side of midline to the vertebral skeleton [22]. The multiple muscle attachments might not be so surprising if the head were involved in the fine motor control and variety of motions found in the hand and fingers. Motions of the head,

however, are primarily directed toward orienting and stabilizing the position of the eyes in space [14,23]. The quantity of muscles available seems even more extraneous in the light of a recent fluoroscopic study of free head movements in several animals, including cats and rabbits, that demonstrated that only a small number of the available degrees of freedom in the cervical column are used in head movement [24]. In humans, the ligamentum flavum passively stabilizes the head so that it will not succumb to the gravitational pull and fall forward on the chest [22]. Thus head position can easily be restricted structurally and need not be constantly monitored and set by the exertion of muscular force.

In this paper we will examine on two levels how the CNS controls a motor system that has multiple joints and more muscles than there are degrees of freedom of motion. First, studies that measured the coordination of the spatial patterns of action in the neck muscles of cats and humans will be presented. Results from these studies indicate that for tasks eliciting either reflex or voluntarily organized movements, the CNS programs muscles to respond in specific orientations rather than generating an infinite variety of muscle patterns. Then, we will explore the strategies used by human subjects in producing voluntary stabilization of the head. The effect on specific properties of the movement by alterations in sensory feedback suggests that several CNS mechanisms actually participate in changing or maintaining the position of the head in space.

How the CNS programs compensatory muscle activation

Kinematic properties of neck reflexes in cats

The coordination of the directional forces produced by the actions of the multiple neck muscles during the VCR has been examined in decerebrate cats [13]. A best axis of rotation for excitation of given neck muscles was identified in relation to defined spatial orientations of the head in space. The VCR was stimulated by placing the animal on a rotating platform and rotating it in the dark while the head was fixed in relation to the body. EMG responses were recorded from several muscles as the platform was rotated about a large number of vertical and horizontal axes. We have performed a similar experiment to measure the spatial response properties of the VCR in two alert cats. Animals were surgically prepared and electrodes inserted as described by Goldberg and Peterson [14]. Implanted muscles included biventer cervicis, complexus, splenius, occipitoscapularis, and rectus capitis major, all studied bilaterally.

Methods of kinematic analysis

Once collected, the rectified and filtered EMG signals were fitted with a least-squares error sinusoid. The amplitude of the fitted fundamental sinusoid was divided by the angular position amplitude of the turntable to determine EMG responsiveness (*gain*). Gain and response phase, relative to position of the turntable, were determined for each muscle recorded. Optimal response planes for each

muscle were illustrated by calculating a response axis vector from the responses to frontal plane, pitched yaw, and pitch to roll rotations in all orientations. The two gain values for pure pitch, yaw and roll were taken from the sinusoidal function fit to the respective rotation series and averaged (see Fig. 1). The length of the three-dimensional vector composed of these three values was then normalized to one, and displayed on a series of two-dimensional axes (e.g. see Fig. 6 in [13] and Fig. 1 this paper).

Results

As reported previously in decerebrate cats [13], the EMG activity in all of the muscles recorded was sinusoidally modulated by rotation. In Fig. 1, the response gains of one muscle in an alert cat, the left complexus, are plotted as data points against the orientation of the rotation axis with respect to the head during the three series of rotations. Clearly seen is the sinusoidal modulation of the muscle

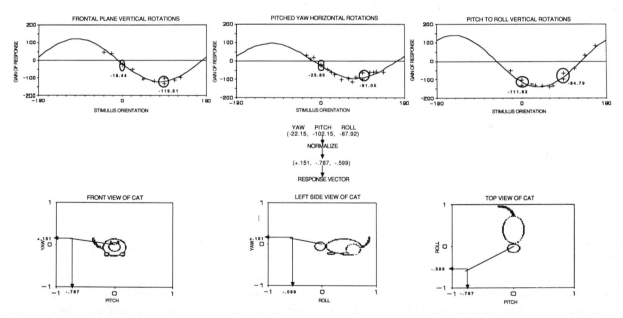

Fig. 1. Calculation of response vectors for the left complexus muscle of an alert cat. Gain of the EMG response is plotted against orientation angle for each series of head rotations. A sinusoidal function is fit to the data, and the values of pitch, yaw and roll are obtained from the fitted curve. These values are averaged, combined, and normalized to a length of 1.0 to produce a vector that represents the axis of the rotation that would maximally excite the muscle. The optimal response vector is displayed on two-dimensional drawings representing three views of the cat. Using the right-hand rule, imagine grasping the vector with your right hand, thumb pointing along the vector away from the cat. Your fingers point in the direction of angular rotation that maximally excites the muscle.

EMG response in all three rotational series. The phase of the VCR response also demonstrates the phase advance expected in a response related to stimulus velocity. Preferred directions of activation were observed in the individual neck muscles of the alert cats during the VCR [25]. These maximal activation directions were quite similar for both decerebrate and alert cats during stimulation of the VCR. In Fig. 2, maximal response vectors are plotted to demonstrate the best direction of excitation for each muscle EMG response in the alert and the decerebrate cats during the VCR tasks. During excitation of the VCR, all of the dorsal neck muscles were excited by downward rotations and inhibited by upward rotations of a turntable. Quantitative comparisons between the vectors indicate small angular differences that averaged about 20° between the decerebrate and alert response vectors, and between the response vectors of the two alert cats in this task. On closer examination of the preferred directions, we find that the biventer muscle was best activated by stimuli that elicit a compensatory response in the upward pitch direction. Complexus demonstrated a preference for roll with some pitch components. Occipitoscapularis and splenius were best activated in the horizontal planes, and the greatest response of rectus major was in pitch with some yaw. As would be expected of a reflex, each muscle was best activated during compensatory motions of the head.

Since the automatic neck reflexes are elicited by excitation of two separate sensory systems (labyrinths in the case of the VCR and neck proprioceptors for the CCR), it is conceivable that each reflex elicits a different pattern of excitation in specific muscles. The spatial patterns of neck muscles during the CCR have undergone preliminary measurements in both decerebrate and alert cats [26]. In this paradigm, the head was fixed in space while the body was rotated about the same 24 axes. The CCR was found to be stronger and more consistently responsive in the decerebrate than in the alert preparation. Preferred directions of activation similar to those of the VCR were characteristic of the muscle responses during CCR stimulation. Angular diffe-

rences between the response vectors of the CCR and the VCR were no greater than those between the alert and decerebrate VCR responses.

Kinematic properties of voluntary head movements in alert cats

The two alert cats that were tested for the VCR were simultaneously tested during a voluntary head tracking task. The animals were trained to follow a water spout as it rotated sinusoidally (0.25 Hz) about the same 24 axes as the turntable. EMG recordings were collected as described above. The responses of the left rectus major during the voluntary and reflex tasks in the pitch to roll series are compared in Fig. 3 where it can be seen that differences exist both in the orientation of the null response (112° in tracking and 67° in the VCR), and in the phase of the response. The VCR demonstrated the phase advance expected in a response related to stimulus velocity, whereas the phase of the response during tracking was related to the position of the head as it tracked the water spout.

Since muscle activity during the VCR serves in a compensatory fashion, and activity during voluntary motion assists the movement of the head, it was expected that the response vectors for matched head movements should occur in equal and opposite directions. This hypothesis was supported in the response vectors of the biventer cervicis muscle (see Fig. 2). Not all of the muscles were organized in this fashion, however. For some of the muscles, reflex and voluntary activity occurred as a more orthogonal relationship (e.g. complexus). In other muscles, the direction of maximal activation was the same for the reflex response, but differed during voluntary motion. For example, splenius exhibited a greater roll component, and occipitoscapularis more yaw in one cat during voluntary tracking while in the other cat the preferred directions of these two muscles were reversed. Also, maximal activation in the direction that would be expected from the anatomical position of the muscle was not always seen. As seen in Fig. 2, right complexus produced its major response component while the head

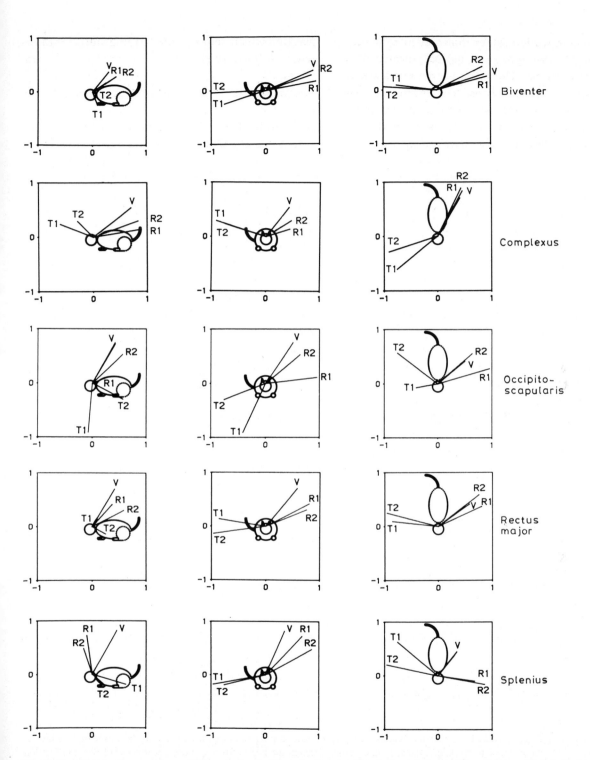

Fig. 2. Averaged response vectors of five muscles during voluntary tracking in two alert cats (T_1 and T_2) and whole-body rotations in alert (R_1 and R_2) and decerebrate (V) cats. Left muscles are inverted to appear as though they are on the right side of the body. The maximal response vectors were derived as shown in Fig. 1.

was rolling to the left rather than assisting the head in turning to the right as would be expected for a right-sided muscle. The response pattern for each muscle was surprisingly consistent within a cat over several months of testing. Overall, muscle response vectors tended to be more alike between the two cats during reflex activity than during voluntary tracking which demonstrated average angular differences as great as 50°.

Spatial patterns of head stabilization in humans

Our results from the experiments with cats suggested that the CNS programs the neck muscles to

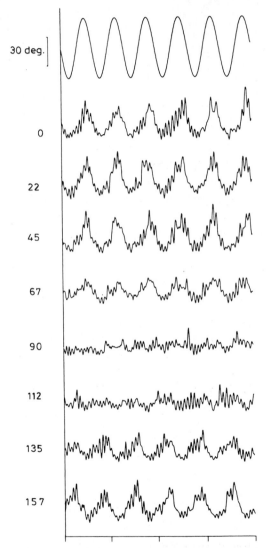
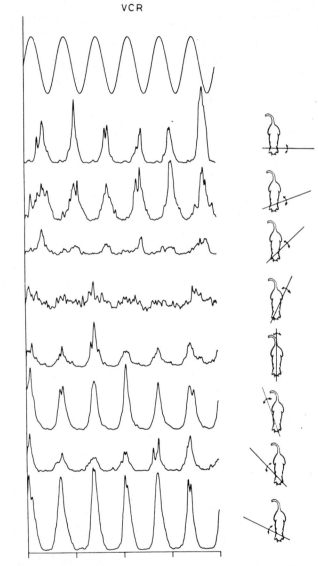

Fig. 3. Rectified and integrated EMG data from the left rectus major muscle during voluntary head tracking and whole body rotations in an alert cat. On the far right of the figure, the solid line passing through the head of the cat indicates the axis of rotation for that set of records. This series of rotations includes pitch (0°) and roll (90°). EMG responses are sinusoidally modulated in both tasks, but the null plane, where the response diminishes and reverses direction, differs for muscle activation during body rotation (VCR) and head tracking.

respond in a unique fashion for each task presented. That preferred response direction could vary, however, between the tasks, or between animals. Preferential activation in human neck muscles was also explored during an isometric head stabilization task [27]. Since this was a task requiring a voluntary response to an applied force, we expected greater variability than had it been a measure of reflex activation.

We used surface EMG recordings of four neck muscles on the right side, including SEMI, SPL, TRAP, and SCM. Electrode placements were later verified with bipolar intramuscular electrode recordings. Subjects were seated and received visual feedback as to the position of their heads at all times. A weight and pulley system applied horizontally directed forces to a specially adapted helmet so that the subjects counteracted a moderate force applied to the centre of mass of the head at 22° intervals. Average amplitude of the EMG response for each muscle appears on a polar plot, illustrating the level of activation in each direction of applied force (see Fig. 4). Zero degrees represents a forward flexion force requiring neck extension to stabilize the head. A force at 90° required rightward lateral rotation (or right roll) of the head, and −90° required left roll. Placing the pulley directly behind the subject resulted in pure flexion (180°).

It is clear from these plots that each muscle had a small area of preferred response with one direction of maximal excitation. A null response of each muscle in the orthogonal directions indicates that the muscles are reciprocally activated during this task. As predicted in standard anatomy and kinesiology texts [28], SEMI works primarily in pitch extension with some lateral rotation (0° to 45°); SCM in flexion with lateral rotation (90° to 180°). An unexpected result, however, was that of SPL. This muscle has always been described as exhibiting a lateral rotation and extension action. Yet half of our subjects presented a strong rightward roll response with flexion (135°) rather than extension (45°); this finding was confirmed with intramuscular recordings (see Fig 4A). TRAP also presented a somewhat confusing picture, probably due to the low levels of activation of this muscle in all of the tested directions. As seen in Fig. 4A, upper TRAP fibres responded primarily in leftward roll with extension (−45°), suggesting that TRAP was actually performing scapular depression in order to stabilize the scapular during head movements. Intramuscular recordings confirmed that a much stronger activation of this muscle occurred during isolated shoulder elevation than during head movements.

The observed levels of activation were very consistent for all of our subjects in each direction (see Fig. 4B). In two subjects, we tested the robustness of the relationship between direction and activation level by gradually increasing the amount of force applied to the head. As a result, linear increases in the EMG response were observed in the previously identified preferred directions of each muscle. When the weight was increased by three to four times the original amount, sudden jumps in EMG response magnitude were observed in directions that exhibited no response at lower forces. Even at maximum loading of the muscle, increases of equal magnitude were not seen in the preferred directions.

Reflex and voluntary contributions to head stabilization

Guitton et al. [17] assessed the influence of mental set and the relative importance of visual and vestibular cues on head stabilization in humans. Normal subjects and patients with bilateral vestibular deficit were tested under three conditions of head stabilization while rotated horizontally using a white noise stimulus with a bandwidth of 0 to 1 Hz. The gunsight condition (GU) required that the subject keep the head coincident with a stationary visual target while the chair was rotated. The imaginary gunsight condition (IGU) had the same requirement, but no visual feedback was available. During mental arithmetic (MA), the subject's attention was removed from the task of stabilization while rotation was ongoing. The role of the visual system was also assessed during a visual tracking (VT) condition in which the target moved but the body remained stationary.

336

Normal subjects were found to stabilize their head best in the GU condition, and had lower but similar head position response gain in IGU and VT. The vestibular deficit patients, however, had comparable gains in GU and VT with much lower gains in IGU and MA (see Fig. 3 in [17]). The apparent lack of head stabilization during the MA condition suggested that the VCR and CCR produced little effective head stabilization in humans at these frequencies. Vestibular inputs provided a necessary input to head stability in the dark as observed in the

difference between the two populations in the IGU condition.

Guitton et al. [17] calculated the responses of their subjects to a rotation step. Responses in GU and IGU had a latency of 150 ms which led them to conclude that longer-latency, reaction time (voluntary) mechanisms were primarily responsible for the head stabilization observed in their subjects. It was hypothesized that at higher frequencies (e.g. 2–4 Hz), inertial mechanisms would play a more important role in head stabilization, and the longer-

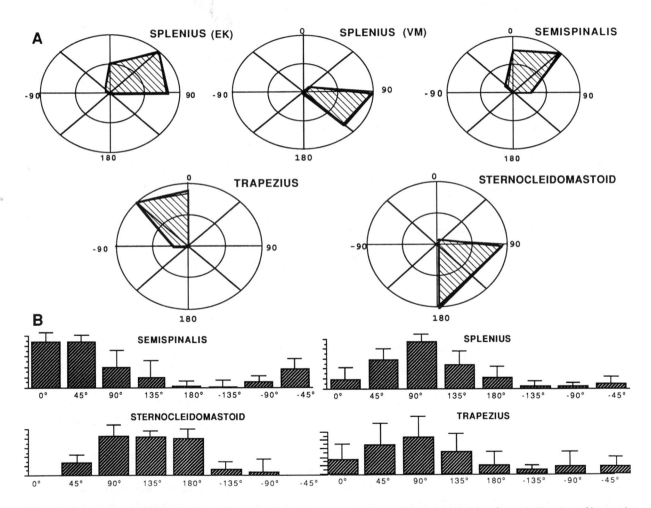

Fig. 4. (A) Polar plots of EMG spike rates recorded with an intramuscular electrode in a single subject for each direction of isometric head stabilization. Points furthest from the origin are the most strongly activated. The different preferential directions of the SPL muscle are demonstrated in the plots of two subjects (EK and VM). (B) Histograms of the average percentage and standard deviations of EMG activation for all subjects in each orientation direction demonstrate consistency in the preferred response of each muscle.

latency mechanisms would present too much of a phase lag to be effective. Thus the reflex mechanisms would be expected to participate at higher frequencies of rotation. We tested this hypothesis by repeating the paradigm of Guitton et al. [17], but with sum-of-sinusoid stimuli at frequencies ranging from 0.35 to 4.55 Hz. Four normal subjects were rotated about the vertical axis at a constant 80°/s using a random sum-of-sinusoids stimulus [29]. Head velocity, chair velocity, and four surface EMG recordings (SEMI, SPL, TRAP and SCM) were collected.

Gains of muscle EMG responses were calculated as in the cat experiments described above. Muscle activity was observed in all four conditions, with the largest gains during GU and VT at frequencies up to 2.65 Hz. The largest EMG response gains were seen in the SEMI and SPL muscles; appropriate behaviour for muscles identified as participating primarily in extension with lateral rotation (see Fig. 4). In fact, SEMI had significantly greater gains in GU and VT than in the other conditions (F $(3,9) = 3.92$, $p < 0.05$) suggesting that, as seen in cats [30], the human visual system has a direct effect on neck motor output.

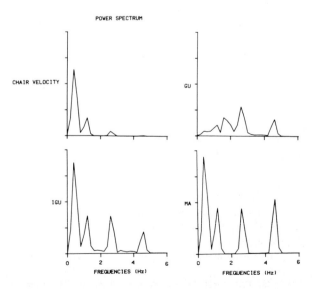

Fig. 5. Power spectrum of chair velocity and of head velocity during the three conditions of head stabilization (GU, IGU, and MA).

The differential effect of visual and vestibular information was most evident in the head velocity power spectrum (Fig. 5). When only vestibular information was available, the spectral response peaked at the stimulus input frequencies, and was not greatly affected by the presence (IGU) or absence (MA) of voluntary processes. Reliance upon visual inputs (GU), however, greatly altered the spectral configuration. The peak at the lowest frequency disappeared, an additional peak appeared around 2 Hz, and all the other peaks were small in comparison with MA and IGU. Apparently, attempting to use a visuomotor system that is too slow for the stimuli they encountered caused the subjects to generate inappropriate responses at frequencies not present in the stimulus. We can conclude that vestibular inputs provide the greatest accuracy for responses to velocity information since response characteristics were in no way improved by the addition of visual or voluntary processes.

Discussion

We have presented studies that attempt to determine how the CNS controls a motor system with multiple joints and more muscles than there are degrees of freedom of motion. First, studies that measured the coordination of the spatial patterns of action in the neck muscles of cats and humans were presented. Results from these studies indicated that for tasks eliciting either reflex or voluntarily organized movements, the CNS programs muscles to respond in specific orientations rather than generating an infinite variety of muscle patterns. Four characteristics of the CNS program for voluntary stabilization of the head have been revealed in the above studies. First, both in cats and humans, the CNS programs the neck musculature to be maximally activated in a unique direction, and that directional preference to be defined by the type of motor program (reflex or voluntary). Thus the pattern of muscle response for the two neck reflexes appears to be very similar, suggesting fixed kinematic properties of the neck motor system even when the pattern of sensory stimuli detected by the CNS differs. Second, during

338

voluntary movements, considerable variability may exist between subjects (e.g. as seen in the SPL muscle), but each individual exhibits a consistent pattern of response to a given task. Third, different parametric requirements of a task require that a different motor program emerge. For example, requiring head stabilization against increased levels of force resulted in a change in the directional properties of the reciprocal activation program to produce cocontraction rather than just a linear increase in the force levels. Finally, analysis of the strategies used by human subjects in producing voluntary stabilization of the head under conditions of altered sensory feedback suggest that the available sensory inputs will determine which of several CNS mechanisms actually participate in changing or maintaining the position of the head in space.

References

[1] Peterson, B.W., Bilotto, G., Goldberg, J. and Wilson, V.J. (1981) Dynamics of vestibulo-ocular, vestibulo-collic and cervico-collic reflexes. *Ann. N.Y. Acad. Sci.*, 374: 395–402.

[2] Keshner, E.A., Allum, J.H.J. and Pfaltz, C.R. (1987) Postural coactivation and adaptation in the sway stabilizing responses of normals and patients with bilateral vestibular deficit. *Exp. Brain Res.*, 69: 77–92.

[3] Nashner, L.M. and Woollacott, M. (1979) The organization of rapid postural adjustments of standing humans: an experimental-conceptual model. In R.E. Talbot and D.R. Humphrey (Eds.), *Posture and Movement*, Raven Press, New York, pp. 243–257.

[4] Jaeger, R.J., Gottlieb, G.L. and Agarwal, G.C. (1982) Myoelectric responses at flexors and extensors of human wrist to step torque perturbations. *J. Neurophysiol.*, 48: 388–401.

[5] Gallistel, C.R. (1980) *The Organization of Action: A New Synthesis*, Lawrence Erlbaum, Hillsdale, 432 pp.

[6] Crago, P.E., Houk, J.C. and Hasan, A. (1976) Regulatory actions of human stretch reflex. *J. Neurophysiol.*, 39: 925–935.

[7] Lee, R.G., Murphy, J.T. and Tatton, W.G. (1983) Long-latency myotatic reflexes in man: mechanisms, functional significance, and changes in patients with Parkinson's disease or hemiplegia. In J.E. Desmedt (Ed.), *Motor Control Mechanisms in Health and Disease*, Raven Press, New York, pp. 489–508.

[8] Easton, T.A. (1972) On the normal use of reflexes. *Am. Sci.*, 60: 591–599.

[9] Hayes, K.C. and Marteniuk, R.G. (1976) Dimensions of motor task complexity. In G.E. Stelmach (Ed.), *Motor Control: Issues and Trends*, Academic Press, New York, pp. 201–229.

[10] Luria, A.R. (1973) *The Working Brain*, Basic Books, New York, 398 pp.

[11] Twitchell, T.E. (1970) Reflex mechanisms and the development of prehension. In K. Connolly (Ed.), Mechanisms of Motor Skill Development, Academic Press, New York, pp. 25–37.

[12] Welford, A.T. (1976) *Skilled Performance: Perceptual and Motor Skills*, Scott, Foresman and Co., Glenview IL, 200 pp.

[13] Baker, J., Goldberg, J. and Peterson, B. (1985) Spatial and temporal response properties of the vestibulocollic reflex in decerebrate cats. *J. Neurophysiol.*, 54: 735–756.

[14] Goldberg, J. and Peterson, B.W. (1986) Reflex and mechanical contributions to head stabilization in alert cats. *J. Neurophysiol.*, 56: 857–875.

[15] Peterson, B.W., Goldberg, J. Bilotto, G. and Fuller, J.H. (1985) Cervicocollic reflex: Its dynamic properties and interaction with vestibular reflexes. *J. Neurophysiol.*, 54: 90–109.

[16] Bizzi, E., Dev, P., Morasso, P. and Polit, A. (1976) Effect of load disturbances during centrally initiated movements. *J. Neurophysiol.*, 41: 542–556.

[17] Guitton, D., Kearney, R.E., Wereley N. and Peterson, B.W. (1986) Visual, vestibular and voluntary contributions to human head stabilization. *Exp. Brain Res.*, 64: 59–69.

[18] Viviani, P. and Berthoz, A. (1975) Dynamics of the head-neck system in response to small perturbations: analysis and modelling in the frequency domain. *Biol. Cybern.*, 19:19–37.

[19] Keshner, E.A. and Allum, J.H.J. (1986) Plasticity in pitch sway stabilization: normal habituation and compensation for peripheral vestibular deficits. In W. Bles and T. Brandt (Eds.), *Disorders of Posture and Gait*, Elsevier, New York, pp. 289–314.

[20] Jeannerod, M. (1984) The contribution of open-loop and closed-loop control modes in prehension movements. In S. Kornblum and J. Requin (Eds.), *Preparatory States and Processes*. Erlbaum New Jersey, pp. 323–338.

[21] Gowitzke, B.A. and Milner, M. (1980) *Understanding the Scientific Basis of Human Movement*, Williams and Wilkins, Baltimore MD, 358 pp.

[22] Sherk, H.H. and Parke, W.W. (1983) Normal adult anatomy. In R.W. Bailey, H.H. Sterk, E.J. Dunn, J.W. Fielding, D.M. Long, K. Ono, L. Penning and E.S. Stauffer (Eds.), *The Cervical Spine Research Society, The Cervical Spine*, J.B. Lippincott, New York, pp. 8–22.

[23] Outerbridge, J.S. and Melvill Jones, G. (1971) Reflex control of head movement in man. *Aerospace Med.*, 42: 935–940.

[24] Vidal, P.P., Graf, W. and Berthoz, A. (1986) The orientation of the cervical vertebral column in unrestrained awake animals. I. Resting position. *Exp. Brain Res.*, 61: 549–559.

[25] Keshner, E.A., Baker, J., Banovetz, J., Peterson, B.W.,

Wickland, C., Robinson, F.R. and Tomko, D.L. (1986) Neck muscles demonstrate preferential activation during voluntary and reflex head movements in the cat. *Soc. Neurosci. Abstr.*, 12: 684.

[26] Banovetz, J.M., Rude, S.A., Perlmutter, S.I., Peterson, B.W. and Baker, J.F. (1987) A comparison of neck reflexes in alert and decerebrate cats. *Soc. Neurosci. Abstr.*, 13: 1312.

[27] Keshner, E.A., Campbell, D. and Peterson, B.W. (1987) Directional preferences of human neck muscles during head

stabilization. *Soc. Neurosci. Abstr.*, 13: 350.

[28] Kapandji, I.A. (1974) *The Physiology of the Joints, Vol. 3, The Trunk and the Vertebral Column*, Churchill Livingstone, New York, 251 pp.

[29] McKinley, P. and Peterson, B.W. (1985) Voluntary modulation of the vestibuloocular reflex in humans and its relation to smooth pursuit. *Exp. Brain Res.*, 60: 454–464.

[30] Vidal, P.P., Roucoux, A. and Berthoz, A. (1982) Eye position related activity in neck muscles of the alert cat. *Exp. Brain Res.*, 46: 448–453.

O. Pompeiano and J.H.J. Allum (Eds.)
Progress in Brain Research, Vol. 76
© 1988 Elsevier Science Publishers B.V. (Biomedical Division)

CHAPTER 30

Tensorial aspects of the multidimensional massively parallel sensorimotor function of neuronal networks

A. Pellionisz

Department of Physiology and Biophysics, New York University Medical Center, 550 First Avenue, New York, NY 10016, U.S.A.

Quantitation and mathematization of experimental neuroscience leads to the establishment of brain theory. Progress is spearheaded by system neuroscience and sensorimotor research, yielding computational paradigms of neural nets, to be utilized by neurocomputing and neurobotics. A mathematical concept and formalism using natural (general) coordinate systems that are intrinsic to the CNS is presented by a detailed elaboration of a computerized tensor network model for the vestibulocollic reflex in the cat, involving the cerebellum. The use of intrinsic coordinates is also shown for the multidimensional frames inherent in neuronal firings, and joint and muscle hyperspaces of the musculoskeletal apparatus of head movements. Tensor theory leads towards a quantitation and geometrization of concepts of motor strategies, trajectories, posture and style.

Introduction

Progress in brain research is characterized today by two main trends. One is the well-known, ceaseless growth of the body of data gathered on the structure and the functioning of the CNS. The other trend is perhaps less noticeable, and is underrepresented in the literature. Experimental neuroscience, just like any other maturing branch of natural science, is irrevocably advancing from a qualitative data-gathering stage (phenomenology) to a disciplined research. Brain science is going to stand on its own philosophical, conceptual, and most of all mathematical–theoretical basis.

Quantitation of the parallel organization of the brain

The progress towards quantitation and mathematization is led by system neuroscience in general, and sensorimotor research in particular. This is the natural proving ground of any mathematical brain theory, since invariants of the external world, such as displacements, directions, forces etc., represented by the CNS in both sensory and motor manner, can be physically measured. This is not necessarily true for higher order but less accessible brain functions, e.g. consciousness. Therefore, in the modern era Hering [29], Mach [42], Helmholtz [28], Högyes [31], Lorente de Nó [40], Szentágothai [82] and others envisioned the understanding of brain function as based on the strategy of first concentrating on simple sensorimotor function (most particularly, the oculomotor reflex), basically following the age-old approach set by Descartes. This cautious and prudent strategy is particularly profitable today as robotics and the emerging neurocomputer industry are looking on neuroscience as the resource of proven natural sensorimotor paradigms for coordinated, vision- and tactile-equipped, and ultimately,

---

Abbreviations: AOS, accessory optic system; CF, climbing fibre; CNS, central nervous system; GC, granule cell; IO, inferior olive; MF, mossy fibre; PC, Purkinje cell; VCR, vestibulocollic reflex.

intelligent organisms [18, 19, 38, 49, 54, 55].

The present task is to make sure that neuroscience's own theoretical concepts and mathematical formalisms facilitate an advancement in experimental brain research. It is not that neuroscience has been without concepts of quantitation or mathematical techniques. The problem is that such approaches have been borrowed from other disciplines (mostly from engineering) and thus were applied to the brain in a manner that is axiomatically not necessarily appropriate. One example of this is that 19th century philosophy considered the brain to be a machine. Thus, feedback control analysis, as used in electrical engineering, was employed until very recently to characterize, by single-dimensional gain–phase description of the amplification, the function of neuronal networks that underlie movements, e.g. oculomotor activity. Lately, the field of eye movement research has rebounded from such a single-dimensional representation and a multidimensional approach has taken hold [30, 58, 76].

The limitations inherent in concepts that consider the brain as an amplifier and thus, in effect, reduce brain theory to a chapter in control engineering are a subject of a newly established field, neurophilosophy [14]. Here, suffice to illuminate them by pointing out two major inadequacies. First, the automatic assumption that the brain is a machine, implies that the underlying laws are based on the well-known Newtonian classical mechanics with a separation of the space and the time domain (e.g. [12]). It is a fact, however, that lacking a simultaneity agent in the CNS, space and time information cannot be separated, and thus the brain uses non-Newtonian mechanics [59]. A second automatic, but not at all necessarily true assumption is that the brain is a serial processor–a computer. This belief is an undue generalization of the fact that virtually all man-made (electronic) machines are serially organized (they perform one operation at a time, albeit in ultra-fast sequence). As a result, concepts taken from engineering without scrutiny often imply that the CNS is also a serially organized machine, or at most, a device where several (e.g. x, y, and z) processors work in parallel, but are separable to independent systems (e.g. horizontal, vertical and torsional).

Modern scientists, especially computer experts [84] emphasize, however, that the serially organized computers (so-called von-Neumann machines) created by them are very much unlike the CNS, since the brain is a massively parallel system (high number of neurons perform their operations at once). This notion, which is an axiomatic understanding in neurocomputer research [18, 19] was, in fact, well expressed already in Sherrington's intuition [77] which characterized the CNS as an 'enchanted loom', where flickerings of myriads of neurons in parallel express the operandum. The same idea of parallelism is inherent in a number of other classic concepts. 'Synergies' [6] describe movements in terms of co-activation of several muscles. 'Schemas' [72] also imply that the CNS expresses its action by collective terms. 'Patterns' and 'assemblies' [21, 27, 48] are also terms introduced to represent a parallel action of arrays of neurons.

Formalisms for parallel sensorimotor function

Today, the belated acceptance of the fact that the CNS is a massively parallel processor necessitates multidimensional approaches both to represent and interpret multichannel EMG signals [39], multi-unit electrophysiological recordings of neurons [11, 54, 75], and ultimately also to conceptualize highly intuitive but hitherto qualitative notions implying multicomponent action, such as 'motor strategies', 'trajectories', or 'posture', in a quantitative and formal mathematical manner.

Given the virtual concensus today that CNS function is expressed by parallel action of a multitude of components, it is only natural that oculomotor research, as one of the most advanced sensorimotor fields where the arrays of individual motor elements (eye muscles) and sensory detectors (vestibular canals) are plainly visible, has embraced multidimensional approaches [30]. Beyond this major conceptual advancement, a key technical issue concerns the question of suitable mathematical formalism. Since the time of Pitts and McCulloch [73] and

Wiener [85], vector–matrix formalism, using multidimensional arrays, has been extensively applied in particular in the research of posture and gaze [3, 5, 46, 49–51, 53, 56, 58, 63–68, 76, 79] and in sensorimotor research in general [22, 25, 26]. One central issue that is presently still unsettled about such vector–matrix formalisms concerns the nature of the coordinate systems in which CNS vectors are expressed. While the choice of convenience of frames is the well-known Cartesian (3-dimensional orthogonal x, y, z) system, it is an undeniable fact that the CNS is not limited to the use of such special frames. In fact, brain function is expressed in coordinate systems that are intrinsic to the organism [58] and our task is simply 'letting the brain speak in its own terms' [78].

The multidimensional approach to the CNS that explores parallel function in terms of intrinsic coordinate systems presents two main classes of problems. One is the anatomical establishment of coordinate systems. This field of activity, originated by Helmholtz' [28] measurement of the rotational axes of human extra-ocular muscles has produced a good number of quantitative data lately on the vestibular system [8, 9, 15], oculomotor apparatus [16, 17, 20, 80] and neck musculature [4, 71]. Eventually, this new field of quantitative computerized anatomy is expected to grow into a major area of research with its own computerized (graphical) data-gathering technology and retrieval system.

The second major item on the agenda is research establishing how to mathematically interpret the CNS' use, by means of neuronal networks, of the intrinsic coordinates. Both issues will be exposed in this paper through the example of a tensorial model of the vestibulocollic reflex in the cat [61, 62, 64–69].

Sensorimotor function by multidimensional transformations of intrinsic coordinates: a tensorial model of the VCR in the cat

The problem faced by sensorimotor systems is how to transform information about the environment, measured by a diverse set of sensors, into appropriate responses executed by multiple muscles acting in concert. When one focuses attention to the spatial (kinematic) properties of the transformation, the geometrical arrangement of sensors and muscles are critical since they define the intrinsic biological coordinate frames in which the stimulus and response are expressed. The nervous system in turn must transform stimuli expressed in one frame into responses expressed in the other, perhaps by stages involving additional coordinate frames (cf. section 'Generalized functional intrinsic coordinates').

The basis of tensorial modelling of the VCR

As for data by quantitative anatomy, such intrinsic frames of reference are shown in Fig. 1. The sensory apparatus is shown in Fig. 1B: the rotational axes of vestibular semicircular canals were established by Blanks et al. [8]. The anterior, horizontal and posterior (pairs of) semicircular canals constitute a three-dimensional frame in which head movements are physically measured as the orthogonal projections of the head movement to these axes. A compensatory head movement is physically generated by the motor apparatus, using a 30-axis motor frame, in the form of the sum of the motor vector components. Having such a dual expression, both in a sensory and motor frame, of a physical entity, the VCR can be analysed as a primary sensorimotor system. This is unlike the vestibulo-ocular reflex, where reflex output is not directly sensed by the semicircular canals [51]. Moreover, for the VCR both the tenfold overcompleteness of the motor intrinsic frame over the sensory (from three components to thirty) and the nonorthogonality of the frames (especially that of the motor axes) are self-evident.

As for the basic mathematical concepts of how to represent such intrinsic vectorial expressions and their transformations by networks, a key consideration is that Nature's frames of reference and transformations between and among them can be described by generalized vectorial (tensorial) formalism. The proposal that neuronal networks should be considered as tensors [57] was based upon the conceptual definition that tensors are mathematical operators expressing entities (i.e. the event that the sensory inputs arise from and the response that the motor activity generates) in any possible frame of reference in a generalized mathematical manner (cf. [7, 36]). Tensorial operations which, in simplest cases, take the form of matrices, could thus express, via neuronal networks, the stages of transformation of stimulus to response. Fig. 1A shows a general scheme (valid any case of sensory and motor frame [50]), applicable for a set of

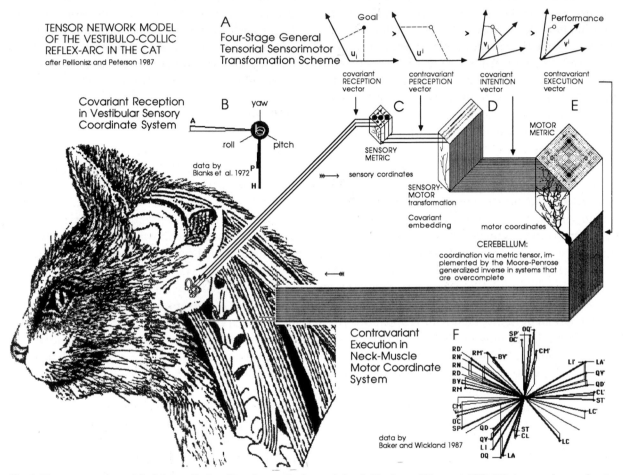

TENSOR NETWORK MODEL
OF THE VESTIBULO-COLLIC
REFLEX-ARC IN THE CAT
after Pellionisz and Peterson 1987

A
Four-Stage General
Tensorial Sensorimotor
Transformation Scheme

Goal

Performance

u_i u^i v_i v^i

covariant RECEPTION vector   contravariant PERCEPTION vector   covariant INTENTION vector   contravariant EXECUTION vector

Covariant Reception
in Vestibular Sensory
Coordinate System

B   yaw

A

roll   pitch

data by
Blanks et al. 1972 P
H

C

SENSORY
METRIC

sensory cordinates

SENSORY-
MOTOR
transformation

Covariant
embedding

D

MOTOR
METRIC

E

motor coordinates

CEREBELLUM:
coordination via metric tensor, implemented by the Moore-Penrose generalized inverse in systems that are overcomplete

Contravariant
Execution in
Neck-Muscle
Motor Coordinate
System

F

data by
Baker and Wickland 1987

Fig. 1. Tensor network model of the vestibulocollic reflex arc in the cat (after Pellionisz and Peterson [62]). (A) A general sensorimotor transformation scheme of the vectorial expression of a goal in a nonorthogonal sensory system to an overcomplete, nonorthogonal motor frame. The sequence is an orthogonal projection-to-parallelogram component transformation in the sensory frame, projection of the motor axes on the sensory, and projection-to-parallelogram components in the exemplary motor frame, which will yield a performance of the goal. (B) Neuronal networks of this head-stabilization reflex use coordinates intrinsic to the structure of vestibular semicircular canals (A, anterior; P, posterior; H, horizontal). The rotational axes of these canals have been anatomically measured [8] and the paired canal directions are displayed here in a pitch–roll–yaw frame. (F) For the head-movement system, the rotational axes of neck muscles have been measured [4] and displayed here in the same pitch–roll–yaw frame as the vestibular directions. Data and abbreviations of the 15 muscles (of each side) follow the nomenclature of [62]. (C, D, E) Tensor network modules, schematically displaying tensor transformation matrices implemented by neuronal networks. Arrays of patches display the tensor-matrix elements (corresponding to strengths of connections among input and output lines). One cell in a 'stack' of output neurons is visualized. Such a module multiplies the vector of firing frequencies arriving through the input lines by the tensor matrix implemented by the patch interconnections, to yield the vector of firing frequencies of the output neurons. The 3×3 sensory metric tensor (C), 3×30 sensorimotor covariant embedding transformation (D) and 30×30 motor metric tensor (E) have been calculated from data shown in B and F, according to the method shown in detail in [51].

three transformations with four different vectorial expressions. Fig. 1C, D, E show the tensor matrices, shown by dot diagrams, that represent the transformations implemented by means of neuronal networks.

Adoption of this general formalism enables one to discern an important difference between the types of vectorial representations of sensory input and motor output in their respective coordinate frames (even if these frames were identical). The response of a sensor, such as a semicircular canal (see Fig. 1A, stage 1), to a stimulus is independent of the responses of other sensors and is proportional to the cosine of the angle between the sensor's axis of maximum sensitivity and the axis of the applied stimulus (or equivalently to the projection of the stimulus vector upon the sensor axis). On the other hand, the muscle activations that generate the motor response are not independent of one another since the forces or torques they generate must sum in a parallelogram fashion to produce the desired movement (see Fig. 1A, stage 4). The projection-type vectorial representations are termed covariant in tensorial nomenclature, while the parallelogram-type representations are termed contravariant (cf. Fig. 1 in [7]). The CNS can thus be conceived of as a neuronal network performing tensorial transformations converting a covariant sensory input in one frame into a contravariant motor output in another frame [58].

When constructing a tensorial model of the VCR, one must consider an additional conceptual problem raised by the overcompleteness in sensorimotor systems. A system is overcomplete when the number of independent effectors (muscles) exceeds the number of controlled degrees of freedom of the apparatus they control. The simplest example of overcompleteness of a motor system is shown in Fig. 1A, where the exemplary motor frame is 3-dimensional, compared to the 2 sensory axes in the two-dimensional plane. The difficulty posed by an overcomplete motor system is that it can generate the same movement using an infinite number of different patterns of muscle activation. The modeller must then find the type of criterion that the CNS

uses in 'choosing' the particular pattern observed experimentally. The tensorial modelling scheme [50], utilizes the difference between covariant intention and contravariant execution representations of the desired movement. These vectorial versions, both given in the motor frame, are determined by the muscle geometry. The covariant presentation can always be found uniquely by projecting an invariant to the axes of a frame. The problem is then to find a unique contravariant representation. In a non-overcomplete system this is just the inverse of the covariant metric tensor. In an overcomplete system the problem is not that such an inverse does not exist but that there are an infinite number of inverses. It was hypothesized [49, 50] that the nervous system chooses a unique solution equivalent to the Moore-Penrose generalized inverse of the covariant metric [1]. Beyond the fact that this inverse minimizes the sum of squares of activity of the muscles during any movement, it should be noted that it may be implemented by a network (matrix) that could be constructed by the plausible biological process of reverberative oscillations in the developing nervous systems [60]. As it is shown in detail elsewhere [62], it is this choice of an optimal inverse that gives the VCR model its predictive power. Related models have been prepared for the vestibulo-ocular reflex [79] and tested in the case of voluntary arm movements [23]. The deviation of maximal EMG directions from muscle rotation axes can be calculated from the Moore-Penrose generalized inverse, and this allows one to make predictions of patterns of motor activation, on the basis of the geometry of the receptors and effectors. In fact, this tensor model predicts the actual VCR activation of the 6 neck muscles tested within the range of experimental precision [62].

Sensorimotor tensor transformations

The above-characterized theoretical solution is based on the four-stage (three-tensor) scheme of sensorimotor transformation shown in Fig. 1A. The transformation tensors are not shown in this figure by matrices, but schematically by 'tensor network modules' (C, D, E). In such modules, elements of the calculated matrices are represented by patches, symbolizing the strengths of connections among input and output arrays of axons. The firing frequencies of such a bundle of n axons are mathematically represented as n-dimensional vectors. The task performed in this scheme is threefold: *(a)* to change the sensory frame into motor, *(b)* to change the measured, covariant type vector to an executable contravariant version, and *(c)* to increase dimensions from three to thirty. The central, covariant embedding tensor (Fig. 1D) accomplishes both *(a)* and *(c)*, simply by projecting the 3 sensory (*i* subscripts) upon the 30 motor axes (*j* subscripts) which can be mathematically expressed as

$$\mathbf{c}_{ij} = \mathbf{u}_i \cdot \mathbf{v}_j,$$

where **u** and **v** are the coordinates of the (normalized) sensory and motor axes, respectively, and each matrix element of $\mathbf{c}_{ij}$ is the inner (scalar) product of the vectors of coordinates of the ith and jth axis.

The reason that the $\mathbf{c}_{ij}$ covariant embedding tensor is necessary but not sufficient in converting the covariant sensory reception vector $\mathbf{u}_i$ into contravariant motor execution $\mathbf{v}^j$ is that $\mathbf{c}_{ij}$ is a projective tensor. It turns a physical-type (contravariant) input vector into an output that is provided in its projection components (covariants). However, our task is the opposite; to turn the available sensory input (which is covariant), into the output required (which should be contravariant). This is why the other two conversions in the tensorial sensorimotor scheme are necessary. The sensory metric tensor $\mathbf{g}^{ii}$ (Fig. 1C) converts the covariant sensory reception into contravariant sensory perception, and the motor metric $\mathbf{g}^{ij}$ (Fig. 1E) turns covariant motor intention into contravariant motor execution. This general function of transforming covariant nonorthogonal versions into contravariant ones by metric tensors can be accomplished for any given set of axes by a matrix implemented by a divergent–convergent set of neuronal connections, often reporting on different sensory modalities, so characteristical for the CNS, e.g. among primary and secondary vestibular neurons [2, 3, 44, 74], and among brainstem premotor neurons and neck motoneurons.

Mathematically, the required contravariant tensor $\mathbf{g}^{ii}$ can be established as the inverse of the covariant metric tensor ($\mathbf{g}_{ii}$):

$$\mathbf{g}^{ii} = (\mathbf{g}_{ii})^{-1}$$

where components of $\mathbf{g}_{ii}$ are the inner (scalar) products of the arrays of coordinates of the (normalized) axes:

$$\mathbf{g}_{ii} = \mathbf{u}_i \cdot u_i$$

Two important questions arise regarding such metric transformations; a biological and a mathematical one. First of all, even if such transformations are implemented by matrices of neuronal networks, the CNS does not arrive at them by mathematical computation, but by some procedure feasible for a biological system. The question relates to the nature of this unknown procedure. Second, at the level of pure mathematics, a problem occurs with overcomplete coordinate systems. In such cases $\mathbf{g}_{ii}$ is singular (its determinant is zero), thus $\mathbf{g}_{ii}$ has an infinite number of inverses. The question is how CNS neuronal can arrive at a unique covariant-to-contravariant transformation (even in case of overcompleteness).

An attempt, aimed at answering both questions jointly, led to the proposal of a metaorganization principle and procedure which utilizes the Moore-Penrose generalized inverse [49, 50, 60]. Biologically, the proposed solution is based on arriving at special vectors whose covariant and contravariant expressions have identical directions (so-called eigenvectors of the system). This can be performed by the CNS in the form of a reverberative oscillatory procedure, where muscle proprioception recurs as motoneuron output, setting up tremors stabilizing in the eigenvectors. These special activation vectors would imprint a matrix of neural connections that can serve as the proper coordination device (implemented, for example, by the cerebellar neuronal circuit). Mathematically, this unique inverse of $\mathbf{g}_{jj}$ can be obtained from the outer (dyadic matrix) product (symbolized by $><$) of the eigenvectors $\mathbf{E}_m$, weighted by the inverses of the eigenvalues $\mathbf{L}_m$, where $1/\mathbf{L}_m = 0$ if $\mathbf{L}_m$ was 0:

$$\mathbf{g}^{ij} = \Sigma_m \, 1/\mathbf{L}_m \cdot (\mathbf{E}_m > < \mathbf{E}_m)$$

Once the Moore-Penrose generalized inverse is calculated by the above formula for the third transformation, the model predicts for each neck muscle a unique direction of head rotation for which that muscle should be maximally activated. Muscle activation during rotation about other axes is predicted to decline as the cosine of the angle between these axes and the optimal axis. As shown in detail elsewhere [62] the predicted optimal activation direction should typically differ quite significantly from muscle pulling directions, but can be readily tested experimentally with confirmatory results [62, 70].

Although pulling and activation directions are quite widely separated in this nonorthogonal system, the model predicts the activation directions within 4 to 11°. Thus the hypothesis that the CNS determines neck-muscle activation patterns in a manner corresponding to the Moore-Penrose generalized inverse is supported by the fact that the model predicts the pattern of muscle activity, produced by the VCR in decerebrate cats, within the limitations of experimental error.

Elaborations: tensor network models

The modelling approach described here opens avenues for substantial developments. First, while the data used in this paper are for the VCR of a traditional experimental animal, the cat, the problem addressed is applicable to many forms of motor control in a broad range of species including humans. Software is now available to construct similar models for any sensory–motor system where the geometry of sensors and muscles is made available by quantitative anatomical studies.

Second, investigators may wish to experimentally evaluate some quantitative predictions of such simple tensorial models. Gielen and Zuylen [23] have recently reported successful prediction of patterns of human arm muscle activation using a tensorial model. The experimental approach of recording EMG responses to multidirectional stimuli is also broadly applicable and could yield useful information about principles underlying motor control in a variety of species.

A third possibility is to further explore the neuronal network embodiments of such general coordinate transformations. The manner of how this challenge is addressed is indicated in Fig. 2. This multidimensional network scheme is the neuroanatomical elaboration of the rudimentary four-stage sensorimotor transformation shown in Fig. 1. The scheme in Fig. 2 introduces two refinements. One is based on the fact that the motor metric transformation is not implemented in a simple throughout manner (as shown in Fig. 1) but via an 'add-on' organ, the cerebellum (cf. [10]. This principle of organization is presented in detail elsewhere [50–52, 60].

The parallelly organized multidimensional neuronal network shown in Fig. 2 performs the motor metric function via the connection matrix of PCs with MFs collaterals to the cerebellar nuclei. Given that the execution vectors (PC projections) are inhibitory, the nucleofugal output will be the difference of motor intention and execution vectors, which will yield in the neck motor nuclei the required execution-vector output. The second aspect of elaboration is the path of multidimensional visual error signals to the PCs (via the AOS to the IO and to CF analogous to [43, 81]). As elaborated in [52] the CF vector, by projecting to the cerebellar nuclei both directly (through collaterals) and indirectly (via the PCs), in effect changes the motor metric tensor function of the cerebellum: altering the curvature of the motor functional space in an ongoing manner. While the rapprochement of such multidimensional quantitative parallel network models to neuroanatomical realities will require much further studies, it seems evident already at this stage that representation of such circuits as loops of single axons with nuclei merely serving as relay stations will no longer suffice.

A fourth important direction of studies is the ex-

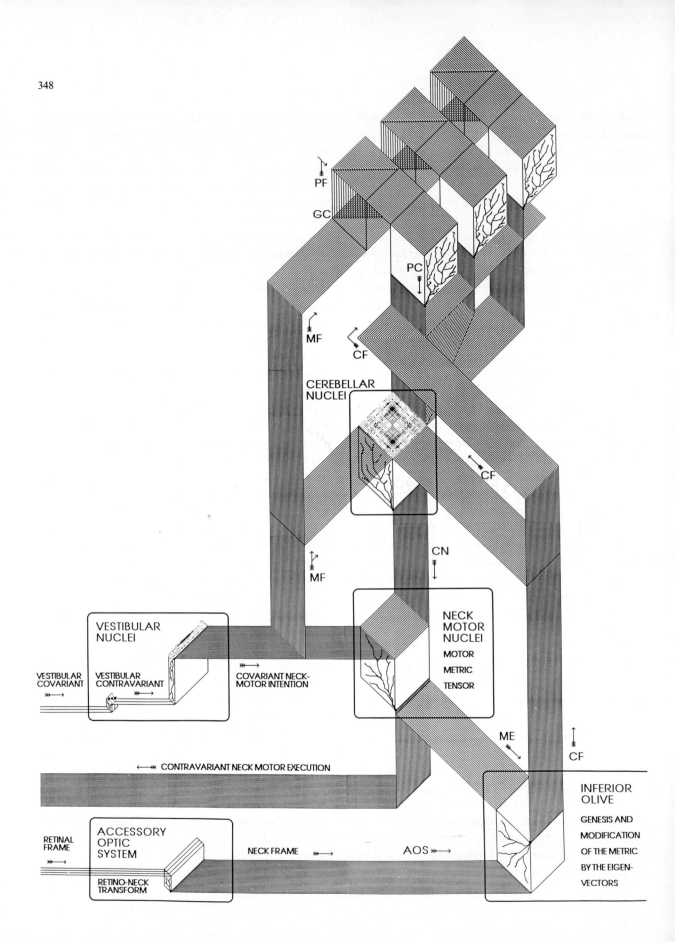

PF

GC

PC

MF

CF

CEREBELLAR
NUCLEI

CF

CN

MF

NECK
MOTOR
NUCLEI

MOTOR

METRIC

TENSOR

VESTIBULAR
NUCLEI

VESTIBULAR
COVARIANT

VESTIBULAR
CONTRAVARIANT

COVARIANT NECK-
MOTOR INTENTION

ME

CF

CONTRAVARIANT NECK MOTOR EXECUTION

INFERIOR
OLIVE

GENESIS AND

MODIFICATION

OF THE METRIC

BY THE EIGEN-

VECTORS

RETINAL
FRAME

ACCESSORY
OPTIC
SYSTEM

NECK FRAME

AOS

RETINO-NECK
TRANSFORM

ploration of intrinsic coordinates of more abstract nature than those embedded in skeletomuscular structure.

Generalized functional (other than structural) intrinsic coordinates

The fact that brain function is expressed by multidimensional intrinsic coordinates is most obvious in the case of anatomically explicit sensory and motor systems. Neurons connected to the peripheries of sensorimotor systems (e.g. vestibular canals and neck muscles) must use structural frames. Their rotational axes have been quantitatively established for several species. Typically, they are nonorthogonal overcomplete multidimensional frames (Fig. 1). In this light it is surprising to find claims in the literature that central neurons of this system apparently use an orthogonal frame: the paramedian pontine reticular formation reportedly contains medium-lead burst cells, whose firing rate is tightly related to eye velocity in either horizontal or vertical saccades [13, 24, 32, 33, 41].

The possibility that the CNS employs intrinsic coordinate systems in its operation that are different from the ones at the sensory and motor ends, of course, cannot be excluded. In fact, it has been shown that functionally and not structurally determined directional preferences (in our terms, intrinsic coordinates) do exist in the visual system, both at the retina [47] and in its relayed form to the cerebellum [43]. There are two main tasks: one is to experimentally identify such internal intrinsic frames, and the other is to theoretically interpret their functional significance. It is shown below that this paradox between a nonorthogonal structural frame and an orthogonal functional frame may receive an explanation in tensor theory with important implications to both theory and experimentation.

Tensorial relationship between structural and functional reference frames of brain function: saccade neurons in the monkey utilize frames composed of the eigenvectors of the frame of extra-ocular muscles

Tensor network theory of the CNS centers around the general question of transformations among intrinsic coordinates [50]. An even more profound problem is, however, how different (structural and functional) geometries are connected [60]. When attempting to relate the nonorthogonal structural frame with the apparently orthogonal functional frame, the question emerged as to whether the apparently orthogonal functional frame is, in fact, aligned with the eigenvectors of the nonorthogonal extra-ocular structural frame [53].

Availability of the rhesus monkey oculomotor frame (Fig. 3A; data from [80]) permits calculation of its eigenvectors (Fig. 3B). The procedure of this calculation is given in [51, 56, 60]. Comparison of

Fig. 2. Neuroanatomically realistic multidimensional network diagram of the tensor model of VCR in the cat. This scheme incorporates the simplified network model shown in Fig. 1. into a circuitry accounting for the cerebellar 'add-on' architecture, following the detailed model in [52, 60]. The input to the system is the vestibular 3-component vector, which is transformed through a 3 × 3 'tensor network module' of a vestibular sensory metric and a 3 × 30 sensorimotor covariant embedding module into a 30-dimensional output vector leaving the vestibular nuclei. This nucleofugal signal carries a covariant motor intention vector. This vector (without the cerebellum) would actuate via the neck motor nuclei a dysmetric head movement (by means of the 30 neck muscles). The tensor network module of the motor metric is embodied by the PC–cerebellar nuclear connection system (cf. Fig. 1E). Thus, the ascending MF–GC–PF intention vector (which is covariant) will be transformed by this metric into a contravariant execution vector. As the PC vector is inhibitory, this will result– with the MF collaterals into the cerebellar nuclei–a nucleofugal vector that is the difference of motor intention and execution. This nucleofugal vector adding to the direct intention vector will yield the exact contravariant execution signal for the compensatory head movement. The visual signal, reporting on the performance in retinal frame (a 3-dimensional vectors) enters through the AOS, where it is transformed into a vector expressed in the neck frame.This route is shown analogously to those in [81], although for neck muscles the path of error-vector may involve an indirect AOS to IO connection via a hitherto unexplored pathway through the interstitial nucleus of Cajal. Thus, the IO, as a comparator, will emit a CF vector that is the difference of execution and performance. This 'error' vector, projecting to the array of cerebellar nuclear cells both directly (via collaterals) and indirectly (via PCs) will generate ongoing dyadic product corrections with the error vector, in effect altering the metric properties of the cerebellar transformation.

Figs. 3A and B reveals that the above hypothesis meets an affirmative answer: Functional and structural geometries are connected in a manner that the frame in one utilizes the eigenvectors of the frame in the other. This finding may have both important theoretical and experimental implications. From a theoretical viewpoint, it was shown in the meta-organization of networks [60], that neurons must utilize the eigenvectors of the metric tensor of the motor frame to enable independent adaptive modifications, since eigenvectors form an orthogonal set. Experimentation could help by further investigating this issue. Data would be desirable in other species that have different motor frames and eigenvectors (see [51, 56], where such eigendirections are calculated for the human and the cat). Quantitative

properties of adaptive coordination along eigenvectors could also be experimentally explored. The paradigm of eigenvector connection of structural and functional frames therefore illustrates that a theory of CNS function expressed with multidimensional intrinsic coordinates can provide not only mathematical explanation of certain features of parallel brain function, but also yield specific suggestions for experimental investigation.

Geometrization of complex descriptions of sensorimotor function: motor strategies, trajectories, posture

Tensorial modelling of the CNS's use of structural and functional intrinsic coordinates is likely to pre-

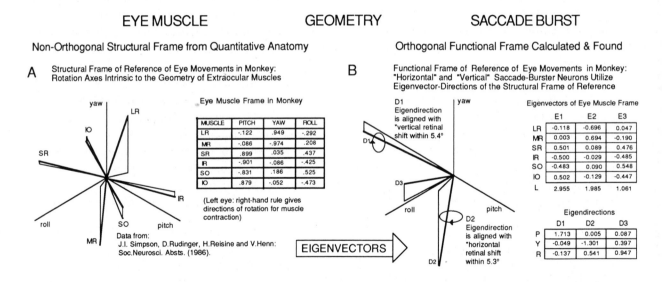

Fig. 3. Saccadic burster neurons in the monkey may use a functional frame of reference that is the eigenvector system of the structural frame of reference of the oculomotor muscles (after [53]). (A) Data by quantitative morphology (from [80]) showing the rotational axes, in a pitch–roll–yaw frame, of the six extra-ocular muscles in the rhesus monkey. Data refer to the left eye, data and visualization uses the right-hand rule. LR, lateral rectus; MR, medial rectus; SR, superior rectus; IR, inferior rectus; SO, superior oblique; IO, inferior oblique. This diagram is used here to display obvious features of this structural frame: (*a*) the overcompleteness, (*b*) the non-orthogonality, (*c*) the gross deviation of the axes from pure horizontal and vertical directions. (B) The eigendirections, calculated from the structural frame presented in A. The table of E1-E3 eigenvectors (with L1-L3 eigenvalues) has been calculated as shown in [51, 56]. The D1-D3 eigendirections are both tabulated and displayed in a frame identical to the one in panel A. As shown, the D2 and D1 eigendirections (preferred functional directions, since they are orthogonal, and thus separable) are aligned with an almost pure vertical and horizontal retinal shift, within 5.4° precision. Thus, the experimentally observed 'vertical' and 'horizontal' saccadic burster neurons [13, 24, 32, 33, 41] may well utilize an abstract functional intrinsic frame that is the eigenvector frame of the structural intrinsic coordinate system.

sent both major difficulties and new possibilities. One of the biggest hindrances at present is the meager availability of quantitative data on intrinsic structural frames (and the shortage is even more serious for functional neuronal frames). While quantitative computerized anatomy is likely to become an abundant source of data in the future, techniques are already explored that could alleviate the present shortage of quantitation. For instance, anatomical measurements of cat neck muscles [4] are only available for a fixed-head animal (where it is a good approximation that the head rotates around the single C1/C2 joint-point). However, with more complex head movements this approximation is not satisfactory, and thus data gathered by the 'Helmholtz method' (fixed origin and insertion points of muscles, fixed single rotational centre) no longer yield sufficient approximation.

A graphics-based computer software technique has been developed [34, 35, 37, 54] that removes the above bottlenecks, although this new method is not without limitations itself and is extraordinarily labor-intensive. Once a graphical rendering of the skeletomuscular system is available in the form of photographs, X-rays, drawings, etc., this information is scanned into a graphical computer. Fig. 4 provides examples of the display of the cat's head skeletomuscular system (cf. [71, 83]). Once (any number of) joint rotation points, relative stiffness values, muscle origin and insertion points are established by the operator, relative to the (movable) skeletal parts, the intrinsic movement coordinates belonging to individual muscles are computed, together with the covariant metric tensor (table of cosines among muscle axes) and its Moore-Penrose generalized inverse. This computation can be re-

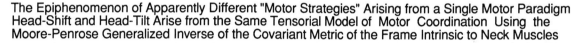

The Epiphenomenon of Apparently Different "Motor Strategies" Arising from a Single Motor Paradigm Head-Shift and Head-Tilt Arise from the Same Tensorial Model of Motor Coordination Using the Moore-Penrose Generalized Inverse of the Covariant Metric of the Frame Intrinsic to Neck Muscles

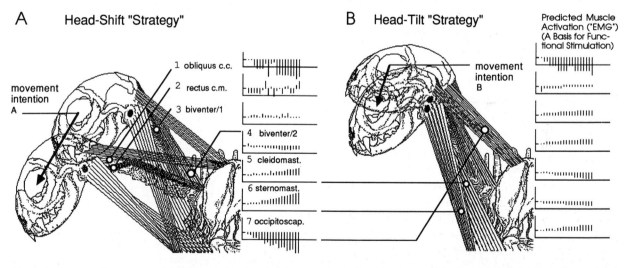

Fig. 4. Still pictures from a tensorial model movie of the head movements in the cat, using graphics-based establishment of the intrinsic coordinates of the skeletomuscular system consisting of the skull, all cervical vertebrae and 7 exemplary neck muscles. The head-shift *movement strategy* and head-tilt *strategy* arise from an identical model, where only the command of the movement is different (an 'intention' specified by the operator). While the movement intentions are straight displacements, the model predicts curved *trajectories* (an expression of the curved geometry of the functional motor space). Also, both the head-movement display as well as the predicted activations of 7 muscles with time (right side of panels) can be dramatically different with somewhat different intentions. Software that extracts the structural intrinsic coordinates from graphical input and calculates the Moore-Penrose generalized inverse of the motor metric in a dimension-free (tensorial) manner can be applied to several sensorimotor systems of many species.

freshed during a movement if desired. Thus, to any intention movement specified by the operator, the corresponding execution components of the muscles are computed, and the resulting movement is displayed (also by a computer movie). Motor behaviour of such systems can be studied restricted to the joint space (without muscles), or in muscle space and, with high enough resolution in the future, approximating the motoneuron space. Some applications of this model, capable of quantitating the functional behaviour of complex skeletomuscular systems, already yielded insights to sensorimotor function.

The display shown in Fig. 4 demonstrates that the identical model may yield remarkably different 'motor strategies' (a shift in A, utilizing several cervical rotational points, while a tilt in B basically around a single rotation point) if somewhat different motor intention is imposed by the operator. Thus, it is expected that this method will be helpful for studies by quantitative modelling also those hip–ankle–knee 'motor strategies' that seem to arise in experimental conditions [45]. A similar complex characterization of movements uses trajectories (curved paths) of movements that can be readily observed in most experimental conditions. It is, therefore, worth comparing the curved movements of appendages used in such tensorial skeletomuscular models even though the imposed intentions are straight lines. Since in the model such curvature is the direct consequence of the position-dependence of the intrinsic coordinate system (and the position-dependence of the functional geometry and the metric tensor of the motor space), the trajectories arise in the model in a manner characterizing the underlying geometry. (Using a metaphor: trajectories of flowing water on a mountain surface reveal the geometry of the structure of a mountain). Thus, it is expected that future studies by using advanced versions of tensorial models shown in this paper will be useful not only for revealing the neuronal networks that produce them, but also for quantitating high-level complex motor behaviour patterns as 'motor strategies', 'trajectories' and, perhaps, even 'posture' and 'style'.

Acknowledgement

This research was supported by the Grant NS 22999 from NINCDS

References

[1] Albert, A. (1972) *Regression and the Moore-Penrose Pseudoinverse.* Academic Press, New York.

[2] Allum, J.H.J., Graf, W., Dichgans, J. and Schmidt, C.L. (1976) Visual-vestibular interactions in the vestibular nuclei of the goldfish. *Exp. Brain Res.* 26: 463–485.

[3] Baker, J., Goldberg, J. and Peterson, B. (1985) Spatial and temporal response properties of the vestibulocollic reflex in decerebrate cat. *J. Neurophysiol.*, 54: 735–756.

[4] Baker, J. and Wickland, C. (1988) Kinematic properties of the vestibulocollic reflex. In B.W. Peterson and F.J. Richmond (Eds.), *Control of Head Movement*, Oxford Univ. Press, New York, pp. 167–177.

[5] Berthoz, A. and Melvill-Jones, G. (1985) *Adaptive Mechanisms in Gaze Control, Reviews in Oculomotor Research, Vol. 1*, Elsevier, Amsterdam.

[6] Bernstein, N.A. (1947) *O Postroyenii Dvizheniy (On the Construction of Movements)*, Medgiz, Moscow.

[7] Bickley, W.G. and Gibson, R.E. (1962) *Via Vector to Tensor*, John Wiley and Sons, New York.

[8] Blanks, R.H.I., Curthoys, I.S. and Markham, C.H. (1972) Planar relationships of semicircular canals in the cat. *Am. J. Physiol.*, 223: 55–62.

[9] Blanks, R.H.I., Curthoys, I.S. and Markham, C.H. (1975) Planar relationships of semicircular canals in man. *Acta Otolaryngol. Stockholm*, 80: 185–196.

[10] Bloedel, J.R., Dichgans, J. and Precht, W. (1985) *Cerebellar Functions*, Springer Verlag, Berlin.

[11] Bower, J. and Llinás, R. (1983) Simultaneous sampling of the responses of multiple, closely adjacent Purkinje cells responding to climbing fiber activation. *Soc. Neurosci. Abstr.*, 9: 607.

[12] Braitenberg, V. and Onesto, N. (1961) The cerebellar cortex as a timing organ. Discussion of an hypothesis. *Proc. 1st Int. Conf. Med. Cybernet.*, Giannini, Naples, pp. 1–19.

[13] Büttner, U., Waespe, W. and Henn, V. (1976) Duration and direction of optokinetic afternystagmus as a function of stimulus exposure time in the monkey. *Arch. Psychiatr. Nervenkr.*, 222: 281–291.

[14] Churchland, P.S. (1986) *Neurophilosophy: Toward a Unified Science of the Mind–Brain.* MIT Press, Cambridge MA.

[15] Curthoys, I.S., Blanks, R.H.I., and Markham, C.H. (1977) Semicircular canal functional anatomy in cat, guinea pig and man. *Acta Otolaryngol. Stockholm*, 83: 258–265.

[16] Daunicht, W. and Pellionisz, A. (1986) Coordinates intrinsic to the semicircular canals and the extra ocular muscles in the rat. *Soc. Neurosci. Abstr.*, 12: 1089.

[17] Daunicht, W. and Pellionisz, A. (1987) Spatial arrangement of the vestibular and the oculomotor system in the rat. *Brain Res.*, 435: 48–56.

[18] Denker, J.S. (Ed.) (1986) *Neural Networks for Computing*, AIP Conf. Proc. 151, New York.

[19] Eckmiller, R. and Malsburg, C. (Ed.) (1988) *Neural Computers*, Springer Verlag, Berlin.

[20] Ezure, K. and Graf, W. (1984) A quantitative analysis of the spatial organization of the vestibuloocular reflexes in lateral and front-eyed animals. *Neuroscience*, 12: 85–93.

[21] Farley, B.G., and Clark, W.A. (1954) Simulation of self-organizing system by digital computer. *IRE Trans. Inf. Theor.*, 4: 76.

[22] Georgopoulos, A.P., Schwartz, A.B. and Kettner, R.E. (1986) Neuronal population coding of movement direction. *Science*, 233: 1416–1419.

[23] Gielen, C.C.A.M. and Van Zuylen, E.J. (1986) Coordination of arm muscles during flexion and supination: application of the tensor analysis approach. *Neuroscience*, 17: 527–539.

[24] Van Gisbergen, J.A.M., Robinson, D. and Gielen, S. (1981) A quantitative analysis of generation of saccadic eye movements by burst neurons. *J. Neurophysiol.*, 45: 417–442.

[25] Grossberg, S. and Kuperstein, M. (1986) *Neural Dynamics of Adaptive Sensory-Motor Control. Ballistic Eye Movements*, Elsevier/North Holland, Amsterdam.

[26] Gurfinkel, V.S. (1987) Robotics and biological motor control. *Proc. II IBRO World Congr. Neuroscience Suppl.*, 22: S381.

[27] Hebb, D.O. (1949) *The Organization of Behaviour*, John Wiley, New York.

[28] Helmholtz, H. von (1896) *Handbuch der Physiologischen Optik*, 2nd Edn., Voss, Leipzig.

[29] Hering, E. (1868) *Die Lehre vom binocularen Sehen*, Engelmann, Leipzig.

[30] Henn, W. and Cohen, B. (Eds.) (1988). *Representation of 3-Dimensional Space in the Vestibular, Oculomotor and Visual Systems. Ann. N.Y. Acad. Sci.*, in press.

[31] Högyes, E. (1880-1884) Az associált szemmozgások idegmechanismusáról. Ertekezések a természettudományok köréböl. X, 18, 1–62 (1880), XI, 1–100 (1881); XIV, 9, 1–84 (1884). German translation: Högyes, A. (1912) Über den Nervenmechanismus der assoziierten Augenbewegungen. *Mschr. Ohrenheilk.*, 46: 685–740; 809–841; 1027–1083; 1353–1413; 1554–1571.

[32] Keller, E.L. (1974) Participation of medial pontine reticular formation in eye movement generation in monkey. *J. Neurophysiol.*, 37: 316–332.

[33] King, W.M. and Fuchs, A.F. (1979) Reticular control of vertical saccadic eye movements by mesencephalic burst neurons. *J. Neurophysiol.*, 42: 861–876.

[34] Laczkó, J., Pellionisz, A.J. Peterson, B.W. and Buchanan, T.S. (1987) Multidimensional sensorimotor 'patterns' arising from a graphics-based tensorial model of the neck-motor system. *Soc. Neurosci. Abstr.*, 13: 372.

[35] Lestienne, F., Liverneaux, Ph. and Pellionisz, A. (1987) Role of the superficial and deep neck muscles in the control of monkey head movement: application of the tensor analysis approach. *Soc. Neurosci. Abstr.*, 13: 372.

[36] Levi-Civita, T. (1926) *The Absolute Differential Calculus (Calculus of Tensors)*, Dover, New York.

[37] Liverneaux, Ph., Pellionisz, A.J. and Lestienne, F.G. (1987) Morpho-anatomy and muscular synergy of sub-occipital muscles in *Macaca mulatta*: study of head–trunk coordination. *Proc. II IBRO World Congr. Neurosci. Suppl.*, 22: S847.

[38] Loeb, G.E. (1983) Finding common ground between robotics and physiology. *Trends Neurosci.*, 5: 203–204.

[39] Loeb, G.E. and Richmond, F.J.R. (1986) Synchronization of motor units in and among diverse neck muscles during slow movements in intact cats. *Soc. Neurosci. Abstr.*, 12: 687.

[40] Lorente de Nó, R. (1933) Vestibulo-ocular reflex arc. *Arch. Neurol. Psychiatr.*, 30: 245–291.

[41] Luschei, E.S. and Fuchs, A.F. (1972) Activity of brainstem neurons during eye movements of alert monkeys. *J. Neurophysiol.*, 35: 445–461.

[42] Mach, E. (1886) *Beiträge zur Analyse der Empfindungen*. Fisher, Jena. (English translation by C.M. Williams, revised and supplemented by Sydney Waterlow, 1959, Dover, New York.)

[43] Maekawa, K. and Simpson, J.I. (1973) Climbing fiber responses evoked in the vestibulo-cerebellum of rabbit from visual system. *J. Neurophysiol.*, 36: 649–666.

[44] Markham, C.H. and Curthoys, I.S. (1972) Convergence of labyrinthine influences on units in the vestibular nuclei of the cat. II. Electrical stimulation. *Brain Res.*, 43: 383–396.

[45] Nashner, L.M. (1977) Fixed patterns of rapid postural responses among leg muscles during stance. *Exp. Brain Res.*, 30: 13–24.

[46] Ostriker, G., Pellionisz, A. and Llinás, R. (1985) Tensorial computer model of gaze. I. Oculomotor activity is expressed in non-orthogonal natural coordinates. *Neuroscience*, 14: 483–500.

[47] Oyster, C.W., Takahashi, E. and Collewijn, H. (1972) Direction selective retinal ganglion cells and control of optokinetic nystagmus in the rabbit. *Vision Res.*, 12: 183–193.

[48] Palm, G. (1982) *Neural Assemblies*, Springer, Berlin.

[49] Pellionisz, A. (1983) Brain theory: connecting neurobiology to robotics. Tensor analysis: utilizing intrinsic coordinates to describe, understand and engineer functional geometries of intelligent organisms. *J. Theor. Neurobiol.*, 2: 185–211.

[50] Pellionisz, A. (1984) Coordination: a vector-matrix description of transformations of overcomplete CNS coordinates and a tensorial solution using the Moore-Penrose generalized inverse. *J. Theor. Biol.*, 110: 353–375.

[51] Pellionisz, A. (1985) Tensorial aspects of the multidimensional approach to the vestibulo-oculomotor reflex and gaze. In A. Berthoz and G. Melvill-Jones (Eds.), *Adaptive Mechanisms in Gaze Control, Reviews of Oculomotor Research, Vol. 1*, Elsevier, Amsterdam, pp. 281–296.

[52] Pellionisz, A. (1985) Tensorial brain theory in cerebellar

354

modeling. In J. Bloedel, J. Dichgans and W. Precht (Eds.), *Cerebellar Functions*, Springer, Heidelberg, pp. 201–229.

[53] Pellionisz, A. (1986) Tensorial relationship found for structural and functional reference frames of brain function: saccade neurons in monkey utilize frames composed of the eigenvectors of the frame of extraocular muscles. *Soc. Neurosci. Abstr.*, 12: 1186.

[54] Pellionisz, A. (1987) Vistas from tensor network theory: a horizon from reductionalistic neurophilosophy to the geometry of multi-unit recordings. In R. Cotterill (Ed.), *Computer Simulation in Brain Science*, Cambridge University Press, Cambridge, pp. 44–73.

[55] Pellionisz, A. (1987) Sensorimotor operations: a ground for the co-evolution of brain theory with neurobotics and neurocomputers. *Proc. IEEE 1st Annu. Int. Conf. Neural Networks*, Vol. IV, pp. 593–600.

[56] Pellionisz, A. and Graf, W. (1987) Tensor network model of the 'three-neuron vestibulo-ocular reflex-arc' in the cat. *J. Theor. Neurobiol.*, 5: 127–151.

[57] Pellionisz, A. and Llinás, R. (1979) Brain modeling by tensor theory and computer simulation. The cerebellum: distributed processor for predictive coordination. *Neuroscience*, 4: 323–348.

[58] Pellionisz, A. and Llinás, R. (1980) Tensorial approach to the geometry of brain function. Cerebellar coordination via a metric tensor. *Neuroscience*, 5: 1761–1770.

[59] Pellionisz, A. and Llinás, R. (1982) Space–time representation in the brain. The cerebellum as a predictive space–time metric tensor. *Neuroscience*, 7: 1949–2970.

[60] Pellionisz, A. and Llinás, R. (1985) Tensor network theory of the metaorganization of functional geometries in the CNS. *Neuroscience*, 16: 245–273.

[61] Pellionisz, A. and Peterson, B.W. (1985) Tensor models of primary sensorimotor systems, such as the vestibulo-collic reflex (VCR) and of the metaorganization of hierarchically connected networks. *Soc. Neurosci. Abstr.* 11: 83.

[62] Pellionisz, A. and Peterson, B.W. (1988) A tensorial model of neck motor activation. In B.W. Peterson and F.J. Richmond (Eds.), *Control of Head Movement*, Oxford University Press, New York, pp. 178–186.

[63] Pellionisz, A.J., Soechting, J.F., Gielen, C.C.A.M., Simpson, J.I., Peterson, B.W., Georgopoulos, A.P. (1986) Multidimensional analyses of sensorimotor systems. *Soc. Neurosci. Abstr.* 12: 1.

[64] Peterson, B., Baker, J., Goldberg, J. and Wickland, C. (1985) Kinematic organization of the cat vestibulo-ocular reflex (VOR). *Soc. Neurosci. Abstr.*, 10: 162.

[65] Peterson, B.W., Baker, J., Wickland, C. and Pellionisz, A. (1985) Relation between neck muscle pulling directions and activity by the VCR: experimental test of a tensor model. *Soc. Neurosci. Abstr.* 11: 83.

[66] Peterson, B.W., Baker, J., Wickland, C., and Pellionisz, A. (1988) Sensorimotor transformation in oculomotor and neck-motor control systems. In *Proc. Annu. Conf. Engineering in Medicine and Biology.*, in press.

[67] Peterson, B.W., Baker, J.F., and Pellionisz, A.J. (1987) Comparison of spatial transformation in vestibulo-ocular

and vestibulo-spinal reflexes. *Ann. N.Y. Acad. Sci.*, in press.

[68] Peterson, B.W., Baker, J.F., and Pellionisz, A.J. (1987) Multidimensional analysis of vestibulo-ocular and vestibulo-collic reflexes (VOR and VCR). *In Proc. Int. Symp. Basic and Applied Aspects of Vestibular Function, Hong Kong*, in press.

[69] Peterson, B.W. and Pellionisz, A.J. (1986) A tensorial model of the kinematics of head movements in the cat. *Soc. Neurosci. Abstr.*, 12: 684.

[70] Peterson, B.W., Pellionisz, A.J., Baker, J.A. and Keshner, E.A. (1987) Functional morphology and neural control of neck muscles in mammals. *Proc. Symp. Axial Movement Systems: Biomechanics and Neural Control*, in press.

[71] Peterson, B.W. and Richmond, F. (1988) *Control of Head Movement*, Oxford University Press, Oxford.

[72] Piaget, J. (1980) *Structuralism*, Basic Books, New York.

[73] Pitts, W.H. and McCulloch, W.S. (1947) How we know universals: the perception of auditory and visual forms. *Bull. Math. Biophys.*, 9: 127–147.

[74] Pompeiano, O. (1975) Vestibulo-spinal relationships. In R.F. Noughton (Ed.), *The Vestibular System*, Academic Press, New York, pp. 147–180.

[75] Reitböck, H.J.P. (1983) A 19-channel matrix drive with individually controllable fiber microeleetrodes for neurophysiological applications. *IEEE Trans. System, Man Cybernetics*, SMC-13/5: 677–682.

[76] Robinson, D.A. (1982) The use of matrices in analyzing the three-dimensional behaviour of the vestibulo-ocular reflex. *Biol. Cybern.*, 46: 53–66.

[77] Sherrington, C. (1906) *The Integrative Action of the Nervous System*, Scribner, New York.

[78] Simpson, J.I. and Graf, W. (1985) The selection of reference frames by nature and its investigators. In A. Berthoz and G. Melvill-Jones (Eds.), *Adaptive Mechanisms in Gaze Control. Facts and Theories. Reviews of Oculomotor Research Vol. 1*, Elsevier, Amsterdam, pp. 3–20.

[79] Simpson, J.I. and Pellionisz, A. (1984) The vestibulo-ocular reflex in rabbit, as interpreted using the Moore-Penrose generalized inverse transformation of intrinsic coordinates. *Soc. Neurosci. Abstr.*, 10: 909.

[80] Simpson, J.I., Rudinger, D., Reisine, H. and Henn, V. (1986). Geometry of extraocular muscles of the rhesus monkey. *Soc. Neurosci. Abstr.*, 12: 1186.

[81] Simpson, J.I., Soodak, R.E. and Hess, R. (1979) The accessory optic system and its relation to the vestibulo-cerebellum. In R. Granit and O. Pompeiano (Eds.), *Reflex Control of Posture and Movements. Progress in Brain Research, Vol. 50*, Elsevier, Amsterdam, pp. 715–724.

[82] Szentágothai, J. (1950) The elementary vestibulo-ocular reflex arc. *J. Neurophysiol.*, 13: 395–407.

[83] Vidal, P.P., Graf, W. and Berthoz, A. (1986) The orientation of the cervical vertebral column in unrestrained awake animals. I. Resting position. *Exp. Brain Res.*, 61: 549–559.

[84] Von Neumann, J. (1958) *The Computer and the Brain*, Yale University Press, New Haven CT.

[85] Wiener, N. (1949) *Cybernetics*, MIT Press, Cambridge MA.

Compensation of Vestibulospinal Deficits

O. Pompeiano and J.H.J. Allum (Eds.)
Progress in Brain Research, Vol. 76
© 1988 Elsevier Science Publishers B.V. (Biomedical Division)

Overview

M. Lacour

Laboratoire de Psychophysiologie, Université de Provence, Centre de Saint-Jérôme, Rue H. Poincaré, F-13397 Marseille CEDEX 13, France

A basic property of the central nervous system seems to be its capability to produce active reorganization when sensorimotor systems lesions occur. These reorganizations, which lead to a total or partial recovery of function, may involve specific plastic structural changes and/or more global functional rearrangements of the neuronal networks, which are generally considered as the main processes underlying behavioural adaptations.

Unilateral lesion of the vestibular system produces a classical syndrome characterized by dramatic impairments of postural and oculomotor functions. These deficiencies occurring after hemilabyrinthectomy or unilateral vestibular neurectomy are often compensated for to a large extent during the following days, weeks or months, according to the species. This functional recovery, referred to as vestibular compensation, has been extensively studied in many species since the end of the last century. In a more recent past, vestibular compensation has been used as a model to study the plastic and adaptive mechanisms of the central nervous system, and particularly those concerning lesion-induced plasticity. The actual knowledge in this field is considerable. Synaptic changes have been demonstrated in the partially deafferented vestibular nuclei. The contribution of the remaining labyrinth input, of the visual (optokinetic) signals and of proprioceptive afferents in the reestablishment of a balanced resting firing rate in the bilateral nuclei and in the recalibration of dynamic vestibular reflexes has been analysed. The role of many central nervous structures interfering in the recovery process and of various factors controlling the adaptive reorganizations has also been reported. Different concepts or models dealing with particular aspects of the recovery process have been elaborated from these results, but the attempt to conciliate them in a more general theory of the vestibular compensation remains rather unsuccessful at present.

The aim of this section on vestibular compensation was not to propose such a theory. Maybe it does not exist. But it was first to summarize the recent advances in the understanding of the mechanisms leading to functional recovery and to present some new experimental evidence concerning the positive effects of physical exercise and neuropeptides in vestibular compensation. The second interesting point in this section was the critical reflexion which has been developed around the theoretical models and the new hypotheses emerging from the most recent investigations.

The utilization of procedures capable of accelerating functional recovery actually constitutes a field of research with important clinical implications. It is now well established that physical exercise and active movement can assist behavioural locomotor balance function and oculomotor function. This significant contribution of sensorimotor activity in the recovery process, as initially shown by our observations on the locomotor balance of unilateral vestibular neurectomized monkeys [1] and cats [2] has also been reported after two-stage bilateral labyrinthectomy in the squirrel monkey (Chapter 34).

The first two weeks appear to constitute a critical time-period for exercise to organize repairs or to facilitate the recovery mechanisms. The cerebellum, which receives various spinal ascending inputs, seems to be particularly involved in the sensorimotor recalibration. Moreover, physical exercise may help the dynamic rearrangement of neural transmitters at the vestibular nuclei level, or in other nervous structures. A second way of influencing vestibular compensation is neuropharmacological. Positive effects of $ACTH_{4-10}$ were seen on locomotor deviation and slow phase velocity of spontaneous nystagmus in the squirrel monkey (Chapter 34). $ACTH_{4-10}$-like neuropeptides also accelerate considerably the compensation of head postural asymmetry in the frog (Chapter 37), as they influence learning and memory processes, i.e. all forms of behavioural plasticity. If we consider lesion-induced plasticity as a relearning process, we can probably postulate the existence of common basic mechanisms which, however, remain unclear at present. As for the application of physical exercise, neuropeptide treatment has better effects when applied during the early stages of compensation, which could represent a similar sensitive period for functional recovery. This period may be crucial for achieving well-adapted behaviour.

Many theoretical considerations were put forward during this session, leading to very stimulating discussions on the real nature of the recovery process after vestibular lesion. The main topics which were briefly, but critically discussed, are summarized in the following questions:

(a) Is the recovery process a unitary one?

(b) Is it mainly restricted to the vestibular nuclei or more widely distributed?

(c) Is it achieved by means of restitution or of substitution mechanisms?

(d) Is vestibular compensation a good model to study plasticity of the nervous system?

Since different aspects of recovery can be dissociated, it appears that vestibular compensation does not act like a single process. In the guinea-pig, for instance, the process of postural compensation may go on independently of nystagmus (Chapter 32).

This point was discussed in the general frame of the Galiana model based on the hypothesis that restoration of symmetry in bilateral resting activity within the vestibular nuclei is achieved by changes of neural gain in closed commissural loops. Placing the site of vestibular compensation in pathways linking the vestibular nuclei is still rather controversial at present. First, the dynamics of the vestibulo-ocular reflex is poorly recovered in frog, cat and guinea-pig (Chapters 32 and 35) as shown at the neuronal level by a normal type II cell distribution but abnormal type I cell repartition in the partially deafferented vestibular nuclei. Secondly, there is no intervestibular nuclear coupling between the Deiters' nuclei on both sides [3] and, therefore, recovery of the vestibulospinal reflexes dynamics cannot be accounted for by the Galiana model [4]. Thirdly, vestibular compensation results from the combined activity of many brainstem and cerebral structures as already pointed out in the rat [5] and in the frog [6] and also evidenced in this session in the cat (Chapter 33). The compensation process would imply a broad distribution of functional modifications, including the vestibular nuclei.

In fact, depending on:

(a) the function–structure relationship which may vary from one species to another,

(b) the tested function (posture, locomotion, vestibulospinal or vestibulo-ocular reflexes, static versus dynamic characteristics), and

(c) the specific or more diffuse role normally played by the vestibular system in these different functions, one can expect either rather localized plastic or functional changes (in the vestibular nuclei, for instance), or modifications more widely distributed in complex circuitries able to recalibrate the vestibular reflexes. The demonstration of central cholinergic and noradrenergic mechanisms, located in the dorsal aspect of the pontine tegmentum and regulating the gain of the vestibulospinal reflexes (Chapter 31), illustrates this latter point.

Finally, what is important for the nervous system is to produce adaptive reorganizations. In this way, both restitution and substitution processes may assist functional recovery. Permanent or long-term deficiencies do not necessary signal the absence of plasticity within the central nervous system, but some limitation in the restitution processes which can be compensated for by substitution mechanisms or behavioural strategies. The observation in the frog that saccades compensate for parts of the missing slow phase movement of the vestibular reflexes is in agreement with this conception (Chapter 35). The missing vestibulocollic reflex is substituted acutely immediately after lesion by a saccadic subsystem. This corroborates a new hypothesis proposed in this meeting (Chapter 36), indicating that gaze control and corollary discharge from eye-position signals, rather than vision, would be important during the acute stage, as a complementary active process.

It is well known that restitution mechanisms (structural and plastic changes) predominate in lower species and are particularly well developed in the young, while substitution processes are more frequently observed in higher vertebrates and when lesion is made at adult age. They probably co-exist and act together with different gradients of efficacy, leading to a total or only partial functional recovery. They would represent two different modes of plasticity, defined in its wide acceptation, i.e. all of the processes involved in behavioural adaptations. In this context, the vestibular lesion model is a good experimental paradigm to study nervous plasticity.

References

[1] Lacour, M., Roll, J.P. and Appaix, M. (1976) Modifications and development of spinal reflexes in the alert baboon (*Papio papio*) following a unilateral vestibular neurotomy. *Brain Res.*, 113: 255–269.

[2] Xerri, C. and Lacour, M. (1980) Compensation des déficits posturaux et cinétiques après neurectomie vestibulaire unilatérale chez le chat. Rôle de l'activité sensorimotrice. *Acta Otolaryngol. Stockholm*, 90: 414–424.

[3] Pompeiano, O., Mergner, T. and Corvaja, N. (1978) Commissural, perihypoglossal and reticular afferent projections to the vestibular nuclei in the cat. An experimental anatomical study with the method of the retrograde transport of horseradish peroxidase. *Arch. Ital. Biol.*, 116: 130–172.

[4] Galiana, H.L., Flohr, H. and Melvill Jones, G. (1984) A reevaluation of intervestibular nuclear coupling: its role in vestibular compensation. *J. Neurophysiol.*, 51: 258–275.

[5] Llinas, R. and Walton, K. (1979) Vestibular compensation: a distributed property of the central nervous system. In H. Asanuma and V.J. Wilson (Eds.), *Integration in the Nervous System*, Igaku-shoin, Tokyo, pp. 145–166.

[6] Flohr, H., Bienhold, H., Abeln, W. and Macskovics, I. (1981) Concepts of vestibular compensation. In H. Flohr and W. Precht (Eds.), *Lesion-Induced Neuronal Plasticity in Sensorimotor Systems*. Springer, Berlin, pp. 153–172.

O. Pompeiano and J.H.J. Allum (Eds.)
Progress in Brain Research, Vol. 76
© 1988 Elsevier Science Publishers B.V. (Biomedical Division)

CHAPTER 31

Noradrenergic and cholinergic mechanisms responsible for the gain regulation of vestibulospinal reflexes

P. D'Ascanio, O. Pompeiano and G. Stampacchia

Dipartimento di Fisiologia e Biochimica, Università di Pisa, Via S. Zeno 31, 56100 Pisa, Italy

Experiments performed in precollicular decerebrate cats have shown that dorsal pontine structures, including the LC and the related dorsal pRF, play an important role not only in the control of posture but also in the gain regulation of the VS reflexes. The LC neurons, which are not only noradrenergic but also NE-sensitive due to the existence of self-inhibitory synapses acting on α_2-adrenoceptors, send inhibitory afferents to the dorsal pRF; on the other hand, these pontine reticular neurons, which are presumably cholinergic as well as cholinoceptive due to the existence of self-excitatory synapses, project excitatory afferents to the medullary inhibitory RS system. The increased discharge of these pontine reticular neurons and the related inhibitory RS neurons following local injection of cholinergic agonists into the dorsal pRF decreased the postural tonus in the ipsilateral limbs but greatly enhanced the amplitude of the EMG modulation and thus the response gain of ipsilateral limb extensors to labyrinth stimulation. This finding did not depend on the decreased postural activity, since it was still observed when the EMG activity was reflexly maintained by an increased static stretch of the muscle. Similar results were also obtained when the discharge of the pontine reticular neurons and the related inhibitory RS neurons was raised after local injection of an α_2-adrenergic agonist into the LC, leading to functional inactivation of the noradrenergic LC neurons. On the other hand, an increased postural activity in the ipsilateral limbs as well as a reduced gain of the corresponding VS reflexes were obtained when the discharge of the pontine reticular neurons and the related inhibitory RS neurons was reduced, as shown after local injection

of cholinergic agonists into the LC leading to activation of the noradrenergic neurons. There was also evidence that cholinergic excitatory afferents to the LC originated from the ipsilateral dorsal pRF. The effects described above were dose-dependent as well as site-specific, as shown by histological controls. In conclusion, the pontine structures described above operate as a *variable-gain regulator* acting at the motoneuronal level during the VS reflexes. Since the same structures are also responsible for the spontaneous fluctuations in posture related to the sleep–waking cycle, they may well intervene as a control system in order to adapt to the animal state the response gain of limb extensors following labyrinth stimulation.

Introduction

Experiments performed in decerebrate cats have shown that the postural tonus depends not only on excitatory VS volleys originating from the lateral vestibular nucleus [66], but also on inhibitory RS volleys originating from the medial aspect of the mRF, where the nucleus reticularis magnocellularis is located [35, 48, 50, 64].

These inhibitory RS neurons, which display a very low discharge rate in decerebrate animals [52, 74], are under the tonic excitatory control of the lateral tegmentoreticular tract originating from the dorsal pRF [37, 83]; for references see [81, 84], where presumably cholinergic and self-excitatory cholino-

---

Abbreviations: ACh(e), acetylcholine(esterase); EMG, electromyogram; LC, locus coeruleus; NE, norepinephrine; (m/p)RF, (medullary/pontine) reticular formation; (m)RS, (medullary inhibitory) reticulospinal; SC, locus subcoeruleus; VS, vestibulospinal.

ceptive neurons are located [4, 68, 70, 92, 95], as shown also by histochemical [41, 42, 62, 63] and electrophysiological studies [10, 89]. On the other hand, the activity of this dorsal pontine area is under the tonic inhibitory control of NE-containing LC-complex (i.e. LC and SC) neurons [68, 81, 84, 92], which send afferent projections to the underlying reticular neurons [37, 82, 85], as shown also by the presence of NE-containing varicosities in the pRF [36]. These LC-complex neurons are not only noradrenergic but also NE-sensitive, due to the existence of self-inhibitory synapses which act on α_2-adrenoceptors by utilizing mechanisms of recurrent and/or lateral inhibition [3, 11–13, 24, 26, 93, 94]. The connections between these noradrenergic and cholinergic neurons are illustrated schematically in Fig. 1.

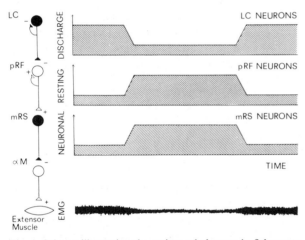

Fig. 1. Scheme illustrating the reciprocal changes in firing rate of the two populations of LC neurons and dorsal pRF neurons, leading to changes in tonic activity of ipsilateral limb extensor muscles. *Left side*: Inhibitory or excitatory neurons are indicated by filled or empty symbols, respectively. The NE-containing LC neurons, which are self-inhibitory, also inhibit the cholinergic pRF neurons located immediately ventral to them (see Fig. 2A). On the other hand, the latter neurons, which are self-excitatory, also excite the medullary inhibitory reticulospinal (mRS) neurons, whose increased discharge reduces the activity of ipsilateral limb extensor motoneurons (αM). *Right side*: A reduced discharge of LC neurons releases from inhibition the activity of the cholinergic pRF neurons and the related mRS neurons, thus reducing the contraction of ipsilateral limb extensor muscles. (From [77]).

In intact animals during waking, as well as in acute decerebrate animals, the postural activity is present in so far as the LC neurons show a regular discharge, which keeps under their inhibitory control the dorsal pRF neurons and the related medullary inhibitory RS neurons. However, as soon the discharge of the LC neurons decreased, as shown during desynchronized sleep in intact animals [24, 38, 57, 81, 84, 92] or after systemic injection of an anticholinesterase in decerebrate cats [68, 71, 72], the activity of the dorsal pRF neurons and the related inhibitory RS neurons increased, thus leading to a decrease or suppression in postural activity [3].

In addition to these changes in posture, the neuronal system described above may also play an important role in the control of the VS reflexes. It is known that an increased contraction of the limb extensor motoneurons occurs during side-down roll tilt of the animal leading to stimulation of macular labyrinth receptors [23, 51, 86]. This contraction depends on both an increased discharge of excitatory VS neurons [7, 8, 54, 87] and a reduced discharge of medullary inhibitory RS neurons [52, 74] while just the opposite results occur for the other direction of animal orientation [69]. However, in spite of the good physiological conditions of the decerebrate cat and the detectable modulation of a large proportion of VS and medullary RS neurons to animal tilt, the gain of the VS reflexes was quite small in forelimb extensors [51] and actually not measurable in hindlimb extensors [9, 53, 75].

In order to account for these findings we postulated that for a given amount of labyrinth input the amplitude of the EMG modulation of limb extensors depends on the background discharge of the dorsal pRF neurons and the related inhibitory RS neurons, so that if the firing rate of these RS neurons is very low as in the decerebrate preparations [52], a small amount of disinhibition would affect the limb extensor motoneurons during side-down animal tilt. These motoneurons would then respond less efficiently to the excitatory VS volleys elicited by given parameters of animal displacement, giving rise to a small-amplitude modulation of the EMG activity and thus to a small gain of responses of limb extensors to labyrinth stimulation. On the other hand, just the opposite effect would occur if the background discharge of the pRF neurons and the related medullary RS neurons increases. Indeed, there is evidence that the increased discharge of these pontine [32] and medullary RS neurons [90] following systemic injection of small doses of an anticholinesterase, while decreasing the postural activity (for references see [68]), greatly increased the gain of the VS reflexes [53, 73, 75].

The main aim of the present experiments was to find out whether local injection in dorsal pontine structures of substances leading either to activation of the cholinergic pRF neurons or to inactivation of the NE-containing LC neurons could not only decrease the postural activity, but also increase the response gain of limb extensors to sinusoidal stimulation of labyrinth receptors.

Vestibular reflexes in limb-extensor muscles of decerebrate cats

The experiments were performed in precollicular decerebrate cats. In particular, the multiunit EMG activity of a forelimb extensor, i.e. the medial head of the triceps brachii, was sampled by a digital signal averager during roll tilt of the animal at 0.15 Hz, $\pm$ 10°, leading to sinusoidal stimulation of labyrinth receptors. A computer analysis of the responses allowed the evaluation of the base frequency (mean firing rate of the multiunit activity recorded during each test in imp./s), the gain (imp./s/deg) and the phase angle (deg) of the first harmonic of the output with respect to the peak of the side-down stimulus displacement ipsilateral to the recording side, following the method described previously [51]. These responses were characterized by an increased activity during side-down and a decreased activity during side-up tilt of the animal. Moreover, the peak of the responses was closely related to the extreme animal displacement, thus being attributed to stimulation of position-sensitive macular (utricular) receptors. Groups of 6 averaged EMG responses were obtained at regular intervals of 5–10 min for several hours before and after mi-

croinjection with a vertically oriented stainless-steel cannula of various transmitter agonists or antagonists either into the dorsal pRF (P3.0, L2.5 or 2.8, H$-$2.5 or $-$3.5) or into the LC complex (P2.0 or 3.0, L2.5 or 2.8, H$-$2 or $-$2.5). Usually, 0.10–0.25 μl of solutions of active substances at different concentrations in sterile saline (pH 7.4 $\pm$ 0.2) marked with 5% pontamine were injected into dorsal pontine structures of one side. At the end of the experiments the tip of the cannula used for each penetration, as well as the extent of the nerve tissue stained with the blue dye, were identified on serial frozen sections of the brainstem, mounted on glass slides and stained with neutral red.

Increase in response gain of limb extensors after injection of cholinergic agonists into the pontine reticular formation

Experiments performed by Barnes et al. [5] have shown that injection into the dorsal aspect of the pRF of 0.1–0.2 μl of a solution of the cholinergic agonist carbachol at the concentration of 0.01–0.2 μg/μl, while decreasing the decerebrate rigidity as well as the myotatic stretch reflex in the ipsilateral fore- and hindlimb, greatly increased the amplitude of modulation of thus the response gain of the ipsilateral triceps brachii to animal tilt at 0.15 Hz, $\pm$ 10°. Moreover, a decrease in phase lead and actually a slight phase lag of the response was observed. These findings were not attributed to a decreased postural activity following the injection, since they were still observed when the postural EMG activity was reflexly maintained by an increased static stretch of the muscle. The changes in posture as well as in response gain produced by the carbachol injection appeared suddenly, and persisted after a partial decline up to 3 hours following the injection. No changes in the dynamic characteristics of the responses were observed in the contralateral triceps brachii.

Since carbachol is a mixed nicotinic and muscarinic agonist, experiments were performed to ascertain whether the cholinoceptive pontine structures utilized muscarinic receptors. Injection of 0.25 μl of

364

a solution of bethanechol, which is a pure muscarinic agonist, at the concentration of 0.1 μg/μl produced changes in posture as well as in the response gain of the VS reflexes similar to those induced by carbachol injection (Fig. 2B and C). Moreover, injection of 0.25 μl of a solution of the muscarinic blocker atropine sulphate at the concentration of 6 μg/μl not only produced a recovery in the postural activity of the ipsilateral limbs, but also suppressed the increased gain and the phase lag of the responses produced by the cholinergic substances, returning them to control values.

The effects described above were not due to mechanical stimulation of the pontine neurons following injection of the fluid, since neither changes in posture nor in gain of the VS reflexes were observed following administration of an equal volume of saline prior to the injection of the active drugs; moreover, the effects were dose-dependent. Histological controls made at the end of the experiments showed that the structure which was critically responsible for the postural and reflex changes described above was located in the dorsal aspect of the pontine tegmentum, immediately ventral to the LC. This area corresponds to the periLC region and the surrounding pRF, from which a tegmentoreticular tract exciting the medullary inhibitory RS neurons originates (see Fig. 2A).

We postulated that cholinergic activation of dorsal pRF neurons increased the background discharge of the medullary inhibitory RS neurons, so that the higher the firing rate of these RS neurons in the animal at rest the greater the disinhibition that affected the limb-extensor motoneurons during side-down animal tilt. This increased disinhibition would then enhance the response of these motoneurons to the excitatory VS volleys elicited by given parameters of labyrinth stimulation. The opposite result would occur following inactivation of the dorsal pontine tegmental region by atropine sulphate, decreasing the resting discharge of the inhibitory RS neurons.

In conclusion, it appears that local activation of dorsal pontine reticular neurons, which are probably not only cholinergic but also cholinoceptive due to

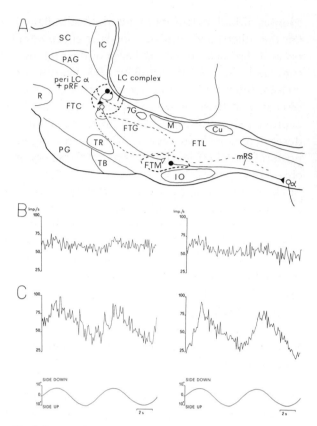

Fig. 2. Increase in the response gain of the triceps brachii to animal tilt after local injection of the muscarinic agonist bethanechol in the ipsilateral dorsal pRF. (A) Schematic sagittal section of the brainstem, showing anatomical connections between the noradrenergic LC neurons and the cholinergic neurons located in the periLC area and the dorsal aspect of the pRF; this structure projects to the magnocellular tegmental field (MTF), from which the medullary inhibitory reticulospinal (mRS) system ending on extensor α-motoneurons (α) originates. Both LC and pRF neurons give rise to self-inhibitory and self-excitatory recurrent collaterals, respectively; inhibitory and excitatory neurons are indicated by filled or empty symbols. (B and C) Decerebrate cat. Sequential pulse density histograms (SPDHs) showing averaged multiunit responses of the left triceps brachii to roll tilt of the animal at 0.15 Hz, $\pm$ 10° (average of 6 sweeps); the lower traces monitor the animal displacement. (B) Control records showing an average base frequency of 59.3 imp./s, a response gain of the first harmonic of 0.42 imp./s/deg and a phase lag of $-3.5°$ with respect to the ipsilateral side-down tilt. (C) Responses to the same parameters of animal tilt recorded 1 and 3 min after local injection in the ipsilateral dorsal pRF (at P3, L2.8, H-3) of 0.25 μl of a bethanechol solution at the concentration of 0.1 μg/μl of saline. In this instance, the average base frequency corresponded to 57.0 imp./s, the gain was 1.93 imp./s/deg, while the phase angle corresponded to a lag of $-32.7°$. (From [5].)

the existence of muscarinic receptors, decreased the postural activity in the ipsilateral limbs but greatly enhanced the amplitude of modulation of the ipsilateral limb extensors to labyrinth stimulation, thus exerting a critical role in the gain regulation of the corresponding VS reflex.

Increase in response gain of limb extensors after injection of the α_2-adrenergic agonist clonidine into the locus coeruleus complex

Since the pRF neurons and the related medullary inhibitory RS system are under the tonic inhibitory control of NE-containing neurons located in the LC complex, i.e. the LC and the SC, experiments were designed to find out whether inactivation of the LC neurons could modify the postural activity as well as the response gain of limb extensor muscles to labyrinth stimulation, as shown after direct activation of the cholinergic pontine reticular system. It is well known that iontophoretic application of NE or epinephrine [12, 13], as well as of the α_2-adrenergic agonist clonidine [26, 93], into the LC inhibits the activity of the corresponding NE-containing neurons. Moreover, histoimmunochemical observations have shown the existence of both adrenergic terminals [30, 36] and α_2-adrenergic receptors within the LC [98]. These and other data have led to the suggestion that the activity of LC cells is dampened by a self-inhibitory circuit represented by *recurrent* collaterals from the LC axons themselves [1, 12–14]. Another possibility, however, is that the NE contained in proximal dendrites and somata of the LC and the SC neurons is released as a consequence of impulse activity [44] and, due to dendrodendritic and dendrosomatic contacts between neighbouring LC neurons [88] leads to *lateral* suppression of LC cells activity [24].

Experiments by Pompeiano et al. [76, 77] have shown that local injection of 0.25 μl of clonidine solution at the concentration 0.012–0.15 μg/μl into the LC complex of one side decreased the decerebrate rigidity particularly in the ipsilateral limbs, but greatly increased the amplitude of modulation and thus the response gain of the ipsilateral triceps bra-

chii to labyrinth stimulation (at 0.15 Hz, $\pm$ 10°); moreover, a slight decrease in phase lead of the responses was observed (Fig. 3A and B). These results were obtained even when an increased EMG activity following passive flexion of the ipsilateral forelimb compensated for the reduced EMG discharge following clonidine injections. The effects described above were first observed 10–15 min after injection of clonidine in the ipsilateral LC, reached the highest value in about 30–60 min and persisted for more than 2 hours after the injection.

It is of interest that clonidine increased the amplitude of modulation and thus the response gain not only of the ipsilateral but also of the contralateral triceps brachii. There was, however, a slight increase in phase lead of the responses with respect to the control values which contrasted with the decrease in phase lead of the responses recorded ipsilaterally to the side of the injection. These reflex changes usually followed the same time course as that obtained from the ipsilateral triceps brachii.

The effects of clonidine were not due to irritative phenomena, since no postural and reflex changes were observed following local injection of saline into the LC complex. On the other hand, the amount of these changes depended on the dose of clonidine injected.

Histological controls demonstrated that both the dorsocaudal and the ventrolateral part of the LC were involved; the effective area, however, also included the SC area and the surrounding dorsal pRF. This finding can easily be explained, since in the cat NE-containing neurons are located not only in the LC but also in the SC and the neighbouring pRF; moreover, clonidine may act on α_2-receptors located not only on the cell body, but also on terminals of NE-containing neurons.

Inactivation of the LC complex neurons following clonidine injection released from inhibition the activity of the related cholinergic and cholinoceptive pRF neurons. In fact, the postural and reflex changes which involved the triceps brachii following clonidine injection into the dorsal aspect of the pRF were greatly reduced or suppressed after local administration into the same pontine region of atropine sulphate at the concentration of 6 $\mu g/\mu l$. This last effect, however, was strictly ipsilateral.

In conclusion, the present experiments have shown that local injection of the α_2-adrenergic agonist clonidine into the LC complex of one side as well as in the surrounding pRF decreased the postural activity, particularly in the ipsilateral limbs, but greatly increased the response gain of the VS re-

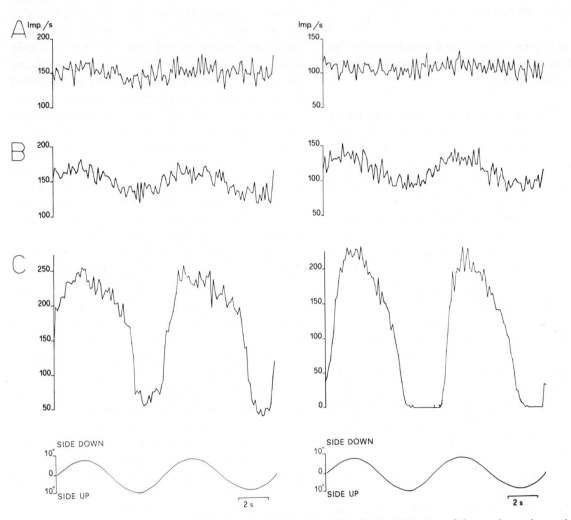

Fig. 3. Increase in the response gain of the triceps brachii to animal tilt after local injection of the α_2-adrenergic agonist clonidine in the ipsilateral LC and its further enhancement after injection of the muscarinic blocker atropine sulphate in the ipsilateral pontine reticular structures. Decerebrate cat. SPDHs showing the averaged multi-unit responses of the right triceps brachii to roll tilt of the animal at 0.15 Hz, $\pm$ 10° (average of 6 sweeps); the lower traces monitor the animal displacement. (A) Control records showing an average base frequency of 128.9 imp./s, a response gain of the first harmonic of 0.44 imp./s/deg and a phase lead of $+16.2°$ with respect to the ipsilateral side-down tilt. (B) Responses to the same parameters of animal tilt recorded 44 min and 1 hour and 55 min after local injection in the right LC (at P3, R2.8, H−2.1) of 0.25 μl of a clonidine solution at the concentration of 0.015 $\mu g/\mu l$ of saline. In this instance the average base frequency corresponded to 133.0 imp./s, the gain was 1.88 imp./s/deg, while the phase angle corresponded to a lead of $+4.5°$ with respect to the peak of the ipsilateral side-down tilt. (C) Responses recorded 8 and 10 min after local injection in the lateral tegmental field of the right side (at P3, R2.2, H−4.4) of 0.25 μl of an atropine sulphate solution at the concentration of 6 $\mu g/\mu l$ of saline. The average base frequency was 142.0 imp./s, the gain 10.35 imp./s/deg, while the phase angle corresponded to a lag of $-27.4°$ with respect to the peak of the ipsilateral side-down tilt. (From [31].)

flexes acting on the forelimb extensors of both sides. These effects were attributed to an increased discharge of the pontine tegmental neurons and the related medullary inhibitory RS neurons, which were disinhibited on both sides following unilateral inactivation of the NE-containing LC-complex neurons. These neurons may thus play a critical but permissive role in the control of posture as well as in the gain regulation of the VS reflexes.

Decrease in response gain of limb extensors after injection of cholinergic agonists into the locus coeruleus complex

The discharge of LC neurons and the consequent liberation of NE from their terminals is under the influence not only of inhibitory transmitters like NE, but also of excitatory transmitters like ACh. Histochemical studies in the rat have in fact shown that both somata and proximal dendrites of LC neurons stain positively for AChe activity [2, 34, 41–43, 47, 49, 59, 61]. Moreover, AChe activity has also been located in some presynaptic terminals impinging on LC cells [33]. This finding is consistent with the presence of cholinergic fibres [78] and terminals in the LC [17, 42]. These fibres are probably excitatory on LC neurons, as shown by iontophoretic experiments [3, 6, 21, 22, 24, 26–28, 45]. Moreover, there is evidence that cholinergic transmission in the LC is muscarinic in nature [21, 22, 28, 46, 79, 96].

Experiments were performed by Stampacchia et al. [91] to determine whether activation of the NE-containing LC neurons could modify the postural activity as well as the gain of the VS reflexes. In particular, injection in precollicular decerebrate cats of 0.1–0.4 μl (usually 0.25 μl) of carbachol at the concentration of 0.02–0.1 μg/μl into the LC complex of one side, which slightly increased the extensor rigidity of the ipsilateral limbs, decreased the amplitude of modulation and thus the response gain of the extensor triceps brachii to roll tilt of the animal at 0.15 Hz, $\pm$ 10°; this occurred even when the limb position was adjusted so as to produce the same background discharge of the muscle as in the con-

trol experiments. A significant increase in phase lag of the responses was also observed and appeared at a threshold dose lower than that required to decrease the response gain of this extensor muscle. The effects described above, which involved mainly if not exclusively the limbs ipsilateral to the side of the injection, began a few minutes after the injection, became most prominent within the first 20–30 min and persisted for a few hours following the injection. Moreover, the observed changes increased in magnitude by increasing the dose of carbachol.

Histological controls indicated that the structure responsible for the postural and reflex changes described above corresponded to the LC. The site-specificity of the responses was shown by the fact that just the opposite effects were obtained in the same experiments when an equal amount of carbachol was injected into the dorsal aspect of the pRF located immediately ventral to the LC.

It was previously reported that the LC exerts an inhibitory influence on the dorsal pRF, thus reducing the discharge of the related medullary inhibitory RS system. The reduced discharge of these RS neurons following cholinergic activation of the LC neurons would first increase the postural activity; moreover, the lower the firing rate of these RS neurons in the animal at rest, the smaller the disinhibition that would affect the extensor motoneurons during side-down animal tilt. These motoneurons would then respond less efficiently to the same excitatory VS volleys elicited by given parameters of stimulation, thus leading to a reduced gain in the EMG response of limb extensors to labyrinth stimulation.

Pontine reticular origin of the cholinergic excitatory afferents to the locus coeruleus controlling the gain of the vestibulospinal reflexes

Since the self-excitatory pRF neurons, which create the steady background discharge of the medullary inhibitory RS system, can be driven not only by carbachol, which acts on both muscarinic and nicotinic receptors, but also by bethanechol, which acts on pure muscarinic receptors [5, 95], and the cholinergic receptors located in the LC are also muscarinic in origin (see previous section), we postulated that dorsal pontine reticular neurons contribute cholinergic afferents to the LC neurons, thus providing the pRF with a negative feedback system via the LC. In this case, functional inactivation of this cholinergic afferent system to the LC following appropriate injection of the muscarinic blocker atropine sulphate in pontine reticular structures might reduce the discharge of the LC neurons, a finding which, on the basis of clonidine experiments, should lead to a decreased postural activity in the ipsilateral limbs as well as to an increased gain of response of forelimb extensors to labyrinth stimulation.

Experiments performed in precollicular decerebrate cats by Horn et al. [31] have shown that injection of 0.25 μl of a solution of atropine sulphate at the concentration of 6 μg/μl into the dorsal aspect of the pRF modified neither the postural activity in the ipsilateral limbs nor the gain and the phase angle of the first harmonic component of the multiunit EMG response of the triceps brachii to roll tilt of the animal at 0.15 Hz, $\pm$ 10°. However, if the same dose of atropine sulphate was injected into the dorsal pRF after injection of the α_2-adrenergic agonist clonidine in the ipsilateral LC, the decrease in postural activity as well as the increase in amplitude of modulation and thus in response gain of the ipsilateral triceps brachii to labyrinth stimulation following clonidine injection further increased (see Fig. 3B and C). Moreover, an additional decrease in phase lead of the responses with respect to that obtained after clonidine injection and actually a phase lag was observed after atropine injection. The effects described above persisted even when the decrease in spontaneous EMG activity following injections of clonidine and atropine was compensated by an increased muscular activity following static stretch of the muscle.

It is of interest that while injection of clonidine into the LC of one side increased the gain of the VS reflex of both sides, the successive injection of atropine into the corresponding dorsal pRF increased the gain of the VS reflex only of the ipsilateral side, while that of the contralateral side was either unmodified or slightly reduced, and was associated with an average increase in phase lead of the responses. The structure whose selective inactivation, following injection of the muscarinic blocker, increased the response gain of the triceps brachii to labyrinth stimulation corresponded to the pontine tegmental field located ventromedially rather than ventrolaterally to the LC.

Discussion

It was reported in the introduction that in the dorsal aspect of the pontine tegmentum, namely in the periLC area and the surrounding dorsal pRF, there are cholinergic and cholinoceptive neurons which exert a tonic excitatory influence on the medullary inhibitory RS neurons. We have recently shown that in decerebrate cats these neurons play an important role in the control of posture as well as in the gain regulation of the VS reflexes. In fact, microinjection into these pontine structures of small doses of cholinergic agonists, like carbachol which acts on both muscarinic and nicotinic receptors, or bethanechol which acts on pure muscarinic receptors, not only decreased the postural activity in the ipsilateral limbs but also enhanced the response gain of the triceps brachii to labyrinth stimulation [5]. The conclusion that mechanisms responsible for the postural and reflex changes described above are cholinergically mediated is supported by the results of several experiments showing the following:

(1) Electrolytic lesion of dorsal pontine reticular structures of one side, which increased the postural activity in the ipsilateral limbs due to a reduced discharge of the medullary inhibitory RS system, not only decreased the amplitude of the EMG responses of the triceps brachii to labyrinth stimulation in decerebrate cats, but also suppressed the increased gain of these responses after systemic injection of small doses (0.03–0.05 mg/kg) of the anticholinesterase eserine sulphate [20, 70].

(2) The increased gain of response of the triceps brachii to labyrinth stimulation following local injection of carbachol into the dorsal pRF was sup-

pressed by local injection into the same pontine reticular area of minute doses of the muscarinic blocker atropine sulphate [5].

(3) The increased gain of the VS reflexes following systemic injection of eserine sulphate was suppressed by administration of atropine sulphate (0.25–0.50 mg/kg, i.v.) [73].

In order to understand the influence that the cholinergic system exerts on the static and dynamic control of posture, it is worth mentioning that cholinergic activation of the dorsal pRF neurons [32] tonically excites the medullary inhibitory RS neurons [90] as shown after systemic injection of the anticholinesterase. The increased discharge of these inhibitory RS neurons would first exert a tonic inhibitory influence on extensor motoneurons, thus decreasing the extensor rigidity [39, 55, 56, 67, 68].* Moreover, for a given labyrinth signal, the higher the firing rate of these RS neurons in the animal at rest, the greater the disinhibition affecting the extensor motoneurons during side-down animal tilt. These motoneurons would then respond more efficiently to the same excitatory VS volleys elicited by given parameters of stimulation, resulting in an increased gain of the EMG responses of forelimb extensor muscles to labyrinth stimulation. The low discharge rate of the dorsal pRF neurons [32] as well as of the medullary RS neurons in the control experiments [52, 74] explains why the response gain of the triceps brachii to animal tilt was quite low after decerebration [51]; moreover, a suppression of the residual activity of the cholinergic pontine structures following injection of the muscarinic blocker into the dorsal pRF may lead to a complete abolition of the EMG responses [5].

Since the pontine reticular neurons as well as the related medullary RS neurons are under the tonic inhibitory control of the LC, it was obviously to be expected that inactivation of the NE-containing LC neurons would lead to changes in posture as well as in gain of the VS reflexes comparable to those elicited by direct activation of the cholinergic pontine reticular system [76]. Indeed, injection into the LC complex or else in the dorsal aspect of the surrounding pRF of small doses of the α_2-adrenergic agonist clonidine, not only reduced the postural activity in the ipsilateral limb extensors, but also increased the amplitude of modulation and thus the gain of the multiunit EMG responses of the ipsilateral triceps brachii to labyrinth stimulation.

The decreased postural activity in the ipsilateral limbs following injection of clonidine into the LC complex of one side can be attributed in part at least to inactivation not only of the direct coeruleospinal neurons [97], which exert an excitatory influence on extensor motoneurons [25], but also of the LC neurons which exert an inhibitory influence on the dorsal pRF neurons and the related inhibitory RS neurons of the medulla. The resulting increase in discharge rate of both these pontine and medullary reticular neurons led also to an increased gain of the VS reflexes, which utilized the cholinergic mechanism. In fact, when the clonidine effects were elicited by local injection of the α_2- adrenergic agonist into the dorsal aspect of the pRF, they were suppressed by administration in the same structures of the muscarinic blocker atropine sulphate.

It is of interest that the LC of one side keeps under its tonic inhibitory control the pontine tegmental region not only of the ipsilateral but also of the contralateral side. The crossed effect was usually not so prominent as to decrease the postural activity on that side, but it was strong enough to enhance the response gain of the corresponding triceps brachii to labyrinth stimulation.

The results described above represent a phenomenon of deficit, since the same postural and reflex changes following functional inactivation of the NE-containing LC complex neurons were also obtained in decerebrate cats after electrolytic lesion of the LC of one side [19].

In addition to inhibitory transmitters like NE, the LC neurons are also subjected to the direct influence of excitatory transmitters like acetylcholine [6, 21, 22, 26–28]. This finding is consistent with the presence of cholinergic fibres [78] and terminals in

---

*Indeed, spinal cord motoneurons can be postsynaptically inhibited following pontine administration of carbachol [58].

the LC [17], where they act on muscarinic receptors [3, 21, 22, 24, 28, 46, 79]. These excitatory cholinergic afferents ending on the LC neurons would then counteract the inhibitory influences exerted on the same neurons by the NE synapses. In fact, in contrast to the results obtained by inactivation of the LC by the α_2-adrenergic agonist clonidine, activation of the LC following local injection of the cholinergic agonist carbachol not only increased the postural activity in the ipsilateral limbs, but also reduced the response gain of the corresponding triceps brachii to labyrinth stimulation [91]. Obviously, the increased postural activity in the ipsilateral limbs can be attributed to cholinergic activation of the direct coeruleospinal neurons, which exert an excitatory influence on extensor motoneurons, as well as of the LC neurons exerting an inhibitory influence on the dorsal pRF neurons and the related inhibitory RS neurons of the medulla, as indicated schematically in Fig. 1. The reduced discharge of the dorsal pRF neurons and the medullary inhibitory RS neurons would also decrease the response gain of the ipsilateral triceps brachii to labyrinth stimulation. In fact, the lower the firing rate of these RS neurons in the animal at rest, the smaller the disinhibition which affects the limb extensor motoneurons during side-down animal tilt. These motoneurons would then respond less efficiently to the same excitatory VS volleys elicited by given parameters of labyrinth stimulation, thus leading to a reduced gain of the EMG response of limb extensors to animal tilt.

It is of interest that the same cholinergic pRF region which drives the RS inhibitory system may also send cholinergic excitatory afferents to the LC. Indeed, there is evidence that the LC receives afferents from the dorsolateral pRF [15, 18, 37, 60, 80, 85], which are likely to be cholinergic in nature, acting on muscarinic receptors (see page 367).

It was previously shown that local injection of atropine sulphate produces its blocking effect on the pRF neurons, thus reducing the gain of the VS reflexes, only when the firing rate of the corresponding reticular neurons was *locally* raised either by injection of cholinergic agonists, which excite the cholinoceptive pontine neurons, or by local administration of the α_2-adrenergic agonist clonidine, which blocks the inhibitory influence exerted by the noradrenergic terminals on the dorsal pontine reticular neurons. However, when clonidine was not injected into the pRF but directly within the LC, thus leading to a prominent disinhibition of the pRF, a successive injection of atropine sulphate into the medial aspect of the pontine reticular area greatly increased the gain of the VS reflexes. This finding can be attributed to the fact that inactivation by atropine sulphate of the cholinergic pontine reticular neurons acting on the LC further reduced the discharge rate of the LC neurons originally attenuated by clonidine injection, as well as their inhibitory influence on the dorsal pRF and the related medullary RS neurons, thus enhancing the gain of the VS reflexes. The fact that in normal decerebrate cats injection of atropine sulphate into the same pontine reticular area did not modify the gain of the VS reflexes can easily be explained, since in this preparation the activity of the self-excitatory cholinergic pontine reticular neurons [32] and the related medullary RS neurons [52, 69, 74] is very low, due to the prominent inhibitory influence exerted on them by the spontaneously firing LC neurons [71, 72].

All these findings taken together indicate that the background discharge of the LC neurons exerting a regulatory influence on posture as well as on the gain of the VS reflexes results in part at least upon a balance between noradrenergic inhibitory influences and cholinergic excitatory volleys. However, while the former influences originate from the same NE-containing neurons located in the LC, which are not only self-inhibitory, due to recurrent or lateral inhibition, but also inhibitory on the cholinergic pRF neurons, the latter influences probably originate from the dorsal pRF neurons which are not only self-excitatory (in fact they are cholinoceptive), but also excitatory on the inhibitory RS neurons (Fig. 1).

It is of interest that a reciprocal interaction between the self-inhibitory LC neurons and the self-excitatory pRF neurons, similar to that postulated above, is apparently responsible for the episodes of postural atonia which occur either during desynchronized sleep in unrestrained, unanaesthetized cats [24, 39, 65, 81, 84, 92] or after administration of high doses of an anticholinesterase in decerebrate cats [39, 55, 56, 67, 68]. In particular, the arrest of the tonic discharge of LC neurons which occurs in these two experimental conditions (see Introduction) is associated with an increase in firing rate of both dorsal pontine reticular neurons [29, 32, 68, 81, 84, 92] and medullary inhibitory RS neurons [16, 40, 84, 90], which act prominently by suppressing posture [65, 67, 92].

Acknowledgements

This study was supported by the NIH grant NS 07685-19 and a grant from the Ministero della Pubblica Istruzione, Roma, Italy.

References

[1] Aghajanian, G.K., Cedarbaum, J.M. and Wang, R.Y. (1977) Evidence for norepinephrine-mediated collateral inhibition of locus coeruleus neurons. Brain Res., 136: 570–577.

[2] Albanese, A. and Butcher, L.L. (1980) Acetylcholinesterase and catecholamine distribution in the locus coeruleus of the rat. Brain Res. Bull., 5: 127–134.

[3] Amaral, D.G. and Sinnamon, H.M. (1977) The locus coeruleus: neurobiology of a central noradrenergic nucleus. Progr. Neurobiol., 9: 147–196.

[4] Baghdoyan, H.A., McCarley, R.W. and Hobson, J.A. (1985) Cholinergic manipulation of brainstem reticular systems: effects on desynchronized sleep generation. In A. Wauquier, J.M. Gaillard, J.M. Monti and M. Radulovacki (Eds.), Sleep: Neurotransmitters and Neuromodulators, Raven Press, New York, pp. 15–27.

[5] Barnes, C.D., D'Ascanio, P., Pompeiano, O. and Stampacchia, G. (1987) Effects of microinjection of cholinergic agonists into the pontine reticular formation on the gain of vestibulospinal reflexes in decerebrate cats. Arch. Ital. Biol., 125: 71–105.

[6] Bird, S.J. and Kuhar, M.J. (1977) Iontophoretic application of opiates to the locus coeruleus. Brain Res., 122: 523–533.

[7] Boyle, R. and Pompeiano, O. (1980) Reciprocal responses to sinusoidal tilt of neurons in Deiters' nucleus and their dynamic characteristics. Arch. Ital. Biol., 118: 1–32.

[8] Boyle, R. and Pompeiano, O. (1981) Convergence and interaction of neck and macular vestibular inputs on vestibulospinal neurons. J. Neurophysiol., 45: 852–868.

[9] Boyle, R. and Pompeiano, O. (1984) Discharge activity of spindle afferents from the gastrocnemius-soleus muscle during head rotation in the decerebrate cat. Pflügers Arch., 400: 140–150.

[10] Bradley, P.B. and Wolstencroft, J.H. (1967) Effects of acetylcholine, nicotine and muscarine on brain stem neurons. Ann. N.Y. Acad. Sci., 142: 15–20.

[11] Bunney, B.S. and Aghajanian, G.K. (1975) Evidence for drug actions in both pre- and postsynaptic catecholamine receptors in the CNS. In E. Usdin and W.E. Bunney, Jr. (Eds.), Pre- and Postsynaptic Receptors, Marcel Decker, New York, pp. 89–122.

[12] Cedarbaum, J.M. and Aghajanian, G.K. (1976) Noradrenergic neurons of the locus coeruleus: inhibition by epinephrine and activation by the alpha-antagonist piperoxane. Brain Res., 112: 413–419.

[13] Cedarbaum, J.M. and Aghajanian, G.K. (1977) Catecholamine receptors on locus coeruleus neurons: pharmacological characterization. Eur. J. Pharmacol., 44: 375–385.

[14] Cedarbaum, J.M. and Aghajanian, G.K. (1978) Activation of locus coeruleus neurons by peripheral stimuli: modulation by a collateral inhibitory mechanism. Life Sci., 23: 1383–1392.

[15] Cedarbaum, J.M. and Aghajanian, G.K. (1978) Afferent projections to the rat locus coeruleus as determined by a retrograde tracing technique. J. Comp. Neurol., 178: 1–16.

[16] Chase, M.H., Enomoto, S., Murakami, T., Nakamura, Y. and Taira, M. (1981) Intracellular potential of medullary reticular neurons during sleep and wakefulness. Exp. Neurol., 71: 226–233.

[17] Cheney, D.L., LeFevre, H.F. and Racagni, G. (1975) Choline acetyltransferase activity and mass fragmentographic measurement of acetylcholine in specific nuclei and tracts of rat brain. Neuropharmacology, 14: 801–809.

[18] Clavier, R.M. (1979) Afferent projections to the self-stimulation regions of the dorsal pons, including the locus coeruleus, in the rat as demonstrated by the horseradish peroxidase technique. Brain Res. Bull., 4: 497–504.

[19] D'Ascanio, P., Bettini, E. and Pompeiano, O. (1985) Tonic inhibitory influences of locus coeruleus on the response gain of limb extensors to sinusoidal labyrinth and neck stimulations. Arch. Ital. Biol., 123: 69–100.

[20] D'Ascanio, P., Bettini, E. and Pompeiano, O. (1985) Tonic facilitatory influences of dorsal pontine reticular structures on the response gain of limb extensors to sinusoidal labyrinth and neck stimulations. Arch. Ital. Biol., 123: 101–132.

[21] Egan, T.M. and North, R.A. (1985) Acetylcholine acts on m_2-muscarinic receptors to excite rat locus coeruleus neurons. Br. J. Pharmacol., 85: 733–735.

[22] Engberg, G. and Svensson, T.H. (1980) Pharmacological analysis of a cholinergic receptor mediated regulation of brain norepinephrine neurons. J. Neural Transm., 49: 137–150.

[23] Ezure, K. and Wilson, V.J. (1984) Interaction of tonic neck

372

and vestibular reflexes in the forelimb of the decerebrate cat. *Exp. Brain Res.*, 54: 289–292.

[24] Foote, S.L., Bloom, F.E. and Aston-Jones, G. (1983) Nucleus locus coeruleus: new evidence of anatomical and physiological specificity. *Physiol. Rev.*, 63: 844–914.

[25] Fung, S.J. and Barnes, C.D. (1984) Locus coeruleus control of spinal cord activity. In Barnes C.D. (Ed.), *Brain Stem Control of Spinal Cord Function, Research Topics in Physiology, Vol. 6,* Academic Press, Orlando, pp. 215–255.

[26] Guyenet, P.G. (1980) The coeruleospinal noradrenergic neurons: anatomical and electrophysiological studies in the rat. *Brain Res.*, 189: 121–133.

[27] Guyenet, P.G. and Aghajanian, G.K. (1977) Excitation of neurons in the nucleus locus coeruleus by substance P and related peptides. *Brain Res.*, 136: 178–184.

[28] Guyenet, P.G. and Aghajanian, G.K. (1979) ACh, substance P and met-enkephalin in the locus coeruleus: pharmacological evidence for independent sites of action. *Eur. J. Pharmacol.*, 53: 319–328.

[29] Hobson, J.A., McCarley, R.W., Pivik, R.T. and Freedman, R. (1974) Selective firing by cat pontine brain stem neurons in desynchronized sleep. *J. Neurophysiol.*, 37: 497–511.

[30] Hökfelt, T., Fuxe, K., Goldstein, M. and Johansson, O. (1974) Immunohistochemical evidence for the existence of adrenaline neurons in the rat brain. *Brain Res.*, 66: 235–251.

[31] Horn, E., d'Ascanio, P., Pompeiano, O. and Stampacchia, G. (1987) Pontine reticular origin of cholinergic excitatory afferents to the locus coeruleus controlling the gain of vestibulospinal and cervicospinal reflexes in decerebrate cats. *Arch. Ital. Biol.*, 125: 273–304.

[32] Hoshino, K. and Pompeiano, O. (1976) Selective discharge of pontine neurons during the postural atonia produced by an anticholinesterase in the decerebrate cat. *Arch. Ital. Biol.*, 114: 244–277.

[33] Ishii, S. (1981) Morphological studies on the mechanism of adrenergic transmission in the central nervous system. I. Granulated vesicles. In O. Eränkö (Ed.), *Histochemistry of Nervous Transmission. Progress in Brain Research, Vol. 34,* Elsevier, Amsterdam, pp. 187–206.

[34] Ishii, Y. (1957) The histochemical studies of cholinesterase in the central nervous system. I. Normal distribution in rodents. *Arch. Histol. Jpn.*, 12: 587–612.

[35] Jankowska, E., Lund, S., Lundberg, A. and Pompeiano, O. (1968) Inhibitory effects evoked through ventral reticulospinal pathways. *Arch. Ital. Biol.*, 106: 124–140.

[36] Jones, B.E. and Friedman, L. (1983) Atlas of catecholamine perikarya varicosities and pathways in the brainstem of the cat. *J. Comp. Neurol.*, 215: 382–396.

[37] Jones, B.E. and Yang, T.-Z. (1985) The efferent projections from the reticular formation and the locus coeruleus studied by anterograde and retrograde axonal transport in the rat. *J. Comp. Neurol.*, 242: 56–92.

[38] Jones, G., Segal, M., Foote, S.L. and Bloom, F.E. (1979) Locus coeruleus neurons in freely moving rats exhibit pronounced alterations of discharge rate during sensory stimulation and stages of the sleep-wake cycle. In E. Usdin, I.J. Kopin and J. Barchas (Eds.), *Catecholamines: Basic and Clinical Frontiers,* Pergamon Press, New York, pp. 643–645.

[39] Jouvet, M. (1972) The role of monoamines and acetylcholine-containing neurons in the regulation of the sleep–waking cycle. *Ergebn. Physiol.*, 64: 166–307.

[40] Kanamori, N., Sakai, K. and Jouvet, M. (1980) Neuronal activity specific to paradoxical sleep in the ventromedial medullary reticular formation of unrestrained cats. *Brain Res.*, 189: 251–255.

[41] Kimura, H. and Maeda, T. (1982) Aminergic and cholinergic systems in the dorsolateral pontine tegmentum. *Brain Res. Bull.*, 9: 493–499.

[42] Kimura, H., McGeer, P.L., Peng, J.H. and McGeer, E.G. (1981) The central cholinergic system studied by choline acetyltransferase immunohistochemistry in the cat. *J. Comp. Neurol.*, 200: 151–201.

[43] Knight, D.P. (1970) Histochemical demonstration of catecholamines and acetylcholine esterase in the same cell bodies in the locus coeruleus (rat hind brain). *Proc. R. Microsc. Soc.*, 6: 26.

[44] Koda, L.Y., Aston-Jones, G. and Bloom, F.E. (1980) Small granular vesicles in the locus coeruleus may indicate dendritic release of norepinephrine. *Soc. Neurosci. Abstr.*, 6: 446.

[45] Kuhar, M.J., Atweh, S.F. and Bird, S.J. (1978) Studies of cholinergic-monoaminergic interactions in rat brain. In L.L. Butcher (Ed.), *Cholinergic-Monoaminergic Interactions in the Brain,* Academic Press, New York, pp. 211–227.

[46] Lewander, T., Joh, T.J. and Reis, D.J. (1975) Prolonged activation of tyrosine hydroxylase in noradrenergic neurones of rat brain by cholinergic stimulation. *Nature*, 258: 440–441.

[47] Lewis, P.R. and Schon, F. (1975) The localization of acetylcholinesterase in the locus coeruleus of the normal rat and after 6-hydroxydopamine treatment. *J. Anat. London*, 120: 373–385.

[48] Llinás, R. and Terzuolo, C.A. (1964) Mechanisms of supraspinal actions upon spinal cord activities. Reticular inhibitory mechanisms on alpha extensor motoneurons. *J. Neurophysiol.*, 27: 579–591.

[49] Maeda, T. and Gerebtzoff, M.A. (1969) Recherches sur le development du locus coeruleus. II. Étude histoenzymologique. *Acta Neurol. Psychiat. Belg.*, 69: 11–19.

[50] Magoun, H.W. and Rhines, R. (1947) *Spasticity. The Stretch-Reflex and Extrapyramidal Systems.* C.C. Thomas, Springfield, IL, 59 pp.

[51] Manzoni, D., Pompeiano, O., Srivastava, U.C. and Stampacchia, G. (1983) Responses of forelimb extensors to sinusoidal stimulation of macular labyrinth and neck receptors. *Arch. Ital. Biol.*, 121: 205–214.

[52] Manzoni, D., Pompeiano, O., Stampacchia, G. and Srivastava, U.C. (1983) Responses of medullary reticulospinal neurons to sinusoidal stimulation of labyrinth receptors in dece-

rebrate cat. *J. Neurophysiol.*, 50: 1059–1079.

[53] Manzoni, D., Pompeiano, O., Srivastava, U.C. and Stampacchia, G. (1984) Gain regulation of vestibular reflexes in fore- and hindlimb muscles evoked by roll tilt. *Boll. Soc. Ital. Biol. Sper.*, 60 Suppl. 3: 9–10.

[54] Marchand, A.R., Manzoni, D., Pompeiano, O. and Stampacchia, G. (1987) Effects of stimulation of vestibular and neck receptors on Deiters neurons projecting to the lumbosacral cord. *Pflügers Arch.*, 409: 13–23.

[55] Matsuzaki, M. (1969) Differential effects of sodium butyrate and physostigmine upon the activities of para-sleep in acute brainstem preparations. *Brain Res.*, 13: 247–265.

[56] Matsuzaki, M., Okada, Y. and Shuto, S. (1968) Cholinergic agents related to para-sleep state in acute brain stem preparation. *Brain Res.*, 9: 253–267.

[57] McGinty, D.J., Harper, R.M. and Fairbanks, M.K. (1974) Neuronal unit activity and the control of sleep states. In E.D. Weitzman (Ed.), *Advances in Sleep Research, Vol. 1.* Spectrum, Flushing/New York, pp. 173–216.

[58] Morales, F.R., Engelhardt, J.K., Soja, P.J., Pereda, A.E. and Chase, M.H. (1987) Motoneuron properties during motor inhibition produced by microinjection of carbachol into the pontine reticular formation of the decerebrate cat. *J. Neurophysiol.*, 57: 1118–1129.

[59] Mori, S., Maeda, T. and Shimizu, N. (1964) Electron microscopic histochemistry of cholinesterases in the rat brain. *Histochemie*, 4: 65–72.

[60] Nauta, W.J.H. and Kuypers, H.G.J.M. (1958) Some ascending pathways in the brain stem reticular formation. In H.H. Jasper, L.D. Proctor, R.S. Knighton, W.C. Noshay and R.T. Costello (Eds.), *Reticular Formation of the Brain*, Little and Brown, Boston, pp. 3–30.

[61] Palkovitz, M. and Jacobowitz, D.M. (1974) Topographic atlas of catecholamine and acetylcholinesterase-containing neurons in the rat brain. II. Hindbrain (mesencephalon, rombencephalon). *J. Comp. Neurol.*, 157: 29–42.

[62] Papp, M. and Bozsik, G. (1966) Comparison of the cholinesterase activity in the reticular formation of the lower brainstem of cat and rabbit. *J. Neurochem.*, 13: 697–703.

[63] Pavlin, R. (1965) Cholinesterase in reticular nerve cells. *J. Neurochem.*, 12: 515–518.

[64] Peterson, B.W., Pitts, N.G. and Fukushima, K. (1979) Reticulospinal connections with limb and axial motoneurons. *Exp. Brain Res.*, 36: 1–20.

[65] Pompeiano, O. (1967) The neurophysiological mechanisms of the postural and motor events during desynchronized sleep. *Res. Publ. Ass. Nerv. Ment. Dis.*, 45: 351–423.

[66] Pompeiano, O. (1975) Vestibulo-spinal relationships. In R.F. Naunton (Ed.), *The Vestibular System*, Academic Press, New York/San Francisco/London, pp. 147–180.

[67] Pompeiano, O. (1976) Mechanisms responsible for spinal inhibition during desynchronized sleep: experimental study. In C. Guilleminault, W.C. Dement and P. Passouant (Eds.), *Narcolepsy, Advances in Sleep Research, Vol. 3*, Spectrum, New York, pp. 411–449.

[68] Pompeiano, O. (1980) Cholinergic activation of reticular and vestibular mechanisms controlling posture and eye movements. In J.A. Hobson and M.A.B. Brazier (Eds.), *The Reticular Formation Revisited, IBRO Monograph Series, Vol. 6*, Raven Press, New York, pp. 473–512.

[69] Pompeiano, O. (1984) A comparison of the response characteristics of vestibulospinal and reticulospinal neurons to labyrinth and neck inputs. In C.D. Barnes (Ed.), *Brainstem Control of Spinal Cord Function, Research Topics in Physiology, Vol. 6*, Academic Press, New York, pp. 87–140.

[70] Pompeiano, O. (1985) Cholinergic mechanisms involved in the gain regulation of postural reflexes. In A. Wauquier, J.M. Gaillard, J.M. Monti and M. Radulovacki (Eds.), *Sleep: Neurotransmitters and Neuromodulators*, Raven Press, New York, pp. 165–184.

[71] Pompeiano, O. and Hoshino, K. (1976) Central control of posture: reciprocal discharge by two pontine neuronal groups leading to suppression of decerebrate rigidity. *Brain Res.*, 116: 131–138.

[72] Pompeiano, O. and Hoshino, K. (1976) Tonic inhibition of dorsal pontine neurons during the postural atonia produced by an anticholinesterase in the decerebrate cat. *Arch. Ital. Biol.*, 114: 310–340.

[73] Pompeiano, O., Manzoni, D., Srivastava, U.C. and Stampacchia, G. (1983) Cholinergic mechanism controlling the response gain of forelimb extensor muscles to sinusoidal stimulation of macular labyrinth and neck receptors. *Arch. Ital. Biol.*, 121: 285–303.

[74] Pompeiano, O., Manzoni, D., Srivastava, U.C. and Stampacchia, G. (1984) Convergence and interaction of neck and macular vestibular inputs on reticulospinal neurons. *Neuroscience*, 12: 111–128.

[75] Pompeiano, O., Wand, P. and Srivastava, U.C. (1985) Influence of Renshaw cells on the gain of hindlimb extensor muscles to sinusoidal labyrinth stimulation. *Pflügers Arch.*, 404: 107–118.

[76] Pompeiano, O., d'Ascanio, P., Horn, E. and Stampacchia, G. (1987) Effects of local injection of the α_2-adrenergic agonist clonidine into the locus coeruleus complex on the gain of vestibulospinal and cervicospinal reflexes in decerebrate cats. *Arch. Ital. Biol.*, 125: 225–269.

[77] Pompeiano, O., Stampacchia, G., Horn, E. and d'Ascanio, P. (1987) The role of the locus coeruleus in the gain regulation of vestibulospinal reflexes. *Acta Otolaryngol., Stockholm*, 103: 404–409.

[78] Raichle, M.E., Hartman, B.K., Eichling, J.O. and Sharpe, L.G. (1975) Central noradrenergic regulation of cerebral blood flow and vascular permeability. *Proc. Natl. Acad. Sci. USA*, 72: 3726–3730.

[79] Rotter, A., Birdsall, N.J.M., Field, P.M. and Raisman, G. (1979) Muscarinic receptors in the central nervous system of the rat. II. Distribution of binding of [3H]-propylbenzilylcholine mustard in the midbrain and hindbrain. *Brain Res.*

Rev., 1: 167–183.

[80] Russell, G.V. (1955) The nucleus locus coeruleus. *Tex. Rep. Biol. Med.*, 13: 939–988.

[81] Sakai, K. (1980) Some anatomical and physiological properties of ponto-mesencephalic tegmental neurons with special reference to the PGO waves and postural atonia during paradoxical sleep. In J.A. Hobson and M.A.B. Brazier (Eds.), *The Reticular Formation Revisited. IBRO Monograph Series, Vol. 6*, Raven Press, New York, pp. 427–447.

[82] Sakai, K., Touret, M., Salvert, D., Leger, L. and Jouvet, M. (1977) Afferent projections to the cat locus coeruleus as visualized by the horseradish peroxidase technique. *Brain Res.*, 119: 21–41.

[83] Sakai, K., Sastre J.-P., Salvert, D., Touret, M., Tohyama, M. and Jouvet, M. (1979) Tegmentoreticular projections with special reference to the muscular atonia during paradoxical sleep in the cat: an HRP study. *Brain Res.*, 176: 233–254.

[84] Sakai, K., Sastre, J.-P., Kanamori, N. and Jouvet, M. (1981) State-specific neurons in the ponto-medullary reticular formation with special reference to the postural atonia during paradoxical sleep in the cat. In O. Pompeiano and C. Ajmone-Marsan (Eds.), *Brain Mechanisms of Perceptual Awareness and Purposeful Behavior, IBRO Monograph Series, Vol. 8*, Raven Press, New York, pp. 405–429.

[85] Scheibel, M.E. and Scheibel, A.B. (1973) Discussion. In *Brain Information Service Conference Report No. 32*, Brain Information Service/Brain Research Institute UCLA, Los Angeles, pp. 12–17.

[86] Schor, R.H. and Miller, A.D. (1981) Vestibular reflexes in neck and forelimb muscles evoked by roll tilt. *J. Neurophysiol.*, 46: 167–178.

[87] Schor, R.H. and Miller, A.D. (1982) Relationship of cat vestibular neurons to otolith-spinal reflexes. *Exp. Brain Res.*, 47: 137–144.

[88] Shimizu, N., Katoh, Y., Hida, T. and Satoh, K. (1979) The fine structural organization of the locus coeruleus in the rat with reference to noradrenaline contents. *Exp. Brain Res.*, 37: 139–148.

[89] Shiromani, P. and McGinty, D.J. (1986) Pontine neuronal response to local cholinergic infusion: relation to REM sleep. *Brain Res.*, 386: 20–31.

[90] Srivastava, U.C., Manzoni, D., Pompeiano, O. and Stampacchia, G. (1982) State-dependent properties of medullary reticular neurons involved during the labyrinth and neck reflexes. *Neurosci. Lett.*, 10: S461.

[91] Stampacchia, G., Barnes, C.D., D'Ascanio, P. and Pompeiano, O. (1987) Effects of microinjection of a cholinergic agonist into the locus coeruleus on the gain of vestibulospinal reflexes in decerebrate cats. *Arch. Ital. Biol.*, 125: 107–138.

[92] Steriade, M. and Hobson, J.A. (1976) Neuronal activity during the sleep-waking cycle. *Progr. Neurobiol.*, 6: 155–376.

[93] Svensson, T.H., Bunney, B.S. and Aghajanian, G.K. (1975) Inhibition of both noradrenergic and serotonergic neurons in brain by the α-adrenergic agonist clonidine. *Brain Res.*, 92: 291–306.

[94] Van Dongen, P.A.M. (1981) The central noradrenergic transmission and the locus coeruleus: a review of the data, and their implications for neurotransmission and neuromodulation. *Progr. Neurobiol.*, 16: 117–143.

[95] Vivaldi, E., McCarley, R.W. and Hobson, J.A. (1980) Evocation of desynchronized sleep signs by chemical microstimulation of the pontine brainstem. In J.A. Hobson and M.A.B. Brazier (Eds.), *The Reticular Formation Revisited, IBRO Monograph Series, Vol. 6*, Raven Press, New York, pp. 513–529.

[96] Wamsley, J.K., Lewis, M.S., Young, W.S. and Kuhar, M.J. (1981) Autoradiographic localization of muscarinic cholinergic receptors in rat brainstem. *J. Neurosci.*, 1: 176–191.

[97] Westlund, K.N., Bowker, R.M., Ziegler, M.G. and Coulter, J.D. (1984) Origins and terminations of descending noradrenergic projections to the spinal cord of monkey. *Brain Res.*, 292: 1–16.

[98] Young, W.S. III and Kuhar, M.J. (1980) Noradrenergic α_1 and α_2 receptors: light microscopic autoradiographic localization. *Proc. Natl. Acad. Sci. USA*, 77: 1696–1700.

O. Pompeiano and J.H.J. Allum (Eds.)
Progress in Brain Research, Vol. 76
© 1988 Elsevier Science Publishers B.V. (Biomedical Division)

CHAPTER 32

Postural compensation in the guinea pig following unilateral labyrinthectomy

I.S. Curthoys, P.F. Smith and C.L. Darlington

Vestibular Research Laboratory, Department of Psychology, University of Sydney, Sydney 2006, N.S.W. Australia

Recent behavioural and neural studies of vestibular compensation in guinea pigs are reviewed. Vestibular compensation is not a unitary process in that ocular motor and postural symptoms recover at different rates. Selective section of the horizontal canal nerve alone, rather than total unilateral labyrinthectomy, produces the usual spontaneous nystagmus in light (without roll head tilt or maintained yaw head tilt) which compensates faster than after total unilateral labyrinthectomy. Commissural connections between the guinea-pig vestibular nuclei are not necessary for the compensation of the postural symptoms. Neuronal recordings in compensating animals show a return of resting activity to horizontal canal neurons in the medial vestibular nucleus on the lesioned side which parallels the behavioural recovery. There are permanent neuronal gain changes. It is hypothesized that resting activity returns by virtue of changes in the membrane excitability of neurons in the medial vestibular nucleus, just as it has been demonstrated to occur in deafferented neurons in the lateral cuneate nucleus. Vestibular compensation is probably an unusual and inadequate example of 'plasticity' in the central nervous system.

Introduction

Over the last five years we have conducted a series of experiments on guinea pigs documenting the behavioural consequences of unilateral labyrinthectomy and the time course of compensation of the ocular motor and postural symptoms observed immediately after the labyrinthectomy. The neural correlates of these behavioural changes have also been studied by quantifying the response characteristics of populations of neurons in the vestibular nuclei at various times after the labyrinthectomy. The present report summarizes the major results of all these studies.

The guinea pig was selected for this research because other species (such as the frog) do not show the full range of behavioural symptoms following ULD shown by mammals (see [1] for review) and also because other species (such as the frog) have functionally excitatory commissural connections between the vestibular nuclei [2] unlike mammals which have functionally inhibitory commissural connections [3]. This important species difference makes interpretation of neural and behavioural studies of vestibular compensation in the frog difficult and the applicability of neural results in frogs to mammals is questionable. (In unpublished experiments we have confirmed that the vestibular commissures are functionally inhibitory in the guinea pig, just as they are in the cat.) Furthermore, the guinea pig has the distinct advantage that much is known about the anatomy and physiology of the inner ear and the inner structures are readily accessible [4].

Abbreviations: HRP, horseradish peroxidase; RA, resting activity; ULD, unilateral labyrinth deafferentation

Some previous studies of vestibular compensation in the guinea pig have used a chloroform injection into the middle ear to produce the labyrinth destruction (e.g. [5]). The precise extent of the labyrinthine damage produced by such a procedure is unknown and, based on our own explorations with the chloroform method, we suspect that the labyrinthine damage produced may vary considerably from animal to animal (see also [6]). Because of such uncertainties we have used a direct surgical approach with visualization of the receptor structures prior to their surgical destruction. In our experiments the surgical labyrinthectomy is complete and its completeness is routinely confirmed by visual inspection or histological procedure.

Results

Behavioural changes after total ULD

Pigmented guinea pigs were anaesthetized with the short-acting anaesthetic combination of Ketamine (100 mg/kg, i.m.) and Rompun (4 mg/kg, i.m.) and a surgical labyrinthectomy performed. Following recovery from this ULD, measurements were made at regular hourly intervals of spontaneous nystagmus in light and the postural symptoms. In this report we wish to use new terms to replace the previous confusing terminology for the postural symptoms observed after ULD: yaw head tilt to replace 'lateral head deviation' and roll head tilt to replace 'longitudinal twist'. Fig. 1 illustrates the definitions of these terms as applied to a guinea pig after a right-sided ULD and shows how the angles defining these tilts were measured.

After recovery from anaesthesia the animals show vigorous spontaneous nystagmus in light (approximately 20 beats/15 seconds) which diminishes over time and disappears by about 52 hours after the operation [7]. Likewise, the postural symptoms of roll head tilt and yaw head tilt are largest immediately after recovery from anaesthesia and diminish over time, but the recovery of these symptoms, especially roll head tilt, follows distinctly different time courses to the recovery of spontaneous nystag-

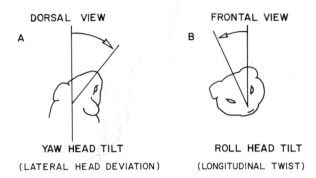

Fig. 1. Illustration of the definitions of yaw head tilt (A) and roll head tilt (B). Yaw head tilt is defined as the angle in degrees between the line passing through the midscapular point and sacrum and the line from the midscapular point to the centre of the guinea pig's snout. Yaw head tilt refers to a head rotation about the z axis of the skull. The term yaw head tilt is proposed to replace the term 'lateral head deviation'. Roll head tilt is defined as the angle in degrees between the line passing through the centre of the guinea pig's head and the line perpendicular to the floor. Roll head tilt refers to a rotation about the X axis of the skull. The term roll head tilt is proposed to replace the term 'longitudinal twist'.

mus. A strong piece of evidence in support of this statement is that at 4 months after the operation the animals still have a roll head tilt of 14.6° on average ($\pm$ 3.9° S.D) which is significantly different from 0°, whereas the other symptoms have entirely disappeared by this time.

We conclude from this dissociation of the recovery rates of different symptoms, that vestibular compensation is not a single unitary process as has apparently been assumed in some previous studies [8]. Instead it seems that the different symptoms recover at different rates and most probably different neural mechanisms are governing the various ocular motor and postural compensation processes. As further support for this conclusion it should be noted that vision affects the different processes of compensation differently. If animals are maintained in darkness during the recovery period it is found that spontaneous nystagmus recovers at the same rate as it does when the animal is kept in light; however, recovery of roll head tilt is significantly delayed by this procedure [7].

A recent theoretical account has explained vesti-

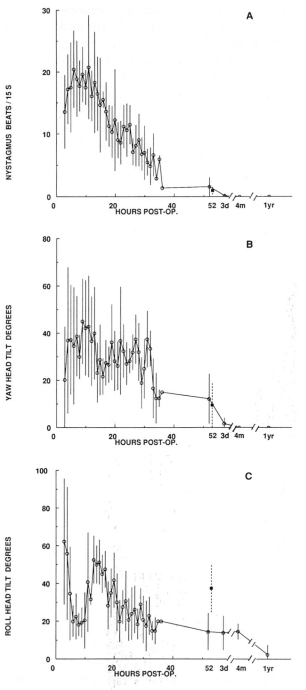

Fig. 2. Compensation of spontaneous nystagmus in light (A), yaw head tilt (lateral head deviation) (B) and roll head tilt (longitudinal twist) (C). Dashed lines and solid data points represent those animals maintained in complete darkness for 52 hours following ULD. Bars represent ± 1 S.D. (d, days; m, months; yr, year.) (Modified from [7].)

bular compensation in terms of changes in the synaptic efficacy of the commissural fibres between the vestibular nuclei [8]. In this model the emphasis is upon these commissural fibres forming a *closed* feedback loop as opposed to an *open* loop (see Fig. 3). Evidence for this model has been adduced from ocular motor and postural compensation in both mammals and frogs. For example, it has been briefly reported that cutting brainstem commissural fibres in frogs causes permanent decompensation [9]. It seemed that a direct test of this model would be to establish whether, in mammals, cutting these commissural fibres prevented vestibular compensation taking place.

In 4 guinea pigs the brainstem commissural fibres were cut at the time of the labyrinthectomy [10]. The operation involved very gently elevating the cerebellum to visualize the floor of the fourth ventricle and then using a fine iris knife to cut the commissural fibres to at least a depth of 2 mm from a level rostral to the abducens nucleus to a level caudal to the descending vestibular nucleus. Very great care was taken not to damage the cerebellum during this operation since there are reports of cerebellar damage alone producing decompensation [11, 12]. The histology confirmed that cerebellar damage was minimal. It was reasoned that if the commissural fibres are the basis for compensation then cutting these fibres should prevent compensation.

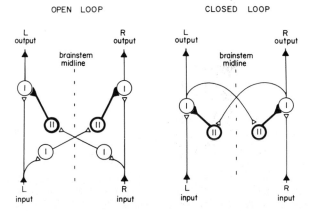

Fig. 3. Schematic examples of open- and closed-loop commissural interaction systems between the vestibular nuclei.

378

In fact the postural symptoms in all these guinea pigs compensated at approximately normal rates despite the absence of dorsal brainstem commissural fibres between the vestibular nuclei (see Fig. 4). It should be noted that in these commissurectomized animals we could only measure the postural symptoms of roll head tilt and yaw head tilt since there was no horizontal spontaneous nystagmus. The reason for the absence of spontaneous nystagmus is that the commissure sectioning not only cuts fibres between the vestibular nuclei but also cuts the axons of neurons from the vestibular nucleus to the con-

tralateral abducens nucleus and the axons of internuclear neurons from one abducens nucleus to the contralateral oculomotor nucleus (see [13] for review). Both abducens nuclei will thus be deprived of the excitatory input from the contralateral vestibular nuclei and so no horizontal slow phases (and no horizontal quick phases) will be produced. In a previous study [14] in the monkey it has been reported that horizontal nystagmus could still be observed after section of the commissural fibres; however, this is almost certainly due to the commissural section in that study sparing the axons of vestibular nucleus neurons projecting to contralateral abducens (and probably also sparing some commissural fibres as well). Our recent intracellular HRP injections into physiologically identified type I neurons in the medial vestibular nucleus have shown that some of these axons project to contralateral abducens and contralateral vestibular nucleus via a rostral pathway, in some cases the axon passes through the centre of the ipsilateral abducens nucleus [15, 16].

The demonstration of postural compensation in guinea pigs without dorsal brainstem commissural connections between the vestibular nuclei implies that brainstem commissural connections are not necessary for the compensation of the postural symptoms of ULD as is postulated in the Galiana model [8]. This conclusion is supported by the results of recent experimental anatomical studies using HRP which show that, at least in the cat, direct commissural connections are present between different vestibular nuclei which control ocular motor activity, but not between the lateral vestibular nuclei which control posture [17]. However, the demonstration that postural compensation occurs in the guinea pig without dorsal brainstem commissures is inconsistent with the finding that transsection of the dorsal brainstem commissures produces postural decompensation in the frog [9]. We suggest that the reasons for the discrepancy may be either a species difference, or inadvertent cerebellar damage in the frog, or the fact that the commissural section in frogs was performed *after* compensation had taken place and produced permanent decom-

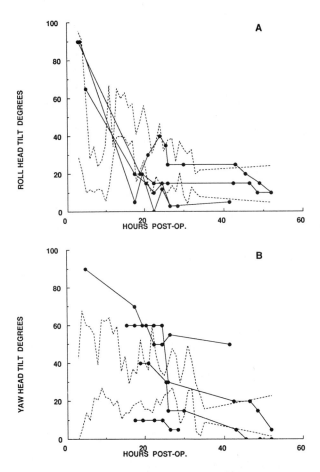

Fig. 4. Compensation of roll head tilt (longitudinal twist) (A) and yaw head tilt (lateral head deviation) (B) in 4 guinea pigs following ULD *and* sectioning of the dorsal brainstem commissures (●—●). Dashed lines represent ± 1 S.D. for data in Fig. 2 where animals received a right labyrinthectomy only. (Modified from [10].)

pensation. It is possible that commissural section in compensated animals may have different effects compared to commissural section in animals at the time of labyrinthectomy.

This dissociation between ocular motor and postural symptoms of vestibular compensation is even more clearly shown by some recent studies in which we have selectively lesioned only the nerve to the horizontal canal ampulla, rather than performing an entire unilateral labyrinthectomy. The same species, strain, anaesthesia, measurement procedures and observers were used to compare the effects of such selective nerve section with the effects of total ULD. In 9 animals the nerve to the horizontal canal crista was surgically sectioned leaving the membranous labyrinth intact, and in 8 animals the entire horizontal crista was removed at operation to completely ensure that there was no afferent input from the horizontal canal during the period of the behavioural measures of compensation. The behavioural results from both groups of animals were similar and are shown in Fig. 5. The combined group ($n = 17$) was compared with the results of total ULD. After selective lesion of just the nerve to the horizontal canal ampulla the animals show spontaneous nystagmus in light but show no roll head tilt. There was a modest fluctuating yaw head tilt which was qualitatively completely unlike the maintained rigid 'locked up' yaw head tilt observed after total ULD. The selectively lesioned animals could voluntarily move their heads in yaw to either side and showed an intermittent head nystagmus which is rarely seen after a total ULD in guinea pigs because of the maintained, fixed yaw head position produced by the total ULD. In other animals selective lesion of the saccule receptors (using a direct lateral surgical approach via the oval window) resulted in a brief (2 hour) roll head tilt but no horizontal nystagmus. Control experiments in which either the surgical exposure only was performed, or the middle ear was opened, or the inner ear was opened but the membranous labyrinth was not disturbed, showed at most a brief (2 hour) horizontal nystagmus (see Fig. 6).

After selective lesion of the horizontal canal

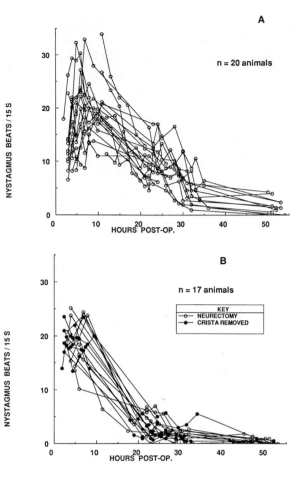

Fig. 5. Spontaneous nystagmus in light (in number of nystagmus beats per 15 second interval) at varying times after total ULD (A) or selective lesion of the horizontal canal nerve (B). Each line shows the result for an individual guinea pig. In B, the open circles are data points for animals where the horizontal canal nerve was cut but the membranous labyrinth was not opened, whereas filled circles are for animals where the entire horizontal canal ampulla and crista was removed. There was no detectable difference between the results of these two groups.

nerve, guinea pigs showed horizontal spontaneous nystagmus in light which was not significantly different from that found after total ULD; however, it compensated at a significantly faster rate (see Fig. 6). By 25 hours the nystagmus in the selective lesioned group was significantly less that that found in the total ULD group. These selective lesioned animals had no *maintained* yaw head tilt, unlike the total ULD group, and some experiments by Petto-

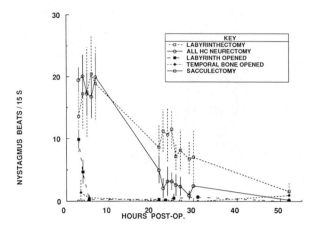

Fig. 6. Average spontaneous nystagmus in light at varying times after operation: for total ULD (□—□), horizontal canal neurectomy (○—○). Each data point shows the average of measurements from different animals in the given 1-hour time interval. The vertical bars show ± 1 standard deviation. Also shown are the average results from animals receiving a unilateral sacculectomy and the average result of animals in the sham operated control groups.

rossi and Petrosini [18] suggest that under such conditions they should have compensated more *slowly* than the total ULD group since they lacked the neck input produced by the maintained yaw head tilt. Instead, we observed that they compensated more *quickly* than the total ULD group. The full role of neck afferent input and input from the contralateral intact otolithic receptors responding to the roll head tilt [19] remains to be established but on the basis of the present results it would appear that neither of them has a major role.

Neural changes

To understand the neural changes correlated with these behavioural changes, we have used acute extracellular unit recording to record from popula-

tions of single neurons responding to horizontal angular accelerations in the rostral medial vestibular nuclei of anaesthetized guinea pigs before, immediately, after, 52 hours after and about 1 year after ULD (20–22). These animals were labyrinthectomized and allowed to recover (in these latter two categories) in light before the unit recording session. Both type I and type II neurons were studied in the vestibular nuclei on both the side of the intact labyrinth and on the side of the labyrinthectomy. For unit recording the animals were anaesthetized with Nembutal (30 mg/kg, i.m.) and Innovar (0.75 ml/kg = 0.30 mg/kg Fentanyl and 15.0 mg/kg Droperidol, i.m) and artificially respired with very close attention to EEG to ensure the level of anaesthesia was not too deep. The midline cerebellum was aspirated to expose the floor of the fourth ventricle and glass microelectrodes were inserted into the vestibular nucleus under visual control. Fig. 7 provides an overall summary of the averaged quantitative data from the neural experiments. The major variables which were measured were resting activity (RA, spikes/s), the gain of the neural response to a standardized sinusoidal horizontal angular acceleration stimulus of 0.2 Hz, and the phase of the neural response re. the peak stimulus velocity. In addition we sought to obtain some measure of the relative frequency of occurrence of neurons by recording the number of neurons per animal. This is a very coarse measure but it provides an approximate index of how frequently cells of the various categories were encountered.

Prior to labyrinthectomy, type I neurons were more frequently encountered than type II neurons. Immediately after the labyrinthectomy type I neurons were rare on the lesioned side but frequent on the intact side. In contrast, type II neurons were frequent on the lesioned side but rare on the intact side. Because of the coarseness of this measure of

Fig. 7. Neuronal changes in the medial vestibular nucleus up to 1 year following ULD (based on a sample of 897 neurons). The size of the circle at the top of each histogram provides an index of the frequency of occurrence of neurons in animals where unbiassed searches of the vestibular nuclei were undertaken. The vertical bars show two-tailed 95% confidence intervals. The sample size for each mean is shown adjacent to the data point. The one set of control data are shown on both the intact and lesioned sides for the purpose of comparison.

INTACT SIDE

LABYRINTHECTOMIZED SIDE

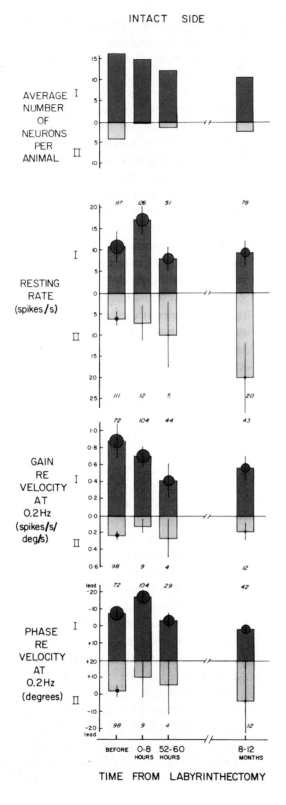
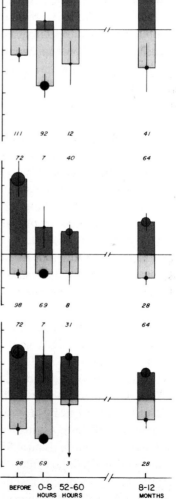

AVERAGE
NUMBER
OF
NEURONS
PER
ANIMAL

RESTING
RATE
(spikes/s)

GAIN
RE
VELOCITY
AT
0.2 Hz
(spikes/s/
deg/s)

PHASE
RE
VELOCITY
AT
0.2 Hz
(degrees)

BEFORE 0-8 52-60 8-12
HOURS HOURS MONTHS

TIME FROM LABYRINTHECTOMY

BEFORE 0-8 52-60 8-12
HOURS HOURS MONTHS

TIME FROM LABYRINTHECTOMY

cell frequency and the biasses to which it is subject, no statistical analysis of these figures have been undertaken.

Of great interest for understanding the rapid behavioural compensation described earlier is the fact that in recordings in the vestibular nucleus on the lesioned side in animals 52 hours after the labyrinthectomy, type I neurons could again be recorded with approximately normal RA although they were not as frequently encountered as type I neurons in bilaterally intact animals. The gain of these type I neurons on the lesioned side to rotational stimulation was reduced in comparison to control values and in fact the average gain of such type I neurons remained significantly below control values even in animals studied one year after the labyrinthectomy. In addition to those neurons responsive to horizontal angular acceleration, there were many other neurons with moderate RA which were unresponsive. These other nonresponsive neurons may have been horizontal canal type I neurons prior to the labyrinthectomy which had recovered their RA by 52 hours but which could not be driven via the commissural fibres from the intact vestibular nucleus sufficiently to demonstrate a type I response to rotation. The relatively active vestibular nucleus on the lesioned side in animals at 52 hours is in sharp contrast to the relatively silent vestibular nucleus on the lesioned side (apart from the type II responses) immediately after the ULD. It may be that some neurons are permanently silenced by the unilateral labyrinthectomy. We have not been able to answer this question yet.

In type I neurons there seem to be comparatively modest changes in frequency, RA, gain or phase from 52 hours to 1 year after the ULD.

It is our hypothesis (following Precht, Shimazu and Marklam [23]) that during the first 52 hours RA returns to the deafferented neurons in the vestibular nucleus on the lesioned side and as this RA returns it can be modulated via the commissural fibres from the vestibular nucleus on the intact side.

We have sought the mechanisms responsible for the rapid return of RA in the vestibular nucleus on the lesioned side. It is unlikely to be from activity of surviving primary afferent cells in Scarpa's ganglion on the lesioned side since attempts at recording activity in this ganglion showed an almost complete absence of spikes, in contrast to the vigorous response of Scarpa's ganglion on the intact side under comparable conditions (see also [24, 25]). Furthermore, in some long-term animals which had shown normal compensation, Scarpa's ganglion on the lesioned side had entirely atrophied.

It is unlikely that the commissural fibres themselves are responsible for the return of RA since cutting the fibres either in normal animals or in animals 52 hours after labyrinthectomy causes an almost identical increase in average RA. If the commissural fibres had been responsible for the return of RA, for example by causing a reduction of inhibition exerted on type I neurons, then one would expect a significantly smaller increase in RA following commissurectomy in 52-hour animals (corresponding to reduced disinhibition). There was no evidence for such a process. Furthermore, if disinhibition by the brainstem commissures were responsible for the return of type I RA on the lesioned side, it might be expected that type II neurons on the lesioned side would have a lower than normal RA. Instead the RA of type II neurons on the lesioned side was not significantly different from normal both at 52 hours and 1 year after ULD. Furthermore, the recovery of type I RA by 52 hours is too fast to be produced by axonal sprouting [8]: functional re-innervation by sprouting has been reported to take somewhere around 9 days at a minimum [26].

We hypothesize that in the vestibular nucleus, as in other brainstem nuclei such as the lateral cuneate nucleus [27], deafferentation by ULD results in changes in membrane excitability of individual neurons and that it is this mechanism by which 'denervation supersensitivity' allows the return of resting activity. These cell membrane excitability changes are well documented in the lateral cuneate nucleus and we suggest that the same processes occur in cells in the vestibular nuclei, complicated by the presence of commissural input from the contralateral (intact) vestibular nucleus. This hypothesis places vestibular compensation in the general framework of recovery of neural activity after lesion rather than being a 'special' and particularly good example of plasticity in the central nervous system. In fact there may be very little neural *plasticity* in vestibular compensation: the gain of guinea pig type I neurons remains significantly below control values in both vestibular nuclei, even one year after labyrinthectomy, and the gain of the behavioural vestibulo-ocular response in man [28], shows a permanent asymmetry when the appropriate pure vestibular tests, uncontaminated by prediction, are performed (e.g. using unpredictable head impulses to test vestibular function rather than predictable sinusoidal rotation).

The guinea pigs in these neural studies were anaesthetized and the midline cerebellum was aspirated. Both of these procedures have been shown to abolish vestibular compensation [11, 12] (i.e. to produce decompensation) and so it might be expected that such decompensation would also occur in the present study, particularly in the animals studied only 52 hours following the labyrinthectomy. In neural terms one would expect that decompensation would cause the results of recording on the lesioned side to be similar to the results obtained immediately after labyrinthectomy (e.g. few type I's with low RA, many type II's, etc). In fact there are very clear differences between the neural results of the immediate and the 52-hour groups and so we suggest any decompensation which was produced by the anaesthesia or the midline cerebellar removal was modest. The anaesthesia is light and particular attention was paid to animals in the 52-hour group to ensure (from the EEG) that the depth of anaesthesia was light. Aspiration of the midline cerebellum may predominantly affect the postural responses after ULD, via its effects on the bilateral lateral vestibular nuclei, rather than the responses of the medial vestibular nucleus neurons which we recorded.

Conclusion

The behavioural results point to separate and different processes of compensation for ocular motor and postural symptoms following ULD. It is likely that these different processes are governed by different neural processes in different regions of the vestibular nuclei. The available evidence suggests that the neural changes governing ocular motor compensation occur within the medial and superior vestibular nuclei whereas the neural changes governing postural compensation are more likely to occur within the lateral vestibular nucleus [29]. The former site is characterized by strong and direct commissural connections to the contralateral medial and superior vestibular nuclei whereas direct commissural connections between the lateral vestibular nuclei are lacking [17] or minor [30]. Interconnections between the lateral vestibular nucleus on each side are more indirect and may be achieved via the transcerebellar pathways. In particular, there is evidence that the macular input of one side may influence the lateral vestibular nucleus of the opposite side by utilizing the lateral vestibulospinal tract acting on neurons of the crossed spino–reticulocerebellar pathway [31]. In both cases we hypothesize that the labyrinthectomy either silences or severely reduces neural activity in the various vestibular nuclei on the lesioned side and that the various behavioural symptoms are either direct or indirect manifestations of the consequences of such deafferentation. In a fairly short time RA returns, possibly because of changes in membrane excitability or some other such realization of 'denervation supersensitivity' and as RA returns so the ocular motor and postural symptoms decline.

References

[1] Precht, W. and Dieringer, N. (1985) Neuronal events paralleling functional recovery (compensation) following peripheral vestibular lesions, In A. Berthoz and G. Melvill Jones (Eds.), *Adaptive Mechanisms in Gaze Control. Facts and Theories*, Elsevier, Amsterdam, pp. 251–268.

[2] Ozawa, S., Precht, W. and Shimazu, H. (1974) Crossed effects on central vestibular neurons in the horizontal canal system of the frog. *Exp. Brain Res.*, 19: 394–405.

[3] Shimazu, H. and Precht, W. (1966) Inhibition of central vestibular neurons from the contralateral labyrinth and its mediating pathway. *J. Neurophysiol.*, 29: 467–492.

384

[4] Curthoys, I.S. (1982) The response of primary horizontal semicircular canal neurons in the rat and guinea pig to angular acceleration. *Exp. Brain Res.*, 47: 286–294.

[5] Schaefer, K.-P. and Meyer, D.L. (1973) Compensatory mechanisms following labyrinthine lesions in the guinea pig. A simple model of learning. In H.P. Zippel (Ed.), *Memory and Transfer of Information*, Plenum Press, New York, pp. 203–232.

[6] Jensen, D.W. (1979) Reflex control of acute postural asymmetry and compensatory symmetry after a unilateral vestibular lesion. *Neuroscience*, 4: 1059–1073.

[7] Smith, P.F., Darlington, C.L. and Curthoys, I.S. (1986) The effect of visual deprivation on vestibular compensation in the guinea pig. *Brain Res.*, 364: 195–198.

[8] Galiana, H.L., Flohr, H. and Melvill Jones, G. (1984) A re-evaluation of intervestibular nuclear coupling: its role in vestibular compensation, *J. Neurophysiol.*, 51: 258–275.

[9] Bienhold, H. and Flohr, H. (1978) Role of commissural connections between vestibular nuclei in compensation following unilateral labyrinthectomy, *J. Physiol. London*, 284: 178.

[10] Smith, P.F., Darlington, C.L. and Curthoys, I.S. (1986) Vestibular compensation without brainstem commissures in the guinea pig. *Neurosci. Lett.*, 65: 209–213.

[11] Carpenter, M.B., Fabrega, H. and Glinsmann (1959) Physiological deficits occurring with lesions of labyrinth and fastigial nuclei. *J. Neurophysiol.*, 22: 222–234.

[12] Azzena, G.B. (1969) Role of the spinal cord in compensating the effects of hemilabyrinthectomy, *Arch. Ital. Biol.*, 107: 43–53.

[13] Shimazu, H. (1983) Neuronal organization of the premotor system controlling horizontal conjugate eye movements and vestibular nystagmus. In J.E. Desmedt (Ed.), *Motor Control Mechanisms in Health and Disease*, Raven Press, New York, pp. 565–588.

[14] Vianney De Jong, J.M.B., Cohen, B., Matsuo, V. and Uemura, T. (1980) Midsagittal pontomedullary brainstem section: effects on ocular adduction and nystagmus, *Exp. Neurol.*, 68: 420–442.

[15] Oghaki, T., Curthoys, I.S. and Markham, C.H. (1986) Intracellular injection of HRP in eye movement-related pause neurons in the cat. *Soc. Neurosci. Abstr.*, 12(1): 457.

[16] Oghaki, T., Curthoys, I.S. and Markham, C.H. (1987) HRP morphology of functionally identified vestibular type I neurons in the cat, *Proc. Bárány Society Meeting, Bologna*, p. 7.

[17] Pompeiano, O., Mergner, T. and Corvaja, N. (1978) Commissural, perihypoglossal and reticular afferent projections to the vestibular nuclei in the cat. An experimental anatomical study with the method of retrograde transport of horseradish peroxidase, *Arch. Ital. Biol.*, 116: 130–172.

[18] Pettorossi, V.E. and Petrosini, L. (1984) Tonic cervical influences on eye nystagmus following hemilabyrinthectomy: immediate and plastic effects. *Brain Res.*, 324: 11–19.

[19] Fluur, E. and Siegborn, J. (1973) Interaction between the utricles and the horizontal semicircular canals. I. Unilateral selective sectioning of the horizontal ampullar nerve followed by tilting around the longitudinal axis. *Acta Otolaryngol. Stockholm*, 75: 17–20.

[20] Curthoys, I.S., Harris, R.A. and Smith, P.F. (1987) Effect of unilateral labyrinthectomy on neural activity in the guinea pig vestibular nuclei. In M.D. Graham and J.L. Kemink, (Eds.), *The Vestibular System: Neurophysiologic and Clinical Research*, Raven Press, New York, pp. 677–687.

[21] Smith, P.F. and Curthoys, I.S. (1987) Neuronal activity in the contralateral medial vestibular nucleus of the guinea pig following unilateral labyrinthectomy. *Brain Res.*, in press.

[22] Smith, P.F. and Curthoys, I.S. (1987) Neuronal activity in the ipsilateral medial vestibular nucleus of the guinea pig following unilateral labyrinthectomy. *Brain Res.*, in press.

[23] Precht, W., Shimazu, H. and Markham, C.H. (1966) A mechanism of central compensation of vestibular function following hemilabyrinthectomy, *J. Neurophysiol.*, 29: 996–1010.

[24] Jensen, D.W. (1983) Survival of function in the deafferented vestibular nerve, *Brain Res.* 273: 175–178.

[25] Sirkin, D.W., Precht, W. and Courjon, J.H. (1984) Initial, rapid phase of recovery from unilateral vestibular lesion in rat not dependent on survival of central portion of vestibular nerve. *Brain Res.*, 302: 245–256.

[26] Cotman, C.W. and Nadler, J.V. (1978) Reactive synaptogenesis in the hippocampus. In C.W. Cotman (Ed.), *Neuronal Plasticity*, Raven Press, New York, pp. 227–271.

[27] Calvin, W.H. (1980) Normal repetitive firing and its pathophysiology. In J.S. Lockard and A.A. Ward (Eds.), *Epilepsy: A Window to Brain Mechanisms*, Raven Press, New York, pp. 97–120.

[28] Cremer, P.D., Henderson, C.J., Curthoys, I.S. and Halmagyi, G.M. (1987) Horizontal vestibulo-ocular reflex changes following unilateral vestibular neurectomy, *Neurosci. Lett., Suppl.* 27, S64.

[29] Xerri, C., Gianni, S., Manzoni, D. and Pompeiano, O. (1983) Compensation of central vestibular deficits. I. Response characteristics of lateral vestibular neurons to roll tilt after ipsilateral labyrinth deafferentation. *J. Neurophysiol.*, 50: 428–448.

[30] Ito, J., Matsuoka, I., Sasa, M. and Takaori, S. (1985) Commissural and ipsilateral internuclear connection of vestibular nuclear complex of the cat. *Brain Res.*, 341: 73–81.

[31] Pompeiano, O. (1979) Neck and macular labyrinthine influences on the cervical spinoreticulocerebellar pathway. In R. Granit and O. Pompeiano (Eds.), *Reflex Control of Posture and Movement, Progress in Brain Research, Vol. 50*, Elsevier, Amsterdam, pp. 501–514.

O. Pompeiano and J.H.J. Allum (Eds.)
Progress in Brain Research, Vol. 76
© 1988 Elsevier Science Publishers B.V. (Biomedical Division)

CHAPTER 33

Mechanisms of vestibular compensation in the unilateral labyrinthectomized cat

M. Maeda

Department of Neurosurgery and Casualty Center, School of Medicine, Juntendo University, 2-1-1 Hongo, Bunkyo-ku, Tokyo 113, Japan

The autoradiographic [^{14}C]deoxyglucose method for quantitative determination of LCGU was used to study the compensatory process following hemilabyrinthectomy in adult cats. In the critical stage when the cats were not compensated, glucose utilization in the deafferented vestibular nuclei was well below that of the intact side. The increased LCGU was seen in nucleus reticularis parvocellularis, nucleus pontis on both sides, ipsilateral abducens nucleus and its ventral parts. Activity levels in the inferior olive were not much changed. In the cerebellum, the posterior vermis and the nodulofloccular lobe were very active. LCGU in the cerebellar nuclei was not noticeably changed. In the compensatory stage, the rate of LCGU in the deafferented vestibular nuclei had increased to that of the intact side. The increased LCGU was evident in the nucl. reticularis parvocellularis, gigantocellularis and lateralis, and superior colliculus. Posterior vermis, nodulus and cerebellar nuclei were active. Destruction of the vermis, fastigial nuclei and surrounding white matter produced a marked imbalance during walking and a tremor of the head while the animals were feeding. These signs subsided very gradually. In addition to the above lesions, the interruption of the transreticular vestibular crossed connection produced severe motor disturbances on standing, walking and feeding. A restoration of normal functioning was not found to occur. These findings may suggest that vestibular compensation results from the combined activity of many brainstem and cerebellar structures, where intervestibular crossed pathways are seen to be one of important factors in compensation.

Introduction

After hemilabyrinthectomy, men and animals exhibit a characteristic behavioural pattern. Recovery of function following unilateral destruction occurs rapidly and is remarkably complete. This compensatory process, which is basically similar in all vertebrates, has been well known [1, 2] since the early investigations of Bechterew [3]. In these studies this process can be divided into three distinct stages as defined by the presence of characteristic behavioural patterns [4]. In the critical stage, beginning immediately after hemilabyrinthectomy, the animals exhibit severe symptoms of imbalance including rapid spontaneous nystagmus, severe head deviation and forced circling or rolling toward the deafferented side. The acute stage is marked by a rapid partial recovery of asymmetry. Restoration of normal functioning occurs during the compensatory stage.

In cats, lesion-induced symptoms of ocular and postural imbalance recover almost to control values within the first postoperative week. Essentially similar results were obtained from other species although the time courses of recovery vary considerably. Compensation of head tilt in the rat takes only a matter of hours [5]. Ocular imbalance abates with similar time courses in rats [5], guinea pigs [6] and cats.

According to electrophysiological investigations of the vestibular nucleus of the cat, the most salient characteristics are both a decrease in spontaneous activity in the deafferented vestibular nuclei which begins immediately after unilateral labyrinthectomy and lasts for several days in the cat [7, 8] and a recovery of normal activity in the compensatory stage. Although changes in the properties of neurons within the deafferented vestibular nuclei may play a role in compensation [9–12], structures other than the vestibular nuclei may play a role in the rapid and complete acquisition of compensation such as the spinal cord [13], the cerebellum [14, 15], the cerebellar nuclei [16] and the visual system [17]. Concerning the role of the cerebellar system in the vestibular compensation, Llinas and Walton [5] conclude that the cerebellar nuclei and the integrity of the inferior olive are important in achieving and maintaining the compensatory states. Most recently, Galiana et al. [18] demonstrated that commissural pathways interconnecting the two sides of the brainstem represent a powerful putative site for adaptive modulation of the static characteristics of vestibular responses.

To examine this area further, two types of experiments were done. The first approach was to use the autoradiographic [^{14}C]deoxyglucose method for quantitative determination of LCGU [19, 20]. This was used as a marker for the plastic changes generating vestibular compensation. The second approach was to elucidate the effects of interruption of crossed vestibular nuclear coupling via transreticular [21] and transcerebellar [22] pathways on vestibular compensation using chronically hemilabyrinthectomized cats. In the first part of this chapter, we shall describe changes occurring in the various nuclei of the brainstem and the cerebellum. In the second part, we shall deal with the importance of vestibular crossed pathways involving both the brainstem and the cerebellum. Part of the results in this paper has previously appeared in brief form [23].

Methods

Labyrinthectomy was performed in halothane-anaesthetized cats by a ventral, extracranial approach. Two hours, 24 hours, 4 weeks, and 10 months after hemilabyrinthectomy, LCGU was measured in the above cats sitting in a partial restraining bag.

Autoradiographic [^{14}C]deoxyglucose method

2-[^{14}C]deoxyglucose (125 μCi/kg) was given as an intravenous pulse. Its concentration and that of the glucose was subsequently monitored in the plasma. The animals were sacrificed after 45 min and the brain was dissected out, frozen in Freon 12, mounted with embedding medium and sectioned 20 μm in thickness using a cryostat for quantitative autoradiography. Densitometric measurement of [^{14}C] concentration from autoradiographs was performed. From the optical density values, plasma variables and kinetic constant, rates of glucose utilization were calculated by the equation as originally described by Sokoloff et al. [19]. LCGU was compared in normal, uncompensated and compensated animals.

Lesions in the cerebellum and the brainstem

To begin with, the behaviour of four cats which had been hemilabyrinthectomized and which had fully recovered were observed. Posterior vermis, fastigial nuclei and surrounding white matter were aspirated by suction after suboccipital craniectomy. In the second type of experiment, six cats were used. After removal of the vermis, fastigial nuclei and surrounding white matter, and visualizing the fourth ventricle, the brainstem was cut longitudinally along the midline from the caudal end of the inferior colliculus to near the obex. The longitudinal incision was not extended to the ventral surface of the brainstem, but to the depth of 4.0–5.0 mm from its dorsal surface along the midline. The extent of the cerebellar and brainstem lesions was investigated histologically using Klüver Barrera stained serial sections. To document observations the animals were filmed at various stages in the course of the study.

Results

Normal cats

Autoradiographs of selected regions of the brainstem and the cerebellum of the normal unanaesthetized cat are illustrated in Fig. 1. A coronal section taken through the cerebellar cortex reveals that the radioactivity is concentrated in the granular and Purkinje cell layers. In this figure, the cerebellar nuclei, i.e. the fastigial, interpositus and dentate nuclei, can be distinguished very clearly. Within the brainstem several cell groups were clearly observed: the vestibular nuclei, the inferior olive and the colliculi. In the present studies, the rates of glucose utilization were measured in the following structures of the brainstem: vestibular nuclei (medial, lateral, inferior v.n.), nucl. reticularis parvocellularis, gigantocellularis and lateralis, formatio reticularis mesencephali, inferior olive, abducens nucleus and its vicinity, superior colliculus, and nucl. reticularis pontis. In the cerebellum the anterior and posterior vermis, hemisphere, nodulofloccular lobe and cerebellar nuclei (fastigial, interpositus and dentate) were investigated.

The values for the rates of glucose utilization in the brainstem and the cerebellum of the unanaesthetized cat are listed in Table 1. The rates in gray matter were much higher than those in white matter. The values for LCGU in the unanaesthetized cat were considerably below those observed in the rat [19]. The rates in the vestibular nuclei, the inferior olive, the colliculi and nodulofloccular were relatively high. The highest value was in the inferior colliculus, as has also been reported in the rat and the monkey [19, 20].

Uncompensated cats

Two hours after right hemilabyrinthectomy, during the critical stage when the cats are uncompensated, distribution of activity within the brainstem and the cerebellum was significantly different from that seen in the normal cat. Fig. 2 shows the percentage effects of the rates of glucose utilization in the lesioned cat (2 hours after right hemilabyrinthectomy) compared with the control cat. The most noticeable change from the control was seen in the vestibular nuclei (medial, lateral and inferior vestibular nucleus) themselves, where glucose utilization

TABLE I

Values for local cerebral glucose utilization (μmol/100 g/min) of the brainstem and the cerebellum in the normal unanaesthetized cat, in comparison with the albino rat [19] and the monkey

Structures	Cat (control)	Rat [19]	Monkey
Brainstem:			
Vestibular nucleus			
Medial	56.7	128 ± 5	66 ± 3
Lateral	52.3		
Inferior	47.1		
Nucleus reticularis			
parvocellularis	24.7		
gigantocellularis	28.4		
lateralis	27.5		
Formatio reticularis	21.5		
Inferior olive	70.7		
Nucleus abducens and ventral part	21.5		
Inferior colliculus	118	197 ± 10	103 ± 6
Superior colliculus			
superficial layer	55.5	95 ± 5	55 ± 4
intermediate and deep	42.6		
Formatio reticularis mesencephali	26.1		
Nucleus reticularis pontis	29.6		
Nucleus pontis	32.0		
Cerebellar cortex:		57 ± 2	31 ± 2
Anterior lobe			
vermis	39.7		
paramedian	44.8		
Posterior lobe			
uvula	45.7		
pyramid tuber	47.4		
hemisphere	40.4		
Nodulofloccular			
nodulus	50.5		
flocculus	61.5		
Cerebellar nuclei		100 ± 4	45 ± 2
fastigii	37.2		
interpositus	43.7		
dentate	45.9		
White matter	12.3	37 ± 2	12 ± 1

in the deafferented nucleus was well below (62% of the control value) that of the intact side (101% of the control value). The increased LCGU could be seen in nucl. reticularis parvocellularis (125%), nucl.

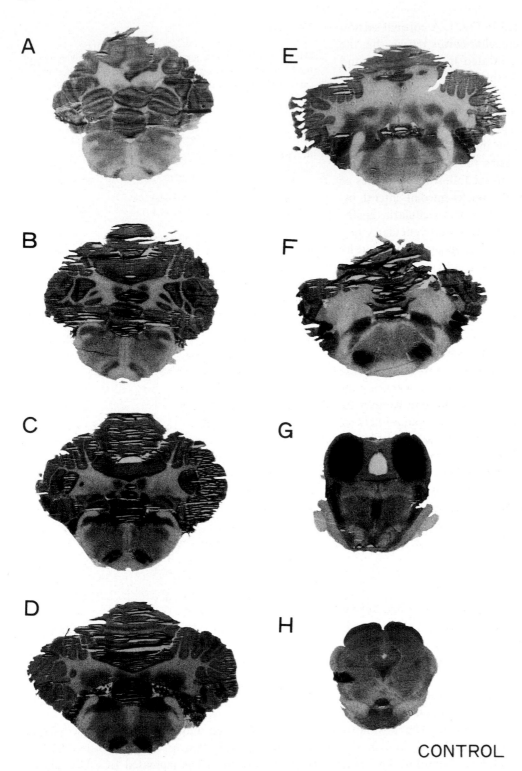

A

E

B

F

C

G

D

H

CONTROL

Fig. 1. Autoradiographs of coronal sections of the brainstem and the cerebellum in the intact, unanaesthetized cat (control).

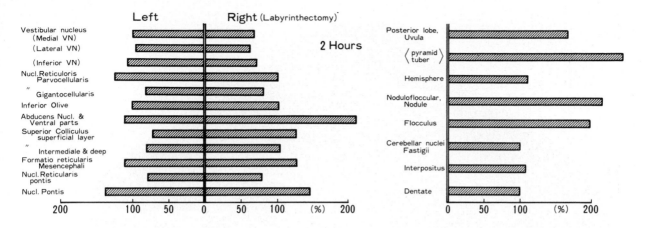

Fig. 2. Percentage change in local cerebral glucose utilization in an uncompensated cat 2 hours after right hemilabyrinthectomy compared with normal control values.

reticularis pontis (150%) on both sides, ipsilateral abducens nucleus and its ventral parts (as much as 212%), and ipsilateral superior colliculus (127%). LCGU in the contralateral superior colliculus was found to be reduced to 73% of the control value [23]. Activity levels in the inferior olive did not change much during the critical stage (102% of the control value). In the cerebellum, the posterior vermis and the noduloflocular were very active. LCGU in the cerebellar nuclei was not considerably modified.

Twenty-four hours after right hemilabyrinthectomy, the changes of the values for the rates of glucose utilization are very similar to those found 2 hours after operation. Decreased activity was observed in the deafferented vestibular nuclei (Fig. 3). Increased LCGU was seen in nucl. reticularis parvocellularis, formatio reticularis mesencephali and nucl. reticularis pontis. The inferior olive was also slightly active. In the cerebellum, the posterior vermis and the noduloflocular lobe were also seen to be active (Fig. 4).

Compensated cats

Four weeks after hemilabyrinthectomy, in the compensatory stage, the most important feature was that the value for glucose utilization in the deaffe-

rented vestibular nucleus (85–95%) increased so as to equalize that of the intact side (95%). Moderately increased activity was seen in the nucl. reticularis parvocellularis. On the other hand, LCGU in the inferior olive was almost equal to the control value (101–111%). In the cerebellum, the posterior vermis was very active (as much as 160%), and increased LCGU was also observed in the fastigial, interpositus and dentate nuclei.

Ten months after hemilabyrinthectomy, when the cat was completely compensated, the rates of glucose utilization were very similar to those of previously described four weeks after the deafferentation (Fig. 5). No asymmetric change in glucose utilization was observed in the vestibular nuclei of both sides. An increased LCGU could be seen in the nucl. reticularis parvocellularis (140% of the control), gigantocellularis (115%), lateralis (157–167%) and superior colliculus (130%). Posterior vermis (160%), nodulus (179%) and cerebellar nuclei (fastigial 150%, interpositus 130%, dentate 130%) were active as well.

In the completely compensated cat (three months after right hemilabyrinthectomy), destruction of the contralateral (left) labyrinth produced a distinct nystagmus, its quick component being directed toward the first operated labyrinth as if it were still intact. This phenomenon is called Bechterew's com-

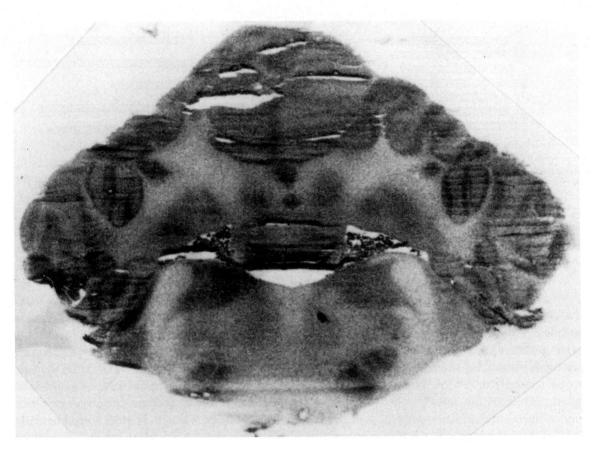

Fig. 3. Autoradiographs of the brainstem and the cerebellum in an uncompensated cat 24 hours after right hemilabyrinthectomy.

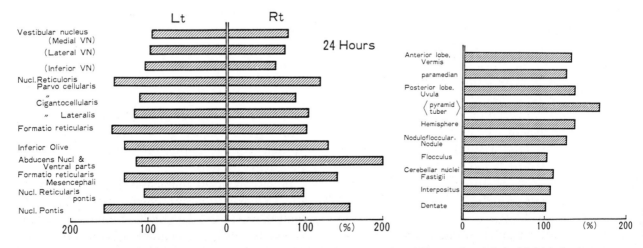

Fig. 4. Percentage change in local cerebral glucose utilization in an uncompensated cat 24 hours after right hemilabyrinthectomy compared with normal control values.

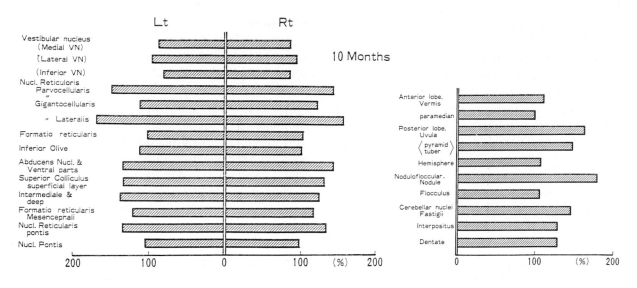

Fig. 5. Percentage change in local cerebral glucose utilization in a compensated cat 10 months after right hemilabyrinthectomy compared with normal control values.

pensatory nystagmus. The second labyrinthine destruction was also accompanied by head rotation and ocular deviation as if the first labyrinth were still intact. Two hours after the second labyrinthectomy (left), the rates of LCGU were quite similar to those of the previously presented two-hour (uncompensated) cat. Glucose utilization in the left

vestibular nucleus (the second labyrinthectomy side) was well below (66–86% of the control value) that on the firstly deafferented vestibular nucleus (80–100%) (Fig. 6). An increased activity was seen in nucl. reticular parvocellularis, lateralis, formatio reticularis mesencephali, nucl. reticularis pontis, posterior vermis and noduloflocular.

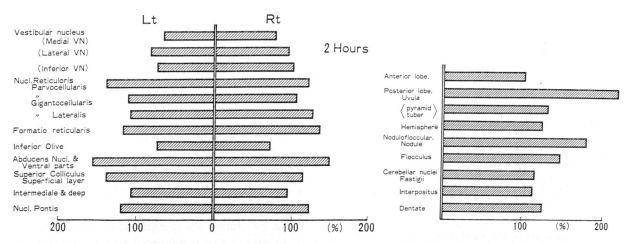

Fig. 6. Percentage change in local cerebral glucose utilization in the cat (accompanied with Bechterew phenomenon) compared with normal control. During compensatory stages, three months following right hemilabyrinthectomy, the left labyrinth was destroyed. LCGU was measured two hours after the second labyrinthectomy.

Effect of cerebellar lesions

Destruction of the vermis, bilateral fastigial nuclei and surrounding white matter in four animals subjected to hemilabyrinthectomy 1, 2 or 3 months previously and fully compensated produced marked imbalance during walking and a tremor of the head during feeding. These signs subsided very gradually.

Effect of interrupting transreticular and transcerebellar crossed pathways linking bilateral vestibular nuclei

Destruction of the vermis, fastigial nuclei and the transreticular crossed connections between bilateral vestibular nuclei (Fig. 7) in six animals hemilabyrinthectomized 2 to 6 months previously and fully compensated produced tilting of the head toward the hemilabyrinthectomized side. These animals showed severe motor disturbances during standing, walking and feeding and in fact were almost unable to stand and walk. A very pronounced head tremor was observed in all animals. This tremor subsided when the animal was at rest, but was always present during feeding. The severe motor disturbance did not abate during the 2- to 6-month observation period.

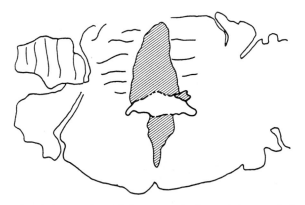

Fig. 7. Destruction of the transreticular and transcerebellar crossed connections between bilateral vestibular nuclei: line drawing of histological section of the brainstem and cerebellum showing the lesion (shaded area).

Discussion

Rates of local glucose utilization in the cat vary over a wide range as found in the rat [19]. The values found in the gray matter were generally three to five times those found in the white matter. The components of the auditory system are metabolically the most active structures of the brain with the highest rate of glucose utilization in the inferior colliculus, similarly found in the rat.

The values for LCGU in the intact unanaesthetized cat were considerably below those observed in the rat, and were almost identical to those obtained in the monkey [20].

In the critical stage, two hours after hemilabyrinthectomy, glucose utilization in the deafferented vestibular complex (62%) was well below that of the intact side. This is consistent with electrophysiological findings of decreased spontaneous activity following acute peripheral vestibular lesion [4, 7, 10, 11, 25]. Increased activities were seen in nucl. reticularis parvocellularis, the ventral part of abducens nucleus, the posterior vermis, and the noduloflocular lobe. These changes in the rates of LCGU in particular regions could be related to the generation of a vestibular nystagmus and the marked abnormalities, and they could also be involved in the compensation processes. The value for the rate of glucose utilization in the flocculus was very high (121 μmol, 197% of the control value) in the uncompensated stage, but not so much in the compensatory stage. This result may indicate that the flocculus is required for initiating rather than maintaining the compensatory process following peripheral lesions. Courjon et al. [26] reported that normal cats submitted to hemilabyrinthectomy compensate from the effects of the lesion in about two months, whereas cats previously submitted to a hemiflocculectomy still present a very poor compensation 2-3 months after hemilabyrinthectomy.

Four weeks to ten months after hemilabyrinthectomy, i.e. during the compensatory stage, the rate of LCGU in the deafferented vestibular nuclei increased so as to equalize that of the intact side. In the compensatory stage of the vestibulo-ocular function, frequencies of spontaneous discharges of type I neurons on the destroyed side were still lower than those on the intact side [25]. A major question is to define the systems and mechanisms by which vestibular balance is restored. The reappearance of spontaneous discharges of type I neurons after degeneration of the main excitatory sensory input may be caused by biochemical sensitization of deafferented type I neurons or by sprouting of other afferent fibres such as those related to reticulovestibular connections which are clearly present in cats [27]. Dieringer and Precht [28] reported that neurons in the chronically but partially deafferented vestibular complex (hemilabyrinthectomized frogs) showed an increased excitability and an increased synaptic efficacy in commissural transmission. More recently, Galiana et al. [18] demonstrated that commissural pathways connecting the two sides of the brainstem represent a powerful putative site for adaptive modulation of the static characteristics of vestibular responses.

Our observations of behaviour in the present study showed that, in fully compensated cats, interruption of the vestibular crossed connections through reticular and cerebellar pathways [21, 22] resulted in tilting of the head toward the hemilabyrinthectomized side and severe motor disturbances during standing, walking and feeding. Bienhold and Flohr [29] reported similar observations after commissurectomy in fully compensated frogs. On the other hand, Smith et al. [30] studied the effects of the commissurectomy in the hemilabyrinthectomized guinea pigs with an intact cerebellum. They demonstrated that postural symptoms were compensated in the absence of the (transreticular) vestibular commissures. In the present study, the vermis, fastigial nuclei and surrounding white matter were aspirated to interrupt the transcerebellar inhibitory interaction between the bilateral vestibular nuclei. Thus, both the transreticular and transcerebellar crossed pathways linking the bilateral vestibular nuclei were interrupted. With only cerebellar lesions, vestibular compensation is greatly delayed when the vermis and fastigial nuclei are involved. Therefore, further study is required to determine

whether these cerebellar areas contribute to the overall system of crossed pathways linking the bilateral vestibular nuclei or whether they make another contribution to the compensatory process.

The compensatory stage is marked by increased activity in nucl. reticularis parvocellularis, gigantocellularis and lateralis, superior colliculus, posterior vermis, nodulus and cerebellar nuclei. This supports the hypothesis that vestibular compensation results from the combined activity of many brainstem and cerebellar structures. Following acute labyrinthine deafferentation the level of spontaneous activity in the vestibular nuclei is severely decreased and symmetry of function is lost. As the animal returns to normal functioning, there is a proportionate increase in activity in the deafferented vestibular nucleus and in other structures. In vestibular compensation, input from the intact labyrinth may contribute to this reconstruction, and information derived from other sensory system may also be important. Information from muscle, joint and cutaneous afferents would first be integrated in brainstem nuclei, and then process to the vestibular and cerebellar nuclei [5]. Descending inputs from the cerebral cortex and visual centres including the visuotectal system would influence the activity of vestibular neurons as well. According to Putkonen et al. [31], static visual input is a necessary condition for compensation of the postural deficits of hemilabyrinthectomy in the cat. Maintenance of stable head position also depends upon continuous availability of visual input. All of these systems may modulate the output of vestibular neurons by increasing activity in such a way as to correct for the postural and oculomotor abnormalities.

References

[1] Fluur, E. (1960) Vestibular compensation after labyrinthine destruction. *Acta Otolaryngol. Stockholm*, 52: 367–375.
[2] Pfaltz, C.R. and Kamath, R. (1970) Central compensation of vestibular dysfunction. I. Peripheral lesions. *Pract. Otorhinolaryngol.*, 32: 335–349.
[3] Bechterew, W. (1883) Ergebnisse der Durchaschneidung des N. acusticus, nebst Erörterung der Bedeutung der semicirculären Canäle für des Karpergleichgewicht. *Pflüger's Arch.*, 30: 312–347.

[4] McCabe, B.F. and Ryu, J.H. (1969) Experiments on vestibular compensation. *Laryngoscope*, 79: 1728–1736.

[5] Llinas, R. and Walton, K. (1979) Vestibular compensation: a distributed property of the central nervous system. In H. Asanuma and V.I. Wilson (Eds.), *Integration in the Nervous System*, Igaku-shoin, Tokyo. pp. 145–166.

[6] Jensen, D.W. (1979) Vestibular compensation: tonic spinal influence upon spontaneous descending vestibular nuclear activity. *Neuroscience*, 4: 1075–1084.

[7] Gernandt, B.E. and Thulin, L.H. (1952) Vestibular connections of the brainstem. *Am. J. Physiol.*, 171: 121–127.

[8] McCabe, B.F., Ryu, J.H. and Sekitani, T. (1972) Further experiments on vestibular compensation. *Laryngoscope*, 82: 381–396.

[9] Precht, W. (1974) Characteristics of vestibular neurons after acute and chronic labyrinthine destruction. In H.H. Kornhuber (Ed.), *Handbook of Sensory Physiology, Vol. 6(1), Vestibular Mechanisms*, Springer, Berlin, pp. 451–462.

[10] Xerri, C., Gianni, S., Manzoni, D. and Pompeiano, O. (1983) Central compensation of vestibular deficits. I. Response characteristics of lateral vestibular neurons to roll tilt after ipsilateral labyrinth deafferentation. *J. Neurophysiol.*, 50: 428–448.

[11] Pompeiano, O., Xerri, C., Gianni, S. and Manzoni, D. (1984) Central compensation of vestibular deficits. II. Influences of roll tilt on different-size lateral vestibular neurons after ipsilateral labyrinth deafferentation. *J. Neurophysiol.*, 52: 18–38.

[12] Lacour, M., Manzoni, D., Pompeiano, O. and Xerri, C. (1985) Central compensation of vestibular deficits. III. Response characteristics of lateral vestibular neurons to roll tilt after contralateral labyrinth deafferentation. *J. Neurophysiol.*, 54: 988–1005.

[13] Azzena, G.B. (1969) Role of the spinal cord in compensating the effects of hemilabyrinthectomy. *Arch. Ital. Biol.*, 107: 43–53.

[14] Schaefer, K.P. and Meyer, D.L. (1973) Compensatory mechanisms following labyrinth lesions in guinea pigs. A simple model of learning. In H.P. Zippel (Ed.), *Memory and Transfer of Information*, Plenum, New York, pp. 203–232.

[15] Schaefer, K.P. and Meyer, D.L. (1981) Aspects of vestibular compensation in guinea pigs. In H. Flohr and W. Precht (Eds.), *Lesion-Induced Neuronal Plasticity in Sensorymotor systems*. Springer, Berlin, pp. 197–205.

[16] Carpenter, M.B., Fabrega, H. and Glinsman, W. (1959) Physiological deficits occuring with lesions of labyrinth and fastigial nuclei. *J. Neurophysiol.*, 22: 222–234.

[17] Lacour, M., Roll, J.J.P. and Appaix, M. (1976) Modification and development of spinal reflexes in the alert baboon (*Papio papio*) following a unilateral vestibular neurotomy. *Brain Res.*, 113: 255–269.

[18] Galiana, H.L., Flohr, H. and Melvill Jones, G. (1984) A reevaluation of intervestibular nuclear coupling: Its role in vestibular compensation. *J. Neurophysiol.*, 51: 242–259.

[19] Sokoloff, L., Reivich, M., Kennedy, C., Des Rosier, M.H., Patlak, C.S., Pettigrew, K.D., Sakurada, O. and Shinohara, M. (1977) The [^{14}C]deoxyglucose method for the measurement of local cerebral glucose utilization: theory, procedure, and normal value in the conscious and anesthetized albino rat. *J. Neurochem.*, 28: 897–916.

[20] Sokoloff, L. (1978) Mapping cerebral function activity with radioactive deoxyglucose. *Trends Neurosci.*, 1: 75–79.

[21] Shimazu, H. and Precht, W. (1966) Inhibition of central vestibular neurons from the contralateral labyrinth and its mediating pathway. *J. Neurophysiol.*, 29: 467–492.

[22] Furuya, N., Kawano, K. and Shimazu, H. (1976) Transcerebellar inhibitory interaction between bilateral vestibular nuclei and its modulation by cerebellocortical activity. *Exp. Brain Res.*, 25: 447–463.

[23] Maeda, M., Miyaoka, M., Ito, E. and Ishii, S. (1985) Local cerebral glucose utilization in the hemilabyrinthectomized cat during uncompensated and compensated stages. *J. Cerebral Blood Flow Metab.*, 5: s215–s216.

[24] Maeda, M., Shibazaki, T. and Yoshida, K. (1979) Labyrinthine and visual inputs to the superior colliculus neurons. In R. Granit and O. Pompeiano (Eds.), *Reflex Control of Posture and Movement, Progress in Brain Research, Vol. 50*, Elsevier, Amsterdam, pp. 735–743.

[25] Precht, W., Shimazu, H. and Markham, C.H. (1966) A mechanism of central compensation of vestibular function following hemilabyrinthectomy. *J. Neurophysiol.*, 29: 996–1010.

[26] Courjon, J.H., Flandrin, J.M., Jeannerod, M. and Schmid, R. (1982) The role of the flocculus in vestibular compensation after hemilabyrinthectomy. *Brain Res.*, 239: 251–257.

[27] Pompeiano, O., Mergner, T. and Corvaya, N. (1978) Commissural, perihypoglossal and reticular afferent projection to the vestibular nuclei in the cat. An experimental anatomical study with the method of the retrograde transport of horseradish peroxidase. *Arch. Ital. Biol.*, 116: 130–172.

[28] Dieringer, N. and Precht, W. (1977) Modification of synaptic input following unilateral labyrinthectomy. *Nature*, 269: 431–433.

[29] Bienhold, H. and Flohr, H. (1978) Role of commissural connections between vestibular nuclei in compensation following unilateral labyrinthectomy. *J. Physiol. London*, 284: 178.

[30] Smith, P.F., Darlington, C.L. and Curthoys, I.S. (1986) Vestibular compensation without brainstem commissures in the guinea pig. *Neurosci. Lett.*, 65: 209–213.

[31] Putkonen, P.T.S., Courjon, J.H. and Jeannerod, M. (1977) Compensation of postural effects of hemilabyrinthectomy in the cat. A sensory substitution process? *Exp. Brain Res.*, 28: 249–257.

O. Pompeiano and J.H.J. Allum (Eds.)
Progress in Brain Research, Vol. 76
© 1988 Elsevier Science Publishers B.V. (Biomedical Division)

CHAPTER 34

Physical exercise and balance compensation after total ablation of vestibular organs

M. Igarashi, K. Ishikawa, M. Ishii and H. Yamane

Department of Otorhinolaryngology and Communicative Sciences, Baylor College of Medicine, One Baylor Plaza, Houston, TX 77030-3498, U.S.A.

Unlike the situation after UL, squirrel monkeys after two-stage BL exhibited an extreme difficulty in regaining the pre-lesion level of locomotor balance function (as tested in the task of behaviourally trained overground straight-line running; the squirrel monkey platform runway test), in contrast to the rapid oculomotor balance compensation (i.e. reduction of spontaneous nystagmus). Nonetheless, the enhancement from the application of physical exercise was significant, and all exercised animals eventually (even though after a long time) achieved the pre-lesion level of locomotor balance function.

Introduction

For vestibular compensation, it is known that sensory inputs from various modalities must be mobilized and integrated so that sufficient sensory–motor homeostasis can be achieved. In our previous study [17], it was documented that behaviourally trained squirrel monkeys failed to re-attain their capability to traverse a rotating rail ('squirrel monkey rail test') even 190 days after BL. The necessity of vestibular organs for such an advanced form of dynamic equilibrium function, which requires good sensory–motor coordination with good goal-directed navigation, was thus established. Accordingly, the first objective of this behavioural study was to examine how postBL squirrel monkeys perform a task of an overground straight-line run [19], which

requires less agility and skill, and how much balance function can be regained eventually.

The effectiveness of physical exercise application to patients after labyrinthine injury has been known empirically [7, 9]. A series of squirrel monkey studies has demonstrated the positive effect of physical exercise application following UL [20, 22, 23]. As the second objective of this study, the effectiveness of the application of physical exercise in conjunction with (two-stage) BL was evaluated in squirrel monkeys by characterizing the locomotor balance and oculomotor balance functions.

Methods

In order to measure the extent and direction of gait deviation during a straight overground run, the squirrel monkey platform runway test was used [19]. Squirrel monkeys (*Saimiri sciureus*) of both genders, of approximately 2 years of age (adults) and weighing about 700 grams were used. Three animals each were assigned to the exercise (E) and control (C) groups. When the animals reached the pre-operative performance criterion of locomotor balance function, the animals in the E group were given, after daily runway test, voluntary running exercise [23] for three months. The cumulative time for daily exercise was three hours, in the mode of

---

Abbreviations: ACTH, adrenocorticotropic hormone; BL, bilateral labyrinthectomy; POC, postoperative criterion day; SN, spontaneous nystagmus; SPEV, slow-phase eye velocity; UL, unilateral labyrinthectomy.

minute runs and 2.5 minute rest periods in a motor-driven rotating cage. The animals in the C group received no exercise, but were tested following the same schedule.

Thereafter, all animals underwent UL. Postoperatively the animals in the E group continually received exercise for another three month period, even though they regained locomotor balance compensation earlier. The animals in the C group received no exercise, but were tested in the same way. Postoperatively, in addition to the analysis of total deviation counts, the first calendar day when the animal reached the pre-operative performance level was termed the postoperative criterion day 1 (POC-1). The calendar day when the animal achieved eight uninterrupted trial days with such a performance level was termed the postoperative criterion day 2 (POC-2). The tests were continued until the end of three months.

Then, all the animals underwent contralateral labyrinthectomy (now BL). Thereafter, both groups were treated in an exactly identical way to the post-UL condition. The test continued for as long as 300 days postoperatively.

The horizontal SN was recorded in the dark for three minutes basically every other day, prior to the platform runway test, through a standard DC electronystagmography, and the daily maximum SPEV was manually calculated. The eye speed calibration was done using the pre-operative optokinetic nystagmus, evoked by a 30°/s stimulus.

For statistical comparison, locomotor deviation counts (data from 28 postoperative days) and SPEVs of SN were analysed by two-way analysis of variance. The t-test was also used to compare the time constants of the decays of these two functions.

At the end of all functional data acquisition, the animals were perfused transcardially and the temporal bones were processed in celloidin for histological examination.

Results

Locomotor balance function

After UL, the averaged number of days to reach the POC-1 in the E and C groups was 7.3 and 13.7, respectively (nonsignificant difference). Regarding the POC-2, the E group showed significantly faster acquisition ($p < 0.005$). When the number of days between POC-1 and POC-2 were compared, the difference was also significant ($p < 0.01$). The results suggested that the application of exercise could contribute more to test-to-test performance stability. When the SPEVs of SN on the POC-2 days were compared between the groups, the difference was significant ($p < 0.01$). Thus, in the C group, even on such later days, the animals still had SN with high SPEV.

When the total deviation counts were compared between the groups, a significant difference ($p < 0.05$) was found. Moreover, the time constants of decay functions showed a statistically significant difference between the groups ($p < 0.05$).

After BL, all monkeys showed severe difficulty in regaining locomotor balance (Fig. 1). Large variabilities indicated the existence of a variable degree of dysequilibrium. However, both in the total deviation counts and the time constants of deviation decay functions, the statistical analysis showed a significant difference between the two groups

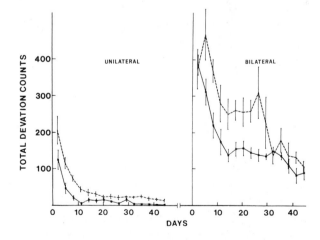

Fig. 1. Graphic displays of total deviation counts (3 days pooled data, for 7 weeks) after unilateral and two-staged bilateral labyrinthectomy, measured by squirrel monkey platform runway test. Solid line, exercise group; dashed line, control group. Error bars: ± SEM.

($p<0.05$). On the other hand, to reach POC-1, an average of 62 days was needed for the E group, and 81 days for the C group (no significant difference). To achieve POC-2, it took an average of 118 days for the E group. In the C group, one animal could not reach the POC-2 level even 300 days after BL, while two other animals needed 126 and 168 days, respectively.

Spontaneous nystagmus

When the number of days after UL before SPEV of SN reached the level of 10°/s were compared between two groups, a significant difference was found ($p<0.05$). The average was 12.3 for the E group, and 55.0 for the C group. When the time constants of SPEV decay functions were compared, the difference was also statistically significant ($p<0.05$). This finding indicated that the E group required less time in reducing SPEV to a set lower SPEV level. This result agrees with that in our previous exercise study [20].

In both groups, the initial SPEVs of SN after BL were low and reached to the lower SPEV level faster than those after UL (Fig. 2). The across-subject variability of SPEV was similar in the two groups, and

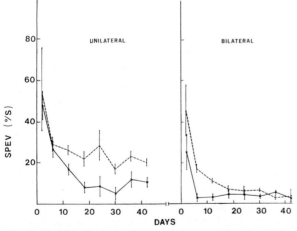

Fig. 2. Graphic displays of slow phase eye velocities (°/s) of spontaneous nystagmus (6 days pooled data, except for the first postoperative points: 2 days pooled data, for 7 weeks) after unilateral and two-staged bilateral labyrinthectomy. Solid line, exercise group; dashed line, control group. Error bars = ± SEM.

it was less than that after UL. After BL, the average number of days to reach the 10°/s level was 4.3 for the E group and 12.5 for the C group, respectively; however, there was no statistically significant difference. Also, when the time constants of SPEV decays were analysed, the difference between the two groups was not significant. Unlike the situation of locomotor balance, the application of physical exercise after BL did not produce a clear positive effect on oculomotor balance compensation. This could be due to the low initial SPEVs and relatively fast achievement of the lower levels in both groups.

The completeness of labyrinthectomy was histologically confirmed in all animals.

Discussion

PostBL compensation

In the present study, five of six animals regained the pre-operative performance level of locomotor balance function (measured by the squirrel monkey platform runway test), requiring a long time after BL, but one animal in the C group failed to reattain that level during the 300-day postBL investigation. Even in the postUL situation, in addition to the commissural pathways, the inputs of other neural channels are needed for behavioural improvement.

The postBL situation is highly complex and even though the animals make possible adjustments in behavioural strategies [44], the functional balance compensation in the present test was not easy. However, when the EMG responses from the soleus and tibialis anterior muscles were studied in baboons after bilateral (two-stage) vestibular neurectomy, Bechterew's compensation was found [31]. In the earlier study using the squirrel monkey rail test [17], which required more skilled sensory–motor coordination, no animal could perform the balance task after BL. The difference is obviously based on the different task difficulty, but at the same time, the primacy of characteristics of vestibular afferents for skilled locomotor balance function and spatial (goal-directed) navigation was confirmed. Unlike the postBL condition however, after two-stage bilateral utriculosacculectomy, the squirrel monkeys could eventually regain skilled locomotor balance function [21], thus indicating the sufficiency of semicircular canal afferents for such a balance function.

One of the factors to decide the severity of imbalance and the time required for compensation after BL is the interval between the UL and BL. When Schaefer and Meyer [42] performed bilateral lesions in guinea pigs with an interval of 3 days, neither the head nor the body showed symptoms, but Bechterew's nystagmus was evident. As was found in the present study, eye nystagmus and body imbalance were compensated following different time courses after UL. In the present series of experiments, the two labyrinthectomies were spaced by three months. By the time of the second labyrinthectomy, both the oculomotor balance and locomotor balance were therefore already normal.

Graybiel and Fregly [15] reported that labyrinthine defective human subjects showed poor scores in quantitative ataxia test batteries. In unconditioned squirrel monkeys, due to their active movements, measures of asymmetry such as head deviation are not reliable and quantification is not possible. The behaviourally conditioned locomotor balance test has many advantages and is a reliable way to quantify the system imbalance. In the present study, even though the reduction of horizontal SN after BL was relatively fast, oscillopsia during head movement could influence the compensation of locomotor balance. However, the potentiation of the cervico-oculomotor reflex during active movement takes place simultaneously through the central modulation, and may be a surrogate, at least partially, for an absent vestibulo-oculomotor reflex [8, 28, 47]. According to Dichgans et al. [10] following bilateral vestibulectomy in monkeys, the recovery of compensatory eye movement reached 90% within 7 weeks but only during active head movements.

Deoxyglucose activity has been reported to exhibit a close correlation with functional recovery after unilateral lesion [33, 37]. During Bechterew's compensation, deoxyglucose activity was reduced in the bilateral vestibular nuclei, with a slightly higher activity on the first labyrinthectomy side. When the Bechterew effect had disappeared, the deoxyglucose activity of both sides remained low [32]. This low-level activity of bilateral vestibular nuclei could be the reason for the poor recovery of locomotor balance function and the low SPEV of SN.

Effect of physical exercise

The positive effect of physical exercise on vestibular compensation after BL should be delivered through the spinal ascending system, visual system, etc. Other factors, such as an increase in muscle strength, metabolic activity, alertness, etc. are also involved. The reduction of locomotor deviations after BL was much slower than that after UL. However, even in this situation, physical exercise contributed significantly.

Regarding the spinal ascending influence, the existence of arthrokinetic nystagmus indicates a convergence of the vestibulo-oculomotor system and somatosensory afferents from joint receptors [6]. According to Pompeiano [38] the joint receptors play a prominent role in supplying postural information to the vestibular nuclei. Precht [41] also indicated that many vestibular neurons are influenced (mainly excitatorily) by stimulation of the spinal cord. Thus, there is ample physiological evidence of spinal ascending influences to the vestibular nuclei.

The role of cervical ascending input for the maintenance of body equilibrium has been exhibited in the squirrel monkey model. After the unilateral removal of C1, C2 dorsal root ganglia, gait asymmetry and spontaneous nystagmus were manifested [16, 18]. The imbalance could be due to ipsilateral extensor hypertonia plus contralateral extensor hypotonia derived through uncrossed and crossed spino–reticulo–cerebello–vestibular connections [40].

Also, retardation of vestibular compensation or reappearance of imbalance after the elimination (or reduction) of spinal ascending input has indicated the importance of spinal afferents both in acquisition and maintenance of vestibular compensation [2, 3, 27, 30, 43].

Recovery of vestibulospinal descending function should be responsible for the recalibration of post-urokinetic functions [39]. The deiterospinal tract, which originates in the dorsal portion of lateral vestibular nucleus and delivers descending excitatory signals to the gamma extensor motoneurons, receives excitatory spinal inputs which come from the lumbosacral cord and hindlimbs. Therefore, the running-type exercise used in the present study should have a positive effect, activating the ascending neural connections to enforce compensation.

The activities of ascending spinal inputs projecting directly or indirectly to the deafferentated vestibular neurons increase with time. Dieringer et al. [12] performed an autoradiographic study in frogs by injecting L-methionine into the dorsal root ganglion, and showed that projections into the deafferentated vestibular nuclei were more dense than in control animals.

Among the various spinal ascending connections to the vestibular nuclei, the spino–reticulo–fastigial pathway could be important for global postural and locomotor function, whereas the spino–olivo–cerebellar cortex pathway could be important for refined coordination [4]. In any case, the cerebellum (with its connections to the inferior olive) is no doubt an important neural structure for sensory–motor recalibration, particularly for the balance function which requires accurate timing control, goal-oriented navigation, and motor pattern recognition. Our recent study on the postUL compensation of locomotor and oculomotor balance functions in the squirrel monkey showed evident retardation by the preplacement of cerebellar vermis lesions [24].

According to Amat et al. [1], unitary response recordings from the Purkinje cell layer of the cerebellum in frogs suggested that, after BL, spinal inputs substitute some of the vestibular inputs. The spinal ascending contribution to vestibular compensation may vary between species, but has been confirmed to be important in many species.

In order to re-establish the system balance, the nervous system must equalize the activity levels on the deafferentated side and intact side. Dieringer and Precht [11] reported that neurons in the deafferentated nucleus in chronic preparations had increased excitability. It was assumed that the connections to the vestibular neurons had formed synapses on the vacated soma of the deafferentated side. Indeed, Korte and Friedrich [29] reported a new type of synaptic boutons in the deafferentated superior vestibular nucleus of the cat, 5–6 days after the lesion. The neural sprouts can certainly facilitate the behavioural substitution [14]. Thus, vestibular compensation can be achieved by the actual structural repair; reactive synaptogenesis [5, 46].

But, even more importantly, the modified synaptic efficacy – deafferentation hypersensitivity, which could be based on proliferation of selective neurotransmitter receptors, changes in neurotransmitter synthesis and release, and changes in postsynaptic sensitivity – can mediate the recovery of sensorimotor functions [13, 34], especially in the early compensation stage. In any case, vestibular compensation appears to be enhanced by means of the active movement which provides an important signal for sensory–motor recalibration. From this viewpoint, physical exercise has a definite merit, and it could improve dynamic rearrangement of neurotransmitters at the vestibular nucleus level. Indeed, the dynamics of γ-aminobutyric acid-like immunoreactivity in lateral vestibular nuclei of squirrel monkeys after UL showed a close correlation with the locomotor balance recovery (acute phase) [45].

Visual input reaches the vestibular nucleus and modulates the outputs of vestibular neurons. The visual input, which is enforced by the moving exercise, should contribute to vestibular compensation. Indeed, increased visual dependency was reported when otolith organ afferents were altered in a microgravity environment. However, its importance may not be the same in different animal species, at different compensation stages or under different circumstances. Furthermore, it is not quite understood which element of visual input and what sort of visual enforcement effectively accelerates vestibular compensation.

Physical exercise can contribute in other ways,

e.g. by increasing muscle strength, the body's metabolic activity, alertness, etc. Musculoneural activity can be enhanced, particularly in the early stage of exercise [36]. Increases in regional muscular strength imply a musculoneural adaptation that is some form of motor learning; perhaps learning to disinhibit motor neurons [25, 35]. When training is given more chronically, the muscle's hypertrophic increase becomes more significant. This could be basically due to the hypertrophy of the nuclear chain fibre, which has both group 2 and group 1A afferents. In relation to physical training, the group 2 afferent may be the important one.

Undoubtedly, it is clinically important to utilize a noninvasive safe procedure to accelerate vestibular compensation. In this regard, neuropharmacological supplementation is certainly very useful. We have recently found a positive effect of $ACTH_{4-10}$ administration on Bechterew's compensation [26].

Through a series of squirrel monkey experiments, we evaluated a variety of physical exercise modes. Nonimpulsive, nonstressful but continual, easy moving and running types of exercise were found to be very effective for this purpose. Lastly, through the present experiment of vestibular compensation, we could confirm the significant contribution from the application of physical exercise even after the total loss of peripheral vestibular labyrinth.

Acknowledgements

This study was in part supported by NINCDS grant NS-10940 and NASA grant NAG-2-289. The authors would like to thank C. Castillo, J. Brown, S. MacDonald, J.K. Levy, K. Schmidt and S. Bonvillain for their technical assistance.

References

[1] Amat, J., Matus-Amat, P. and Vanegas, H. (1984) Visual (optokinetic) and somesthetic inputs to the cerebellum of bilaterally labyrinthectomized frogs. *Neuroscience*, 11: 885–891.

[2] Azzena, G.B. (1969) Role of the spinal cord in compensating the effects of labyrinthectomy. *Arch. Ital. Biol.*, 107: 43–53.

[3] Azzena, G.B., Mameli, O. and Tolu, E. (1976) Vestibular nuclei of hemilabyrinthectomized guinea pigs during decompensation. *Arch. Ital. Biol.*, 114: 389–398.

[4] Azzena, G.B., Tolu, E. and Mameli, O. (1981) The lateral reticular nucleus. Role in vestibular compensation. In H. Flohr and W. Precht (Eds.), *Lesion-Induced Neuronal Plasticity in Sensorimotor Systems*, Springer, Berlin, pp. 254–264.

[5] Bjorklund, A. and Stenevi, U. (1979) Regeneration of monoaminergic and cholinergic neurons in the mammalian central nervous system. *Physiol. Rev.*, 59: 62–100.

[6] Brandt, Th., Büchele, W. and Arnold, F. (1977) Arthrokinetic nystagmus and ego-motion sensation. *Exp. Brain Res.*, 30: 331–338.

[7] Cawthorne, T. (1946) Vestibular injuries. *Proc. R. Soc. Med.*, 39: 270–273.

[8] Chambers, B.R., Mai, M. and Barber, H.O. (1985) Bilateral vestibular loss, oscillopsia, and the cervico-ocular reflex. *Otolaryngol. Head Neck Surg.*, 93: 403–407, 1985.

[9] Cooksey, F.S. (1946) Rehabilitation in vestibular injuries. *Proc. R. Soc. Med.*, 39: 273–275.

[10] Dichgans, J., Bizzi, E., Morasso, P. and Tagliasco, V. (1973) Mechanisms underlying recovery of eye–head coordination following bilateral labyrinthectomy in monkeys. *Exp. Brain Res.*, 18: 548–562.

[11] Dieringer, N. and Precht, W. (1977) Modification of synaptic input following unilateral labyrinthectomy. *Nature*, 269: 421–433.

[12] Dieringer, N., Kunzle, H. and Precht, W. (1984) Increased projection of ascending dorsal root fibers to vestibular nuclei after hemilabyrinthectomy in the frog. *Exp. Brain Res.*, 55: 574–578.

[13] Flohr, H., Bienhold, H., Abeln, W. and Macskovics, I. (1981) Concepts of vestibular compensation. In H. Flohr and W. Precht (Eds.), *Lesion-Induced Neuronal Plasticity in Sensorimotor Systems*. Springer, Berlin, pp. 153–172.

[14] Goldberger, M.E. (1977) Locomotor recovery after unilateral hindlimb deafferentation in cats. *Brain Res.*, 123: 59–74.

[15] Graybiel, A. and Fregly, A.R. (1966) A new quantitative ataxia test battery. *Acta Otolaryngol. Stockholm*, 61: 292–312.

[16] Igarashi, M., Alford, B.R., Watanabe, T. and Maxian, P.M. (1969) Role of neck proprioceptors for the maintenance of dynamic bodily equilibrium in the squirrel monkey. *Laryngoscope*, 79: 1713–1727.

[17] Igarashi, M., Watanabe, T. and Maxian, P.M. (1970) Dynamic equilibrium in squirrel monkeys after unilateral and bilateral labyrinthectomy. *Acta Otolaryngol. Stockholm*, 69: 247–253.

[18] Igarashi, M., Miyata, H., Alford, B.R. and Wright, W.K. (1972) Nystagmus after experimental cervical lesions. *Laryngoscope*, 82: 1609–1621.

[19] Igarashi, M. (1974) Squirrel monkey platform runway test – a preliminary report. *Acta Otolaryngol. Stockholm*, 77: 284–288.

[20] Igarashi, M., Alford, B.R., Kato, Y. and Levy, J.K. (1975) Effect of physical exercise upon nystagmus and locomotor dysequilibrium after labyrinthectomy in experimental pri-

mates. *Acta Otolaryngol. Stockholm*, 79: 214–220.

[21] Igarashi, M., Levy, J.K., Kubo, T. and Matsunaga, T. (1978) Effect of otolith deafferentation on physically advanced locomotor performance in the squirrel monkey. *Otorhinolaryngology*, 40: 226–232.

[22] Igarashi, M., Levy, J.K., Takahashi, M., Alford, B.R. and Homick, J.L. (1979) Effect of exercise upon locomotor balance modification after peripheral vestibular lesions (unilateral utricular neurotomy) in squirrel monkey. *Adv. Otorhinolaryngol.*, 25: 82–87.

[23] Igarashi, M., Levy, J.K., O-Uchi, T. and Reschke, M.F. (1981) Further study of physical exercise and locomotor balance compensation after unilateral labyrinthectomy in squirrel monkeys. *Acta Otolaryngol. Stockholm*, 92: 101–105.

[24] Igarashi, M. and Ishikawa, K. (1985) Post-labyrinthectomy balance compensation with preplacement of cerebellar vermis lesion. *Acta Otolaryngol. Stockholm*, 99: 452–458.

[25] Ikai, M. and Steinhaus, A.H. (1961) Some factors modifying the expression of human strength, *J. Appl. Physiol.*, 16: 157–163.

[26] Ishii, M. and Igarashi, M. (1987) Effect of ACTH(4–10) on Bechterew's compensation in squirrel monkeys. *Otorhinolaryngology*, 49: 87–92.

[27] Jensen, D.W. (1979) Vestibular compensation: tonic spinal influence upon spontaneous descending vestibular nuclear activity. *Neuroscience*, 4: 1075–1084.

[28] Kasai, T. and Zee, D.S. (1978) Eye–head coordination in labyrinthine-defective human beings. *Brain Res.*, 144: 123–141.

[29] Korte, G.A. and Friedrich, V.L. Jr. (1979) The fine structure of the feline superior vestibular nucleus: identification and synaptology of the primary vestibular afferents. *Brain Res.*, 176: 3–32.

[30] Lacour, M., Roll, J.P. and Appaix, M. (1976) Modifications and development of spinal reflexes in the alert baboon (*Papio papio*) following an unilateral vestibular neurotomy. *Brain Res.*, 113: 255–269.

[31] Lacour, M., Xerri, C. and Hugon, M.B. (1979) Compensation of postural reactions to fall in the vestibular neurectomized monkey. Role of the remaining labyrinthine afferences. *Exp. Brain Res.*, 37: 563–580.

[32] Llinas, R. and Walton, K. (1979) Vestibular compensation. In H. Asanuma and V.J. Wilson (Eds.), *Integration in the Nervous System*, Igaku-Shoin, Tokyo, pp. 145–166.

[33] Luyten, W.H.M.L., Sharp, F.R. and Ryan, A.F. (1986) Regional differences of brain glucose metabolic compensation after unilateral labyrinthectomy in rats: a [14C]2-deoxyglucose study. *Brain Res.*, 373: 68–80.

[34] Marshall, J.F. (1984) Brain function: neural adaptations and recovery from injury. *Annu. Rev. Psychol.*, 35: 277–308.

[35] Maynard, J.A. and Tipton, C.M. (1971) The effects of exercise training and denervation on the morphology of intrafusal muscle fibres. *Int. Z. Angew. Physiol.*, 30: 1–9.

[36] Moritani, T. and deVries, H.A. (1979) Neural factors versus hypertrophy in the time course of muscle stretch gain. *Am. J. Phys. Med.*, 58: 115–130.

[37] Patrickson, J.W., Bryant, H.J., Kaderkaro, M. and Kutyna, F.A. (1985) A quantitative [14C]-2-deoxy-D-glucose study of brain stem nuclei during horizontal nystagmus induced by lesioning the lateral crista ampullaris of the rat. *Exp. Brain Res.*, 60: 227–234.

[38] Pompeiano, O. (1972) Spino-vestibular relations. Anatomical and physiological aspects. In A. Brodal and O. Pompeiano (Eds.), *Basic Aspects of Central Vestibular Mechanisms*, Elsevier, Amsterdam, pp. 263–296.

[39] Pompeiano, O., Xerri, C., Gianni, S. and Manzoni, D. (1984) Central compensation of vestibular deficits. II. Influences of roll tilt on different-size lateral vestibular neurons after ipsilateral labyrinth deafferentation. *J. Neurophysiol.*, 52: 18–38.

[40] Pompeiano, O. (1985) Experimental central nervous system lesions and posture. In M. Igarashi and F.O. Black (Eds.), *Vestibular and Visual Control on Posture and Locomotor Equilibrium*, Karger, Basel, pp. 218–231.

[41] Precht, W. (1974) The physiology of the vestibular nuclei. In H.H. Kornhuber (Ed.), *Handbook of Sensory Physiology, Vol. VI (2), Vestibular System, Part 1*, Springer, Berlin, pp. 353–412.

[42] Schaefer, K.P. and Meyer, D.L. (1974) Compensation of vestibular lesions. In H.H. Kornhuber (Ed.), *Handbook of Sensory Physiology, Vol. VI (2), Vestibular System, Part 1*, Springer, Berlin, pp. 463–490.

[43] Schaefer, K.P. and Meyer, D.L. (1981) Aspects of vestibular compensation in guinea pigs. In H. Flohr and W. Precht (Eds.), *Lesion-Induced Neuronal Plasticity in Sensorimotor Systems*, Springer, Berlin, pp. 197–207.

[44] Stein, D.G. (1983) Brain damage and recovery: problems and perspectives. *Behav. Neural Biol.*, 37: 185–222.

[45] Thompson, G.C., Igarashi, M. and Cortez, A.M. (1986) GABA imbalance in squirrel monkey after unilateral vestibular end-organ ablation. *Brain Res.*, 370: 182–185.

[46] Tsukahara, N. (1981) Synaptic plasticity in the mammalian central nervous system. *Annu. Rev. Neurosci.*, 4: 351–379.

[47] Xerri, C., Gianni, S., Manzoni, D. and Pompeiano, O. (1983) Central compensation of vestibular deficits. I. Response characteristics of lateral vestibular neurons to roll tilt after ipsilateral labyrinth deafferentation. *J. Neurophysiol.*, 50: 428–448.

O. Pompeiano and J.H.J. Allum (Eds.)
Progress in Brain Research, Vol. 76
© 1988 Elsevier Science Publishers B.V. (Biomedical Division)

CHAPTER 35

Immediate saccadic substitution for deficits in dynamic vestibular reflexes of frogs with selective peripheral lesions

N. Dieringer*

Institut für Hirnforschung, Universität Zürich, August-Forel Strasse 1, CH-8029 Zürich, Switzerland

Immediately after the section of one horizontal canal nerve compensatory head movements in the horizontal plane are unidirectional in the dark but symmetrical in amplitude in the light. Responses towards the 'weak' (intact) side are saccadic. These head saccades are accompanied by smaller ocular quick phases in the opposite direction. Both head saccades and ocular quick phases are still present even after a bilateral section of the horizontal canal nerves or after removal of both labyrinths. The main sequences of eye–head quick phases and of head saccades are very similar in intact and bilaterally lesioned frogs, indicating that vestibulo-ocular and vestibulocollic reflexes must be suppressed during these fast head movements. The occurrence of these head saccades depends on head-velocity-related proprioceptive signals. This input is facilitated after section of the horizontal canal nerve. Head saccades supplement weak but unaltered optokinetic reflexes at higher frequencies to an extent that compensatory head movements in response to sinusoidal table oscillations are symmetrical in spite of acute unilateral reflex deficits. In some of the chronic hemilabyrinthectomized frogs the vestibulocollic reflexes recovered to an extent that the head slow phase was fast enough to trigger head saccades even in the dark.

Introduction

The recovery from functional deficits as observed after the removal of the labyrinthine organs on one side has attracted the interest of neurobiologists ever since the first observations by von Bechterew [22]. With the progress in neurobiology, particularly in the field of vestibular and ocular motor research, this model for sensory–motor adaptation became even more attractive. The gap between sensory input and motor output appears to be small enough for a successful search for changes in the neuronal substrate underlying the observed behavioural plasticity. However, the 'vestibular lesion syndrome' represents the sum of different symptoms that result from the loss of receptors from different sensory organs with different central organizations. This multitude of deficits might be paralleled by a similar multitude of adaptive processes. Even more complicated, 'repair' for a well-defined single deficit such as posture may, for example, conceivably activate a number of different processes each of which contributes a certain aspect to the overall improvement. A reduction of the number of deficits by more restricted lesions is therefore indicated. In frogs the nerve branches to the individual receptor organs in the inner ear can be sectioned selectively under visual control. With this approach it has been shown that the characteristic postural deficits after hemilabyrinthectomy result from the removal of resting activity from the utricular macula [18].

Animals with the HCN sectioned on one side exhibit no postural deficits. This absence of a distorted neck and a concomitant misalignment of the canals on the intact side allows one to study the def-

Present address: Physiologisches Institut, Universität München, Pettenkoferstrasse 12, D-8000 München 2, F.R.G.
Abbreviation: HCN, horizontal canal nerve

404

icits in the dynamics of the horizontal vestibular reflexes in unrestrained frogs directly after the lesion. Data from animals in an acute stage are a prerequisite for an assessment of the functional recovery at later stages. Only in this way is it possible to distinguish between immediate and more time-consuming recovery processes. Studies employing unrestrained animals are of particular relevance. In this situation, the animal is able to use all sensory cues still available and to express whichever of the available subsystems it has actually selected for a substitution. The most conspicuous symptom for a deficit in the dynamic reflexes after hemilabyrinthectomy in frogs is the jerkyness of head movements in the horizontal plane. This disturbance appears about 6–10 days after the operation whenever the animal is oscillated in the light towards the side of the lesion [8,10]. In the following chapter these jerks will be described in more detail in animals with an acute section of the right HCN. Three aspects will be emphasized: (1) head jerks represent true saccades; (2) head saccades result from an unmasked somatosensory input; and (3) head saccades substitute for deficient vestibular reflexes.

Plane-specific head saccades

Compensatory movements of head and gaze (eye in space) were recorded with search coils in a rotating magnetic field by a system based on the phase-detection principle [15]. Electronic subtraction of head movement signals from those of gaze showed the contribution of the eyes. Compensatory movements were evoked by oscillations of a turntable at 0.2 Hz in front of a stationary contrast-rich visual background or in complete darkness. Animals (*Rana temporaria*) were confined to a transparent plexiglass cylinder [9]. Frogs with one horizontal canal nerve sectioned (HCN; here always on the right side) exhibit a normal head and body posture. Compensatory head movements in the horizontal plane are almost unidirectional in the dark (Fig. 1). In the light, larger compensatory head movements are symmetrical in amplitude but jerky (Fig. 1).

These jerks can be present immediately after re-

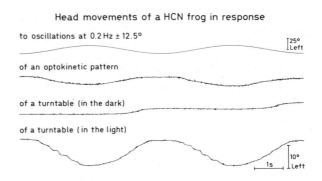

Head movements of a HCN frog in response
to oscillations at 0.2 Hz ± 12.5°

of an optokinetic pattern

of a turntable (in the dark)

of a turntable (in the light)

Fig. 1. Evoked horizontal head movements of a frog with the right horizontal canal nerve sectioned one day before the experiment. The top trace represents a stimulus the direction of which is opposite for pattern and turntable movements.

covery from anaesthesia (less than 1 hour) whenever the lesion involves the horizontal canal nerve or whenever the lumen of this canal is plugged. After the removal of the labyrinthine organs on either side or after sections of the bilateral horizontal canal nerves movements to either side are jerky. However, after a transsection of an anterior or a posterior canal nerve, the utricular or saccular nerve, compensatory head movements in the horizontal plane are smooth, as in intact animals. These results exclude mechanical factors (due to the tilted head posture in hemilabyrinthectomized frogs) or a central interaction of vestibular signals elicited by the turntable and by the abrupt onset of compensatory head movements as a possible origin. Obviously visually driven 'catch up' saccades would be a more likely candidate. The possibility that the jerks represent a sequence of saccades and not a sequence of interruptions of a continuous smooth movement was further studied in animals with both horizontal canal nerves cut.

Head saccades can be assumed to belong to the same class of fast movements as head quick phases. Accordingly, parametric features similar to those already described for head quick phases, i.e. amplitude-dependent peak velocities and amplitude-independent duration [11] may be expected for head saccades. To test these assumptions, resetting head quick phases and head jerks (in the direction of the concomitant slow phase) were evoked by a constant-velocity table rotation (7.5°/s) in front of a patterned visual background. Data from intact and operated frogs (either both horizontal canal nerves sectioned or bilaterally the labyrinthine organs removed) were stored on a computer for later off-line analysis.

The peak velocity of head quick phases of controls increased with amplitude by 5.6°/s per degree in this study and by 6.6°/s per degree in an earlier study [11]. In bilateral HCN frogs peak velocity increased very similarly by 6.4°/s per degree. The duration of these head quick phases was about 200 ms and in both HCN frogs and controls was only slightly dependent on amplitude. These results indicate that vestibulocollic reflexes of intact frogs must be completely suppressed during head quick phases. Most of them reach peak accelerations between 1000 and 3000°/s². The peak velocity of head 'jerks' of controls and of HCN frogs increased with 7.4 and 7.0°/s per degree respectively and the duration was again only slightly amplitude dependent. These similarities in the parameters between head quick phases and head jerks strongly suggest that the observed fast head movements in the direction of the compensatory slow phase are indeed saccades.

Each of these head saccades is accompanied by an ocular quick phase in controls [7], in unilateral (Figs. 2 and 3) and in bilateral HCN, as in bilaterally labyrinthectomized frogs. Therefore, these fast eye movements cannot represent simple vestibulo-ocular reflex responses, even though their onset is delayed by about 20 ms with respect to the onset of a head saccade. This delay is, on the other hand, too short for a visual trigger. It is therefore concluded that these ocular quick phases are coupled to head saccades by a central program. This conclusion is supported by the fact that the peak velocity of these fast eye movements increased similarly with amplitude in controls as in lesioned frogs by 13.5 and 10.2°/s per degree, respectively. These values are again very similar to those measured for ocular quick phases during nystagmus (10°/s per degree).

Release from dynamic vestibular inhibition

The occurrence of these head saccades did not depend on head position but on head velocity. Compensatory slow-phase head movements below 3°/s are as smooth as in controls even though a considerable retinal image slip may exist. The number of these saccades per half cycle increased with an in-

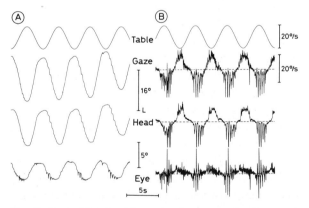

Fig. 2. Evoked horizontal eye–head movements of an acute HCN frog (right horizontal canal nerve sectioned) in response to table oscillation in the light. (A) Simultaneous position records of gaze (eye in space), head and eye (in head). (B) Velocity records of the same responses as in A. Dashed lines indicate zero velocity. Note the saccadic nature of movements towards the left (L).

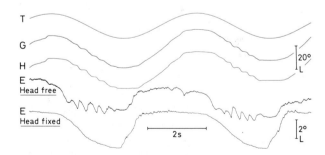

Fig. 3. Evoked horizontal eye–head movements of a HCN frog (right horizontal canal nerve sectioned). Responses were evoked by oscillations of a turntable (T) in the light. After the movements of gaze (G), head (H) and eye (E) had been recorded, the head was restrained. The movements of the eye to the same stimulus as before were now recorded in the absence of a head movement. L indicates evoked movements to the left. Table movements are 180° out of phase with respect to the evoked responses.

crease in the amplitude of the table oscillations. Whenever the responses of an animal to a prolonged sinusoidal oscillation became smaller due to fatigue, the saccades became less frequent and disappeared as the peak velocities of slow-phase head movements declined to values of about 3°/s. With arousal of the animal, slow-phase head velocity improved and head saccades reappeared.

With the head-fixed image stabilization by compensatory eye movements is very limited in frogs [9]. Ocular quick phases can be present (as in Fig. 4A), but typically they occur too infrequently to keep the eye in its working range. During larger amplitudes of table oscillation, eye position appears to

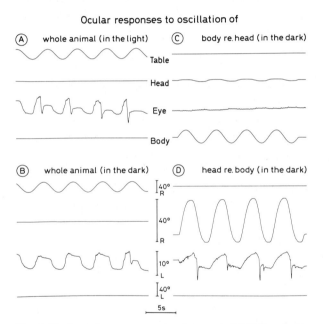

Ocular responses to oscillation of

Fig. 4. Horizontal eye movements of an acute HCN frog in response to different sinusoidal stimuli. In A–C the head was restrained, but not completely in C. The body was moved in C against the head and a coil on the head detected small passive head movements. The barely visible eye movements in C were almost entirely due to these passive head movements. (D) Oscillation of the head against the fixed body in the dark evoked slow and fast eye movements similarly as oscillations of the whole animal in the light (A). However, the fast phases in A are superimposed upon saturated slow phases to the right (see also B) and reset the eye position. In D, however, fast movements are superimposed upon slow phases to the left (intact) side and go in the compensatory direction. Oscillations had a frequency of 0.2 Hz and an amplitude of 20°.

saturate (Figs. 3 and 4B). In actue HCN frogs compensatory eye movements are slightly asymmetrical due to a slowed down response towards the intact (left) side (Figs. 3 and 4A,B). More importantly, these slow phases are devoid of the superimposed small fast phases regularly seen in unrestrained animals. Similarly, in the neck EMG signals of head-restrained frogs, no evidence for attempted saccades can be found. Thus the residual retinal image slip, larger in the head-restrained than in the head-unrestrained situation, does not appear to be directly related with the generation of saccades. Much more so are, apparently, head movements and the associated somatosensory input. The latter input alone, however, is practically ineffective in driving the eyes in intact, acute or even chronic frogs (Fig. 4C; [21]). But passive oscillation of the head in the dark regularly evokes saccades of the eyes towards the intact side (Fig. 4D) whenever peak head velocity towards the side of the lesion exceeds a few degrees/s.

Head saccades of HCN frogs are thus the result of somatosensory inputs that are activated by the head movement. In intact animals this input might be attenuated during a head movement by the concomitantly activated inhibitory vestibulocollic reflex. If so, a section of the horizontal canal nerve or a plug of this canal removes this inhibition and releases the somatosensory input. Consistent with this assumption is the fact that in intact frogs head saccades are not observed during sinusoidal oscillations (when excitatory and inhibitory vestibular reflexes are continuously modulated), but they are regularly seen a few seconds after the onset of a constant-velocity rotation of an optokinetic pattern or of a turntable [7,9]. In the case of a rotation at constant velocity, vestibular reflexes are only initially activated and decline in this species with a time constant of about 3 s. A similar, immediate increase of somatosensory input in the frog has been observed by Amat et al. [2] at the cellular level. They found an increased number of cells in the cerebellum responding to a passive displacement of the limb or of the trunk acutely after the removal of both labyrinths.

Saccadic substitution

These saccades provide an immediate and effective substitute for part of the missing vestibular slow-phase movements of the head. Without these saccades, compensatory reflexes in response to an oscillation of the animal in the light would become the more asymmetric the larger the stimulus amplitude and the higher the frequency of oscillation This asymmetry would result from an increasingly larger predominance of the vestibular over the optokinetic reflex contribution in a combined stimulation situation (i.e. oscillation in the light). Such a gradual shift from optokinetic to vestibular reflex predominance is parallelled on the motor side by a similar gradual shift from the oculomotor to the neck-motor system [7,9].

In acute HCN frogs the gain of compensatory gaze movements to small table oscillations of 0.2 Hz in the light (2.5 and 5°), and the gain to optokinetic stimuli, was practically identical with those recorded in intact frogs. At the largest amplitude tested (20°) the gain during optokinetic stimulation was about 0.2 (as in controls) and during table oscillation in the light about 0.7 (0.8 in intact frogs). The large difference in gain between responses during optokinetic (0.2) and combined stimulation (0.7) shows the increasingly larger contribution of vestibularly driven head slow phases towards the side of the lesion and of head saccades for movements directed towards the intact side (see also Fig. 5). The small difference in gain between responses to combined stimulation in controls (0.8) and in acute HCN frogs (0.7) shows how little the horizontal vestibular reflex from the intact side is reduced after the lesion. This latter observation is at variance with those in mammals but fully compatible with the different functional role of the brainstem commissure in this species [19,20].

Some of the chronic hemilabyrinthectomized frogs exhibit vestibulocollic reflex responses in the dark that are as saccadic and as symmetrical in amplitude as compensatory head movements of acute HCN frogs in the light [8,10]. For the occurrence of these head saccades in the dark, the acutely

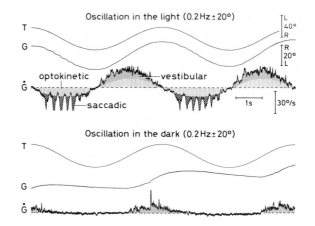

Fig. 5. In the middle frequency range larger oscillations of a right HCN frog in the light evoke compensatory gaze movements of very similar amplitudes to either side, because asymmetric vestibular reflexes (lower part) are substituted by head saccades. T, table; G and Ġ, gaze position and gaze velocity.

missing vestibulocollic slow phase must have recovered sufficiently to move the head fast enough to trigger these saccades. Such a partial recovery of dynamic vestibular reflex function was in fact observed in some chronic hemilabyrinthectomized frogs that were deprived of all nonvestibular inputs when tested [1]. Of course, in addition to the improvement of the deficient vestibulocollic reflex over time the head-velocity-related threshold for the generation of these saccades might also have lowered. Additional evidence suggests in fact that the threshold for these saccades is decreased in a chronic stage.

The presence of saccades in the compensatory head movements of most chronic hemilabyrinthectomized frogs even more than 2 years after surgery suggests that the vestibulocollic reflex never recovers to an extent comparable with controls. It thus appears that most of the 'recovery' from functional deficits in the dynamics of the horizontal vestibulocollic reflex after a horizontal canal nerve lesion or after hemilabyrinthectomy is immediately provided by head saccades that result from a lesion-induced disinhibition of somatosensory inputs. With time the residual vestibular reflex performance of hemilabyrinthectomized frogs improves –

for unknown reasons in some better than in others. These improved slow-phase head movements are then substituted by fewer and smaller saccades which, in a few cases, eventually disappear. The substitution of a compensatory slow-phase movement by a number of saccades is far from ideal in functional terms. Even though dynamic postural stability is improved, visual orientation, restricted to the brief intervals between saccades, becomes increasingly less feasible.

Discussion

A staircase-like sequence of saccades is clinically known to occur whenever the eyes of a patient have to catch up with a moving target, for instance because of a saccadic hypometria or because of a deficient smooth pursuit response. The sequence of small head saccades described here is reminiscent of this symptom, even though quite different in origin. Apart from the fact that frogs use head instead of eye saccades (which is in line with the particular role of compensatory eye and head movements in this species), it appears that the saccadic system is activated to 'catch up' not only for movements in the visual space but, more generally, whenever slow-phase movements are deficient. Such a more general role of the saccadic system as a compensatory subsystem has already been proposed by Berthoz [3] for the vestibulo-ocular reflex. As far as the activation of these saccades is concerned, it is important to note that these head saccades are followed and not preceded by ocular quick phases in the opposite direction, i.e. the head did not follow an eye-position signal nor did the eye follow a head-position signal. Rather the optokinetically driven head movement itself generated a proprioceptive feedback signal that activates the saccade generator. Preprogrammed to these head saccades are 'vestibulo-ocular-like' ocular quick phases which recentre the eye in the orbit even in the absence of vestibular reflexes. Similar 'vestibulo-ocular-like' eye movements were observed in labyrinthine-deficient patients [14] and monkeys [6]. In common with the frog is their presence in the dark, their dependency on actual head movements and, of course, their occurrence in the absence of any vestibular function. These similarities suggest a rather similar mechanism.

The results of this study clearly demonstrate how distributed the deficits in the behaviour are, even after the selective lesion of one canal nerve. This result is in full agreement with observations made with the deoxyglucose method [12,16,17], which emphasize the distributed consequences of a vestibular lesion. Among the various systems which might be particularly involved in the restoration of a new balance as well as in a reduction of the asymmetry in reflex gain have always been proprioceptive signals. In particular, the gain of the colliculo-ocular reflex has been shown to increase in mammals [6,13], including man [5], but not in the frog [21] after bilateral labyrinthectomy. The increased influence of these signals, probably in part an immediate effect as in the case of the head saccades described here, is certainly distributed again and affects a number of other subsystems. In patients devoid of labyrinthine function, somatosensory signals can even cause a strong sensation of rotation [4]. For the more basic aspects of these lesion-induced changes frogs appear to be a useful, even though not simple model.

References

[1] Agosti, R., Dieringer, N. and Precht, W. (1986) Partial restitution of lesion-induced deficits in the horizontal vestibulo-ocular reflex performance measured from the bilateral abducens motor output in frogs. *Exp. Brain Res.*, 61: 291–302.

[2] Amat, J., Matus-Amat, P and Vanegas, H. (1984) Visual (optokinetic) and somesthetic inputs to the cerebellum of bilaterally labyrinthectomized frogs. *Neuroscience*, 11: 735–891.

[3] Berthoz, A. (1985) Adaptive mechanisms in eye–head coordination. In A. Berthoz and G. Melvill Jones (Eds.), *Adaptive Mechanisms in Gaze Control, Reviews in Oculomotor Research, Vol. 1*, Elsevier, Amsterdam, pp. 177–201.

[4] Bles, W., de Jong, J.M.B.V. and de Wit, G. (1984) Somatosensory compensation for loss of labyrinthine function. *Acta Otolaryngol. Stockholm*, 97: 213–221.

[5] Bronstein, A.M. and Hood, J.D. (1986) The cervico-ocular reflex in normal subjects and patients with absent vestibular function. *Brain Res.*, 373: 399–408.

[6] Dichgans, J., Bizzi, E., Morasso, P. and Tagliasco, V. (1973) Mechanisms underlying recovery of eye–head coordination following bilateral labyrinthectomy in monkeys. *Exp. Brain Res.*, 18: 548–562.

[7] Dieringer, N. (1987) The role of compensatory eye and head movements for gaze stabilization in the unrestrained frog. *Brain Res.*, 404: 33–38.

[8] Dieringer, N. and Precht, W. (1981) Functional restitution of static and dynamic reflexes in the frog after hemilabyrinthectomy. In H. Flohr and W. Precht (Eds.), *Lesion-Induced Neuronal Plasticity in Sensorimotor Systems*, Springer, Berlin/Heidelberg, pp. 185–196.

[9] Dieringer, N. and Precht, W. (1982) Compensatory head and eye movements in the frog and their contribution to stabilization of gaze. *Exp. Brain Res.*, 47: 394–406.

[10] Dieringer, N. and Precht, W. (1986) Functional recovery following peripheral vestibular lesions: due to – in spite of – in parallel with – or without synaptic reorganization? In E.L. Keller and D.S. Zee (Eds.), *Adaptive Processes in Visual and Oculomotor Systems*, Pergamon, Oxford, pp. 383–390.

[11] Dieringer, N., Precht, W. and Blight, A.R. (1982) Resetting fast phases of head and eye and their linkage in the frog. *Exp. Brain Res.*, 47: 407–416.

[12] Flohr, H., Bienhold, H., Abeln, W. and Macskovics I. (1981) Concepts of vestibular compensation. In H. Flohr and W. Precht (Eds.), *Lesion-Induced Neuronal Plasticity in Sensorimotor Systems*, Springer, Berlin/Heidelberg, pp. 153–172.

[13] Fuller, J.H. (1980) The dynamic neck–eye reflex in mammals. *Exp. Brain Res.*, 41: 29–35.

[14] Kasai, T. and Zee, D.S. (1978) Eye–head coordination in labyrinthine defective human beings. *Brain Res.*, 144: 123–141.

[15] Kasper, H.J., Hess, B.J.M. and Dieringer, N. (1987) A precise and inexpensive magnetic field search coil system for measuring eye and head movements in small laboratory animals. *J. Neurosci. Methods*, 19: 115–124.

[16] Llinas, R. and Walton, K. (1979) Vestibular compensation: a distributed property of the central nervous system. In H. Asanuma and V.J. Wilson (Eds.), *Integration in the Nervous system*, Igaku-Shoin, Tokyo/New York, pp. 145–166.

[17] Luyten, W.H.M.L., Sharp, F.R. and Ryan, A.F. (1986) Regional differences of brain glucose metabolic compensation after unilateral labyrinthectomy in rats: a [^{14}C]2-deoxyglucose study. *Brain Res.*, 373: 68–80.

[18] McNally, W.J. and Tait, J. (1933) Some results of section of particular nerve branches to the ampullae of the four vertical semicircular canals of the frog. *Q. J. Exp. Physiol.*, 23: 147–196.

[19] Ozawa, S., Precht, W. and Shimazu, H. (1974) Crossed effects of central vestibular neurons in the horizontal canal system of the frog. *Exp. Brain Res.*, 19: 394–405.

[20] Precht, W. and Dieringer, N. (1985) Neuronal events paralleling functional recovery (compensation) following peripheral vestibular lesions. In A. Berthoz and G. Melvill Jones (Eds.), *Adaptive Mechanisms in Gaze Control, Reviews in Oculomotor Research, Vol. 1*, Elsevier, Amsterdam, pp. 117–201.

[21] Rioult-Pedotti, M. and Dieringer, N. (1986) The cervico-ocular reflex (COR) in intact and chronically labyrinthectomized frogs. *Neurosci. Lett. Suppl.*, 26: S549.

[22] Von Bechterew, W. (1983) Ergebnisse der Durchschneidung des N. Acusticus, nebst Erörterung der Bedeutung der semicirculären Kanäle für das Körpergleichgewicht. *Pflugers Arch.*, 30: 312–347.

O. Pompeiano and J.H.J. Allum (Eds.)
Progress in Brain Research, Vol. 76
© 1988 Elsevier Science Publishers B.V. (Biomedical Division)

CHAPTER 36

The role of gaze in compensation of vestibular disfunction: the gaze substitution hypothesis

A. Berthoz

Laboratoire de Physiologie Neurosensorielle, C.N.R.S. 15 rue de l'École de Médecine, F-75006 Paris CEDEX 06, France

This chapter formulates a new hypothesis concerning the mechanisms by which the central nervous system can perform the compensation of labyrinthine lesions. A review of the evidence concerning the influence of gaze-related signals on vestibular mechanisms is first presented. It has been shown that horizontal eye movement signals modulate the activity of the dorsal neck muscles in several species, including man. In addition, gaze signals also considerably modify the various components of the VCR. This influence is mediated via both the vestibulospinal and the reticulospinal tracts. In particular, we have shown that reticulospinal neurons belonging to the medial reticulospinal system and receiving a monosynaptic projection from the superior colliculus, are probably the immediate premotor interneurons in orienting reactions and subserve an eye–ear–head synergy. They probably play an important role in the control of vestibulospinal and possibly vestibulo-ocular reflexes. After vestibular lesions several factors have been proposed as contributing to the compensatory process (vision, cervical proprioception, somatosensory system, etc.). The idea of a possible role of other oculomotor subsystems in the recovery process by the mechanism of substitution has been proposed. The main idea of the hypothesis is that internally generated signals related to gaze can help in the restoration of vestibular tonus in the horizontal plane, and in the replacement of a deficient and noncompensated VOR or VCR by the saccadic or, more generally, the orienting system. Several testable predictions are proposed. A more general value of this hypothesis is suggested in the case of other situations in which there is visual–vestibular or intravestibular conflict.

Introduction

The purpose of this chapter is to present a new hypothesis concerning the mechanisms which may underlie adaptive or recovery processes following vestibular disorders. The main idea is that compensation of vestibular deficits not only involve processes intrinsic to the compensatory VORs or VSRs, as is currently thought, but that other subsystems belonging to the repertoire of the animal, and particularly the gaze-orienting mechanisms, can play a role in short- as well as in long-term vestibular compensation. A general formulation of this idea has been previously published [1]. This hypothesis goes along with the general proposal [2] that gaze plays an important role in posture control.

A simple objection to this point of view could be that it is well known that the brain is clever and can perform a number of complex reorganizations using various strategies. These have been reviewed by Goldberger [3], who makes a clear distinction between (*a*) *sensory substitution*, in which the movement after compensation is identical to the one before lesion but the subject uses a different set of sensory receptors for triggering and control; (*b*)

Abbreviations: COR, cervico-ocular reflex; EMG, electromyogram; VCR, vestibulocollic reflex; VOR, vestibulo-ocular reflex; VSR, vestibulospinal reflex.

functional substitution, in which the neuronal mechanisms subtending the movement have been changed but still belong to the subsystems normally used by the animal; and (*c*) *behavioural substitution*, by which the nervous system calls for new motor behaviours not belonging to its normal repertoire. It is, however, not enough to repeat that the brain has this potential of substitution (which has nicely been demonstrated in the case of tactile substitution of visual deficits in blind patients); it is essential to investigate whether these substitution processes can be operative in particular cases such as vestibular deficits. There is, indeed, abundant evidence that, after a vestibular lesion, sensory receptors from the limbs, or vision, can to an extent substitute for the missing or disturbed vestibular detection of head motion. This important contribution of other reflex loops has to be taken into account. However, the analysis of this role of other sensory cues has been limited to the conceptual frame of multimodal sensory substitution which just suggests the replacement of one sense organ by another. Very few authors have tried to investigate the potential of other active strategies (see review in [1]).

I would like to propose that there are not only external sensory cues which are used in compensation but internally generated signals which specify the direction of gaze. I propose that at least two types of compensatory modifications can be brought about by gaze signals after vestibular lesions:
(*a*) correction of the decrease in resting discharge of the vestibular neurons on the lesioned side, and therefore of the tonic deviation of eye or neck position,
(*b*) substitution of defective dynamic VORs or VSRs by the saccadic system, or eventually by the pursuit system driven by an internal reconstruction of head velocity.

We shall first review the evidence recently accumulated concerning the powerful control exerted by gaze signals on the vestibulo-ocular, vestibulospinal and reticulospinal systems. Then we shall briefly list the main deficits induced by labyrinthine lesions and attempt to show which role actively generated gaze signals play in the compensation process.

Evidence for gaze control of vestibulospinal and reticulospinal mechanisms

Influence of gaze on neck muscle activity: the 'horizontal' ipsiversive eye–head synergy

Relationship between eye position and the tonic component of dorsal neck muscle motoneuron firing rate

A clear relationship between eye position and the tonic component of dorsal neck muscle motoneuron firing rate has been found in the head-fixed cat [4], monkey [5], and human [6] This relationship is valid for muscles involved in horizontal head rotation (longissimus capitis, obliquus capitis, rectus capitis, splenius etc.). By horizontal is meant the plane of the horizontal semicircular canal. This plane is also the plane of the horizontal extra-ocular muscles and it has been shown recently [7] that a large number of species maintain a resting posture which is such that it keeps this privileged plane slightly tilted above the earth horizontal.

The specific property of this eye–head coupling tonic synergy is that it is mainly ipsilateral. In other words, the neck muscles on one side are activated when the eye is deviated towards the ipsilateral side with respect to the primary (straight ahead) position in the orbit. When eye eccentricity increases this increase is achieved by two mechanisms: an increase in firing rate which is linear but saturates for eccentricities above 30 to 45° in humans, and a recruitment of motor units [6].

The influence of eye-position signals on neck muscles is not restricted to the horizontal plane. The biventer cervicis muscles can be activated bilaterally during upward shifts of gaze, for instance. A complete description of these relationships is available (Roucoux et al., in preparation).

Influence of gaze signals on VCRs

These gaze-related signals have been shown to interact with VCRs. In the cat, for example, tilting the animal in the frontal plane induces a contraction of the neck on the ipsilateral side which is clearly dependent upon the vestibular receptors [8]. In the alert head-fixed cat the amplitude of the

VCR is modified according to eye position in the orbit. The EMG of splenius or longissimus capitis in this condition can be considered as resulting from a linear combination of VCR in the frontal plane and horizontal eye–head coupling mechanisms [9].

In the horizontal plane, for low or moderate velocities of head motion, the VCR is nearly absent when the head-fixed cat is really alert. In other words, oscillation of the cat in the horizontal plane at low frequencies does not necessarily evoke a compensatory head movement, but, as is also well known for eye movement, anticompensatory behaviour appears which orients the head in the direction of the ongoing head motion. The relationship between these two mechanisms is obviously complex. A recent attempt to study the modulation of the electrically evoked VCR has provided evidence of this complexity [10].

Influence of horizontal gaze signals on neurons mediating vestibular and reticular control of the VOR and VCR

What is the origin of these eye-position signals in neck muscles and at which level do vestibular reflexes and orienting reactions interact? Only partial answers to these questions are available at present. It is now very obvious that a privileged target for eye-movement signal is the vestibular nucleus. A number of authors have recorded eye-movement-related activity in vestibular nucleus neurons but the first investigation which yielded a definite physiological and morphological identification of second-order vestibular neurons in the alert animal was the one by McCrea et al. [11] and Berthoz et al. [12] It is now clear that the firing rate of second-order medial vestibular nucleus neurons is modulated by eye-position and eye-velocity signals with sensitivity as high as 8 spikes per second/degree for eye position and up to 0.8 spikes per second/degree per second for eye velocity. Increase in firing rate always occurs together with shifts of gaze towards the contralateral side to where the soma of the neuron is.

The second important finding related to our proposal is the fact that axons of a large number of horizontal type I second-order vestibular neurons (at least in the cat), whose soma lie in the medial vestibular nucleus, branch both to the abducens nucleus and to the spinal cord [11,13]. Therefore, a single neuron can subserve both the VOR and the VCR. It can also carry the eye-position signal to neck motoneurons. For instance, an excitatory horizontal crossed type I (Vc) neuron can provide both the excitatory drive for the contralateral neck muscle during ipsilateral head rotation and an increase or decrease of excitation depending upon whether the cat looks to the contralateral or to the ipsilateral side, respectively, with respect to the primary eye position in the orbit. The neck muscle activity will therefore be dependent upon head velocity in space and eye position in the orbit (or gaze space).

Vestibular neurons are, however, not the only candidates for mediating the action of gaze signals on neck motoneurons. Recently, following the extracellular study of Vidal et al. [14], Berthoz and Grantyn [15], Grantyn and Berthoz [16] and Grantyn et al. [17] have shown that pontomedullary reticular neurons whose soma lie in the vicinity of the abducens nucleus and which receive a monosynaptic activation from the contralateral superior colliculus project to abducens nucleus, facial nucleus and neck on the same side. The combined morphological and physiological study of these neurons has demonstrated that they are probably the immediate premotor excitatory interneuron controlling eye, ear and head synergy during ipsilateral orienting reactions. Their firing rate is very close to the EMG of the dorsal neck muscles mentioned above (longissimus capitis, obliquus capitis, splenius) and is also related very closely to the position of the eye in the orbit, but in a way different from vestibular neurons; these reticular neurons only discharge if the eye is on the same side with respect to the primary position and are completely silent otherwise. However, when the eye is at a fixed eccentricity to the ipsilateral side their firing rate is not linearly related with eye position as is the case for vestibular second-order neurons or abducens or neck motoneurons. They tend to 'leak' (their firing rate decreases rapidly with time) when the eye maintains fixation, at least for eccentricities up to about 10° in the head-fixed cat. However, Vidal et al. [14] have reported that some of the neurons may show a tonic eye-position-related activity.

These reticulospinal neurons, in addition to a tectal input, probably receive at least cortical (see Chapter 8) and vestibular inputs [18]. They belong to the tectobulbospinal system and, because they have also been shown to project to the vestibular nuclei, prepositus, and other reticular structures involved in eye and head movement control, they are an important element in the mechanisms underlying eye–head coordination. They may therefore be used in substitution processes when the vestibular neurons undergo a functional deficit.

Vestibular compensation

Let us now review shortly the deficits encountered after hemilabyrinthectomy before attempting to describe the potential role of gaze control mechanisms during compensation. These deficits have been described in number of recent publications [19–28]. All authors agree that there is a strong decrease of the tonic activity in the vestibular nucleus on the lesioned side. This decrease is thought to be responsible for the tonic deviation of the eye and head to the lesioned side. The exact syndrome is: (a) for the eyes, a tonic horizontal component of both eyes towards the lesioned side, downward deviation of the eye which is on the lesioned side and a tonic upward deviation of the eye in the intact side; (b) for the head, a tonic deviation and a head-down tilt towards the lesioned side. These effects are not limited to the eye or head. The recent radiographic studies [29] on the guinea pig describe the distribution of this syndrome in the whole animal.

The mechanisms of recovery from these tonic deficits is, however, a subject of debate. In spite of earlier results indicating a recovery of the balance between the two vestibular nuclei [19,30,31], the observations of Ried et al. [32] indicate that the overall population of type I vestibular neurons responding to horizontal rotation was significantly lower on the deafferented side when compared to the intact side. Precht [27] therefore suggested that 'if many former canal neurons became silent in chronic animals, a strong imbalance would exist between the two vestibular nuclei, and the ocular balance would be brought about by other structures as well' (p. 384). He concluded that 'the remaining sensory systems play an important role in the drive for recovery'. In other words, his view does not favour a decisive role of intrinsic recovery mechanisms. Recent evidence in the guinea pig [33], however, shows that the normal average resting rate is restored in type I neurons within 52 hours postoperation. The authors support the idea of a 'change in ipsi type I neurons themselves'.

A very classical explanation of balance recovery is the idea that the contralateral vestibular nuclei take over the control of the lesioned side by means of the comissural system [30]. This idea is supported by findings of Xerri et al. [25] in the decerebrate cat in the case of vestibular neurons located in Deiters' nucleus and therefore probably involved in the control of head tilt. However, this hypothesis is also under discussion [34]. For example, Smith et al. [35] conclude that for the guinea pig, the postural symptoms compensate in the absence of vestibular comissure and call for 'other factors' in the recovery process.

An intrinsic mechanism which has been proposed is related to sprouting within the deafferented nucleus; however, the time course for the sprouting to develop (several weeks) is too long for this mechanism to be significant in short-term effects.

Another explanation for the compensation of both the tonic and the dynamic deficits of the VOR and VCR is the sensory substitution of various other cues to the perturbed vestibular input. Several sensory systems have been considered as candidates for sensory substitution.

Vision. The contribution of vision has been demonstrated in the monkey during the recovery of VSRs induced by linear vertical acceleration [36]. In the cat, Berthoz et al. [37], Putkonen et al. [38] and Courjon et al. [39] have suggested that compensation of nystagmus, but also of head roll–tilt, was strongly influenced by vision because recovery was delayed when the animal was placed in darkness. In addition, when cats which had compensated their head tilt were put back in the dark, the head would immediately return to the postoperative tilt. It may, however, be unjustified to attribute the compensation to 'vision' on this basis. If, as suggested by the present hypothesis, a centrally generated gaze signal is actively producing compensatory patterns of neuronal discharge, vision is only essential as long it allows a detection of the correct orientation of eye and head in space, allowing thus a computation of a corrective gaze signal. In other words, vision could be used only to provide a spatial reference (visual straight ahead, or visual vertical) to the gaze system but may not directly be instrumental for compensation. The recent results of Smith et al. [40] in the guinea pig show that visual deprivation does not prevent compensation in this animal. Their result is still perfectly compatible with the present hypothesis if one supposes that the animal placed in total darkness still has many ways to determine (from somatosensory cues) the direction of the straight ahead which is necessary to drive gaze mechanisms.

Cervical proprioception. An increase in gain of the COR has been shown in monkeys [41] and in man [42–44]. However, it could very well be that this apparent increase in the 'gain' of the response cannot be attributed strictly to modifications occurring within the pathways of the reflex itself. Bronstein and Hood [44] have noted that the COR gain reverses to an unmodified value if subjects do not engage in a 'considerable conscious effort'. They suggest that 'some element of preprogramming' may be an essential part in this so-called COR gain increase. A similar attempt of monkeys to engage in seemingly programmed compensatory strategies had been observed on the first day after bilateral vestibular lesions by Dichgans et al. [41], before any change in the COR gain could be recorded.

Somatosensory elements have also been shown to contribute to compensation. For instance, Azzena et al. [45] have studied rapid decompensation induced by spinal cord transection. Their results sugest again that active processes are operative in the compensated state.

The idea that many neuronal centres were involved in this complex mixture of automatic and programmed motor reorganization was also suggested by the deoxyglucose study of Llinas and Walton [46]. And the role of activity, particularly in the immediate postoperative days, was underlined following Cawthorne [47], Cooksey [48] and Zuckerman [49] by Igarashi et al. [50], Lacour and Xerri [23] and Precht [27].

Recently, we have suggested that a subsystem-selection mechanism could be used to select among the repertoire of subsystems, one which may have dynamic or geometrical properties suitable for substitution to the defective subsystem [1]. This mechanism has also been suggested to underly some aspects of rapid prism adaptation [51].

The saccadic gaze-substitution hypothesis

The proposed hypothesis is in the line of the previous remarks concerning the role of preprogrammed factors in vestibular compensation. It suggests that at least part of compensation of vestibular deficits is made by active internally generated motor signals produced by the orienting neuronal network controlling gaze. It is compatible with the simultaneous existence of neurochemical mechanisms of vestibular or reticular neurons' plastic modifications. Below are two examples of how this mechanism can operate.

Restoration of vestibular tonus in the horizontal plane by horizontal eye-position signals

Fig. 1 shows in a highly schematic way how a tonic gaze signal could substitute for the missing tone in the medial vestibular nucleus on the lesioned side. If the right labyrinth is lesioned, the right second-order vestibular type I excitatory neu-

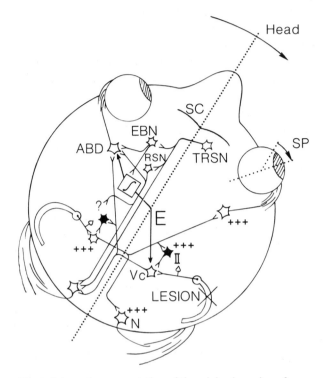

Fig. 1. Schematic representation of the minimal number of neurons may be implied in the saccadic gaze-substitution mechanisms (see text for details). SC, superior colliculus; TRSN, tectobulbospinal neurons; EBN, excitatory burst neuron; RSN, reticulospinal neuron; ABD, abducens motoneuron; Vc, second-order type I excitatory vestibular neuron; II, type II inhibitory vestibular neuron; E, eye-position signal (the integral sign in the square box indicates the neuronal integration network); SP, slow-phase of vestibular nystagmus following a lesion of the right horizontal canal. This schema does not preclude that the action of gaze on the vestibular nucleus comes through other pathways (direct corticoreticulovestibular pathways, for example) than the tectoreticulospinal system which is schematized here. The anatomical location of the various structures within the skull has not been drawn at the correct scale; this scheme being only a functional one. The plus (+) signs indicate the neurons or muscles which exhibit an hyperactivity following unilateral (right) labyrinthectomy. The reticulospinal neuron connections with the gaze generator have not been drawn because they are still hypothetical (for comments see [16,18]) but it is implied in this scheme that the reticulospinal neuron is a pathway fundamental for both the tonic VCR and the dynamic pseudoVOR and -VCR.

rons which mediate both the horizontal angular VOR and VCR are silenced. Slow-phase deviation of the eye occurs to the right under the influence of the left vestibular nucleus whose activity is increased above its normal tonic activity by the lack of inhibition from the lesioned side. At the same time the head is deviated to the right by the excitatory action of the left vestibular neurons on the right neck muscles. If the patient or the animal now directs his eye to the left, the eye-position integration which generates the tonic (E) discharge necessary to maintain the eye on the new eye position will produce an increase of firing rate in second-order vestibular neurons on the lesioned side [12]. The eye-position sensitivity of horizontal type I second-order medial vestibular neurons in the cat ranges between 0.5 and 8 spikes/s/degree. In this animal, one could therefore expect an increase of about 4 to 40 spikes/s in firing rate for a shift of eye position which would bring the eye at 10° eccentricity to the left. In the monkey, eye-position sensitivity of the same type of neurons can be in the order of 4 to 14 spikes/s/degree and a shift of horizontal eye position of 10° may therefore induce a change of vestibular resting rate as high as 140 spikes/s.

A sizable amount of resting rate can thus be recovered by a simple shift of eye position towards the intact side. In addition, this shift of gaze will decrease the activity in the intact (hyperactive) vestibular nucleus, thus also decreasing the slow-phase velocity of the spontaneous nystagmus and relaxing the hypertonic neck muscle on the lesioned (right) side. It could be argued that vestibular patients do not seem to walk around with the eyes deviated to the side contralateral to the lesion, but this has not really been measured. Moreover, it would be enough to adopt a head position slightly deviated to the right in order to obtain the adequate compensation of the vestibular tonus and still have gaze (eye plus head) directed straight ahead. In fact, this could be the very reason for which there can be a great delay of recovery of a straight head position: this delay would not be due to a limited capacity in the recovery process, but to an active choice maintaining the eye deviation.

Another objection to this idea could be that, after compensation, when a hemilabyrinthectomized patient shifts his gaze away from the primary position towards the compensated side, a positional nystagmus may appear. If indeed maintenance of an eccentric eye deviation towards the intact side is a functional problem, another strategy could be adopted by the animal or the patient: the eye could be shifted transiently to the intact side in order to produce transient moments during which a pseudorecovered state would be reached. Such strategies of intermittent compensation are commonly observed during the head-shaking nystagmus with which patients with vestibular deficits actively compensate. Large shifts in eye position towards the intact side and large head shifts have been observed by Denise et al. [52] in the hemilabyrinthectomized cat during the first few days after hemilabyrinthectomy. As suggested above, the role of vision in compensation would then be to provide the necessary reference frame for adjusting the gaze parameters during these active compensatory mechanisms.

It should be clear that the possible contribution of eye-position signals to the recovery of the vestibular resting rate does not preclude the occurrence of other mechanisms based on neuronal plasticity. Previously as proposed [1], long-term compensation of vestibular deficits probably necessitates the replacement of these active substitution mechanisms by plastic changes.

Replacement of the dynamic properties of the VOR and VCR by the saccadic and orienting systems

It has been well documented that patients with total labyrinthine loss can substitute the VOR by a pseudoreflex which can be observed if the patient is asked to imagine a target in front of him [53]. The scheme of Fig. 1 can also be used to indicate very roughly how 'pseudoVOR' and -VCR can be produced through the saccadic generator. If, for instance, the head moves to the right, the activities of the VOR and VCR are low (they only rely upon the disinhibition from the intact left labyrinth). But if the subject can consciously drive the saccadic generator to produce a sequence of saccades to the left,

this signal will not only produce saccades. It will also increase the activity of the right vestibular nucleus neurons as well as the activity of the left reticulospinal neurons subserving the leftward orienting synergy and therefore produce a leftward compensatory eye movement. In this perspective the apparent increase in COR gain observed after labyrinthectomy by several authors (see above) could be interpreted as a substituted saccadic drive of the eye–head coupling synergy; the signals driving the saccadic system may come from neck proprioception (a rightward head movement on the trunk is known to induce a leftward fast phase due to the cervical proprioception). The intact canal could also be used for the detection of head angular position after a neural integration and drive the saccadic system.

The pontine reticular neurons subserving the ipsiversive orienting synergy which have been described above [16], are probably very essential in this creation of a pseudovestibular reflex. They can be driven either by the tectobulbospinal system, if a visual target is present, or by remembered targets. They may also be driven by cortical drive, although the evidence from Sasaki (Chapter 8) suggests a weak cortical influence on reticulospinal neurons belonging to the tectobulbospinal system.

A prediction of the hypothesis is that a close examination of the VOR of hemilabyrinthectomized patients will reveal that when the head is turning towards the lesioned side a pseudo VOR is being formed by blended anticompensatory saccades (or 'quick phases'). This should show particularly well on the eye-velocity traces. Recent results from Dieringer (Chapter 35) indeed confirm the existence of saccades in the oculomotor response of hemilabyrinthectomized frogs during vestibular horizontal stimulation in the dark. The use of saccades as a substitute to deficient vestibular function may therefore not require high cortical mechanisms if it is present in amphibians. It probably belongs to the normal mechanisms of cooperation between the stabilizing and orienting mechanisms. Another prediction is that cortical mechanisms will turn out to be fundamental in vestibular compensation.

418

Use of saccades for substitution of vestibular deficits: a general adaptive mechanism?

This mechanism may be useful not only in the case of vestibular lesions. It could be of a more general value in all cases when there is a conflict within the vestibular system or when there is an intersensory conflict in visual–vestibular interaction. Two examples may illustrate this point. First, in recent space flights in which subjects were deprived of gravity, we measured the VOR during active head movement in darkness. The subjects were instructed to look at an imagined target in darkness and oscillate their head at 0.2 Hz. In one space flight, on the first day, two of the astronauts showed a remarkable pattern of eye movements during VOR in yaw: during sinusoidal oscillation of the head in darkness the eyes moved with saccades in compensatory direction [54]. The gain of the desaccaded slow phase (which corresponded to the real horizontal VOR) was very small (about 0.2). But the total eye displacement (when taking into account the saccades) had a gain of about one. Therefore, given the strong intravestibular conflict due to otolith dysfunction, it seems that the subjects had suppressed the VOR and were performing the task by means of the saccadic system. Similar observations have also been made in the case of prism adaptation by Melvill Jones et al. [51].

References

[1] Berthoz, A. (1985) Adaptive mechanisms in eye head coordination. In A. Berthoz and G. Melvill Jones (Eds.), *Adaptive Mechanisms in Gaze Control*, Elsevier, Amsterdam, pp. 177–201.
[2] Berthoz, A. (1987) Influence of gaze in postural mechanisms. *Neuroscience Suppl.*, 22:S575.
[3] Goldberger, M.E. (1980) Motor recovery after lesions. *Trends Neurosci.*, 3:288–291.
[4] Vidal, P.P., Roucoux A. and Berthoz, A. (1982) Eye position related activity in neck muscle of the alert cat. *Exp. Brain Res.*, 46: 448–453.
[5] Lestienne, F., Vidal, P.P. and Berthoz, A. (1984) Gaze changing behaviour in head restrained monkey. *Exp. Brain Res.*, 55: 215–222.
[6] André-Deshays, C. Berthoz, A. and Revel, M. (1987) Eye head coupling in humans. *Exp. Brain Res.*, in press.

[7] Vidal, P.P., Graf, W. and Berthoz, A. (1986) The orientation of the cervical vertebral column in unrestrained awake animals. *Exp. Brain Res.*, 61: 549–559.
[8] Berthoz, A. and Anderson, J. (1972) Frequency analysis of vestibular influence on extensor motoneurons. III Neck and forelimb activity after hemilabyrinthectomy. *Brain Res.*, 45: 236–240.
[9] Darlot, C., Denise, P. and Droulez, J. (1985) Modulation by eye position of the vestibulo-collic reflex induced by tilting in the frontal plane in the alert cat. *Exp. Brain Res.* 58: 510–519.
[10] Denise, P., Darlot, C., Wilson, V.J. and Berthoz, A. (1987) Modulation by eye position of neck muscle contraction evoked by electrical labyrinthine modulation in the alert cat. *Exp. Brain Res.*, in press.
[11] Mc Crea, R., Yoshida, K., Evinger, C. and Berthoz, A. (1981) The location, axonal arborisation and termination sites of eye movement related secondary vestibular neurons demonstrated by intra axonal HRP injection in the alert cat. In A. Fuchs and W. Becker (Eds.), *Progress in Oculomotor Research, Vol. 12,* Elsevier, Amsterdam, pp. 379–386.
[12] Berthoz, A., Yoshida, K. and Vidal, P.P. (1981), Horizontal eye movement sensitivity in second order vestibular nuclei neurons in the cat. In B. Cohen (Eds.), *Vestibular and Oculomotor Physiology*, Ann. N.Y. Acad. Sci., 174: 144–156.
[13] Isu, N. and Yokota, J. (1983) Morphological study on the divergent projection of axon collaterals of medial vestibular nucleus neurons in the cat. *Exp. Brain Res.*, 53: 151–162.
[14] Vidal, P.P., Corvisier, J. and Berthoz, A. (1983) Eye and neck motor signals in periabducens reticular neurons of the alert cat. *Exp. Brain Res.*, 53:16–28.
[15] Berthoz, A. and Grantyn, A. (1986) Neuronal mechanisms underlying eye head coordination. In H. Freund et al. (Eds.), *The Oculomotor and Skeletomotor Systems: Differences and Similarities, Progress in Brain Research*, Elsevier, Amsterdam, pp. 325–343.
[16] Grantyn, A. and Berthoz, A. (1987) Neuronal mechanisms of orienting movements. I. Reticulospinal neurons coordinating eye head synergy during orienting in the cat. *Exp. Brain Res.*, 66: 339–354.
[17] Grantyn, A., Berthoz, A. and Ong-Meang, V. (1987) Neuronal mechanisms of orienting in the cat. II. Morphological connectivity of pontine reticulo-spinal neurons related to coordination of eye head synergy in the cat. *Exp. Brain Res.*, 66: 355–377.
[18] Peterson, B.W., Anderson, M.E. and Filion, M. (1974) Responses of ponto-medullary reticular neurons to cortical, tectal, and cutaneous stimuli. *Exp. Brain Res.*, 21: 19–44.
[19] Schaefer, K.P. and Meyer, D.L. (1974) Compensation of vestibular lesions. In H.H. Kornhuber (Ed.), *Handbook of Sensory Physiology Vestibular System, Part 2, Psychophysics. Applied Aspects and General Interpretations, Vol 6/2,* Springer, Berlin, pp. 463–490.
[20] Igarashi, M., Levy, J.K., Reshke, M.F., Kubo, T. and Wat-

son, T. (1978) Locomotor disfunction after surgical lesions in the unilateral vestibular nuclei region in squirrel monkeys. *Arch. Oto-Rhino-Laryngol.*, 221: 89–95.

[21] Jensen, D.W. (1979) Reflex control of acute postural asymmetry and compensatory symmetry after a unilateral vestibular lesion. *Neuroscience*, 4: 1059–1073.

[22] Xerri, C. and Lacour, M. (1980) Compensation des déficits posturaux et cinétiques après neurectomie vestibulaire unilatérale chez le chat. Role de l'activité sensorimotrice. *Acta Otolaryngol. Stockholm*, 90: 414–424.

[23] Lacour, M. and Xerri, C. (1981) Vestibular compensation: new perspectives. In H. Flohr and W. Precht (Eds.), *Lesion-Induced Neuronal Plasticity in Sensorimotor Systems*, Springer, Berlin, pp. 240–253.

[24] Maioli, C., Precht, W. and Ried, S. (1983) Short- and long-term modifications of vestibulo-ocular response dynamics following unilateral vestibular nerve lesions in the cat. *Exp. Brain Res.*, 50: 259–274.

[25] Xerri, C., Gianni, S., Manzoni, D. and Pompeiano, O. (1983) Central compensation of vestibular deficits. I. Response characteristics of lateral vestibular neurons to roll tilt after ipsilateral labyrinth deafferentation. *J. Neurophysiol.*, 50, 2: 428–448.

[26] Sirkin, D.W., Precht, W. and Courjon, J.H. (1984) Initial, rapid phase of recovery from unilateral vestibular lesion in rat not dependent on survival of central portion of vestibular nerve. *Brain Res.*, 302: 245–256.

[27] Precht, W. (1986) Recovery of some vestibulo-ocular and vestibulo-spinal functions following unilateral labyrinthectomy. In H.J. Freund et al. (Eds.), *Oculomotor and Skeletalmotor Systems: Differences and Similarities, Progress in Brain Research, Vol. 64*, Elsevier, Amsterdam, pp. 381–391.

[28] Precht, W., and Dieringer, N. (1985) Neuronal events parallelling functional recovery following peripheral vestibular lesions. In G. Melvill Jones and A. Berthoz (Eds.), *Adaptive Mechanisms in Gaze Control*, Elsevier, Amsterdam, pp. 251–268.

[29] De Wael, C., Vidal P.P. and Graf, W. (1987) A quantitative study of head neck geometry in vertebrates. Its consequence for the postural syndrome following hemilabyrinthectomy in the guinea pig. In B. Cohen and V. Henn (Eds.), *Representation of Three Dimensional Space in the Vestibular, Oculomotor and Visual systems, Ann NY. Acad. Sci.*, in press.

[30] Precht, W., Shimazu, H.H. and Markham, C.H. (1966) A mechanism for the central compensation of vestibular function following hemilabyrinthectomy. *J. Neurophysiol.* 29: 996–1010.

[31] Markham, Ch.H, Yagi, T. and Curthoys, I.S. (1977) The contribution of the contralateral labyrinth to second order vestibular neuronal activity in the cat. *Brain Res.*, 138: 99–109.

[32] Ried, S., Maioli, C. and Precht, W. (1984) Vestibular nuclear neuron activity in chronically hemilabyrinthectomised cats. *Acta Otolaryngol. Stockholm*, 98: 1–13.

[33] Smith, P.F. and Curthoys, I.S. (1987) Recovery of resting activity in the ipsilateral vestibular nucleus following unilateral labyrinthectomy: non commissural influences. In E. Pirodda (Ed.), *Proceedings of the Bárány Society Meeting*, Karger, Basle, in press.

[34] Dutia, M.B. (1985) Vestibular control of neck muscles in acute and chronic hemilabyrinthectomised cats. *J. Physiol. London*, 366: 281–290.

[35] Smith, P.F., Darlington, C.L. and Curthoys, I.S. (1986) Vestibular compensation without brain stem commissures in the guinea pig. *Neurosci. Lett.*, 65: 209–213.

[36] Lacour, M., Vidal, P.P. and Xerri, C. (1981) Visual influences on vestibulo-spinal reflexes during vertical linear motion in normal and hemilabyrinthectomised monkeys. *Exp. Brain Res.*, 43: 383–394.

[37] Berthoz, A., Jeannerod, M. Vital-Durand, F. and Oliveras, J.L. (1975) Development of vestibulo-ocular responses in visually deprived kittens. *Exp. Brain Res.*, 23: 425–442.

[38] Putkonen, PT.S., Courjon, J.H. and Jeannerod, M. (1977) Compensation of postural effects of hemilabyrinthectomy in the cat: a sensory substitution process? *Exp. Brain Res.*, 28: 249–257.

[39] Courjon, J.H., Jeannerod, M., Ossuzio, I. and Schmid, R. (1977) The role of vision in compensation of vestibulo-ocular reflex after hemilabyrinthectomy in the cat. *Exp. Brain Res.*, 28: 235–248.

[40] Smith, P.F., Darlington, C.D. and Curthoys, I.S. (1986) Vestibular compensation without brain stem commissures in the guinea pig. *Neurosci. Lett.*, 65: 209–213.

[41] Dichgans, J., Bizzi, E., Morasso, P. and Tagliasco, V. (1973) Mechanisms underlying recovery of eye head coordination following bilateral labyrinythectomy in monkeys. *Exp. Brain Res.*, 18: 548–562.

[42] Barnes, G.R. and Forbat, L.N. (1979) Cervical and vestibular afferent control of oculomotor responses in man. *Acta Otolaryngol. Stockholm*, 88: 79–87.

[43] Leopold, H.C., Doerr, M. and Thoden, U. (1983) Cervico-ocular responses (COR) during slow sinusoidal head movements in subjects with bilateral labyrinthine lesions. *Arch. Psychiat. Nervenkr.*, 223: 439–447.

[44] Bronstein, A.M. and Hood, J.D. (1986) The cervico-ocular reflex in normal subjects and patients with absent vestibular function. *Brain Res.*, 373: 399–408.

[45] Azzena, G.B., Mameli, O. and Tolu, E. (1977) Vestibular units during decompensation. *Experientia*, 33: 234–236.

[46] Llinàs, R. and Walton, K. (1979) Vestibular compensation: a distributed property of the central nervous system. In H. Asanuma and V.J. Wilson (Eds.), *Integration in the Nervous System*, Igaku-Shoin, Tokyo, pp. 145–166.

[47] Cawthorne, T. (1944) The physiological basis for head exercises. *J. Chart, Soc. Physiother.*, 29: 106–107.

[48] Cooksey, F.S. (1946) Rehabilitation in vestibular injuries. *Proc. R. Soc. Med.*, 39: 273–275.

[49] Zuckerman, H. (1967) The physiological adaptation to uni-

420

lateral semicircular canal inactivation. *McGill Med. J.*, 36:8–13.

[50] Igarashi, M., Levy, J.K., Takahashi, M, Alford, B.R. and Hornick, J.L. (1979) Effect of exercise upon locomotor balance modification after peripheral vestibular lesions in squirrel monkeys. *Adv. Oto-Rhino-Laryngol.*, 25: 82–87.

[51] Melvill Jones, G., Guitton, D. and Berthoz, A. (1988) Changing patterns of eye head coordination during 6 hours of optically reversed vision. *Exp. Brain Res.*, 69:531–544.

[52] Denise, P., Corvisier, J. and Berthoz, A. (1988) Relation between oculomotor and neck activity following hemilabyrinthectomy in the cat. *Exp. Brain Res.*, in press.

[53] Kasai, T. and Zee, D.S. (1978) Eye head coordination in labyrinthine defective human beings., *Brain Res.*, 144: 123–141.

[54] Berthoz, A. et al. (1986) Adaptation of the optokinetic and vestibulo-ocular reflexes during exposure to microgravity. In P.R. Sahm, R. Jansen and M.H. Keller (Eds.), *Scientific Results of the German Spacelab Mission D1*, DFVLR, Köln, pp. 481–483.

O. Pompeiano and J.H.J. Allum (Eds.)
Progress in Brain Research, Vol. 76
© 1988 Elsevier Science Publishers B.V. (Biomedical Division)

CHAPTER 37

Effects of melanocortins on vestibular compensation

U. Lüneburg and H. Flohr

Department of Neurobiology, University of Bremen, NW 2, D-2800 Bremen 33, F.R.G.

The effect of ACTH/MSH-like peptides on functional recovery from unilateral labyrinthine lesions was investigated in *Rana temporaria*. The ACTH fragments $ACTH_{4-7}$, $ACTH_{4-10}$, $ACTH_{1-10}$, α-MSH and the synthetic ACTH analogues ORG-2766 and ORG-5041 significantly accelerate the compensation process. [D-Phe7]$ACTH_{4-10}$ inhibits compensation. $ACTH_{1-39}$, $ACTH_{1-24}$, γ_2-MSH – given in equimolar doses – do not influence the rate of compensation. The effects of these peptides on a lesion-induced plastic process are similar to those which they exert on various learning and memory processes.

Introduction

Lesions of the CNS or of its sensory or motor interfaces induce plastic changes that may lead to a recovery of the initially disrupted function. Recovery of function which occurs in the absence of regeneration of the lesioned substrate and which is attributable to a reorganization of remaining structures is usually termed 'compensation'. During the last few years, it has been observed that such compensation processes can be influenced by ACTH/MSH-like neuropeptides (melanocortins) [1–7]. In earlier studies on the effects of ACTH and ACTH-like peptides on CNS damage, attention was focussed on the corticotropic action of these agents and its possible beneficial effects either on events immediately following injury or on scar formation [8–12].

It later became apparent, however, that the above-mentioned effects on compensatory processes can also be achieved by short-chained fragments of ACTH or MSH which are devoid of corticotropic (or melanotropic) properties. It has therefore been proposed that such peptides act specifically on those plastic processes responsible for compensation [13].

Substances with such properties would obviously be of considerable theoretical and practical importance. Accordingly, in the present study the action of ACTH, MSH and a number of their fragments (Fig. 1) on compensatory processes was investigated. The aim of the study was: (*a*) to characterize the amino-acid sequence specifically responsible for the observed effects and (*b*) to evaluate the influence of modifications of the peptide structure on its pharmacological action. The investigations employed the paradigm of *vestibular compensation*, i.e. functional recovery following unilateral vestibular lesions. The experimental subjects were grass frogs (*Rana temporaria*). In this species, unilateral destruction of the labyrinth or vestibular nerve causes two groups of functional deficits: firstly, asymmetries in the tonic influences on posture resulting in, for example, curvature of the longitudinal body axis, head deviation around the longitudinal axis and alterations in extensor/flexor tonus; and secondly, impairment of the dynamic vestibular reflexes dependent on bilateral inputs, such as VOR or VCR. The initial postoperative stage of severe

---

Abbreviations: ACTH, adrenocorticotropic hormone; CNS, central nervous system; MSH, melanocyte-stimulating hormone; VCR, vestibulocollic reflex; VOR, vestibulo-ocular reflex.

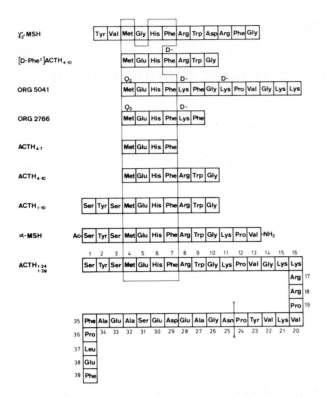

Fig. 1. Primary structure of the ACTH/MSH-related peptides studied.

tained in groups of seven at room temperature in a moist environment and fed with earthworms. Unilateral labyrinthectomy was performed under MS 222 anaesthesia adopting the extracranial approach described by Ewald [15]. Head deviation was measured daily using specially adapted video equipment. The peptides were dissolved in frog Ringer and the various doses were all injected in a volume of 17 ml/kg into the dorsal lymph sac.

Four series of experiments were performed. In the first series, the effects of chronic postoperative treatment with ACTH and ACTH fragments on compensation were investigated. In experimental series 2, a similar treatment was undertaken with two synthetic ACTH analogues, ORG-2766 and ORG-5041. In experimental series 3, the influence of two ACTH/MSH related peptides, [D-Phe7]ACTH$_{4-10}$ and γ_2-MSH was examined, the behavioural activity of which is often opposite to that of the peptides tested in experiment 1 [16]. In experimental series 4, the action of [D-Phe7]ACTH$_{4-10}$ on the compensated state was studied. Details of doses and treatment regimen are presented in the corresponding section of the Results.

Results

Chronic postoperative treatment with ACTH and ACTH fragments

The following peptides were tested: ACTH$_{1-39}$ (300 nmol/kg/day), ACTH$_{1-24}$ (300 and 1200 nmol/kg/day), α-MSH (3, 30, 150 and 300 nmol/kg/day), ACTH$_{1-10}$ (40 and 300 nmol/kg/day), ACTH$_{4-10}$ (6, 40, 300 and 1200 nmol/kg/day) and ACTH$_{4-7}$ (300 and 1200 nmol/kg/day). Treatment consisted of 24 daily injections of the peptide under test (or the vehicle in control animals) beginning on the first postoperative day. The results are shown in Figs. 2, 3, 4 and 9. The latter provides a survey of the effects of all peptides tested, the various treatment groups being compared on the basis of half-compensation times, i.e., the time over which the initial head deviation is reduced by 50%.

α-MSH, ACTH$_{1-10}$ and ACTH$_{4-10}$ accelerate the

symptoms is followed by a partial recovery of functions. The postural symptoms are extensively compensated, whereas the dynamic deficits recover less completely [14].

In the present investigation, compensation of the main postural symptom, head deviation, was chosen as an indicator of pharmacological effects. Unilateral labyrinthectomy in the grass frog leads to an initial head deviation of $33° \pm 4°$ (mean $\pm$ S.D.). The time course of compensation follows an exponential function ($\tau \approx 20$ days). A number of plausible hypotheses have been forwarded concerning the neural mechanisms underlying the compensation of this particular symptom (see Discussion).

Methods

The experiments were carried out on common grass frogs weighing 20–40 g. The animals were main-

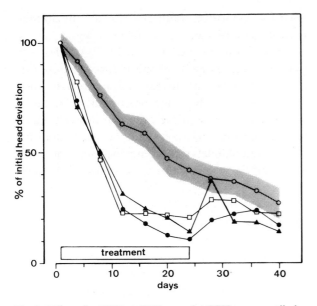

Fig. 2. Effect of α-MSH, ACTH$_{1-10}$ and ACTH$_{4-10}$ on vestibular compensation following unilateral labyrinthectomy in *Rana temporaria*. Peptides were administered daily from the first to the 24th postoperative day in a dose of 300 nmol/kg/day. ○, control (*n* = 261, mean values ± S.D.; shaded area); □, α-MSH (*n* = 15); ▲, ACTH$_{1-10}$ (*n* = 16); ●, ACTH$_{4-10}$ (*n* = 35). Ordinate: mean values of head tilt in percent of initial head deviation measured on the first postoperative day. Abscissa: time in days.

compensation process significantly over a relatively broad dose range. A dose–response relationship is not apparent with the tested doses (Fig. 9). Unlike the above-mentioned peptides, ACTH$_{4-7}$ is not effective in doses up to 300 nmol/kg/day, but it does exert a significant accelerating effect when the dose is increased to 1200 nmol/kg/day (Figs. 3 and 9). ACTH$_{1-39}$ and ACTH$_{1-24}$ given in equimolar doses are inactive or even slightly inhibitory (Figs. 4 and 9).

Chronic treatment with synthetic ACTH analogues

The structure of the two tested analogues (Fig. 1) protects them against proteolytic degradation and they thus have a longer biological half-life than the peptides administered in experiment 1; they exert similar behavioural actions at lower concentrations [17]. The treatment regimen was the same as in ex-

periment 1; ORG-2766 was given at doses of 0.25, 1 and 5 nmol/kg/day and ORG-5041 in doses of 0.0003, 0.3, 3 and 300 nmol/kg/day. The ACTH$_{4-9}$ analogue ORG-2766 (Fig. 5) significantly increases the rate of compensation at extremely low doses, whereas the highest tested dose (5 nmol/kg/day) is ineffective (Fig. 9). The ACTH$_{4-16}$ analogue ORG-5041 is without effect when administered in comparably low doses; a dose of 300 nmol/kg/day, however, accelerates vestibular compensation significantly (Figs. 6 and 9).

Chronic treatment with [D-Phe7]ACTH$_{4-10}$ and γ$_2$-MSH

The amino-acid sequences of these analogues are presented in Fig. 1. [D-Phe7]ACTH$_{4-10}$ was injected daily from the 1st to the 31st postoperative day at doses of 150, 300, 1200 and 4800 nmol/kg/day. γ$_2$-

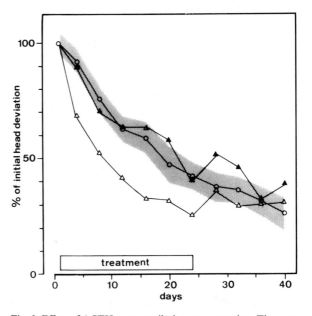

Fig. 3. Effect of ACTH$_{4-7}$ on vestibular compensation. The peptide was administered daily from the first to the 24th postoperative day in two different doses. ○, control (*n* = 261, mean values ± S.D.; shaded area); ▲, ACTH$_{4-7}$ (300 nmol/kg/day, *n* = 14); △, ACTH$_{4-7}$ (1200 nmol/kg/day, *n* = 14). Ordinate: mean values of head tilt in percent of initial head deviation measured on the first postoperative day. Abscissa: time in days.

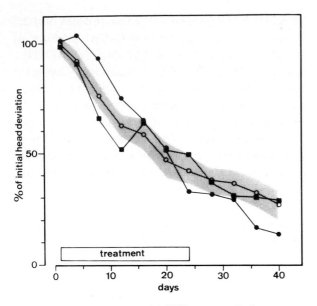

Fig. 4. Effect of ACTH$_{1-39}$ and ACTH$_{1-24}$ on vestibular compensation. Both peptides were given daily in a dose of 300 nmol/kg/day from the first to the 24th postoperative day. ○, control ($n = 261$, mean values $\pm$ S.D.; shaded area); ●, ACTH$_{1-39}$ ($n = 19$); ■, ACTH$_{1-24}$ ($n = 14$). Ordinate: mean values of head tilt in percent of initial head deviation measured on the first postoperative day. Abscissa: time in days.

MSH was given from the 1st to the 21th postoperative day at doses of 0.8, 8, 80, 300 and 1000 nmol/kg/day.

The action of these peptides is shown in Figs. 7 and 9. [D-Phe7]ACTH$_{4-10}$ administered at doses between 300 and 4800 nmol/kg/day strongly inhibits vestibular compensation; 150 nmol/kg/day has no significant effect. γ_2-MSH does not affect the compensation rate at any of the doses tested.

Effect of [D-Phe7]ACTH$_{4-10}$ on the compensated state

The suspected decompensatory action of [D-Phe7]ACTH$_{4-10}$ was studied by administering it chronically to partially compensated animals. In one experiment, treatment was started on the 17th postoperative day and continued for a further 43 days; in a second experiment, treatment commenced after 35 days of compensation and conti-

nued for 25 days. In both experiments the animals received a daily injection of 300 nmol/kg.

Chronic administration of [D-Phe7]ACTH$_{4-10}$ to partially compensated animals induces a temporary decompensation, i.e. the reappearance of symptoms characteristic of the acute postoperative stage including an increase in the degree of head deviation [18]; the decompensatory effect, however, does not appear immediately on commencement of treatment and disappears prior to cessation of the same (Fig. 8).

Discussion

To date only a few investigations have been conducted on the effects of melanocortins on postlesion plasticity; taken as a whole, these results do not yet present a sufficiently consistent picture. Flohr and

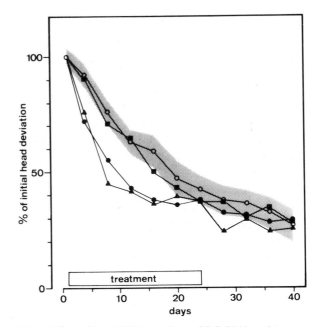

Fig. 5. Effect of the ACTH$_{4-9}$ analogue ORG-2766 on the course of vestibular compensation. The peptide was administered daily in three different doses from the first to the 24th postoperative day. ○, control ($n = 261$, mean values $\pm$ S.D.; shaded area); ●, ORG-2766 (0.25 nmol/kg/day, $n = 26$); ▲, ORG-2766 (1 nmol/kg/day, $n = 27$); ■, ORG-2766 (5 nmol/kg/day, $n = 10$). Ordinate: mean values of head tilt in percent of initial head deviation measured on the first postoperative day. Abscissa: time in days.

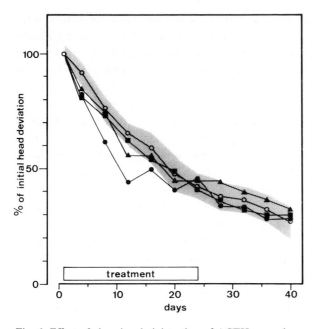

Fig. 6. Effect of chronic administration of ACTH$_{4-16}$ analogue ORG-5041 on vestibular compensation. ORG-5041 was injected daily in three different doses from the first to the 24th postoperative day. ○, control ($n = 261$, mean values $\pm$ S.D.; shaded area); ▲, ORG-5041 (0.0003 nmol/kg/day, $n = 14$); ■, ORG-5041 (3 nmol/kg/day, $n = 15$); ●, ORG-5041 (300 nmol/kg/day, $n = 14$). Ordinate: mean values of head tilt in percent of initial head deviation measured on the first postoperative day. Abscissa: time in days.

Lüneburg [1] observed that ACTH$_{4-10}$ accelerates the rate of vestibular compensation in the frog; Flohr et al. [7] have also shown that similar effects could be obtained with α-MSH and the synthetic ACTH$_{4-9}$ analogue ORG-2766. These results have been confirmed for ACTH$_{4-10}$ by Igarashi and co-workers [6] employing the same paradigm in the squirrel monkey. In the rat, Isaacson and Poplawsky [2,3] used the disappearance of hyperemotionality as a measure of functional recovery from septal lesions. They report that repeated postoperative administration of ORG-2766 enhanced the recovery process, whereas ACTH$_{4-10}$ had no effect. Likewise, in rats, Hannigan and Isaacson [5] found that performance deficits in a food search task induced by hippocampal lesions could be attenuated by ORG-2766 treatment. Such treatment was ineffective,

however, in alleviating the impairment induced in the same task by neocortical lesions. Accelerated recovery of impaired T-maze learning has been observed following chronic postoperative administration of ORG-2766 and α-MSH in rats with parafascicular lesions. γ_2-MSH was without effect in this paradigm [4].

The present findings provide further evidence that ACTH/MSH-like peptides are capable of positively influencing lesion-induced recovery processes. The tetrapeptide ACTH$_{4-7}$ represents the shortest active sequence. With the exception of the long-chained ACTH$_{1-39}$ and ACTH$_{1-24}$, all peptides containing this sequence are effective. Changes in this minimal amino-acid sequence either abolish the effect, as in the case of γ_2-MSH, or exert an antagonistic effect, as with [D-Phe7]ACTH$_{4-10}$. The activi-

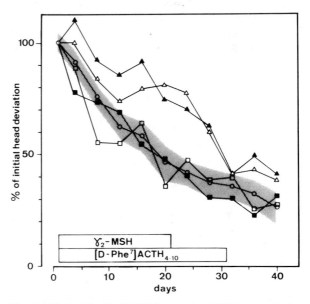

Fig. 7. Effect of [D-Phe7]ACTH$_{4-10}$ and γ_2-MSH on vestibular compensation. [D-Phe7]ACTH$_{4-10}$ was administered daily in two different doses from the first to the 31st postoperative day, whereas γ_2-MSH was given from the first to the 21th postoperative day in two different doses. ○, control ($n = 261$, mean values $\pm$ S.D.; shaded area); △, [D-Phe7]ACTH$_{4-10}$ (300 nmol/kg/day, $n = 21$); ▲, [D-Phe7]ACTH$_{4-10}$ (1200 nmol/kg/day, $n = 34$); □, γ_2-MSH (300 nmol/kg/day, $n = 10$); ■, γ_2-MSH (1000 nmol/kg/day, $n = 12$). Ordinate: mean values of head tilt in percent of initial head deviation measured on the first postoperative day. Abscissa: time in days.

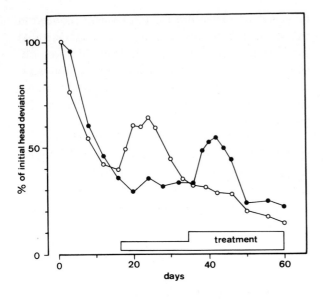

Fig. 8. Effect of [D-Phe7]ACTH$_{4-10}$ on partially compensated animals. The peptide was administered daily in a dose of 300 nmol/kg/day beginning with the 17th (○) or the 35th (●) postoperative day and continued in each case until day 60 ($n = 15$ for both groups). Ordinate: mean values of head tilt in percent of initial head deviation measured on the first postoperative day. Abscissa: time in days.

ty of the minimal sequence can be increased by chain elongation at the C- or N- and C-terminal.

It has long been established that ACTH/MSH-like peptides are capable of influencing learning and memory processes. This has been demonstrated in a number of different learning situations, such as classical and instrumental conditioning, visual discrimination tasks, habituation and imprinting, and in a variety of species, such as fish, amphibians, reptiles, birds and mammals, including man (for recent reviews see [16, 19, 20]). The effects of ACTH/

MSH-like peptides on these forms of behavioural plasticity are strikingly similar to those on lesion-induced plasticity reported in the present paper. In both cases, the shortest active sequence appears to be ACTH$_{4-7}$; longer ACTH fragments containing this sequence are also effective, whilst changes in this sequence lead to ineffective or antagonistically active agents. Since both classes of behavioural plasticity are influenced in the same or similar manner by the same peptides, it is tempting to assume a common underlying mechanism. At the present state of our knowledge, the most likely mode of action of these peptides on adaptive processes could reside in their action on the phosphorylation of cytoplasmic or synaptic proteins (for reviews see [20,21]).

As far as vestibular compensation is concerned, a prerequisite for the recovery of a symmetrical posture is generally assumed to be the restitution of a symmetrical firing rate in the vestibular nuclei of the two sides [22–25]. One hypothesis proposes that the reactivation of neurons in the deafferented nucleus is effected by a *collateral sprouting* of remaining inputs and subsequent formation of new synapses at vacated sites. Such reactive synaptogenesis has been observed as a response to partial denervation in different CNS areas. Indeed, this process has been suggested to be the decisive mechanism in the compensatory rewiring of neuronal circuitry (cf. [26]). Studies in the peripheral nervous system indicate that ACTH – among other trophic effects – may enhance *synaptogenesis* [27–32]. Similar effects on reactive synaptogenesis in the CNS should therefore be considered, in addition to the mechanisms mentioned above, as a possible basis of the peptide action in compensation.

Fig. 9. Survey of activities of melanocortins on vestibular compensation following unilateral labyrinthectomy in *Rana temporaria*. The relative effects of the different peptides and doses are compared on the basis of half-compensation time, i.e. the time over which the initial head deviation is reduced by 50%. The half compensation time of each experimental group is expressed as percent reduction or prolongation ($\pm$ S.E.) relative to the control ($n = 261$; the shaded area is the mean value $\pm$ S.E.). Peptides and doses (nmol/kg/day) are specified below the corresponding bars; numbers of animals are given in brackets. Original data were tested for significance by Welch's t-test (two-tailed analysis): *, $2p < 0.001$, (*), $2p < 0.002$, peptide versus control.

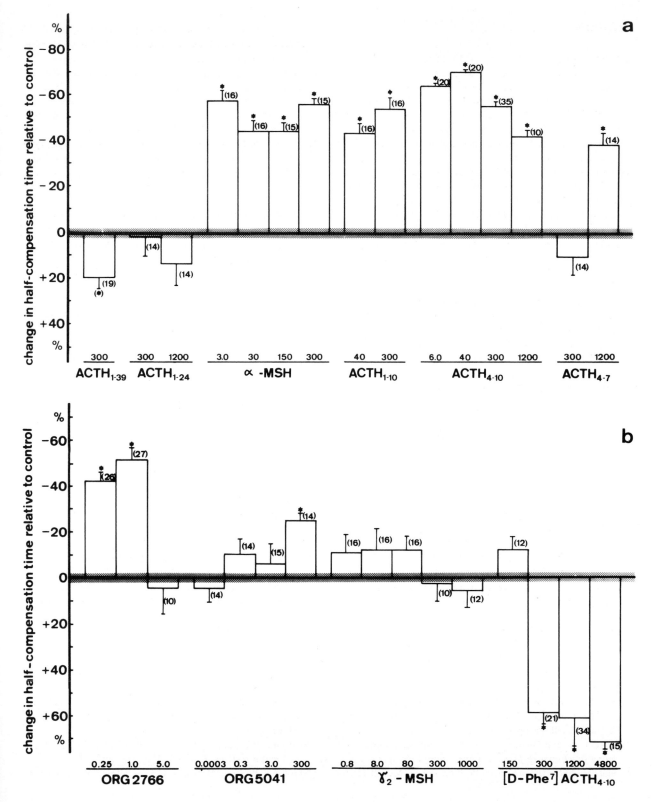

428

References

[1] Flohr, H. and Lüneburg, U. (1982) Effects of ACTH 4–10 on vestibular compensation. *Brain Res.*, 248: 169–173.

[2] Isaacson, R.L. and Poplawsky, A. (1983) An ACTH 4–9 analog (Org 2766) speeds recovery from septal hyperemotionality in the rat. *Behav. Neural Biol.*, 39: 52–59.

[3] Isaacson, R.L. and Poplawsky, A. (1985) ACTH 4–10 produces a transient decrease in septal hyperemotionality. *Behav. Neural Biol.*, 43: 109–113.

[4] Nyakas, C., Veldhuis, H.D. and De Wied, D. (1985) Beneficial effect of chronic treatment with Org 2766 and α-MSH on impaired reversal learning of rats with bilateral lesions of the parafascicular area. *Brain Res. Bull.*, 15: 257–265.

[5] Hannigan, J.H. and Isaacson, R.L. (1985) The effects of Org 2766 on the performance of sham, neocortical, and hippocampal-lesioned rats in a food search task. *Pharmacol. Biochem. Behav.*, 23: 1019–1027.

[6] Igarashi, M., Ishikawa, K., Ishii, M. and Schmidt, K.A. (1985) Effect of ACTH-(4–10) on equilibrium compensation after unilateral labyrinthectomy in the squirrel monkey. *Eur. J. Pharmacol.*, 119: 239–242.

[7] Flohr, H., Lüneburg, U. and Richter-Landsberg, C.(1986) ACTH/MSH-like neuropeptides and lesion-induced plastic processes. In E.L. Keller and D.S. Zee (Eds.), *Adaptive Processes in Visual and Oculomotor Systems, Advances in the Biosciences, Vol. 57*, Pergamon Press, Oxford/New York, pp. 409–416.

[8] Windle, W.F., Clemente, C.D. and Chambers, W.W. (1952) Inhibition of formation of a glial barrier as a means of permitting a peripheral nerve to grow into the brain. *J. Comp. Neurol.*, 96: 359–369.

[9] Clemente, C.D. (1958) The regeneration of peripheral nerves inserted into the cerebral cortex and the healing of cerebral lesions. *J. Comp. Neurol.*, 109: 123–152.

[10] McMasters, R.E. (1962) Regeneration of the spinal cord in the rat. Effects of Piromen and ACTH upon the regenerative capacity. *J. Comp. Neurol.*, 119: 113–121.

[11] Fertig, A., Kiernan, J.A. and Seyan, S.S.A.S. (1971) Enhancement of axonal regeneration in the brain of the rat by corticotrophin and triiodothyrosine. *Exp. Neurol.*, 33: 372–385.

[12] Berry, M., Knowles, J., Willis, P., Riches, A.C., Morgans, G.P. and Steers, A.C. (1979) A reappraisal of the effects of ACTH on the response of the central nervous system to injury. *J. Anat.*, 128: 859–871.

[13] Flohr, H. (1983) Control of plastic processes. In E. Basar, H. Flohr, H. Haken and A.J. Mandell (Eds.), *Synergetics of the Brain, Springer Series in Synergetics, Vol. 23*, Springer, Berlin/Heidelberg, pp. 60–74.

[14] Precht, W. and Dieringer, N. (1985) Neuronal events paralleling functional recovery (compensation) following peripheral vestibular lesions. In A. Berthoz and G. Melvill Jones (Eds.), *Adaptive Mechanisms in Gaze Control. Facts and Theories, Reviews in Oculomotor Research, Vol. 1*, Elsevier, Amsterdam, pp. 251–268.

[15] Ewald, J.R. (1892) *Physiologische Untersuchungen über das Endorgan des Nervus Octavus*, J.F. Bergmann, Wiesbaden.

[16] De Wied, D. and Jolles, J. (1982) Neuropeptides derived from pro-opiocortin: behavioral, physiological, and neurochemical effects. *Physiol. Rev.*, 62: 976–1059.

[17] Greven, H.M. and De Wied, D. (1977) Influence of peptides structurally related to ACTH and MSH on active avoidance behaviour in rats. In T.B. v. Wimersma Greidanus (Ed.), *Frontiers of Hormone Research, Vol. 4*, Karger, Basle, pp. 140–152.

[18] Flohr, H., Abeln, W. and Lüneburg, U. (1985) Neurotransmitter and neuromodulator systems involved in vestibular compensation. In A. Berthoz and G. Melvill Jones (Eds.), *Adaptive Mechanisms in Gaze Control, Facts and Theories, Reviews in Oculomotor Research, Vol. 1*, Elsevier, Amsterdam, pp. 269–277.

[19] Dunn, A.J. (1984) Effects of ACTH, β-lipotropin, and related peptides on the central nervous system. In C.B. Nemeroff and A.J. Dunn (Eds.), *Peptides, Hormones and Behavior*, MTP Press, Lancaster, pp. 273–348.

[20] Gispen, W.H. and Zwiers, H. (1985) Behavioral and neurochemical effects of ACTH. In A. Lajtha (Ed.), *Neurochemical Systems, Handbook of Neurochemistry, Vol. 8*, 2nd edn., Plenum Press, New York/London, pp. 375–412.

[21] Wiegant, V.M., Zwiers, H. and Gispen, W.H. (1981) Neuropeptides and brain cAMP and phosphoproteins. *Pharmac. Ther.*, 12: 463–490.

[22] Dieringer, N. and Precht, W. (1977) Modification of synaptic input following unilateral labyrinthectomy. *Nature*, 269: 431–433.

[23] Dieringer, N. and Precht, W. (1979) Mechanisms of compensation for vestibular deficits in the frog. I. Modification of the excitatory commissural system. *Exp. Brain Res.*, 36: 311–328.

[24] Dieringer, N. and Precht, W. (1979) Mechanisms of compensation for vestibular deficits in the frog. II. Modification of inhibitory pathways. *Exp. Brain Res.*, 36: 329–341.

[25] Flohr, H., Bienhold, H., Abeln, W. and Macskovics, I. (1981) Concepts of vestibular compensation. In H. Flohr and W. Precht (Eds.), *Lesion-Induced Neuronal Plasticity in Sensorimotor Systems*, Springer, Berlin/Heidelberg, pp. 153–172.

[26] Cotman, C. (1978) (Ed.) *Neuronal Plasticity*, Raven Press, New York.

[27] Shapiro, M.S., Namba, T. and Grob, D. (1968) The effect of corticotropin on the neuromuscular junction. *Neurology*, 18: 1018–1022.

[28] Strand, F.L. and Smith, C.M. (1980) LPH, ACTH, MSH and motor systems. *Pharmac. Ther.*, 11: 509–533.

[29] Bijlsma, W.A., Jennekens, F.G.I., Schotman, P. and Gispen,

W.H. (1981) Corticotrophin (ACTH) like peptides stimulate peripheral nerve regeneration. In M.E. van Hof and G. Mohn (Eds.), *Functional Recovery from Brain Damage*, Elsevier, Amsterdam, pp. 411–415.

[30] Edwards, P.M., van der Zee, C.E.E.M., Verhaagen, J., Schotman, P., Jennekens, F.G.I. and Gispen, W.H. (1984) Evidence that the neurotropic actions of α-MSH may derive from its ability to mimick the actions of a peptide formed in degenerating nerve stumps. *J. Neurol. Sci.*, 64: 333–340.

[31] Verhaagen, J., Edwards, P.M., Jennekens, F.G.I., Schot-

man, P. and Gispen, W.H. (1986) α-Melanocyte-stimulating hormone (MSH) stimulates the outgrowth of myelinated nerve fibers after peripheral nerve crush. *Exp. Neurol.*, 92: 451–454.

[32] Verhaagen, J., Edwards, P.M., Jennekens, F.G.I., Schotman, P. and Gispen, W.H. (1987) Early effect of an ACTH 4–9 analog (Org 2766) on regenerative sprouting demonstrated by the use of neurofilament-binding antibodies isolated from a serum raised by α-MSH immunization. *Brain Res.*, 404: 142–150.

Subject Index

432

440

442